Recent Results in Cancer Research 142

E. D. Kreuser P. M. Schlag (Eds.)

New Perspectives in Molecular and Clinical Management of Gastrointestinal Tumors

With 61 Figures and 101 Tables

Springer

Prof. Dr. med. Ernst-D. Kreuser
Freie Universität Berlin
Fachbereich Humanmedizin
Univ.-Klinikum Benjamin Franklin
Medizinische Klinik und Poliklinik
Schwerpunkt Hämatologie und Onkologie
Hindenburgdamm 30
12200 Berlin, Germany

Prof. Dr. med. P.M. Schlag
Robert-Rössle Klinik am
Max-Delbrück-Centrum
Humboldt-Universität
Lindenberger Weg 80
13122 Berlin, Germany

ISBN-13:978-3-642-80037-5

Library of Congress Cataloging-in-Publication Data. New perspectives in molecular and clinical management of gastrointestinal tumors / E.D. Kreuser, P.M. Schlag (eds.). p. cm. – (Recent results in cancer research; 142) Includes bibliographical references and index. ISBN-13:978-3-642-80037-5 e-ISBN-13:978-3-642-80035-1
DOI: 10.1007/978-3-642-80035-1 1. Gastrointestinal system – Cancer – Molecular aspects. 2. Gastrointestinal system – Cancer – Treatment. I. Kreuser, E.D. (Ernst Dietrich), 1945– . II. Schlag, P. (Peter), 1948– . III. Series. [DNLM: 1. Gastrointestinal Neoplasms – diagnosis. 2. Gastrointestinal Neoplasms – therapy. W1 RE106P v. 142 1995/ WI 149 N532 1995] RC261.R35 vol. 142 [RC280.D5] 616.99'4 s – dc20 [616.99'433] DNLM/DLC for Library of Congress 95-39447

Cover design: Design & Production, Heidelberg

Typesetting: Best-set Typesetter Ltd., Hong Kong

SPIN: 10498904 19/3133/SPS – 5 4 3 2 1 0 – Printed on acid-free paper

Springer
Berlin
Heidelberg
New York
Barcelona
Budapest
Hong Kong
London
Milan
Paris
Santa Clara
Singapore
Tokyo

Preface

Over the past few years, a wealth of new insights have been gained and put to use in basic gastrointestinal tumor research, including tumor suppressor genes, oncogenes, cell-cycle control, apoptosis, adhesion receptors, signal transduction, and gene therapy. Similarly, progress has been made in prevention, molecular diagnosis, laparoscopic staging, and antibody-based immunotherapy, and new drugs such as thymidylate and topoisomerase I inhibitors have been developed especially for the treatment of colorectal carcinoma. Despite this burgeoning of knowledge in both basic and clinical research, however, we have just begun to put these results into clinical practice. Therefore, the key goal of this volume is to bring together basic and clinical research findings so as to facilitate the translation of these advances into the clinical management of gastrointestinal tumors.

We hope that this volume, which covers a broad spectrum of research and clinical medicine, will impart new insights and greater understanding to all those interested in the therapy of gastrointestinal tumors and will stimulate further scientific research.

Berlin, January 1996

E.D. Kreuser
P.M. Schlag

Contents

*List of Contributors**

---

* The addresses of the authors are given on the first page of each contribution.
[1] Page on which contribution begins.

I. Basic Research

*The Molecular Biology of Esophageal Carcinoma**

S.J. Meltzer

Univ. of Maryland, Med/GI, N3W62, 22 S. Greene St., Baltimore, MD 21201, USA

Abstract

There have been many new developments in our understanding of esophageal carcinoma biology over the past several years. Information regarding both of the major forms of this disease, adenocarcinoma and squamous cell carcinoma, has accumulated in conjunction with data on precursor conditions such as Barrett's esophagus. Some of the most interesting and promising findings have included aneuploidy (abnormal DNA content), amplification and overexpression of proto-oncogenes, loss of heterozygosity at multiple chromosomal loci, and tumor suppressor gene inactivation. Of particular importance is mutation and deletion involving the tumor suppressor gene p53, but abnormalities in the retinoblastoma, deleted in colon cancer, and adenomatous polyposis coli genes have been described as well. Recently, two important cancer pathways implicated in the genesis of multiple tumor types have also been inculpated in esophageal carcinogenesis: the cyclin kinase inhibitor cascade and the DNA mismatch repair process. Alterations in the p16 and p15 cyclin kinase inhibitors, including point mutation and homozygous deletion, have been reported in primary esophageal tumors and/or tumor-derived cell lines. Microsatellite instability, the hallmark of DNA mismatch repair defects, has been detected in esophageal cancers, particularly those associated with Barrett's metaplasia (where it may represent an early event). Further developments in the field of molecular carcinogenesis of esophageal malignancies promise to yield improvements in the early detection, prognostic categorization, and perhaps eventual gene-based therapy of this deadly disease.

---

* Supported by grants from the American Cancer Society, the Department of Veterans Affairs, NIH Grants DK47717, ES07120, CA67497, and the University of Maryland Designated Research Initiative Fund.

Recent Results in Cancer Research, Vol. 142

Esophageal cancer occurs in two major histologic forms: squamous cell carcinoma and adenocarcinoma. In some respects, these two types of cancer share biological features; in other ways they are distinct. Squamous cell cancer occurs in chronic tobacco smokers and is further potentiated by heavy ethanol use. Adenocarcinoma occurs in patients with Barrett's esophagus, a metaplastic condition in which the normal squamous lining is replaced by columnar mucosa. This condition is caused by chronic gastroesophageal reflux disease, and although families with Barrett's esophagus have been reported (Jochem et al. 1992), the overwhelming majority of Barrett's cases occur sporadically. Similarly, most cases of squamous esophageal cancer are nonfamilial.

Information is rapidly accumulating on the molecular genetic pathophysiology of esophageal carcinoma of both histologic types. The first genetic abnormalities to be described in esophageal cancer were aneuploidy and abnormal chromosome complement. Aneuploidy is defined as abnormal DNA content, usually associated with gross structural and numerical abnormalities involving many chromosomes. This abnormality has been seen in squamous cell carcinoma and its precursor lesion, squamous dysplasia (Robaszkiewicz et al. 1991; Hakura et al. 1994), as well as in all stages of Barrett's-associated carcinogenesis (Rabinovitch et al. 1988). In addition, several studies have addressed specific chromosomal aberrations occurring in Barrett's metaplasia and both types of esophageal cancer. Diverse karyotypic abnormalities including y-chromosome losses, trisomies, and translocations involving chromosomes 7 and 11 have been documented (Garewal et al. 1989; Shimada et al. 1992; L. Rosenblum-Vos et al., unpublished observations). One study described over-representation of chromosome 8, loss of chromosome 17, and loss of the y-chromosome in several cases of Barrett's adenocarcinoma and adjacent metaplastic epithelium (Garewal et al. 1989).

Abnormalities in specific genes were the earliest molecular abnormalities discovered in esophageal cancer. Early studies focused on alterations of proto-oncogenes. Amplification of DNA encoding the epidermal growth factor receptor (EGF-R) (Hunts et al. 1985; Yamamoto et al. 1986; Hollstein et al. 1988; Lu et al. 1988), c-myc (Lu et al. 1988), hst-1 and int-2 (Tsuda et al. 1988; Tsutsumi et al. 1988; Wagata et al. 1991), and cyclin D (Jiang et al. 1992) have all been reported. The cyclin D gene is probably the target of amplification events at the chromosome 11q13 locus, which also includes hst-1 and int-2 (Tsuda et al. 1988; Tsutsumi et al. 1988; Wagata et al. 1991). In addition, overexpression of the EGF receptor has been observed and correlates with lower survival rates (Mukaida et al. 1991). Along similar lines, overexpression of the c-myc proto-oncogene occurs (Tsuboi et al. 1987), and DNA amplification of hst-1 and int-2 are poor prognostic factors (Kitagawa et al. 1991; Shiga et al. 1994).

One feature of both esophageal adenocarcinomas and squamous cell carcinomas distinguishing them from other types of cancer such as colorectal carcinoma is the strikingly low incidence of ras proto-oncogene mutations. In most studies of esophageal neoplasms, these mutations were completely absent (Jiang et al. 1989; Meltzer et al. 1990; Victor et al. 1990; Hollstein et al. 1991). However, c-H-ras mutations occurred in 67% of methylbenzylnitrosamine-induced esophageal papillomas in rats (Barch et al. 1991). The prominent lack of ras proto-oncogene activation in esophageal cancer stands in stark contrast to the more obvious involvement of tumor suppressor genes. In this latter respect, both histologic types of esophageal tumor are similar. Loss of heterozygosity (LOH) involving multiple tumor suppressor gene loci has been reported. These loci include p53 on chromosome 17p (Meltzer et al. 1991), retinoblastoma or Rb on 13q (Boynton et al. 1991), adenomatous polyposis coli (APC) on 5q (Boynton et al. 1992), deleted in colon cancer (DCC) on 18q (Huang et al. 1992), and multiple tumor suppressor 1 (MTS1), also known as p16, on 9p (Tarmin et al. 1994).

Candidate target genes at these chromosomal loci often show point mutations in esophageal cancers of both histologic subtypes. The first target tumor suppressor gene shown to undergo frequent point mutation in primary esophageal squamous tumors and cell lines was p53 (Hollstein et al. 1990). Similar findings were soon reported in noncancerous Barrett's-associated adenocarcinoma and adjacent dysplasia or metaplasia (Casson et al. 1991). The high prevalence of p53 mutations in squamous cancers was confirmed in several subsequent studies (Huang et al. 1993; Bennet et al. 1991; Audrezet et al. 1993; Gao et al. 1994; Chung et al. 1993; Wang et al. 1993). Similarly, p53 mutation was found to be quite frequent in numerous studies of adenocarcinoma (Huang et al. 1993; Greenwald et al. 1992; Blount et al. 1991; Huang et al. 1994). Because p53 mutation was found in premalignant and early malignant tissues in the development of both squamous cancer and adenocarcinoma, multiple investigators concluded that p53 mutation was an early event (Casson et al. 1991; Huang et al. 1993; Gao et al. 1994; Wang et al. 1993; Greenwald et al. 1992). In addition, some investigators found a unique profile of p53 mutations in esophageal cancer, consisting of an unusually high preponderance of nonsense mutations (Huang et al. 1993; Audrezet et al. 1993; Huang et al. 1994).

The probable early timing of p53 inactivation in Barrett's esophageal carcinogenesis was corroborated by two studies that combined flow-cytometric nuclear sorting with 17p-LOH assays (Blount et al. 1993; Blount et al. 1994). The second of these two reports found that 17p-LOH could even occur in the diploid (more grossly normal in terms of DNA content) cells of tumors (Blount et al. 1994). Moreover, since point mutation of p53 often results in p53 protein overexpression, several immunohistochemical studies were performed which also supported the conclusions drawn from earlier DNA analyses, i.e., that p53 inactivation is a common and early event in esophageal carcinogenesis (Blount et al. 1991; Ramel et al. 1992; Flejou et al. 1994a,b; Younes et al. 1993). As is characteristic of other early carcinogenic events (such as ras or APC gene mutation in colorectal cancer), p53 protein overexpression was found to confer no prognostic significance on patient survival in esophageal cancer (Flejou et al. 1994b).

Other candidate genes at regions of frequent LOH are also altered in esophageal carcinoma, including the retinoblastoma (Rb) gene on chromosome 13q (Huang et al. 1993) and the MTS1 or p16 gene on chromosome 9p (Mori et al. 1994; Zhou et al. 1994). The involvement of p16 in esophageal carcinogenesis fits nicely into the cell-cycle-control pathway consisting of Rb, cyclin D1, and the cyclin-dependent kinases such as p16. In this context, as noted above, aberrant transcripts of Rb (Huang et al. 1993) and DNA amplification involving cyclin D or neighboring loci on chromosome 11 (Tsutsumi et al. 1988; Wagata et al. 1991; Tsuda et al. 1988; Jiang et al. 1992; Kitagawa et al. 1991; Shiga et al. 1994) have been noted in esophageal cancer. In this pathway, cyclin D1 is the catalytic subunit of a complex containing the cyclin-dependent kinase p16, which in turn phosphorylates its major substrate, Rb, thus inhibiting entry into the cell cycle. When p16 is mutated or absent, Rb remains unphosphorylated and allows the cell to divide. One notable exception to the pattern of matching LOH and candidate gene inactivation is the adenomatous polyposis coli (APC) tumor suppressor gene on chromosome 5q. Despite rates of LOH on 5q approaching 80% (Boynton et al. 1992), APC mutation within the mutation cluster region of this gene is very rare in both histologic types of esophageal cancer (Powell et al. 1994). This essentially negative finding suggests the presence of another target gene distinct from but in close proximity to APC on chromosome 5q.

One important contrast between the two major histologic types of esophageal cancer concerns the prevalence of microsatellite instability; it is quite frequent and can occur early in Barrett's-associated esophageal adenocarcinoma, but it is rare in esophageal squamous tumors (Meltzer et al. 1994). Finally, another potentially exciting molecular pathogenetic factor is human papillomavirus (HPV) integration (Kulski et al. 1986; Chang et al. 1990; Toh et al. 1992; Furihata et al. 1993; Togawa et al. 1994). It should not come as a surprise that HPV is found in human esophageal cancers, especially since HPV-encoded oncoproteins can interact with and inactivate two esophageal cancer-related tumor suppressor genes, p53 (Scheffner et al. 1990, 1992; Lechner et al. 1992; Dyson et al. 1989) and Rb (Dyson et al. 1992).

References

Audrezet MP, Robaszkiewicz M, Mercier B, Nousbaum JB, Bail JP, Hardy E, Volant A, Lozac'h P, Charles JF, Gouerou H, Ferec C (1993) TP53 gene mutation profile in esophageal squamous cell carcinomas. Cancer Res 53:5745–5749

Barch DH, Jacoby RF, Brasitus TA, Radosevich JA, Carney WP, Iannacone PM (1991) Incidence of Harvey ras oncogene point mutations and their expression in methylbenzylnitrosamine-induced esophageal tumorigenesis. Carcinogenesis 12:2373–2377

Bennett WP, Hollstein MC, He A, Zhu SM, Resau JH, Trump BF, Metcalf RA, Welsh JA, Midgley C, Lane DP, Harris CC (1991) Archival analysis of p53 genetic and protein alterations in Chinese esophageal cancer. Oncogene 6:1779–1784

Blount PL, Ramel S, Raskind WH, Haggitt RC, Sanchez CA, Dean PJ, Rabinovitch PS, Reid BJ (1991) 17p allelic deletions and p53 protein overexpression in Barrett's adenocarcinoma. Cancer Res 51:5482–5486

Blount PL, Meltzer SJ, Yin J, Huang Y, Krasna MJ, Reid BJ (1993) Clonal ordering of 17p and 5q allelic losses in Barrett dysplasia and adenocarcinoma. Proc Natl Acad Sci U S A 90:3221–3225

Blount PL, Galipeau PC, Sanchez CA, Neshat K, Levine DS, Yin J, Suzuki H, Abraham JM, Meltzer SJ, Reid BJ (1994) 17p allelic losses in diploid cells of patients with Barrett's esophagus who develop aneuploidy. Cancer Res 54:2292–2295

Boynton RF, Huang Y, Blount PL, Reid BJ, Raskind WH, Haggitt RC, Newkirk C, Resau JH, Yin J, McDaniel TK, Meltzer SJ (1991) Frequent loss of heterozygosity at the retinoblastoma locus in human esophageal cancer. Cancer Res 51:5766–5769

Boynton RF, Bount PL, Yin J, Brown VL, Huang Y, Tong Y, McDaniel T, Newkirk C, Resau JH, Raskind WH, Haggitt RC, Reid BJ, Meltzer SJ (1992) Loss of heterozygosity involving the APC and MCC genetic loci occurs in the majority of human esophageal cancers. Proc Natl Acad Sci U S A 89:3385–3388

Casson AG, Mukhopadhyay T, Cleary KR, Ro JY, Levin B, Roth JA (1991) p53 gene mutations in Barrett's epithelium and esophageal cancer. Cancer Res 51:4495–4499

Chang F, Syrjanen S, Shen Q, Ji H, Syrjanen K (1990) Human papillomavirus (HPV) DNA in esophageal precancer lesions and squamous cell carcinomas from China. Int J Cancer 45:21–25

Chung KY, Mukhopadhyay T, Kim J, Casson A, Ro JY, Goepfert H, Hong WK, Roth JA (1983) Discordant p53 gene mutations in primary head and neck cancers and corresponding second primary cancers of the upper aerodigestive tract. Cancer Res 53:1676–1683

Dyson N, Howley PM, Munger K, Harlow E (1989) The human papilloma virus-16 E7 oncoprotein is able to bind to the retinoblastoma gene product. Science 243:934–937

Flejou J-F, Paraf F, Potet F, Muzeau F, Fekete F, Henin D (1994a) p53 protein expression in Barrett's adenocarcinoma: a frequent event with no prognostic significance. Histopathol 24:487–489

Flejou J-F, Potet F, Muziau F, Le Pelletier F, Fekete F, Henin D (1994b) Overexpression of p53 protein in Barrett's syndrome with malignant transformation. J Clin Pathol 46:330–333

Furihata M, Ohtsuki Y, Ogoshi S, Takahashi A, Tamiya T, Ogata T (1993) Prognostic significance of human papillomavirus genomes (type-16, -18) and aberrant expression of p53 protein in human esophageal cancer. Int J Cancer 54:226–230

Gao H, Wang L-D, Zhou Q, Hong J-Y, Huang T-Y, Yang CS (1994) p53 tumor suppressor gene mutation in early esophageal precancerous lesions and carcinoma among high-risk populations in Henan, China. Cancer Res 54:4342–4346

Garewal HS, Sampliner R, Liu Y, Trent JM (1989) Chromosomal rearrangements in Barrett's esophagus: a premalignant lesion of esophageal adenocarcinoma. Cancer Genet Cytogenet 42:281–286

Greenwald BD, Huang Y, Baum R, Meltzer SJ (1992) Barrett's carcinoma in a 25-year-old man with point mutation of the p53 tumor suppressor gene. Int J Oncol 1:271–275

Hollstein MC, Smits AM, Galiana C, Yamasaki H, Bos JL, Mandard A, Partensky C, Montesano R (1988) Amplification of epidermal growth factor receptor gene but no evidence of ras mutations in primary human esophageal cancers. Cancer Res 48:5119–5123

Hollstein MC, Metcalf RA, Welsh JA, Montesano R, Harris CC (1990) Frequent mutation of the p53 gene in human esophageal cancer. Proc Natl Acad Sci U S A 87:9958–9961

Hollstein MC, Peri L, Mandard AM, Welsh JA, Montesano R, Metcalf RA, Bak M, Harris CC (1991) Genetic analysis of human esophageal tumors from two high-incidence geographic areas: frequent p53 base substitutions and absence of ras mutations. Cancer Res 51:4102–4106

Huang Y, Boynton RF, Blount PL, Silverstein RJ, Yin J, Tong Y, McDaniel TK, Newkirk C, Resau JH, Sridhara R, Reid BJ, Meltzer SJ (1992) Loss of heterozygosity involves multiple tumor suppressor genes in human esophageal cancers. Cancer Res 52:6525–6530

Huang Y, Meltzer SJ, Yin J, Tong Y, Chang EH, Srivastava S, McDaniel T, Boynton RF, Zou Z-Q (1993) Altered messenger RNA and unique mutational profiles of p53 and Rb in human esophageal carcinomas. Cancer Res 53:1889–1894

Huang Y, Yin J, Meltzer SJ (1994) A unique p53 intragenic deletion flanked by short direct repeats results in loss of mRNA expression in a human esophageal carcinoma. Carcinogenesis 15:1653–1655

Hunts J, Ueda M, Ozawa S, Abe O, Pastan I, Shimizu N (1985) Hyperproduction and gene amplification of the epidermal growth factor receptor in squamous cell carcinomas. Jpn J Cancer Res 76:663–666

Itakura Y, Sasano H, Mori S, Nagura H (1994) DNA ploidy in human esophageal squamous dysplasias and squamous cell carcinomas as determined by image analysis. Modern Pathol 7:867–873

Jiang W, Kahn SM, Guillem JG, Lu SH, Weinstein BI (1989) Rapid detection of ras oncogenes in human tumors: applications to colon, esophageal, and gastric cancer. Oncogene 4:923–928

Jiang W, Kahn SM, Tomita N, Zhang Y-J, Lu S-H, Weinstein IB (1992) Amplification and expression of the human cyclin D gene in esophageal cancer. Cancer Res 52:2980–2983

Jochem VJ, Fuerst PA, Fromkes JJ (1992) Familial Barrett's esophagus associated with adenocarcinoma. Gastroenterology 102:1400–1402

Kitagawa Y, Ueda M, Ando N, Shinozawa Y, Shimizu N, Abe O (1991) Significance of int-2/hst-1 coamplification as a prognostic factor in patients with esophageal squamous carcinoma. Cancer Res 51:1504–1508

Kulski J, Demeter T, Sterrett GF, Shilkin KB (1986) Human papillomavirus DNA in esophageal carcinoma. Lancet 2:683–684

Lechner MS, Mack DH, Finicle AB, Crook T, Vousden KH, Laimins LA (1992) Human papillomavirus E6 proteins bind p53 in vivo and abrogate p53-mediated repression of transcription. EMBO J 8:3045–3052

Lu S-H, Hsieh L-L, Luo F-C, Weinstein IB (1988) Amplification of the EGF receptor and c-myc genes in human esophageal cancers. Int J Cancer 42:502–505

Meltzer SJ, Mane SM, Wood PK, Resau JH, Newkirk C, Terzakis JA, Korelitz BI, Weinstein WM, Needleman SW (1990) Activation of c-Ki-ras in human gastrointestinal dysplasias determined by direct sequencing of polymerase chain reaction products. Cancer Res 50:3627–3630

Meltzer SJ, Yin J, Huang Y, McDaniel TK, Newkirk C, Iseri O, Vogelstein B, Resau JH (1991) Reduction to homozygosity involving p53 in esophageal cancers demonstrated by the polymerase chain reaction. Proc Natl Acad Sci U S A 88:4976–4980

Meltzer SJ, Yin J, Manin B, Rhyu M-G, Cottrell J, Hudson E, Redd JL, Krasna MJ, Abraham JM, Reid BJ (1994) Microsatellite instability occurs frequently and in both diploid and aneuploid cell populations of Barrett's-associated esophageal adenocarcinomas. Cancer Res 54:3379–3382

Mori T, Miura K, Aoki T, Nishihira T, Mori S, Nakamura Y (1994) Frequent somatic mutation of the MTS1/CDK4I (multiple tumor suppressor/cyclin-dependent kinase 4 inhibitor) gene in esophageal squamous cell carcinoma. Cancer Res 54:3396–3399

Mukaida H, Toi M, Hirai T, Yamashita Y, Toge T (1991) Clinical significance of the expression of epidermal growth factor and its receptor in esophageal cancer. Cancer 68:142–148

Powell SM, Papadopoulos N, Kinzler KW, Smolinski KN, Meltzer SJ (1994) APC gene mutations in the mutation cluster region are rare in esophageal cancers. Gastroenterology 107:1759–1763

Rabinovitch PS, Reid BJ, Haggitt RC, Norwood TN, Rubin CE (1988) Progression to cancer in Barrett's esophagus is associated with genomic instability. Lab Invest 60:65–71

Ramel S, Reid BJ, Sanchez CA, Blount PL, Levine DS, Neshat K, Haggitt RC, Dean PJ, Thor K, Rabinovitch PS (1992) Evaluation of p53 protein expression in Barrett's esophagus by two-parameter flow cytometry. Gastroenterology 102:1220–1228

Robaszkiewicz M, Reid BJ, Volant A, Cauvin JM, Rabinovitch PS, Gouerou H (1991) Flow-cytometric DNA content analysis of esophageal squamous cell carcinomas. Gastroenterology 101:1588–1593

Scheffner M, Werness BA, Huibregtse JM, Levine AJ, Howley PM (1990) The E6 oncoprotein encoded by human papillomavirus types 16 and 18 promotes the degradation of p53. Cell 63:1129–1136

Scheffner M, Takahashi T, Huibregtse JM, Minna JD, Howley PM (1992) Interaction of the human papillomavirus type E6 oncoprotein with wild-type and mutant human p53 proteins. J Virol 66:5100–5105

Shiga C, Shiga K, Hirayama K, Kayayama M, Nishihira T, Mori S (1994) Prognostic significance of hst-1 gene amplification in primary esophageal carcinomas and its relationship to other prognostic factors. Anticancer Res 14:651–656

Shimada Y, Imamura M, Wagata T, Yamaguchi N, Takayoshi T (1992) Characterization of 21 newly established esophageal cancer cell lines. Cancer 69:277–284

Tarmin L, Yin J, Zhou X, Suzuki H, Jiang H-Y, Rhyu M-G, Abraham JM, Krasna MJ, Cottrell J, Meltzer SJ (1994) Frequent loss of heterozygosity on chromosome 9 in adenocarcinoma and squamous cell carcinoma of the esophagus. Cancer Res 54:6094–6096

Toh Y, Kuwano H, Tanaka S, Baba K, Matsuda H, Sugimachi K, Mori R (1992) Detection of human papillomavirus DNA in esophageal carcinoma in Japan by polymerase chain reaction. Cancer 70:2334–2338

Togawa K, Jaskiewicz K, Takahashi H, Meltzer SJ, Rustgi AK (1994) Human papillomavirus DNA sequences in esophagus squamous cell carcinoma. Gastroenterology 107:128–136

Tsuboi K, Hirayoshi K, Takeuchi K, Sabe H, Shimada Y, Ohshio G, Tobe T, Hatanaka M (1987) Expression of the c-myc gene in human gastrointestinal malignancies. Biochem Biophys Res Commun 146:699–704

Tsuda T, Nakatani H, Matsumura T, Yoshida K, Tahara E, Nishihara T, Sakamoto H, Yoshida T, Terada M, Sugimura T (1988) Amplification of the hst-1 gene in human esophageal carcinomas. Jpn J Cancer Res 79:584–588

Tsutsumi M, Sakamoto H, Yoshida T, Kakizoe T, Koiso K, Sugimura T, Terada M (1988) Coamplification of the hst-1 and int-2 genes in human cancers. Jpn J Cancer Res 79:428–432

Victor T, Du Toit R, Jordaan AM, Bester AJ, van Helden PD (1990) No evidence for point mutations in codons 12, 13, and 61 of the ras gene in a high-incidence area for esophageal and gastric cancers. Cancer Res 50:4911–4914

Wagata T, Ishizaki K, Imamura M, Shimada Y, Ikenaga M, Tobe T (1991) Deletion of 17p and amplification of the int-2 gene in esophageal carcinomas. Cancer Res 51:2113–2117

Wang L-D, Hong J-Y, Qiu S-L, Gao H, Yang CS (1993) Accumulation of p53 protein in human esophageal precancerous lesions: a possible early biomarker for carcinogenesis. Cancer Res 53:1783–1787

Yamamoto T, Kamata N, Kawano H, Shimizu S, Kuroki T, Toyoshima K, Rikimaru K, Nomura N, Ishizaki R, Pastan I, Gamou S, Shimizu N (1986) High incidence of amplification of the epidermal growth factor receptor gene in human squamous carcinoma cell lines. Cancer Res 46:414–416

Younes M, Lebovitz RM, Lechago LV, Lechago J (1993) p53 protein accumulation in Barrett's metaplasia, dysplasia, and carcinoma: a follow-up study. Gastroenterology 105:1637–1642

Zhou X, Tarmin L, Yin J, Jiang H-Y, Suzuki H, Rhyu M-G, Abraham JM, Meltzer SJ (1994) The MTS1 gene is frequently mutated in primary human esophageal tumors. Oncogene 9:3737–3741

Preventing Colorectal Cancer

E.R. Greenberg

Dartmouth Medical School and the Norris Cotton Cancer Center, Lebanon, NH 03756, USA

Abstract

After decades of little apparent progress against colorectal cancer, we now have the means to avert many of the deaths associated with this malignancy. Earlier diagnosis, either through screening for fecal occult blood or by endoscopy, has been clearly shown to be effective in reducing mortality. There are also prospects for preventing colorectal cancer occurrence through life-style change, since epidemiological studies consistently show that a dietary pattern of high intake of fruits, vegetables, and fiber is associated with a substantially decreased risk of these tumors. A further approach to prevention is the use of pharmacologic agents. Several randomized prevention trials to assess possible preventive drugs or nutrient supplements have focused on patients treated for colorectal adenomas. These trials are feasible, but they pose important challenges in protocol design, recruitment, and patient compliance. Nonsteroidal anti-inflammatory drugs (NSAIDs), especially aspirin, currently appear to be the most promising agents for testing in future trials.

Background

Cancers of the colorectum are among the three most important neoplasms in industrialized countries, as measured by numbers of new cases and deaths (Boyle et al. 1985). In the United States alone, over 150000 patients are diagnosed with colorectal cancer and 60000 deaths are attributed to these tumors each year (Ries et al. 1994). Age-adjusted incidence and death rates for these tumors are somewhat higher among men than women, but the lifetime risks of developing colorectal cancer or dying from it are roughly equal for both sexes, largely because of the longer life span of women (Table 1). Indeed, the burden of colorectal cancer among women seems to receive far less atten-

Recent Results in Cancer Research, Vol. 142

Table 1. Lifetime risk of colorectal cancer, USA (Ries et al. 1994)

	Being diagnosed (%)	Dying (%)
White		
Male	6.3	2.7
Female	6.0	2.7
Black		
Male	4.4	2.0
Female	5.2	2.6

tion than it merits. For example, in a woman aged 65 years, the risk of death from colorectal cancer over the next 20 years rivals that from breast cancer. This fact has been overlooked in discussions of women's health issues, and many women seem to view colorectal cancer as a disease that does not concern them.

After years of little apparent progress in the fight against colorectal cancer, prospects are now better for averting the mortality and morbidity associated with this malignancy. Although the incidence of colorectal cancer had increased moderately in the USA during recent decades, both incidence and death rates now appear to be declining (Table 2). Mortalities from these cancers have clearly fallen in many other industrialized countries as well (Greenwald 1992). Also, a higher proportion of colorectal tumors are being diagnosed at an earlier stage, and more effective methods for treating advanced disease have been developed. Of particular importance is the improvement in our understanding of the molecular mechanisms that underlie colorectal carcinogenesis (Fearon and Vogelstein 1990). These basic scientific findings are made possible by emerging technologies that were not even imaginable a short time ago, and they offer the promise of greatly improved clinical detection and treatment approaches in the coming years. At present, however, the best hope for reducing colorectal cancer deaths is through prevention programs that do not require development of new, or more sophisticated, technology.

Table 2. Annual percentage change in incidence of colorectal cancer among U.S. men and women, 1975–1979 and 1987–1991 (Ries et al. 1994)

	Male	Female
Incidence		
1975–1979	+3.6	+1.3
1987–1991	−4.2	−3.6
Mortality		
1975–1979	+1.2	−1.8
1987–1991	−4.2	−5.9

Table 3. Efficacy of fecal occult blood screening, Minnesota trial (Maudel et al. 1993)

Group	Cases	Deaths	RR (95% CI)[a]
Control	356	121	1.0 (ref)
Biennial screening	323	117	0.94 (0.68–1.31)
Annual screening	323	82	0.67 (0.50–0.87)

[a] Relative risk (95% confidence interval)

Screening

Secondary prevention — i.e., early detection — has received most scrutiny in clinical studies. There now are firm data from a randomized, controlled clinical trial showing that screening by testing for fecal occult blood can reduce mortality from this condition (Mandel et al. 1993). This trial involved over 46000 men and women in Minnesota who were randomized to have fecal occult blood testing, either annually, every 2 years, or not at all. Over an average 13-year follow-up period, the risk of death from colorectal cancer was a third lower in the group assigned to receive annual screening (Table 3). The study provides compelling evidence that early detection programs are feasible and that they can be effective in preventing deaths from colorectal cancer. However, to increase test sensitivity, the Minnesota study investigators used rehydrated slides, and as a consequence the proportion of false-positive tests was large. Over the course of the study, 1002 cases of colorectal cancer were identified, yet more than 12 000 colonoscopies were performed among all trial participants, usually because of positive hemoccult findings. The results are thus encouraging, but they raise questions of whether the cost and inefficiency of occult blood testing warrant its widespread use.

Visual examination of the large bowel, using endoscopy, offers a more direct and specific approach to screening for colorectal neoplasia. Although there are no results from clinical trials, nonexperimental studies strongly suggest that sigmoidoscopy can also reduce the risk of colorectal cancer death. A landmark case-control study, conducted by investigators from the Kaiser-Permanente Group in Oakland, Calif., noted a profound reduction in risk of death from cancers of the distal colon and rectum (but not more proximal tumors) among persons who had had a screening sigmoidoscopy in recent years (Selby et al. 1992) (Table 4). In another case-control study from Wisconsin, the investigators found a similar benefit associated with sigmoidoscopy use, but no benefit for digital rectal examination (Newcomb et al. 1992). The effects of sigmoidoscopy in reducing colorectal cancer deaths presumably resulted primarily from detection and removal of adenomas. Supporting this notion are the results of a follow-up study of patients who were intensively surveyed with endoscopy and polypectomy in the course of a clinical trial testing varying colonoscopy intervals. Among patients enrolled in this trial,

Table 4. Risk of fatal colorectal cancer associated with at least one screening sigmoidoscopy in past 10 years, by location. Case-control data from Kaiser Permanente Medical Care Program of Northern California (Selby et al. 1992)

Site of cancer	Cases	Adj. OR (95% CI)[a]
Within reach of sigmoidoscope	261	0.41 (0.25–0.69)
Above reach of sigmoidoscope	268	0.96 (0.61–1.50)

[a] Adjusted odds ratio (95% confidence interval)

colorectal cancer occurrence and mortality were far less than expected from population rates or from adenoma patient series previously reported (Winawer et al. 1993).

It is important to note that early detection efforts involving fecal occult blood tests or endoscopy do not require sophisticated molecular diagnostic approaches. The precursor lesion for the majority of colorectal tumors appears to be the neoplastic adenoma, a benign neoplasm that is readily identified and removed at endoscopy. Endoscopy can be an expensive procedure, however, and it also involves a slight degree of risk and moderate inconvenience. The cost of colonoscopy is far greater than that for sigmoidoscopy, and the marginal benefit from viewing the entire colon (as opposed to only the distal 60cm) is probably not sufficient to justify routine screening colonoscopy in individuals who are not at very high risk. A strategy of flexible sigmoidoscopy followed by colonoscopy if polyps are seen should, in theory, identify 60–80% of all adenomas. On balance, therefore, flexible sigmoidoscopy seems to be the most practical current means of reducing colorectal cancer mortality, but the cost may still be prohibitive unless the procedure is performed by nonphysicians and not more often than once every 3–5 years. Data from the US National Cancer Institute's ongoing PCLO clinical trial, which involves flexible sigmoidoscopy screening (as well as prostate, ovary, and lung cancer screening tests), should eventually help to clarify the role of this procedure.

Primary Prevention

In contrast to early detection programs, primary prevention efforts are directed at preventing the occurrence of colorectal tumors altogether. Several lines of data indicate that primary prevention may be possible. First, there are profound geographic variations in the occurrence of colorectal cancer, with risks differing by ten times or more between low-rate countries, such as those in Africa, Asia, and South America, and high-rate countries of North America and western Europe (Boyle et al. 1985). Second, migrants to the United States from low-rate countries such as Japan and China rapidly take on the rates of their new home, particularly if they are men (Shimizu et al. 1987; Hanley et al. 1995). Third, an abundance of epidemiological studies indicate that, within a given population, specific lifestyle factors, most notably diet and exercise, are strongly associated with the risk of developing colorectal cancer (Willett 1989).

Dietary factors seem to be the most promising candidates for modifiable causes of colorectal cancer. Two general approaches have been used to describe the relationship between diet and cancer. The first is to identify specific substances within foods (macronutrients or micronutrients) that are associated with increased or decreased risk of cancer. For example, higher consumption of total calories and total fats has been related to higher risk, while intakes of fiber, antioxidant vitamins, and folate have been associated with lower risk. The second approach is to describe patterns of intake of various food groups that are associated with cancer occurrence. Such analyses indicate a higher risk of cancer in people who consume larger quantities of animal products and a lower risk in people whose diets include more plant products. For example, epidemiological studies indicate that risk of colorectal cancer is about 50% lower in people who eat a diet containing greater amounts of vegetables, fruits, and grains compared with those who rarely eat these foods (Steinmetz and Potter 1991b). There are plausible biological mechanisms to explain an anticarcinogenic effect of many substances that occur in plants (Steinmetz and Potter 1991a), and thus, dietary change on a population level conceivably could reduce colorectal cancer deaths by half, or even more.

Nearly all of the information supporting a role of specific dietary factors in colorectal cancer has come from nonexperimental studies. There is widespread opinion that these types of data are insufficient to serve as a basis for public policy recommendations about dietary change to reduce cancer occurrence. First, it is possible that unidentified confounding factors account for the perceived associations between diet and colorectal cancer in epidemiological studies. Second, the dietary information generated in these studies is generally based on self-reports of usual intake and is thus inherently imperfect. Last, these studies cannot readily distinguish between the effects of specific foods (such as vegetables) and the separate ingredients found within these foods (for example, antioxidant vitamins or fiber). In light of this uncertainty, scientists have called for randomized, controlled clinical trials of nutritional interventions as the only way to develop evidence that is convincing and capable of supporting recommendations about dietary change (Hennekens and Buring 1994).

Adenoma Prevention Trials

A randomized trial of a dietary strategy that has reduced colorectal cancer incidence as its goal poses enormous logistical difficulties. Colorectal cancer is a relatively rare occurrence in the United States, with an incidence of roughly one in 1000 persons per year at age 50 and roughly two in 1000 per year at age 65 (Ries et al. 1994). Accordingly, a study with invasive colorectal cancer as its end point would have to enroll enormous numbers of healthy patients to ensure enough future cancer cases for an informative comparison of the trial groups. Also, colorectal cancer appears to result from multiple genetic events which may occur over a period of decades (Fearon and Vogelstein 1990). An intervention that acts early in this process may not produce a measurable decline in invasive cancer incidence within the time frame of any feasible clinical trial. An alternative is to perform clinical trials to prevent invasive cancer among high-risk groups, such as patients with ulcerative colitis or familial polyposis. Often, such trials will not be feasible because of ethical concerns about not using effective preventive measures (e.g., colectomy or endoscopy with polypectomy). Furthermore, there are not many people whose risk of colorectal cancer is known to be very high.

Unlike the large samples required for studies of invasive colorectal cancer, far fewer patients are sufficient for studies focusing on adenomatous polyps. This is because the prevalence of adenomas in adults is relatively high: roughly 50% of mén over the age of 50 in industrialized countries have at least one adenoma found on examination of the entire large bowel (Rickert et al. 1979; Clark et al. 1985). Also, patients who have had an adenoma in the past have a high risk (roughly one in three) of developing at least one new adenoma within the next 3–5 years (Greenberg et al. 1994). Finally, patients with a prior adenoma can be safely observed with intermittent endoscopy and do not require more intensive interventions. Several groups of investigators have, in fact, conducted studies of dietary interventions with adenoma recurrence as the primary end point (McKeown-Eyssen et al. 1988; DeCosse et al. 1989; McKeown-Eyssen et al. 1994; Schatzkin et al. 1994). In their conduct, these trials have entailed many challenges common to virtually all cancer prevention studies. Moreover, the trials pose particular difficulties in their interpretation, since the relationship of adenoma to invasive cancer is not entirely understood.

Our group of investigators has been involved in three large multi-center studies of randomized interventions to reduce adenoma occurrence. Our experience in the first of these studies, a randomized trial of antioxidant vitamins, provides some illustrations of the major issues posed by these types of trials (Greenberg et al. 1994). Briefly, this was a randomized, double-blind, two-by-two factorial study testing whether beta-carotene (25 mg/day) or combinations of the vitamins C (1 g/day) and E (400 mg/day) would be effective in preventing the recurrence of adenomas in the large bowel among patients who previously had one of these polyp tumors resected. The study was conducted at six clinical site): Cleveland Clinic Foundation, Dartmouth-Hitchcock Medical Center, The Lahey Clinic, University of California, Los Angeles/Kaiser-Sunset, University of Iowa, and the University of Minnesota. To be eligible, patients must have had at least one adenomatous polyp removed from the large bowel within 3 months prior to enrollment and must have had a colonoscopy showing no further polyps. They also had to be in general good health and under the age of 80 years. The study called for a 4-year intervention with follow-up colonoscopy 1 year and 4 years after the index polypectomy. The occurrence of at least one adenoma during the last 3 years of the study was the primary end point (Greenberg et al. 1994).

A particularly important challenge in this study was the need to recruit adequate numbers of patients. Our initial estimate of available patients was based on endoscopy and pathology reports; however, largely because of prior invasive cancer and other disqualifying conditions, this group proved to be far larger than those who were found to be eligible once the study started. Also, among the 2029 potentially eligible patients we eventually identified from chart review, only 981 agreed to enter our study. A second major challenge was ensuring compliance with the study regimen. We first tested each patient's adherence to taking study agents using a 3-month period in which they were given placebo pills and capsules only. Of the 981 patients who entered this phase of the study, only 864 reliably took their pills and capsules during these first 3 months and ended up being randomized into the trial. Even with these efforts at careful selection of participants, maintaining compliance still proved to be difficult, particularly among patients who became seriously ill over the course of the trial and lost interest in continuing.

Uniform assessment of study end points also was a challenge. Our collaborating endoscopists agreed not to fulgurate any suspicious lesions but to submit them all for pathological examination. For some of them, this was a change in their usual practice and involved a shift in office procedures to accommodate the study. Also, they agreed to follow a schedule of repeat colonoscopies 1 year and 4 years after the colonoscopy and polypectomy performed immediately before the patient entered the study. Adhering to this schedule became particularly difficult during the later years of the study, when evidence began to accrue suggesting that a less frequent follow-up schedule was sufficient.

The primary result of our study was that there was no reduction in risk of new adenoma associated with either beta-carotene supplementation or with supplements of vitamins C and E (Table 5). Interpretation of these results was not entirely straightforward, however (Schatzkin et al. 1994). Our study focused on adenomas rather than on invasive cancer, so we could not rule out the possibility that the interventions would have prevented progression of adenomas to cancer. It was also conceivable that the interventions affected only the very earliest stages of carcinogenesis and that a longer period of observation was necessary to reveal a change in adenoma. Finally, antioxidant interventions possibly have activity only against the small subset of adenomas that will eventually go on to become cancer. At present, we cannot identify these more dangerous adenomas from among the much larger group of adenomas that will not progress. Thus, we could not say that antioxidant vitamins had no preventive activity in colorectal cancer, only that no benefit was demonstrated in our study.

Table 5. Risk of new adenoma according to treatment assignment (vitamins C and E, beta-carotene) among participants in the Polyps Prevention Study I (Greenberg et al. 1994)

Treatment	Adj RR (95% CI)[a]
Vitamins C and E	1.08 (0.91–1.29)
Beta-carotene	1.01 (0.85–1.20)

[a] Adjusted relative risk (95% confidence interval) for patients receiving the designated antioxidant supplement compared with those not receiving that particular supplement

Other investigators have used similar approaches in testing the effects of nutritional supplementation or dietary supplements in preventing colorectal adenomas. Interventions tested include calcium carbonate, a combination of vitamins C and E (McKeown-Eyssen et al. 1988), and dietary modification to a low-fat, high-fiber intake (McKeown-Eyssen et al. 1994; Schatzkin et al. 1994). None of these studies has yet provided conclusive results. Some have entailed relatively small samples and cannot exclude a moderate protective effect of the intervention. The larger studies have not been completed and reported. Thus, the ultimate value of the adenoma prevention trial as a test of colorectal cancer prevention strategies is still to be demonstrated.

There have been some intriguing ancillary findings from adenoma prevention studies, however. For example, in the course of our first trial we collected information about risk factors that may be relevant to adenoma occurrence. These included questionnaire data on dietary intake, family history, and medication use. A particularly interesting result emerged from our analysis of the use of aspirin among participants. Preliminary studies from both case-control and cohort investigations have suggested that persons who regularly consume aspirin have a 40–50% reduction in risk of invasive colorectal cancer. There are also data from laboratory studies and small-scale clinical trials indicating that other non-steroidal anti-inflammatory drugs can prevent adenoma occurrence or even cause these tumors to disappear (Heath et al. 1994). We therefore examined the relationship between aspirin use and adenomas detected at the follow-up colonoscopy examination, conducted about 9 months after entry to the study. We found that risk of having an adenoma was approximately 40% lower among patients who reported that they took aspirin on both of the questionnaires administered between study entry and the follow-up examination (Greenberg et al. 1993). We later extended this analysis to examine the relationship between aspirin use and adenoma occurrence over the entire 4-year study period. The results of these analyses were consistent with our earlier results and support the notion that aspirin may prevent colorectal tumor formation. On the basis of these and other data, our group and others have now undertaken further clinical trials of colorectal polyp prevention. A new trial from our group involves two doses of aspirin, 360 mg and 80 mg per day, and it also includes a folate arm.

Conclusions

There now are excellent prospects for reducing colorectal cancer deaths in the United States and in other industrialized countries. Screening by fecal occult blood testing or by endoscopy should effectively reduce mortality by a third or more if widely applied in the adult population. Dietary change towards consumption of more plant-based foods seems to be a prudent course, although the benefits for colorectal cancer prevention are still speculative. Chemopreventive strategies also hold promise for the future, and aspirin is a particularly intriguing possible agent for study.

References

Boyle P, Zaridze D et al (1985) Descriptive epidemiology of colorectal cancer. Int J Cancer 36:9–18

Clark JC, Collan Y et al (1985) Prevalence of polyps in an autopsy series from areas with varying incidence of large-bowel cancer. Int J Cancer 36:179–186

DeCosse J, Miller H et al (1989) Effect of wheat fiber and vitamins C and E on rectal polyps in patients with familial adenomatous polyposis. J Natl Cancer Inst 81:1290–1297

Fearon ER, Vogelstein B (1990) A genetic model for colorectal tumorigenesis. Cell 61:759–767

Greenberg ER, Baron JA et al (1993) Reduced risk of large bowel adenomas among aspirin users. J Natl Cancer Inst 85:912–916

Greenberg ER, Baron JA et al (1994) A clinical trial of antioxidant vitamins to prevent colorectal adenoma. N Engl J Med 331:141–147

Greenwald P (1992) Colon cancer overview. Cancer [Suppl] 70:1206S–1215S

Hanley AJG, Choi BCK et al (1995) Cancer mortality among Chinese migrants: a review. Int J Epidemiol 24:255–265

Heath CWJ, Thun MJ et al (1994) Nonsteroidal antiinflammatory drugs and human cancer. Cancer 74:2885–2888

Hennekens CH, Buring JE (1994) Contributions of observational evidence and clinical trials in cancer prevention. Cancer 74:2625–2629

McKeown-Eyssen G, Holloway C et al (1988) A randomized trial of vitamins C and E in the prevention of recurrence of colorectal polyps. Cancer Res 48:4701–4705

McKeown-Eyssen GE, Bright-See E et al (1994) A randomized trial of a low-fat high-fibre diet in the recurrence of colorectal polyps. J Clin Epidemiol 47:525–536

Mandel JS, Bond JH et al (1993) Reducing mortality from colorectal cancer by screening for fecal occult blood. Minnesota Colon Cancer Control Study. N Engl J Med 328:1365–1371

Newcomb PA, Norfleet RG et al (1992) Screening sigmoidscopy and colorectal cancer mortality. J Natl Cancer Inst 84:1572–1575

Rickert RR, Auerbach O et al (1979) Adenomatous lesions of the large bowel: an autopsy survey. Cancer 43:1847–1857

Ries LAG, Miller BA et al (1994) Cancer Statistics Review: 1973–1991: Tables and Graphs, National Cancer Institute. Bethesda, MD, NIH publ no 94-2789

Schatzkin A, Freedman LS et al (1994) Interpreting precursor studies: what polyp trials tell us about large-bowel cancer. J Natl Cancer Inst 86:1053–1057
Selby JV, Friedman GD et al (1992) A case-control study of screening sigmoidoscopy and mortality from colorectal cancer. N Engl J Med 326:653–657
Shimizu H, Mack TM et al (1987) Cancer of the gastrointestinal tract among Japanese and white immigrants in Los Angeles county. J Natl Cancer Inst 78:223–228
Steinmetz K, Potter JD (1991a) Vegetables, fruit, and cancer. II. Mechanisms. Cancer Causes Control 2:427–442
Steinmetz KA, Potter JD (1991b) Vegetables, fruit, and cancer. I. Epidemiology. Cancer Causes Control 2:325–357
Willett W (1989) The search for the causes of breast and colon cancer. Nature 338:389–394
Winawer SJ, Zauber AG et al (1993) Prevention of colorectal cancer by colonoscopic polypectomy. N Engl J Med 329:1977–1981

Adhesion Receptors in Malignant Transformation and Dissemination of Gastrointestinal Tumors

M. Streit[1], R. Schmidt[1], R.U. Hilgenfeld[2], E. Thiel[1], and E.D. Kreuser[1]

[1] Dept. of Hematology and Oncology, University Medical Center Benjamin Franklin, Free University of Berlin, Hindenburgdamm 30, 12200 Berlin, Germany
[2] Medical Department I, St. Joseph Hospital, Bäumerplan 24, 12101 Berlin, Germany

Abstract

Adhesion receptors on the surface of cancer cells play an important role in tumor cell migration, invasion, and metastasis. A number of specific cell surface-associated molecules that mediate cell–matrix and cell–cell interactions have been characterized, including the family of integrin receptors, the cadherins, the immunoglobulin (IgG) superfamily, a 67-kDa laminin-binding protein, and the CD44 receptor. Changes in the expression and function of these adhesion molecules are important characteristics in the development of gastrointestinal malignancies and might be used in the future as prognostic factors or as new targets in diagnosis and therapy. In esophageal cancer a downregulation of the E-cadherin receptor and the cytoplasmic protein α-catenin is associated with tumor dedifferentiation, infiltrative growth, and lymph node metastasis. In gastric cancer a reduction of E-cadherin expression due to gene mutations is restricted to diffuse-type tumors. The occurrence of the CD44 standard and the CD44-9v isoform on the surface of gastric cancer cells is significantly related to a higher tumor-induced mortality and a shorter survival time. The CD44-6v isoform is predominantly expressed by intestinal-type gastric carcinomas giving these tumor cells the ability to metastasize in the lymph nodes. In pancreatic cancer the expression of integrin adhesion receptors is significantly altered during the malignant transformation of the pancreatic tissue while a loss of the E-cadherin receptor can generate dedifferentiation and invasiveness of pancreas carcinoma cells. There is increasing evidence that integrin receptors and different isoforms of the CD44 receptor are altered following the malignant transformation of colonic mucosa into adenomas and invasive carcinomas and thus influencing in their metastatic potential. The expression of the CD44-6v isoform seems to be associated with an adverse prognosis in colorectal cancer due to the development of tumor metastases. A strong

Recent Results in Cancer Research, Vol. 142

correlation could be observed between the expression of the 67-kDa laminin receptor and the degree of differentiation, the invasive phenotype, and the metastatic abilities of colorectal cancer cells. Analyzing the expression of the E-cadherin receptor in colorectal carcinomas it has been shown that this receptor may serve as an independent prognostic marker in Dukes' stage Colon cancer to identify patients with poor prognosis and designate them for adjuvant therapy after curative surgical treatment.

Introduction

Adherent cells use specific cell surface receptors to interact with other cells or with the surrounding extracellular matrix. These receptors are of fundamental importance in the organization of tissues and organs. Adhesion receptors not only anchor cells to their proper locations, but also actively mediate the passage of information into the cell and from the cell interior to the surrounding tissue. Many essential cellular functions, including growth, differentiation, migration, and expression of specific genes, can be controlled by signal transduction via matrix adhesion receptors (Albelda and Buck 1990; Hynes 1992; Juliano and Haskill 1993).

The prognosis of cancer patients is influenced mainly by tumor growth, local infiltration, and metastasis. The ability of malignant tumor cells to invade the extracellular matrix and to metastasize is believed to be due in part to the expression of cellular adhesion receptors that interact with components of the extracellular matrix and the basement membrane. Thus, a change in the pattern of adhesion receptor expression could be indicative of malignant transformation. A transformed cell phenotype may contain several alterations in cell adhesion receptors. Receptors assumed to support the normal phenotype can disappear, and concomitantly, receptors needed for tumor invasion and metastasis can be induced (Aznavoorian et al. 1993). Metastatic spread is a multistep process which consists of numerous tumor cell-host cell and cell-matrix interactions (Liotta et al. 1991). Interactions with the extracellular matrix, especially basement membranes, characterizing the process of invasion include the ability of tumor cells to attach and to proteolyze matrix components in order to migrate through the matrix defect. Metastasizing tumor cells also have to traverse vascular basement membranes on the way to tissue invasion from the circulation. None of these functions is unique to tumor cells. The difference between physiological processes and the pathogenic nature of tumor cell invasion and metastasis must therefore be one of regulation (Aznavoorian et al. 1993). Thus, an understanding of the controlling factors in the processes of cellular attachement, matrix proteolysis, and cell migration mediated in part by different families of cell surface receptors may allow the identification of new targets to inhibit malignant transformation and metastasis formation.

Table 1. Families of cell adhesion receptors

Family	Receptor	Ligand	Distribution
Integrins	See Table 2		
IgG superfamily	ICAM-1 (CD54)	αLβ2	Leukocytes
	ICAM-2	αLβ2	Endothelial cells
	ICAM-3	αLβ2	Leukocytes
	LFA-2 (CD2)	LFA-3	T cells
	LFA-3 (CD58)	LFA-2	Widespread
	VCAM-1	α4β1	Activated endothelial cells
	Ca²-independent CAMs		
	N-CAM	Homophilic binding	Brain, muscle, heart, kidney neural and glial cells
	Ng-CAM	Homophilic and heterophilic binding	
Cadherin	N-Cadherin	Homophilic binding	Neural cells, brain, muscle, lens
	E-Cadherin	Homophilic binding	Epithelium
	P-Cadherin	Homophilic binding	Placenta, epithelium, mesothelinm
Lec-CAM (Selectine)	Lec-Cam 1 (Mel-14)	Carbohydrate	Lymphocytes
	ELAM-1 (Lec-CAM 2)	Sialyl-Lewis X	Endothelial cells, neutrophils, tumor cells
	Lec-CAM 3 (GMP-140)	Lewis X (CD 15)	Platelets, neutrophils, monocytes, endothelial cells
CD44	CD44 and variant isoforms	Hyaluronic acid, laminin, collagens, fibronectin	Widespread

A number of specific cell surface-associated molecules that modulate cell-matrix and cell-cell interactions have been characterized (Table 1). These include the family of integrin receptors, the cadherins, the immunoglobulin (IgG) superfamily, a 67-kD laminin-binding protein, and the CD44 receptor. The role of these classes of adhesion molecules in the development, growth, invasion, and metastasis of malignant tumors is under active investigation. Changes in the expression and function of adhesion molecules are important characteristics of gastrointestinal malignancies. The present review thus focuses on the recent results of the role of adhesion receptors in the malignant transformation and dissemination of gastrointestinal tumors.

The Integrins

The integrins (Fig. 1) constitute a large family of heterodimeric transmembrane receptors that mediate both cell-cell and cell-extracellular matrix adhe-

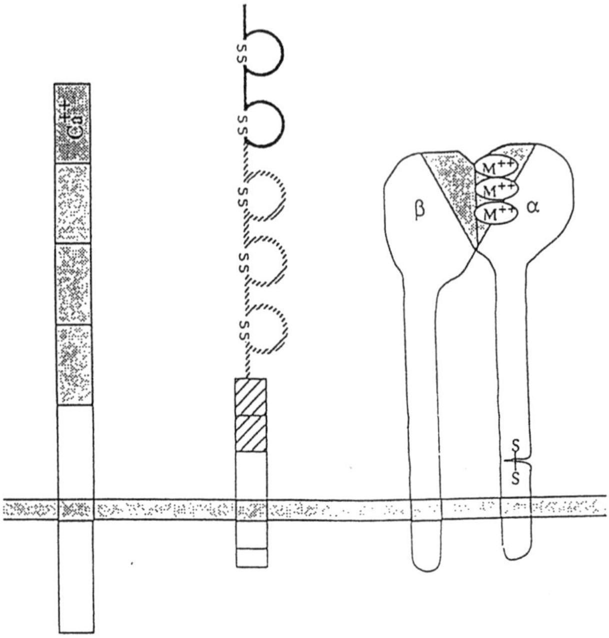

Fig. 1. Major families of cell adhesion receptors. Cadherins are Ca^{2+}-dependent homophilic cell-cell adhesion molecules. Immunoglobulin superfamily adhesion receptors contain immunoglobulin domains (Ω) and, frequently, fibronectin type-II repeats (*cross-hatched boxes*). These cell-cell adhesion receptors are Ca^{2+} dependent and participate in heterophilic and homophilic interactions. Integrins are heterodimeric receptors, some for extracellular matrix proteins and some for immunoglobulin superfamily counter-receptors, and therefore can be involved in both cell-matrix and cell-cell adhesion. Most receptors of all families are transmembrane proteins. Binding domains are indicated by the *shaded areas*

sive interactions (Hynes 1992). Each integrin receptor is composed of a noncovalently linked α and β subunit, each subunit having a large extracellular domain, a transmembrane region, and a short cytoplasmic domain (Albelda and Buck 1990). There are currently 16 α and 8 β subunits identified that combine to form a number of receptors with distinct binding specificities (Table 2). However, the diversity of heterodimeric associations is somewhat restricted, since most α subunits combine with only one β subunit, although $\alpha4$, $\alpha6$, and αv associate with multiple β subunits (Edward 1995). Integrins are the major group of adhesion molecules responsible for mediating cellular interactions with the extracellular matrix, many components of which possess an arginine, glycine, aspartatic acid (RGD) sequence that is recognized by several integrin receptors (Ruoshlahti 1992).

The presence of multiple integrins on the cell surface endows a cell with the capacity to recognize its own extracellular matrix and those matrices secreted

Table 2. Extracellular ligands of integrin receptors

Integrin– β subunit	Integrin – α subunit	Ligands
β1	α1	Collagens
		Laminin
	α2	Collagens
		Laminin
		Fibronectin
		Echovirus 1
	α3	Fibronectin
		Collagen 1
		Epiligrin
	α4	Fibronectin
		Invasin
		VCAMs
	α5	Fibronectin
		RGD sequence
	α6	Laminin
	α7	Laminin
	α8	?
	α9	?
	αv	Fibronectin
		RGD sequence
		Vitronectin
β2	αL	Fibrinogen
		C3bi
		ICAMs
	αM	Fibrinogen
		Factor X
		ICAMs
	αX	Fibrinogen
		C3bi
β3	αIIB	Collagens
		Vitronectin
		Fibronectin
		RGD sequence
		Fibrinogen
		v.Willebrand factor
		Thrombospondin
		Disintegrins
		Borrelia burgdorferi
	αv	Fibronectin
		RGD sequence
		Vitronectin
		Fibrinogen
		Thrombospondin
		Osteopontin
		Cytoactin/Tenascin
		v.Willebrand factor
		Disintegrins
		HIV Tat proteins

Table 2. *Continued*

Integrin – β subunit	Integrin – α subunit	Ligands
$\beta 4$	$\alpha 6$	Laminin
$\beta 5$	αv	Vitronectin
		RGD sequence
		HIV Tat proteins
$\beta 6$	αv	Fibronectin
		Cytoacin/tenascin
$\beta 7$	$\alpha 4$	Fibronectin
		Mucosal ACAM-1
		VCAMs
$\beta 8$	αv	?

ACAM, addression cell adhesion molecule-1; *C3bi*, complement factor C3bi, *VCAM*, vascular cell adhesion molecule

by other cells. This recognition system is responsible for the positional information cells need for anchorage, polarity, differentiation, and directed migration. The ability of tumor cells to invade also seems to depend on the interaction of integrins with their ligands (Juliano and Varner 1993; Heino 1993).

It is becoming increasingly apparent that integrins, and presumably several other adhesion molecules, are expressed on the cell surface in different states of activation, which implies that the expression of a particular adhesion molecule does not necessarily ensure that the cell will adhere to its ligand (Diamond and Springer 1994). A number of signaling events initiated by an extracellular signal may culminate in changes in the activation state of integrins and enhance their binding affinity. Changes in binding affinity are mediated by conformational changes in the integrin structure, resulting in the exposure of the binding site. Following integrin activation, subsequent ligation can lead to changes in gene expression, such as the induction of collagenases and cytokine expression, and affect cellular growth and differentiation (Juliano 1994). As there is a considerable overlap of binding specificities in some of the integrins, it seems that different integrins may bind to the same extracellular matrix protein but transduce different signals into the cell interior (Ginsberg et al. 1992; Juliano and Haskill 1993). The signal transduction mechanism of integrin receptors is mediated in part by protein tyrosine phosporylation. A cytoplasmic protein found to be phosphorylated and activated after integrin clustering and cell adhesion has been identified as a 125-kD protein kinase associated with focal contacts and termed $pp125^{FAK}$ (Schaller and Parsons 1994; Schlaepfer et al. 1994). Integrin ligation resulting in the stimulation of tyrosine phosphorylation of several other proteins has been observed which involves the phosphorylation of key transcription factors and thereby influences gene expression (Juliano 1994). The function of integrins is not restricted to cell adhesion; they are true receptors that can mediate signal transduction processes which may impinge upon gene expression, proliferation, apoptosis, migration, cytokine secretion, and metastasis.

The Cadherins

Cadherins are calcium-dependent cell-cell adhesion receptors that have been identified in vertebrates (Fig. 1). They bind cells by means of homophilic interactions and are responsible mainly for establishing and maintaining intercellular connections (Table 1). Cadherins are therefore important determinants of tissue morphology (Geiger and Agalon 1992; Juna and Hitt 1992). There are at least 12 different known members of the cadherin familiy, which are divided into subclasses sharing a common basic structure. Four subclasses are well characterized at the molecular level: the E-cadherin (epithelial cadherin or uvomorulin), the P-cadherin (placental cadherin), the N-cadherin (neural cadherin, also called A-CAM), and the L-CAM (liver cell adhesion molecule) (Buxton et al. 1993). The important property of cadherins is their binding specificity, since cadherins connect cells to each other by selective binding to identical cadherin types. Each of the cadherin subclasses displays a unique pattern of tissue distribution, and multiple cadherin subclasses are coexpressed in varying combinations in many types of cells. Each cell type can thus be characterized by the expression of one particular cadherin or a set of subclasses (Takeichi 1991). The expression of cadherins is developmentally regulated and correlates with a variety of morphogenetic events that involve cell aggregation and disaggregation. In cancer metastasis, the detachment of cells from the primary tumor is an initial step which is caused by a disruption of mutual cell connections (Van Roy and Mareel 1992). Therefore, the suppression of cadherin activity is necessary and occurs either by a suppression of cadherin gene expression or by a loss of function of the expressed cadherin molecules (Behrens et al. 1989, 1993). Malignant transformation does not necessarily affect cadherin activity, but it was demonstrated that tumor cells with higher and lower activities of spontaneous metastasis often differ in their expression of cadherin receptors (Takeichi 1993; Birchmeier et al. 1993).

The Immunoglobulin Superfamily

The immunoglobulin superfamily (Fig. 1) comprises a wide variety of molecules that share a common structural feature of immunoglobulins: a 70–110 amino acid domain organized into several β-pleated sheets, each stabilized by a single disulfide bond (Springer 1990). The most important member of the immunoglobulin superfamily expressed on gastrointestinal tumor cells seems to be the intercellular adhesion molecule 1 (ICAM-1). ICAM-1 is a cell surface adhesion glycoprotein that is constitutively expressed by endothelial cells and by some leukocytes (Long et al. 1992). ICAM-1 surface expression can be induced in many other cell types both in vivo, in the setting of active inflammation, and in vitro, through the action of inflammatory cytokines (Springer 1990). Cells expressing ICAM-1 can support adhesion of leukocytes, including lymphocytes, by specific interaction with the leukocyte integrins of the $\beta 2$-family (Staunton et al. 1988). ICAM-1 adhesion to the lymphocyte function-associated antigen-1 (LFA-1 or $\alpha L\beta 2$ integrin) is integral to many adhesion-dependent leukocyte functions, including lymphocyte proliferation and cytolytic activity (Makgoba et al. 1989). The potential role of ICAM-1 in lymphocyte carcinoma cell interactions in gastrointestinal tumors has not been clearly defined.

The 67-kD Laminin Receptor

Laminin is a high-molecular-weight glycoprotein and a major component of basement membranes. Laminin has several important biological activities, including the stimulation of cellular attachment, differentiation, proliferation, migration, and neurite outgrowth (Beck et al. 1990). Interactions between cancer cells and laminin have been shown to play a critical role during tumor invasion and metastasis (Hunt 1989). Several different laminin-binding cell surface proteins have recently been described. Among these, a 67-kD, high-affinity, laminin-binding protein has been associated with the invasive and metastatic phenotype of cancer cells (Castronovo 1993; Sobel 1994). The structure of this 67-kD laminin receptor has not been definitely resolved (Castronovo et al. 1991), but it was shown that highly metastatic cancer cells express significantly more 67-kD laminin receptors on their surface than their much less metastatic or benign counterparts (Horan-Hand et al. 1985). To assess the potential diagnostic and prognostic value of detecting the 67-kD receptor in human cancer pathology, several studies examined the expression of this receptor at the protein and mRNA levels in a variety of tumor lesions including breast cancer (Terranova et al. 1983; Castronovo et al. 1990; Daidone et al. 1991) ovarian cancer (D'Errico et al. 1991), and cervical carcinoma (Demeter et al. 1992), as well as gastrointestinal malignancies. The expression of the 67-kD receptor and its precursor was significantly higher in most solid carcinomas analyzed than in the corresponding normal tissue. In colon, breast, ovarian, and gastric cancer there was a direct positive correlation between the expression of the 67-kD receptor in the primary tumor and the metastatic potential of the lesion. These findings suggest that the 67-kD receptor is a gene product whose increased expression might participate in the acquisition of the metastatic phenotype (Castronovo 1993).

CD44 and Variant Isoforms

CD44 is a widely expressed cell surface glycoprotein (Fig. 2) that serves as an adhesion molecule in cell-substrate and cell-cell interactions, including lymphocyte homing, hematopoiesis, cell migration, and tumor metastasis (Lesley et al. 1993). CD44 also has other functions that relate to lymphocyte activation and the binding of certain cytokines to the endothelium (Tanaka et al. 1993). CD44 is a proteoglycan with an NH_2-terminal region that is structurally related to several hyaluronate-binding proteins (Underhill 1992). CD44 is known to bind hyaluronate and collagen, and a chondroitin-sulfated form of CD44 binds fibronectin (Carter and Wagner 1988; Jalkanen and Jalkanen 1992). The numerous functions and molecular interactions of CD44 probably relate to its complex structure. In addition to the standard form (CD44s), there are several larger variant isoforms (CD44v) that are generated by alternative splicing of at

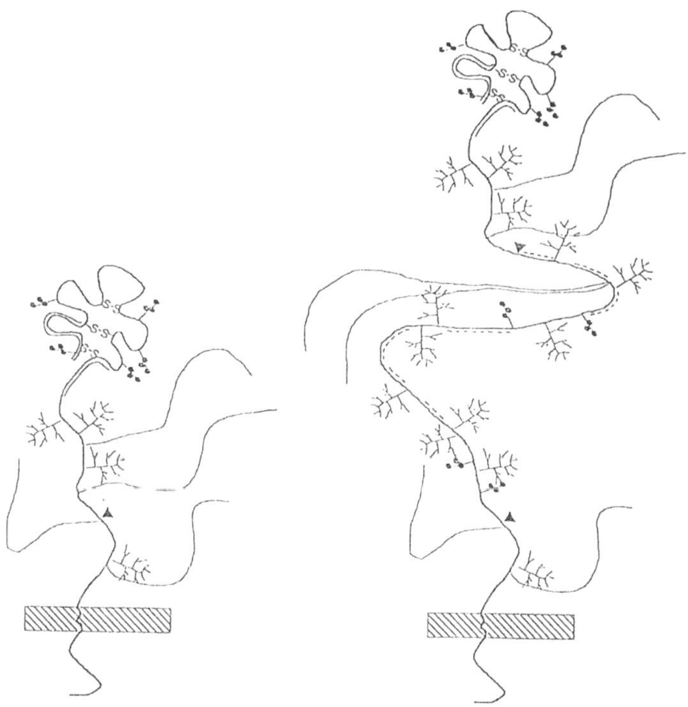

Fig. 2. Structure of the CD44 s and CD44 v receptor. *Left:* Transmembrane glycoprotein CD44 s (standard) with potential N-glycosylations (*bars with dots*), O-glycosylations (*tree structures*), and chondroitin sulfate chains (*thin lines*). The hyaluronate-binding regions in the aminoterminal part are marked by an *additional line*. The position where the variant region can be inserted is indicated by a *triangle*. The cell membrane is represented by a *striped bar*. *Right:* CD44 v (variant isoform). The region *between the triangles* represents the human variant region covering the exons 2v–10v

least 10 exons (Mackay et al. 1994). It was demonstrated that certain combinations of the variant exons are expressed on epithelial cells, carcinomas, and some hematopoietic cells, but little is known about their function or regulation (Günthert et al. 1994). Expression of variant CD44 isoforms in some tissues appears to relate to tumor progression and particularly to the metastatic potential of some carcinomas (Zöller 1995). Günthert et al. (1991) demonstrated that CD44 splice variants sharing the exon v6 promote the metastatic spread of pancreatic carcinoma cells from a subcutaneous injection site in an isogenic animal model. Neither local nor in vitro growth rates seemed to profit from the presence of the v6-splicing variant. Transfecting nonmetastasizing cancer cells lacking the v6 isoform proved that these CD44-v6 transfectants gained the potential to colonize the lungs in an experimental animal model (Seiter et al. 1993). Repeated injection of antibodies specific to the v6 epitope prevents the growth of the v6 transfectants in the draining lymph nodes and the formation of metastases. Thus it appears that the CD44-v6 isoform is needed in the initial phase of lymphogenic tumor cell spread in the animal model explored and may also be important in the metastatic process in man.

Role of Adhesion Molecules in Gastrointestinal Cancer

Esophageal Cancer

E-Cadherin. Little is known about the potential role of cellular adhesion receptors in the pathogenesis and distribution of malignancies of the upper digestive tract. The cell-cell adhesion molecule E-cadherin plays a key role in the establishment and maintenance of epithelial tissue structures. Its down-regulation might be important in the malignant transformation and metastatic spread of carcinomas (Takeichi 1991). Intercellular adhesion of epithelial tissue is regulated mainly by the E-cadherin molecule, as well as by the E-cadherin-associated cytoplasmic protein α-catenin that forms a linkage to the cytoskeleton and regulates E-cadherin function. The investigation of E-cadherin and α-catenin expression in human esophageal cancer demonstrated a reduction of both molecules in most of the tumor samples investigated by Kadowaki et al. (1994). Regarding the clinicopathological features, a reduction in α-catenin as well as in E-cadherin expression was significantly associated with tumor dedifferentiation, infiltrative growth, and lymph node metastasis (Schipper et al. 1991). These findings were supported by in vitro studies investigating the E-cadherin expression in esophageal cancer cell lines. Doki et al. (1993) demonstrated that a down-modulation of E-cadherin leads to a change in cell morphology, to a decrease in intercellular adhesion, and to an increase in tumor cell invasion.

CD44. The CD44 receptor and some of its variant isoforms are differentially expressed in normal epithelia and malignancies of the esophagus (Mackay et al. 1994). The CD44-9v, the CD44-6v, which confers metastatic potential to carcinoma cells in animal models (Günthert et al. 1991), and the CD44-4v splice variants are intensively expressed in stratified squamous epithelium, particularly in the esophagus. While squamous epithelium is the only non-malignant tissue in which the expression of the CD44-4v and the CD44-6v isoform is detectable in squamous cells carcinomas, a down-regulation of CD44-6v expression was observed (Salmi et al. 1993; Terpe et al. 1994).

Gastric Cancer

E-Cadherin. The expression and potential importance of E- and P-cadherin, two calcium-dependent intercellular adhesion molecules, were intensively investigated in the epithelia of stomach and gastric adenocarcinomas (Shimoyama and Hirohashi 1991). E-cadherin is strongly expressed in gastric epithelia from the surface to deep glands. P-cadherin could not be detected in the gastric epithelia, although in part, weak staining was occasionally observed in the proliferative zone of human gastric epithelium. Gastric adenocarcinomas showed a heterogeneous expression and distribution of cadherin receptors, depending on the degree of differentiation. E-cadherin served as the main cadherin molecule responsible for intercellular adhesion in gastric carcinomas, while P-cadherin was unstable in most of them in contrast to the stable expression of E-cadherin. Differentiated carcinomas strongly and uniformly expressed E-cadherin, as did noncancerous gastric epithelia. The adherent type of undifferentiated gastric carcinomas also showed a strong expression of E-cadherin, while most of the scattered-type lesions, such as signet ring carcinomas lacking tight intercellular adhesion, did not express E-cadherin. A study comparing the E-cadherin expression of primary and metastatic gastric carcinomas (Mayer et al. 1993b) showed a significant reduction of E-cadherin expression in primary gastric carcinomas compared with normal mucosa, suggesting that the down-regulation of this adhesion molecule is a common early event in gastric tumorigenesis. In advanced tumors, a significant loss of E-cadherin-positive cells was detected and a correlation between low E-cadherin expression and cellular dedifferentiation and disintegration of tissue architecture was observed. Low E-cadherin expression was associated with a high risk of tumor recurrence and mortality. E-cadherin expression in metastatic lesions also correlated with the degree of glandular differentiation and with the receptor status of primary tumors. In some cases, an increased level of receptor expression in liver metastases of E-cadherin-positive tumors was detected, suggesting a possible regulatory role of the microenvironment. The authors concluded that E-cadherin represents a differentiation marker whose down-modulation might play an important role in early gastric cancer metastasis. The reduced E-cadherin expression in gastric carcinomas could be caused by gene mutations, as shown by in vitro data (Oda et al. 1994). Abnormal mRNA nucleotide sequences were detected in two E-cadherin-positive, poorly differentiated gastric cancer cell lines lacking intercellular adhesion. These findings were caused by DNA mutations around exon-intron junctions, revealing that aberrant RNA splicing was the cause of the mRNA abnormalties. Moreover, in both cell lines the wild-type allele of the E-cadherin locus was lost, suggesting that the E-cadherin gene had been inactivated by a mechanism similar to that for inactivation of tumor suppressor genes.

This concept of E-cadherin as a suppressor of invasion and metastasis in gastric carcinoma has been further substantiated by the in vivo investigations of Becker et al. (1993, 1994). E-cadherin gene mutations could be demonstrated by the reverse transcription polymerase chain reaction in 13 of 26 patients (50%) with diffuse-type gastric cancer and in one of seven (14%) with a mixed gastric carcinoma. The altered forms of E-cadherin mRNA were not present in normal gastric epithelial tissue. In most of the analyzed tumor samples, either exon 8 or exon 9 was missing from the E-cadherin mRNA, which eliminated potential sites determining the adhesive capacity. The authors speculated that E-cadherin molecules lacking either exon 8 or exon 9 were functionally inert, since amino acid substitutions affecting a single calcium-binding site have been shown to abolish the adhesive function (Ozawa 1990). Removal of the complete calcium-binding domain due to a loss of exon 8 or exon 9 would be expected to generate inactive E-cadherin receptors, thus facilitating the scattering of carcinoma cells. Additional point mutations were also found in the E-cadherin cDNA of two diffuse-type and two intestinal-type gastric carcinomas, whereas only the two mutations detected in diffuse-type tumors resulted in a structural change of the E-cadherin molecule. The prevalence of E-cadherin gene mutations in diffuse-type gastric carcinomas provides strong in vivo evidence that E-cadherin alterations play a major role in the development and dissemination of this histological type of gastric cancer. Thus, in addition to previous findings indicating that the E-cadherin-mediated invasion–suppressor role is often inactivated by a down-regulation of the receptor expression, these in vitro and in vivo results impressively demonstrated another mechanism for the initiation of invasion and metastasis in gastric cancer.

Alpha-Catenin. Alpha-catenin is an undercoat protein of adherent junctions which binds to the cytoplasmic domain of E-cadherin, linking E-cadherin to actin-based cytoskeleton. In an investigation of a sample of resected gastric carcinomas, a reduction of alpha-catenin expression was observed (Matsui et al. 1994). This reduction was significantly related to dedifferentiation, depth of tumor invasion, infiltrative growth, and lymph node metastasis. Comparing the co-expression of alpha-catenin and E-cadherin in these gastric carcinomas with their clinical stage showed that alpha-catenin expression is apparently a better predictor of tumor invasion and metastasis than E-cadherin expression in advanced gastric cancer.

CD44. The expression of the CD44 receptor and its variant isoforms seems to be of important prognostic value in gastric carcinomas. While normal gastric mucosa is CD44 negative, the expression of this receptor in benign mucosa is always associated with leukocyte infiltration in the presence of atrophic gastritis and intestinal metaplasia, both being discussed as precancerous lesions (Mackay et al. 1994; Correa and Shiao 1994). In primary gastric carcinomas the expression of CD44 does not seem to be useful as a diagnostic marker, since only half of the investigated tumor samples stained positive (Günthert et al., manuscript in preparation). The most important observation was that the expression of the CD44s and the 9v isoform was significantly related to increased tumor recurrence after curative surgical resection, higher tumor-induced mortality, and shorter survival time (Mayer et al. 1993a). Interesting, in regard to a possible role of CD44 in gastric cancer metastasis, was the finding that the expression of CD44 and the CD44-9v isoform was more common in cardia carcinomas, which have a very poor prognosis, and in advanced tumors with distant metastases (Günthert et al., manuscript in preparation). CD44 expression in metastatic lesions which were highly positive showed no preference for specific metastatic locations (Heider et al. 1993a). While the CD44-9v isoform seems to be of important prognostic relevance, the expression of the CD44-6v isoform is restricted predominantly to intestinal-type carcinomas (Heider et al. 1993a) and may be a means of determining tumor type in gastric carcinomas.

Data recently published by Dämmrich et al. (1995) suggest that the different pattern of lymphogenic spread observed in intestinal-type as opposed to diffuse-type gastric carcinomas might be due to a difference in CD44-6v expression. It was found that CD44-6v-positive intestinal-type carcinomas predominantly involve infiltrative lymph node metastases, whereas sinus carcinosis without infiltrative growth is observed more frequently in CD44-6v-negative diffuse-type tumors. It could be demonstrated that, in lymph nodes, only infiltrative tumor cells expressed CD44-6v. The lymphogenic metastases of intestinal-type tumors were always positive for this isoform, while the cells of diffuse-type carcinomas expressed CD44-v6 only when infiltrative growth had taken place even if the primary tumor lacked this splice variant.

This neoexpression of CD44-6v in lymph node metastases of diffuse-type gastric carcinomas indicates that this isoform plays an important role in tumor cell penetration through the lymphatic vessel by using lymphocytic properties to form lymph node metastases. The expression of the CD44-5v isoform seems to be closely related to gastric tumor differentiation, as shown by Harn et al. (1995). The CD44-5v splicing variant was not seen in normal gastric tissue but could be found in intestinal metaplasia and was strongly stained in tubular and signet ring-cell-type adenocarcinomas as well as in metastatic lymph nodes of gastric adenocarcinomas. Generation of CD44 splice variants may therefore be closely linked with gastric carcinoma tumorigenesis, differentiation, and metastasis. In addition, expression of CD44 standard and CD44-9v seems to be of important prognostic value, while CD55-5v may be used to detect evolving gastric cancer and CD44-6v expression to determine the risk of lymph node metastasis in gastric carcinoma.

Pancreatic Cancer

Integrins. The expression of cell adhesion receptors of the integrin family is significantly altered during malignant transformation of the pancreatic tissue (Weinel et al. 1992; Hall et al. 1991; Rosendahl et al. 1993). The $\alpha 2$- and $\alpha 6$-integrin subunits were moderately to strongly expressed on the basal surface of ductal and acinar cells in normal pancreatic tissue (Table 3), while centro-acinar cells expressed predominantly the $\alpha 3$- and $\alpha 5$-subunits. Islet cells failed to show any expression of integrin subunits. In chronic pancreatitis, the expression of the $\alpha 3$-subunit remained unchanged, and the ductal cells showed the same intensity of $\alpha 2$-integrin expression as the tumor tissue. The integrin expression and distribution was significantly different in pancreatic carcinomas. The $\alpha 2$- and $\alpha 6$-subunits were strongly expressed with a diffuse distribution on the cell surface, and the expression of the $\alpha 3$- and $\alpha 5$-subunits ranged heterogeneously from moderate to weak and was absent in half of the tumors investigated. The functional importance of integrin expression was investigated using pancreatic cancer cell lines. In vitro adhesion assays proved that the $\alpha 2$-subunit was necessary for cell adhesion to collagen type IV, while the $\alpha 6$-subunit served as a laminin receptor, and the adhesion to fibronectin was mediated by the $\alpha 5$-subunit (Weinel et al. 1992). No correlation was found

Table 3. Alterations in the expression of adhesion molecules in gastrointestinal cancer

	Integrin-subunit	Cadherins	IgG superfamily	67-kD laminin receptor	CD44 and variant isoforms
Esophageal cancer		E-cadherin ↓			CD44-6v ↓
Gastric cancer		E-cadherin ↓			CD44s ↑ CD44-6v ↑ CD44-9v ↑
Pancreatic cancer	$\alpha 2$ ↑ $\alpha 6$ ↑ $\alpha 3$ ↓ $\alpha 5$ ↓	E-cadherin ↓	ICAM-1 ↑		
Colorectal cancer	$\alpha 2$ ↓ $\alpha 3$ ↓ $\alpha 5$ ↓ $\alpha 6$ ↓ $\beta 1$ ↓	E-cadherin↓	ICAM-1↑	67 kD↑	CD44s ↑ CD44-6v ↑ CD44-8v ↑ CD44-9v ↑ CD44-10v ↑

between the expression of integrin receptors and the grade of tumor differentiation by analyzing different pancreatic tumor cell lines in vitro (Löhr et al. 1995). Interactions of cells with basement membrane proteins mediated by specific cell adhesion receptors play an important role in the development of malignant epithelial tumors. Initial cell adhesion, spreading, migration, and the modulation of cell differentiation are thought to be regulated by basal laminae and their major cell-binding component, the glycoprotein laminin. It was shown that the degree of malignancy in human pancreatic adenocarcinomas is correlated to the composition and architecture of the surrounding extracellular matrix. The occurrence of an intact basal lamina is restricted to slow-growing and highly differentiated pancreatic tumors, whereas dedifferentiated pancreatic tumors and metastasis with an increasing proliferation are surrounded essentially by interstitial connective tissue (Mollenhauer et al. 1987). In vitro studies using human pancreatic adenocarcinoma cell lines demonstrated that the basement membrane protein laminin promoted the modulation of pancreatic cancer cells from a proliferative to a resting phenotype. Laminin induced a restoration of cell polarity, an increased protein biosynthesis, and glycoprotein secretion due to an enhancement of laminin adhesion receptor expression (Mai et al. 1990).

E-Cadherin. The ability of pancreas carcinomas to invade and metastasize depends largely on the degree of epithelial differentiation within the tumor. Pancreas carcinoma cell lines with an epithelioid phenotype were noninvasive in vitro and expressed the epithelium-specific cell-cell adhesion molecule E-cadherin, whereas carcinoma cell lines with a fibroblastoid phenotype were invasive and had lost the capacity for E-cadherin expression. The invasiveness of these latter cells could be prevented by transfection with E-cadherin cDNA and was again induced by treating the transfected cells with anti-E-cadherin antibodies. These findings indicate that the selective loss of E-cadherin expression can generate dedifferentiation and invasiveness of human pancreas carcinoma cells and, further, that E-cadherin acts as an invasion suppressor (Frixen et al. 1991).

ICAM-1. ICAM-1 is a cell-surface-bound glycoprotein which belongs to the immunoglobulin superfamily and mediates cell-cell adhesion by interacting with its counter-receptors, the integrins αL-$\beta 2$ and $\alpha M \beta 2$. In normal pancreatic tissue no expression of ICAM-1 was found, but strong immunohistochemical staining of ICAM-1 was detected in surgically resected pancreatic tumors. In different pancreatic carcinoma cell lines either ICAM-1 was expressed constitutively, or ICAM-1 receptor expression was induced by treatment with the inflammatory cytokines interferon γ, TGF β, and TNF α (Schwaebele et al. 1993). The potential importance of this ICAM-1 de novo expression on the surface of pancreatic cancer cells in mediating cytolysis by natural killer cells or hematogeneous metastasis by interacting with $\beta 2$-integrin-bearing endothelial cells remains unclear.

Colorectal Cancer

Integrins. Colorectal malignancies develop from benign proliferative lesions according to the model of multistep carcinogenesis (Fearon and Jones 1992; Vogelstein and Kinzler 1993). There is increasing evidence showing that integrin receptors are altered following the malignant transformation of colonic mucosa into adenomas and invasive carcinomas, which thus influences their metastatic potential. The distribution of the α1- to α6-integrin subunit in the human intestine was analyzed by Choy et al. (1990). It was demonstrated that α2-, α3-, and α6-integrin subunits were expressed on all epithelial cells in the small and large bowel, whereas the α1-subunit was expressed on crypt cells of the small and large bowel but only weakly stained or absent on villus epithelial cells of the small bowel and colonic surface epithelial cells. All epithelia were negative for the α4- and the α5-subunits. Intraepithelial lymphocytes were α1 and α4 positive. The α1-, α3-, and α5-subunits were uniformly expressed by muscularis propria, muscularis mucosae, pericrypt cells, and smooth muscle fibers within the villi. In contrast, α2 and α4 were present only in pericrypt cells and fibers within the villi; they were absent from the muscularis mucosae. α1-, α3-, α5-, and α6-subunits were expressed by the endothelium. The malignant transformation of colorectal tissue is accompanied by a change in the expression of different integrin receptors. Pignatelli et al. (1990) observed a progressive loss of the α2-, α3-, and β1-integrin subunits associated with a loss of tumor differentiation in patients with colorectal adenocarcinomas.

In adenomas and well-differentiated adenocarcinomas a strong expression of these subunits was found with no marked difference in intensity compared with normal colonic mucosa. In most of the moderately and all of the poorly differentiated tumors, the expression of these three integrin subunits was significantly altered, showing either a diffuse reduction in staining or a more heterogeneous pattern with a reduced percentage of positive tumor cells. Negative tumor cells were localized mainly to undifferentiated tumor sections, whereas the lining epithelium in direct contract with the stroma showed a strong integrin expression. A significant loss of α3- and α5-subunit expression in tubulovillous adenomas and colorectal carcinomas in comparison to normal colonic mucosa was detected by Stallmach et al. (1991, 1992). In some crypts of the adenomas, the epithelial cells were α3 and α5 positive, whereas in others the cells were completely negative, which may be due to different types of preneoplastic and neoplastic cells in tubulovillous adenomas. Conflicting data were published about a potential decrease in the expression of the α6-integrin subunit in colorectal carcinomas. Stallmach et al. (1991, 1992) described a significant correlation between the reduced expression of the α6-subunit and the transformation of adenomas to invasive carcinomas. Koretz et al. (1991) reported a similar change in the expression and distribution of the α2-subunit in adenomas and a significant loss in the expression of the α2- and β1-subunits during the malignant transformation into invasive colorectal carcinomas. The expression of the $\alpha 6$-integrin subunit on the surface of adenomas and carcinomas resembled that in normal colonic mucosa in this study.

The level of integrin receptor expression and the capacity of colorectal cancer cells to interact with proteins of the extracellular matrix seem to be important in maintaining metastatic capacity and depend on the degree of cellular differentiation (Daneker et al. 1989). Recent data showed that the adhesion, migration, and invasion of colon carcinoma cells to extracellular matrix proteins are mediated mainly by integrin receptors of the $\beta 1$-family (Yamada et al. 1990), whereas the "classical" fibronectin receptor $\alpha 5\beta 1$ is the most important. Stallmach et al. (1994) compared subclones of a colon carcinoma cell line differing in the expression of the $\alpha 5$-$\beta 1$ receptor in their ability to form tumors in nude mice. It was shown that a lack $\alpha 5\beta 1$-integrin expression results in an increase of subcutaneous tumor growth. While adhesion to a fibronectin matrix in vitro was comparable, the deposition of fibronectin in tumor-surrounding stroma was increased in $\alpha 5$-positive colon cancer cells. Herzberg et al. (1996) demonstrated that a stable transfection of $\alpha 5$-mRNA in a human colon adenocarcinoma cell line induced the expression of $\alpha 5\beta 1$-integrin receptor, mediating increased cell adhesion significantly to fibronectin. The transfected cancer cells showed a decrease in cell proliferation both in vitro and when subcutaneously injected into nude mice. Moreover, the $\alpha 5$-transfected colon cancer cells also showed marked inhibition of lung metastasis in comparison to cancer cells lacking the $\alpha 5\beta 1$-integrin receptor. The importance of integrin receptors in regulating cellular growth, differentiation, and the maintenance of cell viability was demonstrated by Bates et al. (1994), using a human colon cancer cell line growing as organized spheroids. An inhibition of cell-to-cell contacts by blocking the αv-integrin receptor resulted in a suppression of spheroid formation and induced apoptosis, or programmed cell death, due to a translocation of the p53 tumor suppressor gene product from the cytosol to the nucleus.

ELAM-1. A key event in the extravasation phase of the metastatic process is tumor cell adhesion to the vascular endothelium. Activation of endothelial cells by inflammatory cytokines strongly promotes tumor cell adhesion and increases the tumor cell entrapment in lung microvasculature, as well as the formation of lung colonies in animal models (Lauri et al. 1990). ELAM-1, a cell surface glycoprotein selectively expressed by cytokine-activated endothelial cells, is the major mediator of colon carcinoma cell adhesion to vascular endothelium (Lauri et al. 1991) and might represent a specific mechanism of colorectal tumor cell recognition of activated endothelial cells.

67-kDa Laminin Receptor. A strong correlation was observed between the expression of specific adhesion receptors of the basement glycoprotein laminin and the degree of differentiation in colorectal carcinomas. Horan-Hand et al. (1985) first described an elevated expression of the 67-kDa laminin receptor in invasive colorectal carcinomas compared with normal colonic mucosa and adenomas of the colon. This increase in laminin receptor expression could be explained by an increase in the mRNA expression of a specific laminin-binding protein in human colon carcinoma tissue but not in adjacent normal colonic epithelium (Yow et al. 1988; Castronovo et al. 1992). The investigation of surgically resected tumor samples and metastases by Mafune et al. (1990) underlined the importance of the increased 67-kDa laminin receptor mRNA in colon carcinomas, suggesting a role of this receptor as a marker of human colorectal cancer progression and biological aggressiveness. It was shown that the degree of laminin receptor mRNA expression correlated with disease progression and Dukes' classification of tumor staging. Furthermore, liver metastses of colon cancers expressed a higher level of mRNA for the 67-kDa receptor than adjacent normal liver tissue. Consistent observations were published by Cioce et al. (1991), which also proved a higher level of laminin receptor expression in colon cancer metastases compared with the primary tumor lesion, suggesting that an increased level of laminin receptor expression is associated with a more invasive phenotype and a higher metastatic potential. Aznavoorian et al. (1990) performed in vitro studies selecting subclones of a human colon carcinoma cell line by their capacity to invade a human amniotic membrane. Highly invasive and noninvasive colon cancer subclones differed mainly in their ability to interact with the basement membrane protein laminin. The highly invasive subclone expressed higher levels of specific laminin receptors and showed a more enhanced laminin-mediated adhesion, spreading, and migration than the noninvasive subclone. Stallmach et al. (1991) detected elevated levels of the 67-kDa laminin receptor as well as a higher expression of laminin-binding integrin receptors on colon carcinoma tissue than on basolateral cell membranes of the adjacent normal colonic epithelium.

In vivo data recently published by Bersalier et al. (1995) showed that inhibition of the 67-kD receptor using a pentapeptide from the laminin-$\beta 1$ chain significantly inhibited liver colonization of human colorectal cancer cells, while a peptide derived from the laminin-$\alpha 1$ chain promoted the formation of liver metastases by stimulating homeotypic cell aggregation into tumor emboli.

ICAM-1. The expression of adhesion molecules on the surface of colorectal carcinomas seems to be important for the infiltrative growth and the metastatic potential of these carcinomas, as well as for chemoresistance and sensitivity to cytotoxic effector cells. Cell-cell adhesion receptors of the IgG superfamily play an outstanding role in mediating interactions between colon carcinoma cells and tumor-infiltrating T cells and lymphokine-activated killer cells (LAK cells). In colorectal cancer a pronounced lymphocytic infiltration is associated with an improved prognosis (Sheperd et al. 1989). The ICAM-1 receptor is one of the specific cell surface receptors required by lymphocytes to adhere to their target cells. Constitutively expressed by endothelial cells, normal colonic epithelium lacked ICAM-1, while colon carcinoma tissue demonstrated a focal ICAM-1 expression. As in pancreatic tissue, ICAM-1 expression was induced by inflammatory cytokines supporting the adhesion of lymphocytes to colonic cancer cells (Kelly et al. 1992). The sensitivity of chemoresistant colon cancer cells to cytotoxic effector cells depends on the level of expression of cell-cell adhesion molecules and is related to the stage of differentiation. Rivoltini et al. (1991) proved an increased expression of the ICAM-1 and LFA-3 receptor on the surface of a chemoresistant colon cancer cell line and an elevated lysability by LAK cells compared with a chemosensitive subline. A reduction of lysis by LAK cells was achieved by blocking the ICAM-1 and LFA-3 receptor with monoclonal antibodies. Treatment with differentiating agents resulted in the decreased expression of cell-adhesion molecules and was accompanied by increased resistance to LAK cell-mediated lysis.

E-Cadherin. Similar to the results found in other gastrointestinal malignancies, the expression of the cell-cell adhesion molecule E-cadherin is significantly down-regulated in moderately to poorly differentiated colorectal carcinomas. A loss of E-cadherin expression is associated with a change in tissue architecture and glandular configuration and relates to the biological behavior of poorly differentiated colorectal carcinomas (Edelmann et al. 1989; Frixen et al. 1991; Kinsella et al. 1993; Nigam et al. 1993).

Hart and colleagues (1993) first demonstrated a good correlation between the presence of E-cadherin on the mRNA and the protein level in Dukes' stage B colorectal carcinomas by using immunohistochemical staining and in situ hybridisation techniques. In a retrospective study of a series of 49 Dukes' stage B colorectal carcinomas resected from patients with known clinical outcomes, in situ hybridisation was performed to measure E-cadherin mRNA (Dorudi et al. 1995). It was apparent from the results of this study that low or absent E-cadherin expression is associated with reduced survival in patients undergoing curative surgical resections for Dukes' stage B colorectal cancer. The authors concluded that a large prospective study is necessary to determine whether levels of E-cadherin expression in colorectal cancer can really yield independent prognostic information to predict the risk of recurrence or metastasis. Since 35% of all colorectal cancers are Dukes' stage B, a group with a 5 year survival rate of approximately 70%, it is of significant clinical and epidemiological importance to identify those patients with a poor prognosis and to thus designate them for protocols of adjuvant therapy.

Pignatelli et al. (1992) demonstrated the importance of E-cadherin and integrin receptors in mediating cell-cell and cell-matrix interactions required for the induction and maintenance of the glandular differentiation of colorectal tumors. Inhibition of E-cadherin as well as of the β1-integrin subunit in vitro resulted in a suppression of glandular differentiation of a colon carcinoma cell line growing in a collagen gel. Pullmann and Bodmer (1992) used the integrin receptor-triggered glandular differentiation of a colon carcinoma cell line on a collagen type-I matrix to select cells with an adhesive phenotype and investigated the regulation of integrin function in these cells. A complementary DNA clone that increases cell adhesion to ECM proteins could be found as could the corresponding gene called CAR (cell-adhesion regulator) located on chromosome 16 were found. This gene encoded an adhesion signal transduction molecule of 142 amino acids that functioned in the suppression of tumor invasion. In conclusion, in vivo and in vitro data revealed that E-cadherin expression is necessary to maintain the glandular configuration of the colorectal tissue and that a loss of E-cadherin is correlated with reduced differentiation and a poor prognosis in patients with colorectal cancer.

CD44. The standard form of the CD44 adhesion receptor is broadly expressed in all epithelial cells of the large bowel mucosa (Mackay et al. 1994) consistently associated with cellular proliferation (Abbasi et al. 1993). While weak expression of the CD44-9v variant isoform is detected in only a few cells of the germinative layer at the basis and the lower part of the tubular crypts (Terpe et al. 1994), none of the other CD44 splicing variants containing exons 3v, 4v, 6v, and 7v is observed. Up-regulation of CD44 seems to be a very early event in colon carcinoma progression, occurring at the time of K-ras as well as p53 mutations (Kim et al. 1994b; Günthert et al. 1994). Even in early adenomas consisting of cells with the same cytological differentiation as normal colorectal mucosa but with a higher mitotic activity there is evidence of a strong increase in the expression of epithelial CD44 variants is already observed. Wielenga et al. (1993) detected an increase in CD44-8v, -9v, and -10v expression in early adenomas. In later-stage adenomas, which consist of dedifferentiated cells with a large mitotic portion but without any evidence of invasion to the lower parts of the colonic wall, CD44-6v expression occurred, continually increasing during tumor progression from Dukes' A to C stages (Heider et al. 1993b; Günthert et al., manuscript in preparation). While Wielenga et al. (1993) observed the highest CD44-6v expression in Dukes' D stage and in the matching distant metastases, Günthert et al. (manuscript in preparation) reported a down-regulation of this isoform, preferentially in distant metastases.

A study performed by the group of Steven T. Pals (1994) correlating the expression of CD44-6v with a survival analysis in 68 patients with colorectal cancer demonstrated an association of this isoform with an adverse prognosis and tumor-related death due to tumor metastases. These data suggested that CD44-6v expression is a valuable additional prognostic marker for identifying patients with a high propensity for developing distant metastases. They concluded that patients in Dukes' stages B and C with CD44-6v-positive colorectal cancer might benefit most from adjuvant chemotherapy and/or radiotherapy after apparently curative radical tumor resection. The results of this study did not correspond with the data published by Koretz et al. (1994), which showed no correlation between CD44-6v expression and the prognosis of colorectal cancer. In 180 patients with colorectal cancer in Dukes' stages A to D the expression of CD44-6v was detected by immunohistochemical methods. All patients in Dukes' stage A to C underwent potentially curative surgical treatment, and the follow-up was documented. The presence of CD44-6v was more frequent in poorly differentiated colorectal carcinomas, but no correlation could be established between the presence of CD44-6v and the Dukes' stage, histological type, or tumor location. Recurrence-free survival in patients who underwent potentially curative resections did not differ, irrespectively of whether CD44-6v was detectable, and the overall survival was not determined by the presence or absence of CD44-6v. As expected, the Dukes' stage, the tumor grade, and the patient's age emerged as independent prognostic factors in a statistical analysis, while no prognostic significance was attributed to the expression of CD44-6v. Steven T. Pals (1995) tried to explain these discrepancies by technical differences due to the fact that the percentage of CD44-6v-positive patients was far lower in the study of Koretz et al. than in his own investigation.

Conflicting data have been published on the use of RT-PCR analysis of colorectal carcinomas to compare the CD44 expression of isolates from malignant regions and neighboring non-malignant tissue. While Tanabe et al. (1993) and Finn et al. (1994) described an increase of CD44-8v, 9v, and 10v, Wielenga et al. (1993) and Günthert et al. (manuscript in preparation) concluded that a quantitative comparison of CD44 variant isoform expression between malignant and adjacent non-malignant colon tissue is not feasible.

Adhesion Receptors As Prognostic Factors in Gastrointestinal Tumors

With increasing emphasis on the early detection of cancer, there is an ongoing search for reliable markers that will be clinically helpful in the diagnosis of small tumors and the assessment of their metastatic potential. There is some evidence that an abnormal pattern of activity of the CD44-adhesion receptor gene is a promising candidate for both of these purposes in various types of malignancies (Herrlich et al. 1993). By a mechanism known as alternative splicing, the CD44 gene can produce different variant isoforms which are detectable on the cell surface as well as in a soluble form in body fluids. In neoplasia, many abnormal variant transcripts are produced (Günthert et al., manuscript in preparation; East et al. 1993; Matsumura et al. 1992). In gastric cancer, the expression of the CD44 standard and the 9v-isoform is significantly related to an increase in tumor recurrence and higher tumor-induced mortality and may serve as an important prognostic marker. The CD44-5v isoform is closely related to gastric tumor differentiation, while the CD44-6v isoform seems to give gastric carcinoma cells the potential to lymph node metastases. In colorectal cancer, and overexpression of the CD44-8v, 9v, and 10v isoform occurred in early adenomas, whereas, in advanced carcinomas, the expression of the CD44-6v isoform increased during tumor progression from Dukes' stages A to D (Wielenga et al. 1993; Tanabe et al. 1993; Günthert 1994).

Therefore the CD44-6v isoform seems to be a valuable, independent prognostic marker for estimating the probability of distant metastases in Dukes' stage B colorectal carcinoma and for identifying those patients who might benefit from adjuvant therapy after surgical tumor resection. Guo et al. (1994) reported that the concentration of soluble CD44 is elevated in the serum of patients with advanced gastric or colorectal cancer. The serum CD44 concentration significantly correlated with tumor burden and tumor metastasis and decreased after complete surgical resection of tumor masses or treatment with chemotherapy. These results demonstrate that the analysis of the CD44 receptor and its isoforms may be applicable in the early detection of metastatic potential in surgical biopsy specimens or readily available body fluids. The detection of CD44 splice variants could be very important in the early diagnosis of gastric and colorectal cancer in screening programs as well as in the assessment of residual disease and in the early detection of tumor recurrence.

Another potentially important prognostic marker might be the cell-cell adhesion receptor E-cadherin. In gastric carcinoma, reduced E-cadherin expression potentially due to gene mutations seems to represent a differentiation marker and is associated with a higher mortality through local tumor recurrence or distant metastases. There is some evidence that E-cadherin expression in Dukes' stage B colorectal cancer can be used as an independent prognostic marker for identifying patients who have poorly differentiated carcinomas with reduced E-cadherin expression and designate them for intensive adjuvant therapy and clinical observation after potentially curative surgical tumor treatment.

Potential Importance of Adhesion Receptors in the Diagnosis and Therapy of Gastrointestinal Tumors

The identification of tumor-cell adhesion molecules and their corresponding ligands in blood vessels, basement membranes, and connective tissues may be useful for both the diagnosis and prevention of malignant tumors and their future metastases (Table 4; Zetter 1993). The repetoire of adhesion molecules detected on the surface of cells removed from a primary tumor at biopsy might be used to predict the probable location of disseminated micrometastases. The predicted site might be considered as a target for diagnostic imaging and possible chemotherapy or radiation therapy. Adhesion receptors on tumor cells may also serve as target antigens for the immunotherapy of minimal residual disease or micrometastases after potentially curative surgical resection (Nassal 1994). Native monoclonal antibodies directed against adhesion receptors can lead to cellular destruction via complement-mediated lysis, antibody-dependent cellular cytotoxicity or opsonization of tumor cells in micrometastases with subsequent phagocytosis. In vitro data reported by Packard et al. (1994) demonstrated that cytotoxic lymphoid immune responses against human tumor cells are inducible by the introduction of bifunctional

Table 4. Adhesion receptors as prognostic markers in gastrointestinal malignancies

	Adhesion receptors	Prognosis
Esophageal cancer	E-cadherin	State of differentiation Infiltrative growth Lymph node metastasis
Gastric cancer	E-cadherin	State of differentiation, tumor recurrence, lymph node metastasis, and mortality
diffuse type	CD44s, CD44-9v	Tumor progression and metastasis
	CD44-5v	Tumor differentiation
intestinal type	CD44-6v	Specific for carcinomas of the intestinal type, lymh node metastasis
Pancreatic cancer	E-cadherin	State of differentiation and infiltrative growth
Colon cancer	$\alpha5\beta1$-fibronectin receptor	Tumor invasion and metastasis
	$\alpha6$-integrin	State of differentiation
	67 kD LR	Invasive and metastatic phenotype
	E-cadherin	Tumor recurrence and metastasis
	CD44-8v, CD44-9v, CD44-10v	Early adenomas
	CD44-6v	Tumor progression and metastasis

antibodies against the $\beta1$-integrin subunit on bone marrow immunocytes and type I mucin glycoproteins on the surface of epithelial tumor cells. Another approach might be the tagging of antibodies against cancer-cell adhesion receptors with radioisotopes, toxins, or drugs. Inflammatory cytokines like interferon-γ or interleukin-1β can support the interaction of cytotoxic leukocytes and cancer cells by induction of the ICAM-1 cell-cell adhesion receptors, as shown in vitro by Kelly et al. (1992). Pauli et al. (1988) have found that specific adhesion molecules can be induced on vascular endothelial cells grown on organ-specific extracellular matrix. Using a monoclonal antibody that blocked tumor-cell adhesion to endothelial cells grown on lung matrix, they isolated a lung-specific adhesion molecule that was preferentially expressed on pulmonary venular endothelial cells and was therefore in a suitable location to mediate adhesion and extravasation of lung-colonizing tumor cells (Zhu et al. 1991). Mice actively immunized against this adhesion receptor termed Lu-ECAM-1 were resistant to metastatic colonization of highly metastatic carcinoma cells (Zhu et al. 1992). These results suggest a novel approach of possible clinical utility in which patients at high risk for certain types of cancer might be "immunized" against adhesion elements at preferred secondary sites for that tumor. The metastatic colonization might be inhibited by not allowing the tumor cells that subsequently develop to specifically adhere and extravasate at that site. The recent molecular characterization of adhesion pathways has led to exploration of their role in a variety of diseases and has opened the door for the development of a new class of pharmaceutics inhibiting cellular adhesion. In order for an antiadhesion therapy to be clinically useful, it must have several characteristics: the ability to inhibit an adhesion interaction that is of sufficiently critical importance to the target disease pathogenesis so that its disruption will lead to clinical benefit; sufficient specificity of an antiadhesion effect to permit other critical adhesion processes to continue; and pharmacokinetik and pharmacodynamic characteristics which permit a convenient dosing schedule suitable for the target disease (Makgoba et al. 1992).

In the therapy of malignant neoplasia, one approach is the targeting of monoclonal antibodies to tumor cells in order to inhibit tumor cell-ligand binding and, thereby intercellular signaling (Makgoba et al. 1992; Agrez and Bates 1994). The disruption of cell-cell contacts by monoclonal antibodies could also prove useful as a means of stimulating apoptosis. Brooks et al. (1994) recently reported that antibodies directed against the $\alpha v\beta 3$ integrin receptor induced rapid regression of human tumors transplanted into an animal model. The antiproliferative effect was caused by the induction of apoptosis of proliferative angiogenic cells during the neovascularization, an important process directly influencing the growth and metastatic properties of solid tumors (Fidler and Ellis 1994). A similar effect could be achieved by the application of high-affinity, cyclic, non-RGID peptide antagonists of the $\alpha v\beta 3$ integrin receptor which binds to the extracellular matrix protein vitronectin. This integrin receptor is strongly expressed on newly growing vascular endothelial cells during tumor angiogenesis and neovascularization (Varner 1995). Seiter et al. (1993) demonstrated that a monoclonal antibody directed against a variant isoform of the CD44 receptor retarded the growth of lymph node and lung metastases of a metastatic tumor cell line in nude mice. The antibody was only effective when given before lymph node colonization and seemed to interfere with the proliferation of metastasizing tumor cells in the draining lymph nodes, most probably by blocking receptor-ligand interactions.

Another therapeutic approach based on the known sequences of adhesion molecules is the use of synthetic peptides to inhibit tumor cell invasion and metastasis (Agrez and Bates 1994). The advantages of small peptides are that they are unlikely to be immunogenic compared to monoclonal antibodies. Adhesion-blocking synthetic peptides containing the Arg-Gly-Asp-Ser (RGDS) sequence have been shown to inhibit tumor cell invasion in vitro and tumor metastasis in animal models (Humphries et al. 1986; Gehlsen et al. 1988). These peptides are capable of inhibiting integrin–receptor-mediated cellular adhesion to extracellular matrix components such as fibronectin and vitronectin. Whalen et al. (1989) have previously demonstrated that the application of GRGDS-synthetic peptides can serve as a prophylaxis against wound contamination during tumor surgery. In a mouse model for wound contamination, GRGDS peptide washing reduced subsequent tumor regrowth. Another synthetic peptide composed of the amino acids Tyr-Ile-Gly-Ser-Arg (YIGSR) derived from the B1 chain of the basement membrane glycoprotein laminin (Graf et al. 1987) has been shown to decrease tumor growth and metastasis in vivo (Iwamoto et al. 1987; Saiki et al 1989; Nomizu et al. 1993; Yamumara et al. 1993) by inhibiting tumor cell attachment and invasion and inducting cellular apoptosis (Kim 1994). An antiangiogenic effect mediated by the inhibition of endothelial cell migration and thus influencing solid tumor growth has been described by Sakamoto et al. (1991). The YIGSR pentapeptide represents the active binding site of the 67-kDa laminin receptor (Graf et al. 1987; Mecham 1991), which showed elevated expression in colorectal cancer and can serve as a potential prognostic marker of tumor progression and biological aggressiveness (Mafune et al. 1990).

It is conceivable that the administration of adhesion-inhibiting therapies using monoclonal antibodies or synthetic peptides at the time of cancer surgery could decrease the incidence of metastasis or prolong the time to onset of clinically evident metastasis by inhibiting the ability of micrometastatic foci of malignant cells to colonize distant tissues.

References

Abbasi AM, Chester KA, Talbot IC, Macpherson AS, Boxer G, Forbes A, Malcom ADB, Begent RHJ (1993) CD44 is associated with proliferation in normal and neoplastic human colorectal epithelial cells. Eur J Cancer 29:1995–2002

Agrez MV, Bates RC (1994) Colorectal cancer and the integrin family of cell adhesion receptors: current status and future directions. Eur J Cancer 30:2166–2170

Albelda SM, Buck C (1990) Integrins and other cell adhesion molecules. FASEB 4:2868–2880

Aznavoorian S, Marphy AN, Stetler-Stevenson WG, Liotta LA (1993) Molecular aspects of tumor cell invasion and metastasis. Cancer 15:1368–1383

Aznavoorian S, Liotta LA, Kupchik HZ (1990) Characteristics of invasive and noninvasive human colorectal adenocarcinoma cells. J Natl Cancer Inst 82:1485–1492

Bates RC, Buret A, vanHelden D, Horton MA, Burns GF (1994) Apoptosis induced by inhibition of intercellular contact. J Cell Biol 125:403–415

Beck K, Hunter I, Engel J (1990) Structure and function of laminin: anatomy of a multidomain glycoprotein. FASEB 4:148–160

Becker KF, Atkinson MJ, Reich U, Becker I, Nekarda H, Siewert JR, Höfler H (1994) E-cadherin gene mutations provide clues to diffuse type gastric carcinomas. Cancer Res 54:3845–3852

Becker KF, Atkinson MJ, Reich U, Huang HH, Nekarda H, Siewert JR, Höfler H (1993) Exon skipping in the E-cadherin gene transcript in metastatic human gastric carcinomas. Hum Mol Genet 2:803–804

Behrens J, Mareel MM, Van Roy FM, Birchmeier W (1989) Dissecting tumor cell invasion: epithelial cells aquire invasive properties after the loss of uvomorulin mediated cell-cell adhesion. J Cell Biol 108:7435–7447

Behrens J, Vakaet L, Winterhager E, Van Roy F, Mareel MM, Birchmeier W (1993) Loss of epithelial differentiation and gain of invasiveness correlates with tyrosine phosphorylation of the E-cadherin/β-catenin complex in cells transformed with a temperature-sensitive v-SRC gene. J Cell Biol 120:757–766

Bersalier RS, Schwartz B, Kim YS, Duh QY, Kleinmann HK, Sullam PM (1995) The laminin $\alpha 1$ chain Ile-Lys-Val-Ala-Val (IKVAV)-containing peptide promotes liver colonization of human colon cancer cells. Cancer Res 55:2476–2480

Birchmeier W, Weidner KM, Hülsken J, Behrens J (1993) Molecular mechanisms leading to cell junction (cadherin) deficiency in invasive carcinomas. Semin Cancer Biol 4:231–239

Brooks PC, Clark RAF, Cheresh DA (1994) Requirement of vascular integrin $\alpha v\beta 3$ for angiogenesis. Science 264:569–571

Brooks PC, Montgomery AMP, Rosenfeld M, Reisfeld RA, Hu T, Klier G, Cheresh DA (1994) Integrin $\alpha v\beta 3$ antagonists promote tumor regression by inducing apoptosis of angiogenic blood vessels. Cell 79:1157–1164

Buxton RS, Cowin P, Franke WW, Garod DR, Green KJ, King IA, Koch PJ, Magee AI, Rees DA, Stanley JR, Steinberg MS (1993) Nomenclature of the desmosomal and other cadherins. J Cell Biol 121:481–483

Carter WG, Wagner EA (1988) Characterization of the class III collagen receptor, a phosphorylated, transmembrane glycoprotein expressed in nucleated human cells. J Biol Chem 263:4193–4201

Castronovo V (1993) Lamininreceptors and laminin-binding proteins during tumor invasion and metastasis. Invasion Metastasis 13:1–30

Castronovo V, Colin C, Claysmith AP, Chen PH, Lifrange E, Lambotte R, Kratzsch H, Liotta LA, Sobel ME (1990) Immunodetection of the metastasis associated laminin-receptor in human breast cancer cells obtained by fine-needle aspriation biopsy. Am J Pathol 137:1373–1381

Castronovo V, Tarboletti G, Sobel ME (1991) Functional domains of the 67 kD laminin receptor precursor. J Biol Chem 226:20440–20446

Castronovo V, Campo E, van den Brule FA, Claysmith AP, Cioce V, Liu FT, Fernandez PL, Sobel ME (1992) Inverse modulation of steady-state messenger RNA levels of two non-integrin laminin-binding proteins in human colon carcinoma. J Natl Cancer Inst 84:1161–1169

Choy MY, Richman PI, Horton MA, MacDonald TT (1990) Expression of the VLA family of integrins in human intestine. Am J Pathol 160:35–40

Cioce V, Castronovo V, Shmookler BM, Garbisa S, Grigioni WF, Liotta LA, Sobel ME (1991) Increased expression of the laminin receptor in human colon cancer. J Natl Cancer Inst 83:29–36

Correa P, Shiao Y (1994) Phenotypic and genotypic events in gastric carcinogenesis. Cancer Res 54:1941–1943

Daidone MG, Silvestrini R, D'Errico A, Di FG, Benini E, Mancini AM, Garbisa S, Liotta LA, Grigioni WF (1991) Laminin receptors, collagenase IC and prognosis in node negative breast cancers. Int J Cancer 48:529–532

Dämmrich J, Vollmers HP, Heider KH, Müller-Hemelink HK (1995) Importance of different CD44 v6 expression in human gastric intestinal and diffuse type cancers for metastatic lymphogenic spreading. J Mol Med 73:395–401

Daneker GW, Piazza AJ, Steele GD, Mercurio AM (1989) Relationship between extracellular matrix interactions and degree of differentiation in human colon carcinoma cell lines. Cancer Res 49:681–686

Demeter LM, Stoler MH, Sobel ME, Broker ME, Chow LT (1992) Expression of high affinity laminin receptor mRNA correlates with cell proliferation rather than invasion in human papilloma virus associated neoplasms. Cancer Res 52:1561–1567

D'Errico A, Garbisa S, Liotta LA, Castronovo V, Stetler-Stevenson SW (1991) Augmentation of type IV collagenase, laminin receptor, and Ki67 proliferation antigen associated with human colon, gastric, and breast carcinoma progression. Mod Pathol 4:239–246

Diamond MS, Springer TA (1994) The dynamic regulation of integrin adhesiveness. Curr Biol 4:506–517

Doki Y, Shiozaki H, Tahara H, Inoue M, Oka H, Iihara K, Kadowski T, Takeichi M, Mori T (1993) Correlation between E-cadherin expression and invasiveness in vitro in a human esophageal cancer cell line. Cancer Res 53:3421–3426

Dorudi S, Sheffield JP, Poulson R, Northover JMA, Hart IR (1993) E-cadherin expression on colorectal cancer: an immunocytochemical and in situ hybridization study. Am J Pathol 142:981–986

Dorudi S, Hanby AM, Poulson R, Northover J, Hart IR (1995) Level of expression of E-cadherin mRNA in colorectal cancer correlates with clinical outcome. Br J Cancer 71:614–615
East JA, Hart IR (1993) CD44 and its role in tumour progression and metastasis. Eur J Cancer 29:1921–1922
Edelman S, Damsky CH, Wheelock MJ, Damjanov I (1989) Expression of the cell-cell adhesion glycoprotein cell-CMA 120/80 in normal human tissues and tumors. Am J Pathol 135:101–110
Edward M (1995) Integrins and other adhesion molecules involved in melanocytic tumor progression. Curr Oncol 7:185–191
Fearon ER, Jones PA (1992) Progression toward a molecular description of colorectal cancer development. FASEB 6:2783–2790
Fidler IJ, Ellis LM (1994) The implications of angiogenesis for the biology and therapy of cancer metastasis. Cell 79:185–188
Finn L, Dougherty G, Finley G, Meisler A, Becich M, Cooper DL (1994) Alternative splicing of CD44 pre-mRNA in human colorectal tumors. Biochem Biophys Res Comm 200:1015–1022
Frixen UH, Behrens J, Sachs M, Eberle G, Voss B, Warda A, Löchner D, Birchmeier W (1991) E-cadherin-mediated cell-cell adhesion prevents invasiveness of human carcinoma cells. J Cell Biol 113:173–185
Gehlsen KR, Argraves WS, Pierschbacher MD, Ruoslahti (1988) Inhibition of in vitro tumor cell invasion by Arg-Gly-Asp-containing synthetic peptides. J Cell Biol 106:925–930
Geiger B, Agalon O (1992) Cadherins. Ann Rev Cell Biol 8:307–332
Ginsberg MH, Xiaoping DU, Flow E (1992) Inside-out integrin signaling. Curr Opin Cell Biol 4:766–771
Graf J, Ogla RC, Robey FA, Saseki M, Martin GR, Yamada Y, Kleinman HK (1987) A pentapeptide from the laminin B1 chain mediates cell adhesion and binds the 67 000 laminin receptor. Biochem 26:6896–6900
Günthert U, Hofmann M, Rudy W, Reber S, Zöller M, Haußmann I, Matzku S, Wenzel A, Ponta H, Herrlich P (1991) A new variant of glycoprotein CD44 confers metastatic potential to rat carcinoma cells. Cell 65:13–24
Guo YJ, Liu G, Wang X, Jin D, Wu M, Ma J, Sy MS (1994) Potential use of soluble CD44 in serum as indicator of tumor burden and metastasis in patients with gastric or colon cancer. Cancer Res 54:422–426
Hall PA, Coates PJ, Lemoine NR, Horton MA (1991) Characterization of integrin chains in normal and neoplastic human pancreas. J Pathol 165:33–41
Harn HJ, Ho LI, Chang JY, Wu CW, Jiang SY, Lee HS, Lee WH (1995) Differential expression of the human metastasis adhesion molecule CD44v in normal and carcinomatous stomach mucosa of chinese subjects. Cancer 75:1065–1071
Heider KH, Dämmrich J, Skroch-Angel P, Müller-Hermelink HK, Vollmers HP, Herrlich P, Ponta H (1993) Differential expression of CD44 splice variants in intestinal- and diffuse-type human gastric carcinomas and normal gastric mucosa. Cancer Res 53:4197–4203
Heider KH, Hofmann M, Hors E, van den Berg F, Ponta H, Herrlich P, Pals ST (1993) A human homologue of the rat metastasis-associated variant of CD44 is expressed in colorectal carcinomas and adenomatous polyps. J Cell Biol 120:227–233
Heino J (1993) Integrin-type extracellular matrix receptors in cancer and inflammation. Ann Med 25:355–342
Herrlich P, Zöller M, Pals ST, Ponta H (1993) CD44 splice variants: metastases meet lymphocytes. Immunol Today 14:395–399
Herzberg F, Schirner M, Schmidt R, Thiel E, Kreuser E-D (1996) De novo expression of the fibronectin receptor subunit α5 reduces proliferation in vitro and

in vivo by increasing skeleton reorganization and signal transduction. Exp Cell Res (in press)

Horan-Hand P, Thor A, Schlom J, Rao CN, Liotta L (1985) Expression of laminin receptor in normal and carcinomatous tissues as defined by monoclonal antibody. Cancer Res 45:2713–2719

Humphries M, Yamada KM, Olden K (1988) Investigations of the biological effects of anti-cell adhesive synthetic peptides that inhibit experimental metastasis of B16-F10 murine melanoma cells. J Clin Invest 81:782–790

Hunt G (1989) The role of laminin in cancer invasion and metastasis. Exp Cell Biol 57:165–176

Hynes RO (1992) Integrins: versatility, modulation, and signaling in cell adhesion. Cell 69:11–25

Hynes RO, Lander AD (1992) Contact and adhesive specificities in the associations, migrations, and targeting of cells and axons. Cell 68:303–322

Iwamoto Y, Robey FA, Graf J, Sasaki M, Kleinman HK, Yamada Y, Martin GR (1987) YIGSR, a synthetic laminin pentapeptide, inhibits experimental metastasis formation. Science 238:1132–1134

Jalkanen S, Jalkanen M (1992) Lymphocyte CD44 binds the COOH-terminal heparin-binding domain of fibronectin. J Cell Biol 116:817–825

Juliano R (1994) Signal transduction by integrins and its role in the regulation of tumor growth. Cancer Metastasis Rev 13:25–30

Juliano RL, Haskill S (1993) Signal transduction from the extracellular matrix. J Cell Biol 120:577–585

Juliano RL, Varner JA (1993) Adhesion molecules in cancer: the role of integrins. Curr Biol 5:812–818

Juna EJ, Hitt AL (1992) Cytoskeleton-plasma membrane interactions. Science 258:955–963

Kadowaki T, Shiozaki H, Inoue M, Tamura S, Oka H, Doki Y, Iihara K, Matsui S, Iwazawa T, Nagafuchi A, Tsukita S, Mori T (1994) E-cadherin and α-catenin expression in human esophageal cancer. Cancer Res 54:291–296

Kelly CP, O'Keane JC, Orellana J, Schroy PC, Yang S, Lamont JT, Brady HR (1992) Human colon cancer cells express ICAM-1 in vivo and support LFA-1 dependent lymphocyte adhesion in vitro. Am J Physiol 263:864–870

Kim H, Yang XL, Rosada C, Hamilton SR, August JT (1994) CD44 expression in colorectal adenomas is an early event occurring prior to K-ras and p53 gene mutation. Arch Biochem Biophys 310:504–507

Kim WH, Schnaper W, Nomizu M, Yamada Y, Kleinman HK (1994) Apoptosis in human fibrosarcoma cells is induced by a multimeric synthetic Tyr-Ile -Gly-Ser-Arg (YIGSR)-containing polypeptide from laminin. Cancer Res 54:5005–5010

Kinsella AR, Green B, Lepts GC, Hill CL, Bowie G, Taylor BA (1993) The role of the cell-cell adhesion molecule E-cadherin in large bowel tumour cell invasion and metastasis. Br J Cancer 67:904–909

Koretz K, Schlag P, Boumsell L, Möller P (1991) Expression of VLA-α2, VLA-α6 and VLA-β1 chains in normal mucosa and adenomas of the colon and in colon carcinomas and their liver metastases. Am J Pathol 138:741–750

Koretz K, Schlag P, Quentmeier A, Möller P (1994) Evaluation of the secretory components as a prognostic variable in colorectal cancer. Int J Cancer 57:365–370

Koretz K, Möller P, Lehnert T, Hinz U, Otto HF, Herrfarth C (1995) Effect of CD44 on survival in colorectal carcinoma. Lancet 345:327–328

Lauri D, Needham L, Martin-Padura I, Dejana E (1991) Tumor cell adhesion to endothelial cells: endothelial leukocyte adhesion molecule-1 as an inducible adhesive receptor specific for colon carcinoma cells. J Natl Cancer Inst 83:1321–1324

Lauri D, Bertomeu MC, Orr FW (1990) Interleukin 1 increases tumor cell adhesion to

endothelial cells through an RGD dependent mechanism: In vitro and in vivo studies. Clin Exp Metastasis 8:27–32
Lesley J, Hyman R, Kincade PW (1993) CD44 and its interaction with extracellular matrix. Adv Immunol 54:271–335
Liotta LA, Steeg PS, Stetler-Stevenson WG (1991) Cancer metastasis and angiogenesis. an imbalance of positive and negative regulation. Cell 64:327–336
Löhr M, Trautmann B, Göttler M, Peters S, Zauner I, Maier A, Klöppel G, Liebe S, Kreuser ED (1996) Expression and function of receptors for extracellular matrix proteins in human ductal adenocarcinomas of the pancreas. Pancreas (in press)
Long MW (1992) Blood cell cytoadhesion molecules. Exp Hematol 20:288–301
Mackay CR, Terpe HJ, Stauder R, Marston WL, Stark H, Günthert U (1994) Expression and modulation of CD44 variant isoforms in humans. J Cell Biol 124:71–82
Mafune K, Ravikumar TS, Wong JM, Yow H, Chen LB, Steele GD (1990) Expression of a M_r32,00 laminin-binding protein messenger RNA in human colon carcinoma correlates with disease progression. Cancer Res 50:3888–3891
Mai M, Brune K, Jacoby B, Kern HF, Mollenhauer J (1990) Laminin interactions with ductal pancreatic adenocarcinoma cells: identification of laminin- and collagen-binding proteins. J Cell Sci 95:65–74
Makgoba MW, Sanders ME, Shaw S (1989) The CD2-LFA3 and LFA-1-ICAM pathways: relevance to T-cell recognition. Immunol Today 10:417–422
Makgoba MW, Bernard A, Sanders MEl (1992) Cell adhesion/signalling: biology and clinical applications. Eur J Clin Invest 22:443–453
Matsamura Y, Tarin D (1992) Significance of CD44 gene products for cancer diagnosis and disease evaluation. Lancet 340:1053–1058
Matsui S, Shiozaki H, Inoue M, Tamura S, Doki Y, Kadowaki T, Iwazawa T, Shimaya K, Nagafuchi A, Tsukita S (1994) Immunohistochemical evaluation of alpha-catenin in human gastric cancer. Virchows Arch 424:375–381
Mayer B, Johnson JP, Leitl F, Jauch KW, Heiss MM, Schildberg FW, Birchmeier W, Funke I (1993) E-cadherin expression in primary and metastatic gastric cancer: down-regulation correlates with cellular dedifferentiation and glandular disintegration. Cancer Res 53:1690–1695
Mayer B, Jauch KW, Günthert U, Figdor CG, Schildberg FW, Funke I, Johnson JP (1993) De novo expression of CD44 and survival in gastric cancer. Lancet 342:1019–1022
Mecham RP (1991) Receptors for laminin mammalian cells. FASEB 5:2538–2546
Mollenhauer J, Röther J Kern HF (1987) Distribution of extracellular matrix proteins in pancreatic ductal adenocarcinoma and its influence on tumor cell proliferation in vitro. Pancreas 2:14–24
Mulder JWR, Krypt PM, Sewnath M, Oosting J, Seldenrijk CA, Weidema WF, Offerhaus GJA, Pals ST (1994) Colorectal cancer prognosis and expression of exon-v6-containing CD44 proteins. Lancet 344:1470–1472
Nassal GJV (1994) Minimal residual disease as the target for immunotherapy of cancer. Lancet 343:1172–1173
Nigam AK, Savage FJ, Boulos PB, Stamp GWH, Liu D, Pignatelli M (1993) Loss of cell-cell and cell-matrix adhesion molecules in colorectal cancer. Br J Cancer 68:507–514
Nomizu M, Yamamura K, Kleinman HK, Yamada Y (1993) Multimeric forms of Tyr-Ile-Gly-Ser-Arg (YIGSR) peptide enhance inhibition of tumor growth and metastasis. Cancer Res 53:3459–3461
Oda T, Kanai Y, Oyama T, Yoshiura K, Shimoyama Y, Birchmeier W, Sugimura T, Hirohashi S (1994) E-cadherin gene mutations in human gastric carcinoma cell lines. Proc Natl Acad Sci 91:1858–1862

Ozawa M, Engel J, Kemler R (1990) Single amino acid substitution in one Ca^{2+} binding site of uvomorulin abolish the adhesive function. Cell 63:1033–1038
Packard BZ, Parry G (1994) Bone marrow activation by immobilized antibodies against tumor cells and immunocytes as a potential cancer immunotherapy. Biochem Biophys Acta 1224:395–400
Pauli BU, Lee CL (1988) Organ preference of metastasis: the role of organ-specifically modulated endothelial cells. Lab Invest 58:379–387
Pignatelli M, Smith MEF, Bodmer WF (1990) Low expression of collagen receptors in moderate and poorly differentiated colorectal adenocarcinomas. Br J Cancer 61:636–638
Pignatelli M, Liu D, Nasim NN, Stamp GWH, Hirano S, Takeichi M (1992) Morphoregulatory activities of E-cadherin and beta-1 integrins in colorectal tumor cells. Br J Cancer 66:629–634
Pullman WE, Bodmer WF (1992) Cloning and characterization of a gene that regulates cell adhesion. Nature 356:529–532
Rivoltini L, Cattoretti G, Arienti F, Mastroianni A, Melani C, Colombo MP, Parmiani G (1991) The high lysability by LAK cells of colon-carcinoma cells resistant to doxorubicin is associated with a high expression of ICAM-1, LFA-3, NCA and a less differentiated phenotype. Int J Cancer 47:746–754
Rosendahl A, Neumann K, Chaloupka B, Rothmund M, Weinel RJ (1993) Expression and distribution of VLA receptors in the pancreas: an immunohistochemical study. Pancreas 8:711–718
Ruoslahti E (1992) Control of cell motility and tumor invasion by extracellular matrix interactions. Br J Cancer 66:239–242
Saiki I, Murata J, Iida J, Nishi N, Sugimura K, Azuma I (1989) The inhibition of murine lung metastasis by synthetic polypeptides [poly (arg-gly-asp) and poly (tyr-ile-gly-ser-arg)] with a core of cell adhesion molecules. Br J Cancer 59:194–197
Sakamoto N, Iwanama M, Tamaka NG, Osada Y (1991) Inhibition of angiogenesis and tumor growth by a synthetic laminin peptide, CDPGYIGSR-NH_2. Cancer Res 51:903–906
Salmi M, Grön-Virta K, Sointu P, Grenman R, Kalimo H, Jalkanen S (1993) Regulated expression of exon v6 containing isoforms of CD44 in man: downregulation during malignant transformation of tumors of squamocellular origin. J Cell Biol 122:431–442
Schaller MD, Parsons JT (1994) Focal adhesion kinase and associated proteins. Curr Biol 6:705–710
Schipper JH, Frixen UH, Behrens J, Unger A, Jahnke K, Birchmeier W (1991) E-cadherin expression in squamous cell carcinomas of head and neck: inverse correlation with tumor dedifferentiation and lymph node metastasis. Cancer Res 51:6328–6337
Schlaepfer DD, Hanks SK, Hunter T, van der Geer P (1994) Integrin-mediated signal transduction linked to RAS pathway by GRB2 binding to focal adhesion kinase. Nature 372:786–791
Schwaebele W, Kerlin M, Meyer zum Büschemfelde KH, Dippold W (1993) De novo expression of intercellular adhesion molecule 1 (ICAM-1, CD54) in pancreas cancer. Int J Cancer 53:328–333
Seiter S, Arch R, Reber S, Komitowski, Hofmann M, Ponta H, Herrlich P, Matzku S, Zöller M (1993) Prevention of tumor metastasis formation by anti-variant CD44. J Exp Med 177:443–455
Sheperd NA, Saraga EP, Love SB, Jass JR (1989) Prognostic factors in colonic cancer. Histopathology 14:129–164
Shimoyama Y, Hirohashi S (1991) Expression of E- and P-cadherin in gastric carcinomas. Cancer Res 51:2185–2192

Sobel ME (1994) Differential expression of the 67kDa laminin receptor in cancer. Semin Cancer Biol 4:311–317
Springer TA (1990) Adhesion receptors of the immune system. Nature 346:425–433
Stallmach A, v. Lampe B, Orzechowski HD, Matthes H, Riecken EO (1994) Increased fibronectin receptor expression in colon carcinoma-derived HT29 cells decreases tumorigenicity in nude mice. Gastroenterology 106:19–27
Stallmach A, v. Lampe B, Matthes H, Bornhöft G, Riecken EO (1992) Diminished expression of integrin adhesion molecules on human colonic epithelial cells during the benign to malign tumour transformation. Gut 33:342–346
Stallmach A, Riese HH, Schuppan D, Bornhöft G, Stein H, Riecken EO (1991) Identification of different laminin binding proteins in basolateral cell membranes of human colorectal carcinomas and normal colonic mucosa. Gut 32:282–286
Staunton DE, Marlin SD, Stratowa C, Dustin ML, Springer TE (1988) Primary structure of ICAM-1 demonstrates interaction between members of the immunoglobulin and integrin supergene families. Cell 52:925–933
Takeichi M (1991) Cadherin cell adhesion receptors as a morphogenic regulator. Science 251:1451–1469
Takeichi M (1993) Cadherins in cancer: implications for invasion and metastasis. Curr Opin Cell Biol 5:806–811
Tanabe KK, Ellis LM, Saya H (1993) Expression of CD44R1 adhesion molecule in colon carcinomas and metastases. Lancet 341:725–726
Tanaka Y, Adams DH, Hübscher S, Hirano H, Siebenlist S, Shaw S (1993) T-cell adhesion induced by proteoglycan-immobilized cytokine MIP-1β. Nature 361:79–82
Terpe HJ, Starck H, Prehm P, Günthert U (1994) CD44 variant isoforms are preferentially expressed in basal epithelia of non-malignant human fetal and adult tissues. Histochem 101:79–89
Terranova V, Rao CN, Kalebic T, Margulies IM, Liotta LA (1983) Laminin receptors on human breast cancer cells. Proc Natl Acad Sci 80:444–448
Underhill C (1992) CD44: the hyaluron receptor. J Cell Sci 103:293–298
Varner JA (1995) Antagonists of the integrin $\alpha v\beta 3$ as potential therapeutics for tumor angiogenesis. ASCO 1995 Educational Book: 378–382
Van Roy F, Mareel M (1992) Tumor invasion: effects of cell adhesion and motility. Trends in Cell Biol 2:163–169
Vogelstein B, Kinzler KW (1993) The multistep nature of cancer. Trends in Genetics 9:138–141
Weinel RJ, Rosendahl A, Neumann K, Chaloupka B, Erb D, Rothmund M, Santoso S (1992) Expression and function of VLA-$\alpha 2$, -$\alpha 3$, -$\alpha 5$ and -$\alpha 6$-Integrin receptors in pancreatic carcinoma. Int J Cancer 52:827–833
Whalen GF, Ingber DE (1989) Inhibition of tumor-cell attachment to extracellular matrix as amethod for preventing tumor recurrence in a surgical wound. Ann Surg 210:75–764
Wielenga VJM, Heider KH, Offerhaus GJA, Adolf GR, van den Berg FM, Ponta H, Herrlich P, Pals ST (1993) Expression of CD44 variant proteins in human colorectal cancer is related to tumor progression. Cancer Res 53:4745–4765
Yamada KM, Kennedy DW, Yamada SS, Gralnick H, Chen WT, Akiyama SK (1990) Monoclonal antibody and synthetic peptide inhibitors of human tumor cell migration. Cancer Res 50:4485–4496
Yamumara K, Kibby MC, Jun SH, Kleinmann HK (1993) Effect of matrigel and laminin peptide YIGSR on tumor growth and matastasis. Semin Cancer Biol 4:259–265
Yow H, Wong JM, Chen HS, Lee C, Steele GD, Chen LB (1988) Increased mRNA expression of a laminin-binding protein in human colon carcinoma: complete se-

quence of a full-length cDNA encoding the protein. Proc Natl Acad Sci USA 85:6394–6398

Zetter BR (1993) Adhesion molecules in tumor metastasis. Semin Cancer Biol 4:219–229

Zhu D, Cheng CF, Pauli BU (1991) Mediation of lung metastasis by a lung-specific endothelial cell adhesion molecule. Proc Natl Acad Sci USA 88:9568–9572

Zhu D, Cheng CF, Pauli BU (1992) Blocking of lung endothelial cell adhesion molecule-1 (Lu ECAM-1) inhibits murine melanoma lung metastasis. J Clin Invest 89:1718–1724

Zöller M (1995) CD44: physiological expression of distinct isoforms as evidence for organ specific metastasis formation. J Mol Med 73:425–438

Human Gene Therapy in Gastrointestinal Diseases: In Vivo and In Vitro Approaches

R. Kaiser, E. Thiel, and E.-D. Kreuser

Department of Hematology and Oncology, University Medical Center Benjamin Franklin, Free University of Berlin, Hindenburgdamm 30, 12200 Berlin, Germany

Abstract

The first clinical trial in human gene therapy began in 1989 with the successful introduction of marker genes into peripheral blood cells as tumor-infiltrating lymphocytes (TIL) in order to investigate the biological behavior of manipulated cells in humans. In further studies, it was possible to ameliorate clinical genetic diseases based on only one single genetic defect such as adenosine deaminase deficiency (ADA) by repeated infusion of manipulated peripheral blood cells. Meanwhile, a multitude of clinical gene transfer studies were initiated. Three main strategies have thus far been applied in human cancer gene therapy: (1) Reinforcement of the body's immune response by gene transfer into immunological cells; (2) reinforcement of the immune response by manipulating tumor cells; and (3) transfer of drug-sensitive genes into tumor cells with subsequent drug treatment. The first clinical trial in gene therapy for gastrointestinal diseases was performed in 1992 with the introduction of the low-density protein receptor gene (LDL) into liver tissue. Human cancer gene therapy of gastrointestinal diseases is still only in the initial phase of research.

Introduction

In its current interpretation, the term human gene therapy stands only for somatic gene therapy, i.e., the specific transfer of a known gene in a specific human somatic cell. This concept might for the first time offer a strategy for correcting the pathobiologic origin of diseases in human beings, rather than treating them with conventional drugs.

The first clinical experience in oncology involving gene transfer, albeit only marker-gene transfer into somatic cells, was gained in 1989, when peripheral blood lymphocytes such as tumor-infiltrating lymphocytes (TIL) were trans-

Recent Results in Cancer Research, Vol. 142

duced with the neomycin-resistance gene obtained from *Escherichia coli* and then reinfused into patients suffering from advanced cancers to examine two primary questions: (a) Is it possible to safely transfer an exogenous gene into patients? (b) Is it possible to demonstrate that the transferred gene will be expressed in cells recovered from the patient? The results in the first five patients showed that gene-marked TIL caused no side effects or pathology attributable to the gene transfer and that they could be detected not only in the blood stream for at least 3 weeks, but also in tumor samples for as long as 9 weeks after infusion (Rosenberg et al. 1990). A great number of other gene-marker protocols using neomycin-resistance gene-transfected cells have been initiated since 1989, as shown in Table 1.

Table 1. Recent gene-marker studies (modified from Cancer Gene Therapy 1995)

Disease	Transfer	Gene	Target cell	Institute
AML, ALL, CML	Retrovirus	Neomycin resistance	T lymphocyte	St. Jude Children's Research Hospital
ALL	Retrovirus	Neomycin resistance	Bone marrow cell	Indiana University
CLL, non-Hodgkin's lymphoma	Retrovirus	Neomycin resistance	Bone marrow cell Peripheral blood cell	MD Anderson Cancer Center
CML	Retrovirus	Neomycin resistance	Bone marrow cell Peripheral blood cell	MD Anderson Cancer Center
CML	Retrovirus	Neomycin resistance	Bone marrow cell Peripheral blood cell	NIH
Multiple myeloma	Retrovirus	Neomycin resistance	Bone marrow cell Peripheral blood cell	Huddinge Hospital Karolinska Institute
Multiple myeloma	Retrovirus	Neomycin resistance	Bone marrow cell Peripheral blood cell	NIH
Breast cancer	Retrovirus	Neomycin resistance	Bone marrow cell Peripheral blood cell	NIH
Melanoma	Retrovirus	Neomycin resistance	TIL	University of Pittsburgh
Advanced melanoma Renal cell cancer	Retrovirus	Neomycin resistance	TIL Peripheral blood cell	University of California
Advanced tumors	Retrovirus	Neomycin resistance	TIL	Centre Régional Léon Bérard
Advanced tumors	Retrovirus	Neomycin resistance	TIL	NIH
Ovary cancer	Retrovirus	Neomycin resistance	TIL	MD Anderson Cancer Center
Bone marrow transplant recipients	Retrovirus	Neomycin resistance	Peripheral blood cell	H.S. Raffaelle Milano
Bone marrow transplant recipients	Retrovirus	Neomycin resistance	Bone marrow cell T-lymphocytes	St. Jude Children's Research Hospital
Lymphoid malignancies Breast cancer	Retrovirus	Neomycin resistance	Peripheral blood cell	Fred Hutchinson Cancer Center
Neuroblastoma	Retrovirus	Neomycin resistance	Bone marrow cell	Baxter Health Care, St. Jude Children's Hospital

TIL, tumor-infiltrating lymphocytes

Human Gene Therapy

In taking the first steps towards a viable human gene therapy aimed at active treatment, it was important to focus on a disease that is due to only one single genetic defect which is, moreover, involved in the mechanisms of cell proliferation, proceeding on the assumption that "gene treatment" could produce corrected cells with a selective growth advantage over untransfected cells (Anderson 1984). Three diseases comply with these conditions: Lesch-Nyhan syndrome or HGPRT (hypoxanthine-guanine phosphoribosyltransferase) deficiency, PNP (purine-nucleoside phosphorylase) deficiency, and ADA (adenosine deaminase) deficiency. ADA deficiency has hitherto been curable by matched bone-marrow transplantation. One year after successful transplantation, the patients normally regenerate all of their own blood cells except the ADA-normal T cells, which were only from the donor. This demonstrates that the transplanted ADA-normal T cells possess not only a normal biologic function but also an important selective growth advantage over the patient's deficient T cells. For these reasons, the first clinical human gene therapy protocol was initiated in 1990 for correction of the ADA deficiency by repeated intravenous infusions of the patient's own gene-transfected T lymphocytes (Culver et al. 1991). After repeated infusions of manipulated cells, two patients showed an improvement of clinical and immunological parameters, with a steady increase in the ADA level of T-cell function, starting at below 1% and reaching nearly 25% after eight infusions. So far, clinical ADA studies indicate that somatic gene therapy is thus far only a substitution therapy limited by the lifetime and transient transfection of the manipulated cells. So the future success of human gene therapy will be determined by the stable integration and expression of transfected genes. Stable gene integration and expression through homologous gene recombination, which might be the best mode of genetic treatment, has hitherto been proven only for embryonic stem cells of mice (Frohmann and Martin 1989). In the meantime, numerous clinical gene therapy protocols have been approved (Table 2).

Human Cancer Gene Therapy and Gastrointestinal Diseases

In contrast to congenital diseases like ADA deficiency with localized genetic defects, the development of cancer represents a multistep process involving a varying loss of gene function. Cancer gene therapy thus pursues three main strategies: The first strategy is aimed at reinforcing the immune response by transfecting cytokine genes to either TIL cells or tumor-specific T cells to make them more effective, and the second strategy involves transfection of cytokine genes or HLA antigens to tumor cells in order to induce the body's immune system to produce more effective TIL cells. These approaches are based on animal studies which showed that immunization with cytokine genes

Table 2. Recent clinical gene-therapy protocols

Disease	Gene	Cell	Institute
Hemophilia B	Factor-9 gene	Autologous skin fibroblasts	Fudan University, Changhai Hospital, China
Familial hypercholesterolemia	LDL receptor gene	Hepatocytes	University of Michigan, Ann Arbor, USA
AIDS	Herpes simplex thymidine kinase gene	Cytotoxic T lymphocytes	Fred Hutchinson Cancer Research Center, University of Washington, USA
ADA-deficient SCID	ADA gene	Peripheral blood T cells	NIH, USA
ADA-deficient SCID	ADA gene	Peripheral blood T cells, Progenitor-enriched bone marrow cells	Scientific Institute, San Raffaele, Italy
ADA-deficient SCID	ADA gene	Bone marrow cells	Institute for Applied Radiobiology and Immunology, University of Leiden, Netherlands

ADA, adenosine deaminase deficiency

like interleukin (IL)-2, IL-4, IL-7, gamma-interferon (IFN), granulocyte-macrophage colony-stimulating factor (GM-CSF), or tumor necrosis factor (TNF)- manipulated tumor cells resulted not only in the killing of unmodified tumor cells but also in a permanent systemic antitumor immunity mediated by T cells (Belldegrun et al. 1993; Tepper et al. 1989; Hock et al. 1991; Gansbacher et al. 1990; Dranoff et al. 1993; Asher et al. 1991). Applying the observations of cytokine-mediated immunization in clinical practice means immunizing cancer patients in their remission interval by injection of autologous cytokine-producing tumor cells to obtain a long-lasting tumor-specific immune response which might protect the patient from a relapse.

Based on the successful approaches with TNF-alpha and IL-2-transfected TIL cells in patients with melanoma, renal cell carcinoma, and bladder cancer (Rosenberg et al. 1990), clinical studies were initiated with IL-2 and IL-4 genes. IL-4-transfected cells produce a considerable antitumor effect through massive attraction of eosinophils and macrophages (Tepper 1989 et al.). IL-2 seems to play an important role even in the induction of a long-term immune response (Foa et al. 1992), as confirmed by animal experiments (Karp et al. 1993). An increased activation of the immune system can also be induced by an improvement of the antigenicity through HLA antigen (e.g., HLA-B7) transfer into tumor cells (Weber and Rosenberg 1990). This approach will be pursued in some clinical protocols for patients suffering from melanoma, renal cell carcinoma, and colon carcinoma by transfection of tumor cells through the lipofectin method. The third strategy mentioned above utilizes the ex vivo transfer of drug-sensitivity genes like the herpes simplex virus-thymidine kinase (HSV-TK) gene or the *E.coli* cytosine-deaminase (CDA) gene in tumor cells (Roemer and Friedmann 1992; Rosenberg 1992; Austin and Huber 1993; Mullen et al. 1992). Drug treatment with gancyclovir for HSV-TK-transfected cells and 5′-fluorocytosine (5′-FC) for CDA-gene-transfected cells leads to tumor-cell-killing metabolites as follows: The CDA enzyme catalyzes the deamination from 5′ FC to toxic 5-fluorouracil. Whereas the HSV-TK converts nontoxic nucleoside analogues such as gancyclovir into phosphorylated compounds, which act as chain terminators through inhibition of the DNA polymerase with a lethal effect on the cell. Clinical studies on gene transfer in gastrointestinal diseases that have been initiated are listed in Table 3.

Hepatic Gene Therapy

The classical strategy for hepatic gene therapy is the ex vivo strategy, in which a segment of the liver is removed by partial hepatectomy in order to isolate,

Table 3. Clinical gene-transfer protocols in gastrointestinal diseases (modified from Cancer Gene Therapy 1995)

Tissue	Gene	Transfer	Author/Institute
Colon, hepatic metastasis	HLA B7 cDNA	Lipofectin	J Rubin, Mayo Clinic, Rochester, USA
Colon cancer	IL-2 cDNA	Retrovirus	R.E Sobol, I. Royston San Diego Cancer Center, USA
Colon cancer	CEA-cDNA	Naked DNA	University of Alabama at Birmingham, AL, USA
Colorectal, hepatocellular liver metastases	p53-cDNA	Adenovirus	University of California, San Francisco, USA
Colon, metastatic colon carcinoma	IL-7 cDNA	Electroporation	I. Schmidt-Wolf , Free University of Berlin, Germany
Liver	LDL receptor cDNA	Retrovirus	D.J. Rader, University of Pennsylvania, USA
Liver	Neomycin resistance	Retrovirus	F.D. Ledley, Texas Children's Hospital, Houston, USA

cultivate, and ultimately transfect the hepatocytes in vitro. Subsequently, these cells are then reimplanted in the liver of the patient. Experiments in animals have demonstrated that transplantation of isolated hepatocytes by injection into the portal vasculature or spleen could be done without causing possible hemodynamic or histologic liver abnormalities, apart from a transient increase in portal pressure (Baumgardner et al. 1988; Grossmann et al. 1992a; Gupta et al. 1993). In the murine model, transplanted cells will survive throughout the lifetime of the animal. More recent distribution studies on transplanted retrovirus-mediated hepatocytes in liver tissue have suggested that labeled hepatocytes do not migrate from the portal space to the previous region, as previously hypothesized. The transplanted hepatocytes were distributed throughout the entire lobule with preponderance in the periportal and mediolobular regions, and, 1 year after transplantation, the pattern distribution of labeled hepatocytes within the lobule was not modified (Bralet et al. 1994).

The two clinical protocols initiated for gene therapy of the liver use this ex vivo approach. The one clinical protocol on retrovirus-mediated LDL receptor introduction is based on animal experiments demonstrating the successful feasibility of hepatocellular transplantation of gene-transfected hepatocytes in LDL receptor-deficient rabbits (Wilson et al. 1988) as well as gene expression in implanted rat hepatocytes following retrovirus-mediated gene transfer (Anderson et al. 1989). Studies on liposomes and retrovirus-mediated gene transfer into human hepatocytes have substantiated these animal experiments (Li et al. 1992; Adams et al. 1992; Grossmann et al. 1992b). But these successful approaches in animal experiments could not be confirmed in the first clinical liver gene transfer protocol for familial hypercholesterolemia. Of five patients, 8–41 years old with different deficiencies of LDL receptor expression, only one showed a significant decrease in hypercholesterolemia after ex vivo LDL receptor gene transfer, whereas one other patient showed no change, and three showed only a minimal decrease (Rader personal communication).

The in vivo strategy of hepatic gene therapy would eliminate the multistep process of the ex vivo strategy by direct infection of hepatic tissue through intravenous injection. In preclinical approaches, it was also possible to temporarily ameliorate the hypercholesterolemia in LDL receptor-deficient rodents by infusion of a DNA/protein complex into the peripheral circulation (Wilson et al. 1992). An adenovirus-mediated in vivo transfer of the LDL-receptor gene by intravenous injection of the recombinant virus in mice demonstrated that, 4 days after virus infection the half-life of plasma LDL was reduced up to tenfold and an estimated 90% of the parenchymal cells in the liver transiently expressed the receptor (Herz and Gerard 1993). On the other hand, the adenovirus-mediated gene transfer of a human apolipoprotein A-1 gene through intravenous injection leads to a transient elevation of the circulating HDL cholesterol concentration (Kopfler et al. 1994).

Cancer therapy approaches have so far been studied only in animal experiments. Thus, retrovirus-mediated in vivo transfer of the drug-sensitive gene

HSV-TK into rats suffering from macroscopic liver metastases by direct intratumoral injection led to a dramatic decrease in the tumor volume. The mean cancer cell mass was reduced approximately 60-fold compared with controls (Caruso et al. 1993). The successful transfection after resection of rat hepatocytes by adenovirus-mediated in vivo transfer of the p53 gene as the key protein of cell-cycle control and apoptosis opens up prospects of a possible, but difficult, use of adenovirus-mediated tumor-suppressor gene as an adjuvant in cancer gene therapy (Drazan et al. 1994). On the other hand, the human liver could be an important target for gene transfer of a multitude of genes confirmed in animal experiments such as factor 8 (Zatlouka et al. 1994), factor 9 (Ferkol et al. 1993; Kay et al. 1993), ornithine transcarbamylase (OTC) (Grompe et al. 1992), or renin (Tomita et al. 1993). Animal experiments under conditions mimicking clinical liver transplantation with retro- and adenovirus-mediated gene transfer into rat liver grafts before orthotopic reimplantation demonstrated the efficient expression of gene products in liver grafts over 2–3 weeks. Thus special gene transfer to liver grafts before transplantation may make it possible to modulate immunogenicity and alter the antigraft immune response (Shaked et al. 1994).

Gene Transfer in Colon Carcinoma

Colorectal carcinogenesis is a multistep process accompanied by the accumulation of genetic changes in proto-oncogenes and tumor-suppressor genes such as p53. The successful in vitro transfer of a normal tumor-suppressor gene copy such as p53 or the retinoblastoma gene into colon carcinoma cells leads to a massive alteration of the malignant phenotype, but unfortunately, these procedures cannot as yet be applied due to their nonspecificity and unimportant effectivity in clinical protocols (Baker et al. 1990; Huang et al. 1988). Gene therapy concepts pursue other approaches, like the immunotherapy of malignancy by gene transfer into tumor cells. Several approaches have been used to increase the natural immune response. Cytotoxic T cells might induce class-I major histocompatibility complex (MHC)-restricted lysis (Kern et al. 1986). Thus, retrovirus-mediated in vivo gene transfer of a foreign MHC gene by direct injection into a subcutaneous tumor of CT26 mouse colon adenocarcinoma cells induced a cytotoxic T-cell response to both MHC-positive cells and MHC-negative cells (Plautz et al. 1993). On the other hand, cytotoxic T lymphocytes expressing a particular T-cell-receptor beta chain were activated by the bacterial superantigen staphylococcal enterotoxin (SEA) binding to MHC class-II molecules on target cells. Based on these approaches, the construction of a recombinant fusion protein of SEA and the Fab region of the C215 monoclonal antibody specific for human colon carcinoma cells led not only to a ten-fold reduction in MHC class-II binding compared with native SEA, but also to an 85–99% inhibition of tumor growth of B16 melanoma cells expressing C215 antigen after transfection in the murine model (Dohlsten et al. 1991, 1994). Lipofectin-mediated in vitro transfection of the cytokine IL-6 gene into the human colon carcinoma cell line HT29 also enhanced tumor antigen expression on tumor cells (Tsang et al. 1993), as did retrovirus-mediated in vitro transfection of the TNF alpha receptor into human colon cancer cells. Subsequent treatment with recombinant TNF led to a massive killing of these transformed cells (Isobe et al. 1994). Subcutaneous injection of TNF-receptor-labeled cells in nude mice resulted in a reduced tumor progression (Walther et al. 1993). A recent approach in the sense of the third strategy mentioned earlier indicates that the introduction of a drug-sensitivity gene such as the CDA gene into cultured human colorectal carcinoma cells can import extraordinary sensitivity to 5-fluorocytosine (Huber and Austin 1993).

Cell-matrix interactions are assumed to be important in regulating differentiation and tumor cell growth. At least 20 different integrins are known to interact with a variety of extracellular matrix components. There is increasing evidence that integrins are altered following malignant transformation. The beta-subunit cytoplasmic domain is required for linking integrins to the cytoskeleton. The beta-6 subunit of the alpha-v beta-6 fibronectin receptor is expressed during fetal development and in a variety of epithelial tumors. Calcium-phosphate-mediated transfection of the alpha-v beta-6 receptor into human colon carcinoma cells enhanced the proliferation capacity of these cells (Agrez et al. 1994). In contrast, transfection of the alpha-5 subunit of the fibronectin receptor into the human colon carcinoma line HT29 led to increased adhesion and migration, as well as to decreased proliferation, in vitro and in vivo. Moreover, pulmonary metastases were significantly reduced in the alpha-5- transfected colon cancer cell line (Herzberg et al. 1996).

Perspectives and Conclusions

As shown, most approaches to gene transfer in colon carcinoma as well as hepatocellular carcinoma have been taken in vitro and in animal models. There have been only a few gene transfer experiments on other gastrointestinal malignancies like pancreatic, gastric, or esophageal cancer. Human gene therapy of cancer and gastrointestinal diseases is only in the initial phase of a long process. Perhaps a few gastrointestinal diseases with special focal genetic defects will be successfully treated in the future. One of the main problems for the clinical development of gene therapy will be to improve gene transfer systems to optimize transfection and long-term stable expression of transfected genes. The safety of retroviral gene transfer represents an important concern, but certainly gene-transfer experiments and gene-transfer approaches in cancer open up prospects of new knowledge in immunological as well as pathophysiological questions.

References

Adams RM, Soriano H, Wang M, Darlington G, Steffen D, Ledley FD (1992) Transduction of primary human hepatocytes with amphotropic and xenotropic retroviral vectors. Proc Natl Acad Sci U S A 89:8981–8985

Agrez M, Chen A, Cone RI, Pytela R, Sheppard D (1994) The alpha-v beta-6 integrin promotes proliferation of colon carcinoma cells through a unique region of the beta-6 cytoplasmatic domain. J Cell Biol 127:547–556

Anderson KD, Thompson JA, Dipietro JM, Montgomery KT, Reid LM, Anderson WF (1989) Gene expression in implanted rat hepatocytes following retroviral mediated gene transfer. Somat Cell Mol Genet 15:215–227

Anderson WF (1984) Prospects for human gene therapy. Science 226:401–409

Asher AL, Mule JJ, Kasid A, Restifo NP, Salo JC, Reichert CM, Jaffe G, Fendly B, Kriegler M, Rosenberg SA (1991) Murine tumor cells transduced with the gene for tumor necrosis factor-alpha. Evidence for paracrine immune effects of tumor necrosis factor against tumors. J Immunol 146:3227–3234

Austin EA, Huber BE (1993) A first step in the development of gene therapy for colorectal carcinoma: cloning, sequencing and expression of *Escherichia coli* cytosine deaminase. Mol Pharmacol 43:380–387

Baker SJ, Markowitz S, Fearon ER, Willson JK, Vogelstein B (1990) Suppression of human colorectal carcinoma cell growth by wild-type p53. Science 249:912–915

Baumgardner GL, Fasola C, Sutherland DE (1988) Prospects for hepatocyte transplantation. Hepatology 8:1158–1161

Belldegrun A, Tso CL, Sakata T, Duckett T, Brunda MJ, Barsky SH, Chai J, Kaboo R, Lavey RS, Mc Bride WH, de Kernion JB (1993) Human renal carcinoma line transfected with interleukin-2 and/or interferon α gene(s): implications of liver cancer vaccines. JNCI 85:207–216

Bralet MP, Branchereau S, Brechot C, Ferry N (1994) Cell lineage study in the liver using retroviral mediated gene transfer. Evidence against the streaming of hepatocytes in normal liver. Am J Pathol 144:896–905

Cancer Gene Therapy (1995) Second European Conference on Gene Therapy of Cancer. Kings College, London, vol 2, pp 225–234

Caruso M, Panis Y, Gagandeep S, Houssin D, Salzmann JL, Klatzmann D (1993) Regression of established macroscopic liver metastases after in situ transduction of a suicide gene. Proc Natl Sci U S A 90(15):7024–7028

Culver KW, Anderson F, Blaese RM (1991) Lymphocyte gene therapy. Hum Gene Ther 2:107–109

Dohlsten M, Hedlund G, Akerblom E, Lando PA, Kalland T (1991) Monoclonal antibody-targeted superantigens: a different class of anti-tumor agents. Proc Natl Acad Sci U S A 88:9287–9291

Dohlsten M, Abrahmsen L, Bjork P, Lando PA, Hedlund G, Forsberg G, Brodin T, Gascoigne NR, Forberg C, Lind P (1994) Monoclonal antibody-superantigen fusion proteins: tumor-specific agents for T-cell-based tumor therapy. Proc Natl Acad Sci U S A 91:8945–8949

Dranoff G, Jaffee E, Lazenby A, Golumbek P, Levitsky H, Brose K, Jackson V, Hamada H, Pardoll D, Mulligan RC (1993) Vaccination with irradiated tumor cells engineered to secrete murine granulocyte-macrophage colony-stimulating factor stimulates potent, specific and long-lasting antitumor immunity. Proc Natl Acad Sci U S A 90:3539–3543

Drazan KE, Shen XD, Csetse ME, Zhang WW, Roth JA, Busuttil RW, Shaked A (1994) In vivo adenovirus-mediated human p53 tumor suppressor gene transfer and expression in rat liver after resection. Surgery 116:197–203

Ferkol T, Lindberg GL, Chen J, Perales JC, Crawford DR, Ratnoff OD, Hanson RW (1993) Regulation of the phosphoenolpyruvate carboxykinase/human factor 9 gene introduced into the livers of adult rats by receptor-mediated gene transfer. FASEB 7:1081–1091

Foa R, Guarini A, Gansbacher B (1992) IL-2 treatment for cancer. From biology to gene therapy. Br J Cancer 66:992–998

Frohmann MA, Martin GR (1989) Cut, paste and save: new approaches to altering specific genes in mice. Cell 56:145–147

Gansbacher B, Bannerji R, Daniels B, Zier K, Cronin K, Gilboa E (1990) Retroviral vector mediated gamma-interferon gene transfer into tumor cells generates potent and long-lasting antitumor immunity. Cancer Res 50:7820–7825

Grompe M, Jones SN, Loulseged H, Caskey CT (1992) Retroviral mediated gene transfer of human ornithine transcarbamylase into primary hepatocytes of spf and spf-ash mice. Hum Gene Ther 3:35–44

Grossmann M, Raper S, Wilson JM (1992a) Towards liver directed gene therapy: retrovirus-mediated gene transfer into human hepatocytes. Somat Cell Mol Genet 17:601–607

Grossmann M, Raper SE, Wilson JM (1992b) Transplantation of genetically modified autologous hepatocytes into nonhuman primates: feasibilty and short-term toxicity. Hum Gene Ther 5:501–510

Gupta S, Y.erneni PR, Vemuru RP, Lee CD, Yellin EL, Bhargava KK (1993) Studies on the safety of intrasplenic hepatocyte transplantation: relevance to ex vivo gene therapy and liver repopulation in acute hepatic failure. Hum Gene Ther 4:249–257

Herz J, Gerard RD (1993) Adenovirus-mediated transfer of low-density lipoprotein receptor gene acutely accelerates cholesterol clearence in normal mice. Proc Natl Acad Sci U S A 90:2812–2816

Herzberg F, Schirner M, Schmidt R, Thiel E, Kreuser ED (1996) Gene transfer of integrin alpha-5 subunit into human tumor cell line induces tyrosine phosphorylation of pp125 FAK and reduces proliferation in vitro and in vivo. Exp Cell Res (in press)

Hock H, Dorsch M, Diamantstein T, Blankenstein T (1991) Interleukin 7 induces CD4+ T-cell-dependent tumor rejection. J Exp Med 174:1291–1298

Huang HJ, Yee JK, Shew JY, Chen PL, Bookstein R, Friedmann T, Lee EY, Lee WH (1988) Suppression of the neoplastic phenotype by replacement of the RB gene in human cancer cells. Science 242:1563–1566

Isobe K, Fan ZH, Emi N, Nakashima I (1994) Gene transfer of TNF receptor for treatment of cancer by TNF. Biochem Biophys Res Commun 202:1538–1542

Karp SE, Farber A, Salo JC, Hwu P, Jaffe G, Asher AL, Shiloni E, Restifo NP, Mule JJ, Rosenberg SA (1993) Cytokine secretion by genetically modified nonimmunogenic murine fibrosarcoma. Tumor inhibition by IL-2 but not tumor necrosis factor. J Immunol 150:896–908

Kay MA, Rothenberg S, Landen CN, Bellinger DA, Leland F, Toman C, Finegold M, Thompson AR, Read MS, Brinkhous KM (1993) In vivo gene therapy of hemophilia B: sustained partial correction in factor 9-deficient dogs. Science 262:117–119

Kern O, Klarnet J, Jensen M, Greenberg PJ (1986) Requirement for recognition of class-II molecules and processed tumor antigen for optimal generation of syngeneic tumor-specific class-I restricted CTL. J Immunol 136:4303–4310

Kopfler WP, Willard M, Betz T, Willard JE, Gerard RD, Meidell RS (1994) Adenovirus-mediated transfer of a gene encoding human apolipoprotein A-I into normal mice increases circulating high-density lipoprotein cholesterol. Circulation 90:1319–1327

Li AP, Myers CA, Kaminski DL (1992) Gene transfer in primary cultures of human hepatocytes. In Vitro Cell Dev Biol 28A:373–375

Mullen CA, Killstrup M, Blaese RM (1992) Transfer of the bacterial gene of cytosine deaminase to mammalian cells confers lethal sensitivity to 5′ fluorocytosine: a negative selection system. Proc Natl Acad Sci U S A 89:33–37
Plautz GE, Yang ZY, Wu BY, Gao X, Huang L (1993) Immunotherapy of malignancy by in vivo gene transfer into tumors. Proc Natl Acad Sci U S A 90:4645–4649
Roemer K, Friedmann T (1992) Concepts and strategies for human gene therapy. Eur J Immunol 208:211–225
Rosenberg SA (1992) Gene therapy of cancer. JAMA 268:2416–2419
Rosenberg SA, Aebersold P, Cornetta K, Kasid A, Morgan RA, Moen R, Karson EM, Lotze MT, Yang JC, Topalian SL (1990) Gene transfer into humans – immunotherapy of patients with advanced melanoma, using tumor infiltrating lymphocytes modified by retroviral gene transduction. N Engl J Med 323:570–578
Shaked A, Csete ME, Shiraishi M, Miller AR, Moen RC, Busuttil RW, Economou JS (1994) Retroviral mediated gene transfer into rat experimental liver transplant. Transplantation 57:32–34
Tepper RL, Pattengale PK, Leder P (1989) Murine interleukin 4 displays potent antitumor activity in vivo. Cell 57:503–512
Tomita N, Higaki J, Kaneda Y, Yu H, Morishita R, Mikami H, Oglihara T (1993) Hypertensive rats produced by in vivo introduction of the human renin gene. Circ Res 73:898–905
Tsang KY, Kashmiri SV, Qi CF, Nieroda C, Calvo B, de Filippi R, Greiner JW, Primus FJ, Schlom J (1993) Transfer of the IL-6 gene into human colorectal carcinoma cell line and consequent enhancement of tumor antigen expression. Immunol Lett 36:179–185
Walther W, Fichtner I, Uckert W (1993) Retrovirus-mediated gene transfer of tumor necrosis factor alpha into colon carcinoma cells generates a growth inhibition. Anticancer Res 13:1565–1573
Weber JS, Rosenberg SA (1990) Effects of murine tumor class-I major histocompatibility complex expression on antitumor activity of tumor infiltrating lymphocytes. J Natl Cancer Inst 82:755–761
Wilson JM, Grossmann M, Wu CH, Chowdhury NR, Wu GY, Chowdhury JR (1992) Hepatocyte-directed gene transfer in vivo leads to transient improvement of hypercholesterolemia in low-density lipoprotein receptor-deficient rabbits. J Biol Chem 267:963–967
Wilson JM, Johnston DE, Jefferson DM, Mulligan RC (1988) Correction of the genetic defect in hepatocytes from the Watanabe heritable hyperlipidemic rabbit. Proc Natl Acad Sci U S A 85:4421–4425
Zatlouka K, Cotten M, Berger M, Schmidt W, Wagner E, Birnstiel ML (1994) In vivo production of human factor 8 in mice after intrasplenic implantation of primary fibroblasts transfected by receptor-mediated adenovirus-augmented gene delivery. Proc Natl Acad Sci U S A 91:5148–5152

Signal Transduction as Target of Gene Therapy

K. Moelling, B. Strack, and G. Radziwill

Institute of Medical Virology, University of Zürich, Gloriastraße 30, 8028 Zürich, Switzerland

Abstract

Cancer development involves multistep events. Therapeutic approaches can be targeted against any of these events individually or in combination. Pancreatic cancer can involve activation of Ki-Ras, overexpression of Myc or ErbB-2, and mutational inactivation of functional p53. Three approaches with nucleic acid-based therapies have been taken. A ribozyme specific for Ki-ras mRNA carrying the activating mutation in codon 12 (GGU to GUU) was designed and shown to be stimulated by interaction with an RNA-binding protein NCp7 of HIV-1. The same protein was targeted to cell-adhesion molecules, which allowed transfer of the ribozyme and an antisense oligodeoxynucleotide (ODN) into the cell. Furthermore, proliferation may be prevented by blocking signal transduction. A transdominant negative mutant of the signaling kinase c-Raf-1 efficiently blocked transmission. A retroviral vector will be used as carrier. Furthermore, the concept of using naked DNA injected intramuscularly as an immunogen against cancer is discussed.

Introduction

Pancreatic cancer leads to almost 100% mortality within a year. Three major cell types can be affected: the neuroendocrine cells forming the islands of langerhans, acinar cells, which produce secretory enzymes, and the duct system. Abnormalities of growth factors and their receptors have been described in pancreatic neoplasia. The epidermal growth factor receptor (EGFR) is overexpressed in nearly all tumors due to enhanced transcription. The transforming growth factor α (TGFα) is expressed and may lead to an autocrine loop. Expression of ErbB-2 and ErbB-3 has been observed. In adenocarcinoma of the pancreas the Ki-ras oncogene is mutated in codon 12

Recent Results in Cancer Research, Vol. 142

in over 80% of cases, involving only a small number of substitutions (Gruenewald et al. 1989). Its oncogenic activation is an early event and may be due to some specific carcinogenic, genetic, or environmental factors (for review see Hall and Lemoine 1993). Furthermore, the tumor-suppressor gene p53 is altered in pancreatic tumors and cell lines; 60% of ductal adenocarcinomas carry p53 point mutations in exons 5, 6, 7, or 8. There are some pathological similarities between pancreatic and colorectal cancer. While chromosomal abnormalities on chromosome 5q, where the APC (adenomatosis polyposis coli) and MCC (mutated in colon cancer) are located, are not seen, involvement of the DCC (deleted in colon cancer) gene on chromosome 18q is possible.

It is interesting to note that the very rare acinus carcinoma exhibits activated myc, which apparently leads to ductal tumors in transgenic myc mice. These were created by expression of c-myc under the acinus-cell-specific elastase promoter (Sandgren et al. 1991). We have recently analyzed mutations of p53 in various pancreatic tumor cell lines and found that in neuroendocrine tumor cell lines of man and rat, expression and detection of p53 by immunofluorescence did not correlate with a detectable mutation (Bartz et al. 1996).

Recent approaches with nucleic acid-based therapies make it feasible to inhibit activated oncogenes or replace defective tumor-suppressor genes. These involve antisense strategies, ribozymes against the Ki-ras mRNA carrying the activating mutation in codon 12, and dominant negative mutants to interrupt the signal cascade leading to cell proliferation. Carriers may involve retroviral vectors or transfer peptides. These could be applied topically, preferably under the control of a tissue-specific enhancer. Furthermore, anticancer vaccination using naked DNA may be worth investigating.

Results

Signal transduction in many proliferating cells involves a pathway from stimulated receptor tyrosine kinases (RTKs) through activation of Ras and activation of the intracellular serine/threonine kinase c-Raf-1 (Fig. 1). The mechanism of activation of c-Raf-1 has not yet been completely resolved. It involves transfer of c-Raf-1 by activated Ras to the membrane, where c-Raf-1 becomes activated (Moodie and Wolfman 1994). Activated c-Raf-1 manifests itself by hyperphosphorylation and reduced electrophoretic mobility in polyacrylamide gel electrophoresis. A target of c-Raf-1 is the mitogen-activated protein kinase kinase (MAPKK) or MEK, which leads via activation of the MAP kinase to phosphorylation of the nuclear transcription factor (TF) c-Jun. Under special conditions, c-Raf-1 can phosphorylate c-Jun directly, bypassing the MAP kinase pathway (Radziwill et al. 1995). Signal transduction through the MAP kinase cascade can be monitored by gel electrophoretic mobility shift of the MAP kinase. Whether other transcription factors such as Myc,

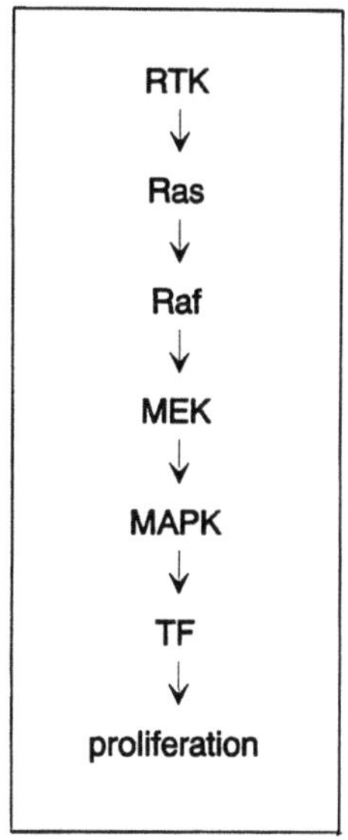

Fig. 1. Signal transduction pathway of receptor tyrosine kinases (*RTK*s). RTK activated by binding of mitogens transduces the signal through Ras to a kinase cascade which involves c-Raf-1, MEK (also named MAPKK), and MAPK. In turn, MAPK can phosphorylate and thereby modulate the activity of certain transcription factors (*TF*), which results in regulation of cell proliferation

Myb, Erb-B2, or Ets are targets of the Ras-Raf-MAPK pathway is unknown. Various stages of this pathway may be relevant as targets for blocking signal transduction and proliferation.

A Ribozyme Against Activated Ki-ras

The oncogenic Ki-ras is constitutively activated by a mutation in codon 12. One of the mutations, GGU to GUU, offers a target for a hammerhead ribozyme. Such a ribozyme was designed and synthesized by using 2′-O-allyl-modified nucleotides at various sites (Fig. 2) (Paolella et al. 1992). A control ribozyme was designed by a deletion which results in loss of catalytic activity. The ribozyme was incubated with in vitro transcribed RNA as substrate, 82 nucleotides in length, which was labeled radioactively (Fig. 2). This substrate comprises 29 nucleotides of the Ki-ras mRNA, including the GUU site. The cleavage of the RNA substrate after incubation with the ribozyme at 37°C was very inefficient. RNA-RNA interaction may depend to a significant degree on the structural conformation. In order to improve the interaction, an RNA-binding protein was added to the cleavage reaction, and this resulted in significant stimulation of the catalytic activity (Fig. 3). The single-stranded RNA-binding protein originated from the HIV-1 retrovirus, namely the nucleocapsid protein NCp7. It serves several functions in retroviral replication. It enhances the interaction of the t-RNA primer to the primer-binding site on the RNA genome. Furthermore, it specifically recognizes a packaging-site PSI which allows packaging of retroviral RNA into the maturing virus particle just prior to budding (Dannull et al. 1994).

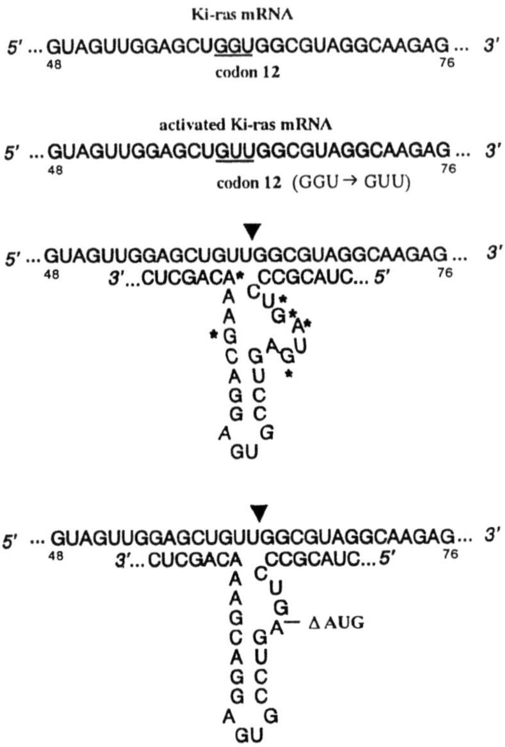

Fig. 2. Sequences of Ki-ras substrate and ribozymes. Activation of Ki-ras is based on a mutation of codon 12. A change from GGT to GTT results in a GUU sequence within the mRNA, which is cleaved by a hammerhead ribozyme. The cleavage site is indicated by a *triangle*. The synthetic ribozymes consist of 2′-O-allyl-modified nucleotides, except for those indicated by *asterisks*. As a control, a ribozyme containing a deletion (*Δ AUG*) within its active core was used, which had been transcribed in vitro

The NCp7 contains two RNA-binding motifs RXXR flanking a zinc-finger-type structure (Fig. 3). This bipartite structure may be the basis for the ability of the protein to melt RNA secondary structures and improve RNA-RNA interactions, and thus lead to stimulation of the ribozyme activity (Mueller et al. 1994). A similar effect has recently been discussed (Tsuchihashi et al. 1993).

A modified version of the NCp7 was designed by fusion to an amino acid sequence which contains the RGD sequence. This sequence specifically interacts with the cell-adhesion molecules of many cells. The complex consisting of this transfer peptide and the ribozyme was transfected into pancreatic tumor cell line Panc-1. The result was no significant reduction of growth properties. In contrast, when the same peptide was used together with an oligodeoxynucleotide (ODN) against the start site of myb-mRNA, proliferation was reduced. It is conceivable that the ribozyme is not effective enough to

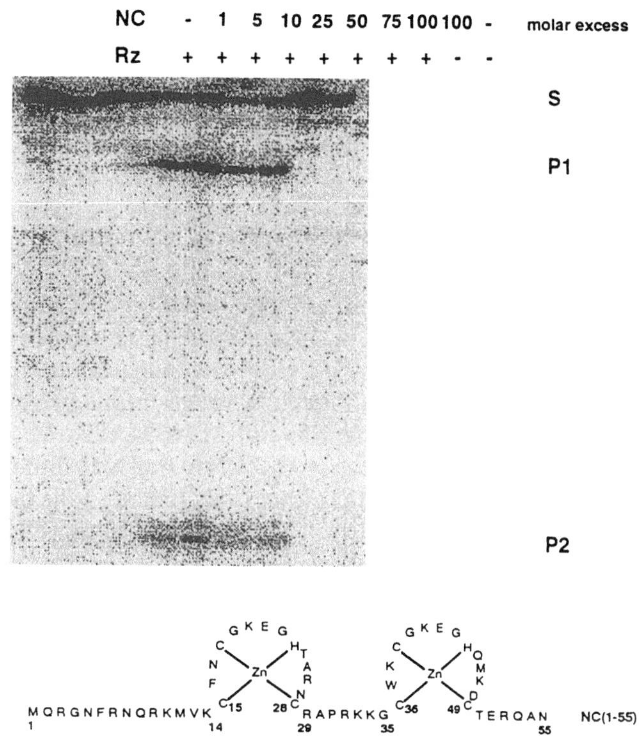

Fig. 3. Effect of NCp7 protein on cleavage of the Ki-ras mRNA substrate. Increasing concentration of a synthetic NCp7 protein (amino acid sequence is shown) were added to the reaction. Cleavage of the 82-nucleotide RNA substrates resulted in two cleavage products P1 (62 nucleotides) and P2 (20 nucleotides), which are indicated. Ribozyme and substrate RNA were used in a 1:1 molar ratio (2.7 pmol each) in the presence of various amounts of NCp7. The *molar excess* of protein over RNA given is related to the total amount of ribozyme and substrate RNA

give rise to biological effects. It may also be true that interruption of a signal cascade is more efficient at the end of the cascade rather than at the beginning, because a network of signals, not a linear transmission, may make it possible to overcome a block of Ras.

Dominant Negative Mutants of c-Raf-1 and Myb

Viruses have evolved as vectors of genetic material from cell to cell. It is therefore conceivable to use viral vectors as carriers of therapeutic genes into malignant cells. The genes transfected may interfere with proliferation of the tumor cell if the signal transduction cascade is disrupted.

One of the possibilities for blocking the signaling pathway is the use of a transdominant negative mutant (Kolch et al. 1991). Such a mutant has been designed against the kinase c-Raf-1. The aminoterminus of c-Raf-1 is a regulatory region which interacts with other proteins such as the Ras-GTP complex or a putative activator (Bruder et al. 1992; Moodie and Wolfman 1994). Overexpression of the aminoterminus without the catalytic domain present at the carboxyterminus functions as a dominant negative mutant presumably by titrating out the putative activator. The block of signal transduction can be determined by analysis of the MAPK, a kinase downstream of c-Raf-1 in the signaling pathway (Fig. 1). MAPK phosphorylation and activation can be determined by a change in electrophoretic mobility. Activation and upshift of the MAPK can be prevented by the addition of the aminoterminus of c-Raf-1. This is shown in Fig. 4, using *Xenopus laevis* oocytes as model system. Development of *Xenopus* oocytes from immature to mature involves a signal cascade which can be stimulated by progesterone or insulin in vitro. Members of this signal pathway are Ras-Raf-MEK-MAPK. Microinjection of in vitro transcribed aminoterminal c-raf-1 RNA (raf-NT) into immature oocytes, followed by treatment with progesterone, inhibited the activation of MAPK, as monitored by the absence of the activated form of MAPK (Fig. 4). Signal transduction is surprisingly well conserved among various species (Blumer and Johnson 1994). Therefore, the result obtained in *Xenopus laevis* can be anticipated to also occur in mammalian cells.

Constructs based on the retroviral vector LNL6 (Miller and Rosman 1989) are being designed and will be packaged in the packaging cell line GP+E-

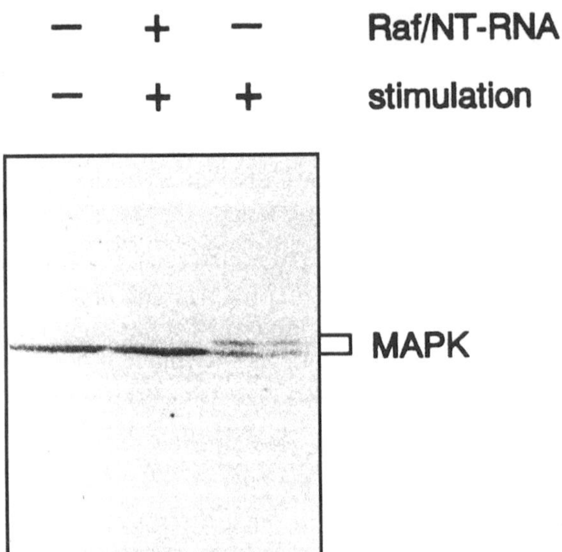

Fig. 4. Dominant negative mutant of c-Raf-1 inhibits MAPK signal transduction pathway. Oocytes were microinjected with 50 ng raf-NT RNA or water. Four hours after injection, the oocytes were treated with progesterone (5 μg/ml) and incubated for a further 8 h. Samples were analyzed by Western blot with antibodies specific for MAPK. A reduction in electrophoretic mobility correlates with activated MAPK

86 (Markowitz et al. 1988) for production of infectious but replication-defective virus particles. These are intended to be applied topically to oncogenic lesions in the pancreas. Inhibition of signal transduction may be most efficient if downstream signals are blocked. Therefore, a dominant negative Myb mutant will also be designed. We expect that the cells will die after such treatment.

Naked DNA

The possibility of circumventing peptide or viral carriers for transfer of genetic material into patients arose after it had been demonstrated that injection of naked plasmid DNA into regenerating muscle resulted in expression of plasmid-encoded genes within cells. The advantages of such a procedure are the low degree of toxicity, stability, and easy production. The amount of protein expressed is low, however. Recent improvements comprise facilitators, such as bupivacaine, which leads to increased expression (Wang et al. 1993), and also the use of particle bombardment by a gene gun (Fynan et al. 1993). Expression of low amounts of protein intracellularly may allow processing and antigenic presentation by the MHC class-I receptor. Therefore, the naked DNA approach may be useful to stimulate cytotoxic T-cell (CTL) response. Various approaches are aimed at using naked DNA as an immunogen to protect against viral infections (Wang et al. 1993; Ulmer et al. 1993). It is conceivable to use activated Ras as an immunogen to raise a CTL-mediated immune response against cancer cells. This is under investigation.

Discussion

Various approaches to preventing the proliferation of pancreatic tumor cells by interfering with the growth factor-stimulated signaling cascade can be envisaged. We have designed a Ki-ras-specific ribozyme and stimulated its activity by addition of an RNA-binding protein. The stimulatory effect was about 17-fold (Mueller et al. 1994). While this work was in progress, a similar report was published to the effect that, under special conditions, a 1000-fold stimulation could be achieved (Tsuchihashi et al. 1993). Intracellularly, RNA-binding proteins functioning as chaperones which bind to RNA and may improve the catalytic effect of a ribozyme. Alternatively, one could envisage expressing the ribozyme RNA from a construct which also contains the packaging-site PSI to which the NCp7 protein binds preferentially. Coexpression of the NC would be required. Otherwise, ribozymes directed against HIV would be activated only in cells harboring NCp7. Therefore, this approach may prove more useful than that described here using pancreatic tumor cells.

Transfer peptides as carriers may prove useful. We used the basic NCp7 protein and fused it to an RGD sequence to target it to integrin receptors.

While efficiency of the transfer of the ribozyme was questionable, the transfer peptide proved to be effective with an antisense. In a known system we were able to inhibit cellular proliferation with up to 50-fold reduced ODN concentrations.

Furthermore, we are designing retroviral vectors with transdominant negative mutants to interfere with the signaling cascade. Such a mutant of c-Raf-1 inhibits signaling. Further downstream within the cascade we may be able to interfere with the action of nuclear oncogenes such as Myc, which indirectly contributes to ductal tumors. Also, a so far unproven approach is the use of naked DNA for vaccination. Such an immunogen has been used against influenza virus or HIV infections in animal studies and has led to protective immunity or cytotoxic T-cell response (Ulmer et al. 1993). On the basis of these results, it may be worth trying to raise an immune response against activated Ki-ras. This is under way.

References

Bartz C, Ziske C, Wiedenmann B, Moelling K (1996) p53 tumor suppressor gene expression in human pancreatic neuroendocrine carcinomas. GUT 38:403–409

Blumer KJ, Johnson GL (1994) Diversity in function and regulation of MAP kinase pathways. Trends Biochem Sci 19:236–240

Bruder JT, Heidecker G, Rapp UR (1992) Serum-, TPA-, and Ras-induced expression from Ap-1/Ets-driven promoters requires Raf-1 kinase. Genes Dev 6:545–556

Dannull J, Surovoy A, Jung G, Moelling K (1994) Specific binding of HIV-1 nucleocapsid protein to PSI RNA in vitro requires N-terminal zinc finger and flanking basic amino acid residues. EMBO J 13:1525–1533

Fynan EF, Webster RG, Fuller DH, Haynes JR, Santoro JC, Robinson HL (1993) DNA vaccines: protective immunizations by parenteral, mucosal, and gene-gun inoculations. Proc Natl Acad Sci U S A 90:11478–11482

Gruenewald K, Lyons J, Frohlich A, Feichtinger H, Weger RA, Schwab G, Janssen JW, Bartram CR (1989) High frequency of Ki-ras codon 12 mutations in pancreatic adenocarcinomas. Int J Cancer 43:1037–1041

Hall PA, Lemoine NR (1993) Models of pancreatic cancer. Cancer Surv 16:135–155

Kolch W, Heidecker G, Lloyd P, Rapp UR (1991) Raf-1 protein kinase is required for growth of induced NIH/3T3 cells. Nature 349:426–428

Markowitz D, Goff S, Bank A (1988) A safe packaging line for gene transfer: separating viral genes on two different plasmids. J Virol 62:1120–1124

Miller AD, Rosman GJ (1989) Improved retroviral vectors for gene transfer and expression. Biotechniques 7:980–990

Moodie SA, Wolfman A (1994) The 3Rs of life: Ras, Raf and growth regulation. Trends Genet 10:44–48

Mueller G, Strack B, Dannull J, Sproat BS, Surovoy A, Jung G, Moelling K (1994) Amino acid requirements of the nucleocapsid protein of HIV-1 for increasing catalytic activity of Ki-ras ribozyme in vitro. J Mol Biol 242:422–429

Paolella G, Sproat BS, Lamond A (1992) Nuclease resistant ribozymes with high catalytic activity. EMBO J 11:1913–1919

Radziwill G, Niehof M, Rommel C, Moelling K (1995) Direct interaction and N-terminal phosphorylation of c-Jun by c-Mil/Raf. Proc Natl Acad Sci USA 92:1421–1425

Sandgren EP, Quaife CJ, Paulovich AG, Palmiter RD, Brinster RL (1991) Pancreatic tumor pathogenesis reflects the causative genetic lesion. Proc Natl Acad Sci U S A 88:93–97

Tsuchihashi Z, Khosla M, Herschlag D (1993) Protein enhancement of hammerhead ribozyme catalysis. Science 262:99–102

Ulmer JB, Donnelly JJ, Parker SE, Rhodes GH, Felgner PL, Dwarki VJ, Gromkowski SH, Deck RR, DeWitt CM, Friedman A et al (1993) Heterologous protection against influenza by injection of DNA encoding a viral protein. Science 259:1745–1749

Wang B, Ugen KE, Srikantan V, Agadjanyan MG, Dang K, Refaeli Y, Sato AI, Boyer J, Williams WV, Weiner DB (1993) Gene inoculation generates immune responses against HIV-1. Proc Natl Acad Sci U S A 90:4156–4160

II. Diagnostic Tools

Prognostic Significance of Molecular Biological and Immunohistological Parameters in Gastrointestinal Carcinomas

J. Rüschoff[1], T. Bocker[1], P. Vogel[2], and J. Schlegel[1]

[1] Institute of Pathology, University of Regensburg, Franz-Josef-Strauss-Allee 11, 93042 Regensburg, Germany
[2] Department of Surgery, University of Regensburg, 93042 Regensburg, Germany

Abstract

Histological type, malignancy grade, and tumor stage are among the most important parameters predicting outcome in cancer patients. Making use of immunocytochemistry as well as polymerase chain reaction-based techniques the demonstration of micrometastatic tumor spread, for example, into bone marrow, lymph nodes, and peritoneal cavity, is a new staging parameter of prognostic significance. In contrast, the prognostic value of different proliferation markers such as Ki67 (Mib 1), PCNA, and AgNOR has not yet been unequivocally established.

A series of genetic change has been described in the development of cancer.

In general, these changes seem to be of predictive value within defined tumor stages and it might be helpful to determine several genetic lesions within one tumor.

Very recently a new mechanism of carcinogenesis closely related to the hereditary nonpolyposis cancer syndrome (HNPCC) was detected. Due to mutations in mismatch repair genes (hMSH 2, hMLH 1, hPMS 1, 2) instabilities in simple repetitive genomic sequences occur, which are the genetic hallmark of most HNPCC tumors. This opens a new field to cancer prevention.

Introduction

During the past decade, extraordinary advances have been made in understanding the mechanisms of carcinogenesis, particularly by applying tech-

Supported by Wilhelm Sander-stiftung (93.055.2)

niques of molecular biology to the field of tumor research. Colorectal cancer (CRC) has provided one of the most useful models of carcinogenesis at the molecular level. Fearon and Vogelstein (1990) examined genetic alterations in CRC at various stages of neoplastic transformation and found that formation of cancer is a multistep process involving successive genetic changes (Fig. 1). This concept is now widely accepted and has been established in different malignomas (Correa and Shiao 1994; Rhyu et al. 1994; Simon et al. 1994). These data raise the question as to whether demonstration of such processes has the potential to serve as a prognostic marker in tumor pathology.

In this article the most recent results regarding the prognostic significance of molecular changes in gastrointestinal tumors will be reviewed, with special reference to CRC. The final judgement about the significance of a new prognosticator will thereby be given in relation to established factors such as tumor grade and stage (Fielding et al. 1992). Finally, recent findings regarding the molecular genetics of familial predisposition to colon cancer will be discussed.

Established Prognostic Factors

Three factors are of central importance for the clinical outcome in cancer patients: (a) the general physical state of the patient, (b) the aggressiveness of the tumor, and (c) the efficacy of the therapy (Ponz de Leon et al. 1992). From the surgical and pathomorphological points of view, prognosis of gastrointestinal carcinomas is primarily determined by curative resection and by the stage of the disease. The first parameter is recorded in the R (residual tumor) classification, the second in the TNM classification according to the UICC (1993). The depth of invasion and the presence or absence of lymph node involvment are the most powerful predictors of whether or not a cancer will recur (Hermanek et al. 1989). Other morphological features which have re-

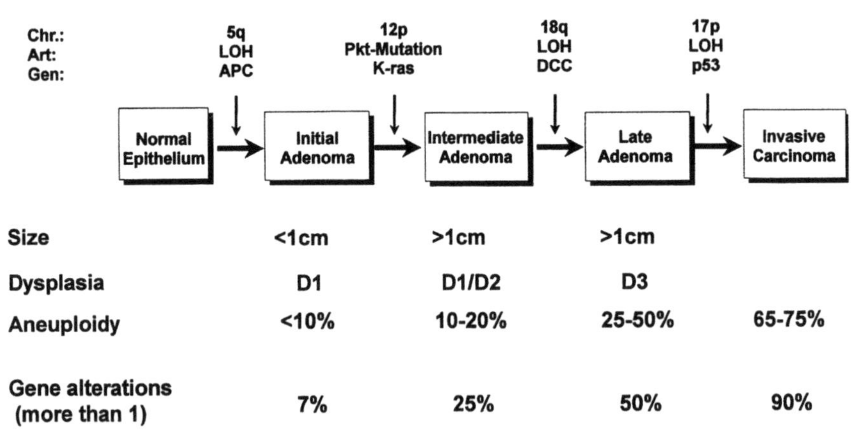

Fig. 1. Multistep carcinogenesis (modified from Fearon and Vogelstein 1990)

cently been shown to be of independent prognostic value are the type of infiltration (expanding vs. infiltrating), venous or lymphatic involvement, and desmoplasia (Graham and Appelman 1990; Jass et al. 1987).

Making use of immunohistochemistry, demonstration of single micrometastatic tumor cells by specific monoclonal antibodies has gained much interest as a potential prognostic factor. The group of Riethmüller (Schlimok et al. 1990) found epithelial cells positive for cytokeratin (CK-18) in bone marrow aspirates of approximately one third of patients with CRC. These patients had a significantly shorter relapse-free 3-year survival rate than those with negative bone marrow aspirates (71% vs. 36%). This was shown to be independent of tumor extension, lymph-node involvement, histological grading, age, and location. Very similar results were obtained in a smaller series of gastric cancers (Schlimok et al. 1991).

The discussion about the clinical significance of occult micrometastases has most recently been extended by Greenson et al. (1994). They searched for CK-positive cells in serial sections of lymph nodes staged as pN0 by routine histology. In 28% of the 568 reevaluated lymph nodes micrometastatic epithelial cells were demonstrated, and this was closely related to a much lower 5-year survival rate (Table 1).

Similarly, we have prospectively studied the prognostic implication of tumor cell spread into the peritoneal cavity in 204 patients with various gastrointestinal malignomas, mostly of the colorectum ($n = 66$) and the stomach ($n = 57$). In 35.5% of the patients a positive cytology was obtained both based on routine cytological criteria and using the epithelial marker HEA125. There was a close relationship to the tumor stage but not to the grade. Most interestingly, relapse-free survival rate within a 21-month follow-up period was approximately 70% in those with negative cytology but only 30% in those who had a positive cytology ($p < 0.01$, Mantel Haenszel-test; Vogel et al. 1994). Since verification of occult micrometastases by specific monoclonal antibodies can easily be performed on routine histological and cytological specimens, this procedure has the potential to become an additional prognostic factor at least

Table 1. Prognostic value of occult micrometastases

	Tumor cells (CK+)	Prognosis (CK+ vs CK–)
Lymph nodes pN0, pT3 (50 patients, 568 nodes) (Greenson et al. 1994)	28%	57% vs 97% (5-year surv.rate)
Bone marrow (156 patients) (Schlimok et al. 1990)	27%	68% vs 32% (relapse <2.5 years)
Peritoneal washouts (204 patients) (Vogel et al. 1994)	35.5%	32.2% vs 67.8% (disease free <21 months)

in colorectal and gastric carcinomas. However, the data have to be confirmed by further multivariate studies.

Prognostic Significance of Proliferation Analysis

Proliferation is one of the most outstanding features characterizing the malignant phenotype and biological behavior of neoplasms. Recently, considerable progress has been achieved in the understanding of cell proliferation and cell-cycle control (Fig. 2). Thereby, numerous genes involved in the regulation of the eukaryotic cell cycle have been identified (for review see Brooks 1992; Kreipe and Pawaresch 1993).

The traditional morphological approach to assessing cell proliferation is to count mitotic figures (Baak 1990). In contrast to other methods, such as in vitro labeling with bromodesoxyuridine and determination of the S-phase fraction by flow cytometry, enumeration of mitotic figures can be done in situ on histological slides. The method lacks reproducibility, however, and standardization requires a large number of cells to be counted.

During the past 10 years much effort has been exerted in the recognition of antigens that are exclusively expressed in cycling cells. Two types of antigens have been delineated. One consists of proteins involved in DNA synthesis such as polymerase alpha, topoisomerase II alpha and proliferating cell nuclear antigen (PCNA). The second group comprises molecules with hitherto unknown functions. The most well established example is the Ki-67 antigen, which is 345-kD and 395-kD in size (Table 2).

One of the most frequently used markers of proliferation in paraffin embedded tissue is PCNA, a 36-kD nuclear auxiliary protein of DNA polymerase delta (Bravo et al. 1987). The prognostic value of PCNA immunostaining

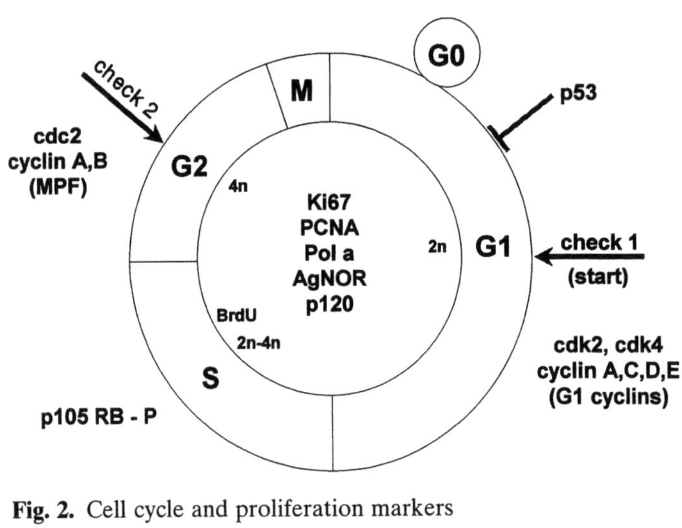

Fig. 2. Cell cycle and proliferation markers

Table 2. Prognostic value of proliferation assessment

	Reference	(*n* =)	Prognosis
Ki-67	Kubota et al. 1992	100	No influence
	Hemming et al. 1992	62	No influence
PCNA	Mayer et al. 1993	82	LI >50% unfavorable
	Al-Sheneber et al. 1993	40	LI↑unfavorable
AgNOR	Griffiths 1989	37	No influence
	Öfner 1990	49	Unfavorable
	Rüschoff et al. 1990	70	Unfavorable
	Joyce 1992	164	Unfavorable
	Rayter 1992	58	No influence
	Öfner et al. 1994	98	Unfavorable

(Table 2) has been shown in a variety of carcinomas including gastric and colorectal cancer (Mayer et al. 1993; Al-Sheneber et al. 1993). Application of this antibody to formalin-fixed and paraffin-embedded tissue, however, revealed conflicting results concerning the specificity in the recognition of proliferating cells. First, the immunostaining is influenced by the fixation procedure. Second, there is evidence that PCNA has a long half-life, leading to labeling of cells that have already left the cell cycle. Finally, there is evidence that PCNA is involved in DNA repair independent of proliferation (Hall et al. 1993). Accordingly, correlation between PCNA, Ki-67, and FCM S-phase fraction proved to be poor (Linden et al. 1993).

In contrast to PCNA, Ki-67 is exclusively expressed in cycling cells outside the G0 phase, resulting in a much better correlation with the ^{3}H-thymidine labeling index. Up to now, however, the prognostic value of Ki-67 growth fraction in gastrointestinal tumors has not been unequivocally documented. In CRC only two large series of at least 100 tumors are available, and they have not proved a prognostic value of Ki-67 growth fraction. One reason for this might be that these studies were performed on frozen-section specimens. Recently, monoclonal antibodies have been introduced that recognize the Ki-67 antigen in paraffin-embedded tissues after microwave antigen retrieval (MIB1-3, Key et al. 1993; Ki-S5, Kreipe et al. 1993). Antigen retrieval has been shown to facilitate analysis of a variety of prognostic markers including proliferation-associated antigens in large series of archive material (Taylor et al. 1994). Thus, much more reliable data about the prognostic significance of Ki-67 staining will be obtained in the very near future.

Besides immunohistochemical demonstration of proliferating cells, another technique has gained much interest during the past 7 years, namely the silver staining of nucleolar organizer regions (AgNORs). This technique shows selectively activated or actively transcribing cristons of ribosomal genes (rDNA or NORs); number, size and distribution of such silver-stained structures are closely related to the duration of the cell cycle and thus to cell proliferation

(Rüschoff 1992). Crocker and Nar (1987) were the first to demonstrate that high-grade and low-grade non-Hodgkin's lymphomas can easily be differentiated by counting of AgNORs. Since then, a series of papers have been published yielding conflicting results about the prognostic significance of this simple and cost-efficient method in tumor pathology. One important reason for contradictory findings is the poor staining quality in formalin-fixed and paraffin-embedded tissue; another is the different methods of evaluation used. In order to overcome these shortcomings, morphometrical analysis was proposed (Rüschoff et al. 1990). Most recently, Öfner et al. (1994) introduced wet autoclave pretreatment of sections prior to silver staining. With this improved method, they were able to show that determination of AgNORs is of prognostic value in colonic carcinomas. Under the guidance of a newly founded international committee on AgNOR quantification, controlled multicenter studies will now be performed in order to evaluate the validity of this technique as a new prognostic factor.

Growth Factors, Oncogenes, and Tumor-Suppressor Genes

Control of cell proliferation depends on a complex interlinked system of intra- and intercellular signaling (Fig. 3). Multiple components are now recognized: growth factors and growth-factor receptors, membrane-associated and cytoplasmic signal transduction molecules, transcription factors, and (proto-)oncogenes and tumor-suppressor genes (Hollywood and Lemoine 1992).

It is largely owing to Vogelstein and his co-workers that human colon cancer has provided the clearest picture to date of how genetic changes correlate with the development of a tumor. They have shown that the accumulation of at least four to five mutations, rather than the order of changes, is required for the development of a malignant colorectal tumor (Fearon and Vogelstein

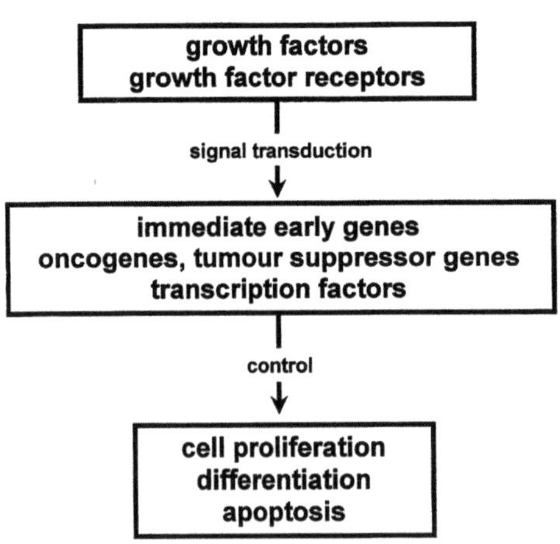

Fig. 3. Control of cell proliferation, differentiation, and apoptosis by intracellular signaling

1990). In general, two types of genetic alterations have been identified, i.e., activation of oncogenes and inactivation of tumor-suppressor genes; the latter changes predominate (see Fig. 1).

To date, studies concerning the prognostic value of such genetic alterations have been performed for K-ras activation and loss of DCC and p53 gene (Table 3). The ras family consists of the three genes H-ras (Harvey), K-ras (Kirsten), and N-ras; each gene encodes a 21-kD membrane-associated protein ($p21^{ras}$) of 188–189 amino acids. This oncoprotein is activated by point mutations, occurring mostly in codons 12, 13, and 61 in approximately half of all human malignancies (Benhattar et al. 1993). The mutated gene product has a reduced or abolished intrinsic GTPase activity, resulting in continuous signaling and thus in cell proliferation. About 40% of primary CRC express mutated K-ras oncogene product p21, with 85% of mutations confined to codons 12 or 13 (Suchy et al. 1992). Very high rates of K-ras mutations of up to 90% have been demonstrated in pancreatic carcinomas, indicating that this alteration may be a useful diagnostic marker for pancreatic cancer; a prognostic significance has not been shown, however (Motojima et al. 1991).

Table 3. Prognostic value of K-ras, DCC, and p53 mutations

K-ras (mutation)	Patients (*n*)	Method	Statistics	Prognosis
Miyahara et al. 1991	45	IH	Univ.	Overexpr: unfavorable
Suchy et al. 1992	109	PCR	Univ.	Mutations increased in metastases
Benhattar et al. 1993	99	PCR	Univ.	Recurrent tumors have more mutations
Finkelstein et al. 1993	119	PCR	Univ.	T3/T4 tumors have more mutations
DCC (LOH)				
Laurent-Puig et al. 1992	109	Southern	Multiv.	LOH: no influence
Jino 1994	71	RF PCR	Univ.	DCC ↓ in liver metastases
Jen et al. 1994	145	PCR	Multiv.	LOH: unfavorable
p53 (LOH)				
Laurent-Puig et al. 1992	109	Southern	Multiv.	LOH: unfavorable
Yamaguchi 1993	203	IH	Univ.	Pos: unfavorable
Jino 1994	98	Southern	Univ.	LOH: vascular invasion
Hamelin et al. 1994	85	PCR	Multiv.	Mut (exons 5–8): unfavorable

IH, Immunohistochemistry; *Univ.*, univariate analysis; *Multiv.*, multivariate analysis; *LOH*, loss of heterozygosity

In other tumors, such as colorectal, breast, and prostate cancer, increased expression of $p21^{ras}$ was noted to be associated with a more aggressive behavior (Miyahara et al. 1991). In CRC demonstration of K-ras mutations is closely related to lymphogenous and hematogenous spread and to more deeply invasive tumors (pT3, pT4). Interestingly, a mutant specific biological behavior of CRC has been observed by Finkenstein et al. (1993). Tumors with mutated codon 13 and those having a valine substitution in codon 12 had significantly lower rates of distant metastases than tumors with the most frequent GGT-to-GAT transition in codon 12. Carcinomas with normal K-ras accounted for most intraperitoneal deposits. Most recently, Benhattar et al. (1993) found K-ras gene mutations at codons 12 and 13 in 25% of nonrecurring and in 71% of patients with recurrent CRC within 5 years of follow-up ($p < 0.0001$). Similar to the findings of Finkenstein et al. (1993), transitions other than GGT to GAT were almost totally restricted to recurrent disease.

In a large multivariate study of 119 CRC, Laurent-Puig et al. (1992) investigated the prognostic value of histological staging, FCM-DNA ploidy, and various molecular genetic alterations such as K-ras mutations, as well as allelic losses on chromosomes 17p (p53), 18q (DCC), 5q (APC, MCC), and 1p. In this setting, demonstration of K-ras mutations, however, was not correlated with the 5-year survival rate, either by univariate or by multivariate analysis. In contrast, histological staging ($p < 0.0001$) and allelic loss of the short arm of chromosome 17 ($p < 0.004$) were found to be independently associated with shorter survival in CRC.

The loss of a large portion of chromosome 17p occurs with high frequency in human malignomas and has been seen in more than 75% of CRC (Fearon and Vogelstein 1990). This region contains the p53 gene, which is one of the most frequently mutated genes in human tumors. The p53 gene encodes a 393 amino-acid nucleoprotein of 53 kD present at low levels in normal cells. The main function of the wild-type protein (wt p53) is regulation of cell cycle; DNA damage induces an overexpression of wt p53, which is followed by cell-cycle arrest to allow DNA repair before the transition to the S-phase (Marshall 1991). Cells without wt p53 have lost their ability to suppress malignant transformation. In general, two mechanisms of p53 inactivation have been described; one refers to loss of one allele (loss of heterozygozity, LOH) and point mutation within the other allele, most frequently (95%) in exons 5–9. Second, p53 can be inactivated by complex formation with viral oncoproteins (e.g., SV40 large T antigen) and several other cellular proteins (e.g., mdm2 gene product) (Burkart 1994). Since the half-life of mutated p53 is 6–10 times longer than that of wt p53 (20 min) accumulation of mutated p53 can be detected by immunohistochemistry. However, the agreement between the frequency of positive immunohistochemistry and the frequency of tumors with mutations detected directly by DNA sequencing varies considerably between different tumor types (Soussi et al. 1994). In CRC a close relationship between high immunohistochemical expression of p53 and gene mutations has been found when the immuno label index was higher than 30% (Baas et al. 1994).

At present, immunohistochemistry is the most widely used approach to searching for p53 alterations in human cancers. Although accumulation of p53 has been shown to correlate with poor prognosis in several cancers, this has not been consistently observed in CRC (Scott et al. 1991; Starzynska et al. 1992; Yamaguchi et al. 1993). In a most recent study conducted by Hamelin et al. (1994) mutations of exons 5–8 demonstrated by PCR and direct sequencing were closely related to prognosis; this was retained as a prognostic factor in multivariate analysis, together with histological staging.

In contrast to p53, only a few studies have been published concerning the prognostic value of mutations at the DCC (deleted in colonic cancer) gene. The DCC gene maps to 18q21, where allelic deletions frequently occur in colorectal cancers. The gene product functions as a cell-adhesion protein (Fearon and Vogelstein 1990). Accordingly, in two studies it was demonstrated that an LOH at 18q was closely related to lymphatic invasion and hepatic metastasis ($p < 0.01$) (Iino et al. 1994). Most recently, Jen et al. (1994) found that allelic loss of 18q as determined by microsatellite markers was closely related to prognosis of stage-II and stage-III CRC. Among patients with stage-II disease without LOH at 18q, the 5-year survival rate was 93%, whereas in patients with LOH the 5-year survival rate was only 54%; among patients with stage-III disease the corresponding values were 52% and 38%, respectively. 18q LOH remained a strong predictive factor even in a multivariate analysis including tumor grade, vein invasion, and TNM stage.

Predisposition to Cancer

Although most CRC are considered to be sporadic, approximately 10–15% are attributed to an inherited predisposition following an autosomal dominant inheritance pattern (Table 4). Familial adenomatous polyposis (FAP) is one of the most well-known inherited colonic cancer syndromes. Localization and isolation of the APC (adenomatous polyposis coli) gene, which is the target gene of FAP, enabled a detailed analysis of this inherited condition, leading to the unambiguous identification of affected persons. FAP accounts for only 1%

Table 4. Characteristics of hereditary and sporadic colorectal carcinoma

	FAP	HNPCC	Sporadic
Incidence	1%	8–15%	85%
Age (years)	30–40	35–45	65–75
Adenomas (*n*)	>100	1–5	<10
Location of Ca	Random	70% proximal	40% rectum

of CRC, however, and the prevalence is thus relatively low (1:10000) (Friedl 1994).

In contrast, Lynch and his co-workers have delineated another colonic cancer predisposition syndome, which is now called "hereditary nonpolyposis colorectal cancer" (HNPCC). This cancer family syndrome is one of the most common genetic diseases of man, affecting as many as 1/200 individuals and accounting for about 8–10% of colorectal carcinomas (Lynch et al. 1993). According to the so-called Amsterdam criteria, HNPCC should be diagnosed if there are (a) three or more first-degree relatives with colorectal cancer and (b) one or more patients diagnosed before the age of 50 (Vasen et al. 1991). Families presenting exclusively with CRC have been called Lynch syndrome I and should be distinguished from families also showing carcinomas of the endometrium and other organs (Lynch II).

Although a series of genes contributing to colon cancer development have been described, none of these was linked to HNPCC families (Fearon and Vogelstein 1990). In May 1993, four publications hailed the discovery of a genetic locus predisposing to HNPCC, suggesting that this new colon cancer gene acts in a novel way, namely by destablizing the genome in widespread simple repetitive microsatellite DNA (Aaltonen et al. 1993; Marx 1993; Peltomäki et al. 1993; Thibodeau et al. 1993). Recently, Strand et al. (1993) have shown that in yeast DNA polymerase causes a very high rate of mismatches on templates containing poly(CA), the most common simple repeat in eukaryotes. The stability of the length of such CA repeats depends thereby on the integrity of specific mismatch repair systems. In *Escherichia coli* there are about 20 known genes involved in DNA replication or repair, so-called mutator genes (Kunkel 1993). Mutations of mismatch repair genes such as mutL and mutS in *E. coli* and pms1, mlh1 (homologues of MutL in *Salmonella*) and msh2 (homologues of MutS in *Salmonella*) in yeast were followed by a 13-fold elevation of tract instability in *E. coli* and a 100- to 700-fold increase of tract instability in yeast. Based on these data, Strand et al. (1993) supposed that instability of the length of simple repeats is a consequence of DNA polymerase slippage on the one hand, and of a decreased efficiency of repair proteins to remove such mismatches on the other.

In fact, screening of human colorectal cancers for mutations in simple repetitive DNA sequences disclosed microsatellite instabilities (Fig. 4) in mono-, di-, and trinucleotide repeats in about 12–20% of sporadic CRC and about 80–90% of HNPCC tumors (Aaltonen et al. 1994). Given the similarity to the aforementioned mutations in bacteria and yeast, the human homologues of mismatch repair genes in *E. coli* (*mutS*, *mutL*) and *Saccharomyces cerevisiae* (MSH, MLH) genes have been cloned and sequenced (hMSH2, hMLH1). One of these mapped to chromosome 2p22-21, and the other (hMLH1) to chromosome 3p21-23. Most recently, two additional genes, hPMS1 and hPMS2 (homologues of prokaryotic *mutL* gene), have been sequenced and localized on chromsome 2q31-33 (hPMS1) and chromsome 7p22 (hPMS2) (Fishel et al. 1993; Nicolaides et al. 1994; Papadopoulos et al. 1994).

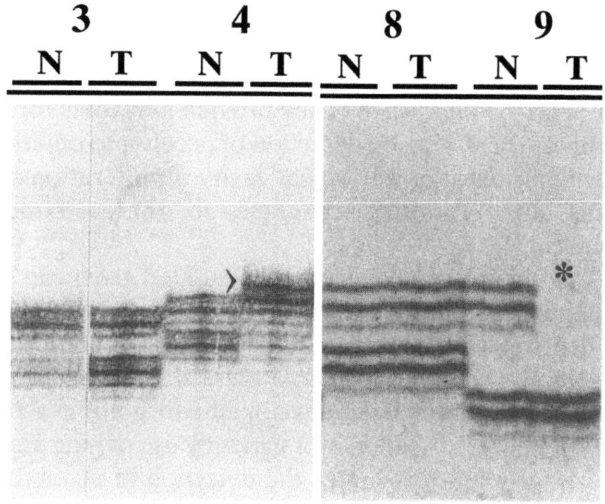

Fig. 4. Analysis of microsatellite instability in colorectal carcinomas. Band shift (>) indicates instability of poly(CA) repeats at the microsatellite locus D10S89; *asterisk*, LOH of chromosome 17p (p53)

Mutations in these genes can be demonstrated in the germline of at least 90% of kindreds meeting the criteria for HNPCC. Thus, it becomes more and more clear that the effect of such mutations is recessive and follows Knudson's two-hit hypothesis given for tumor-suppressor genes (Knudson 1985).

These data are of central importance for both pathologists and clinicians, since they may serve as a new tool for the identification of high-risk individuals before they develop colon cancer or other HNPCC-related carcinomas. For practical purposes, it seems reasonable to screen CRC prospectively for microsatellite instability. We have therefore developed a simple nonradioactive PCR-based method which can be used for routine purposes (Schlegel et al. 1994). At present, however, we do not really know how many patients having a colorectal cancer with microsatellite instability form part of the HNPCC syndrome. For definite molecular diagnosis germline mutations within the human mismatch repair genes have to be demonstrated either in blood or normal tissue.

Conclusion

The tumor's biological properties are determined by an accumulation of changes that usually develop over the span of years and have a cumulative effect on the control of cell differentiation, cell division, and growth. The chance a cancer patient has of surviving depends largely on early diagnosis and prompt administration of the most effective treatment. Thus, determination of the aggressiveness of a tumor and delineation of risk factors predisposing to cancer are major aims of contemporary tumor pathology. Today, a series of specific monoclonal antibodies are available which can reliably be applied to a broad spectrum of routinely fixed specimens, particularly after antigen retrieval by microwave. They provide new tools for an improved assessment of tumor stage, e.g., by detection of occult micrometastases within bone marrow, lymph nodes, or peritoneal cavity. Proliferation markers are thereby one of the most promising techniques for the assessment of prognosis in human cancer.

Although products of single mutated genes can be detected by an increasing number of antibodies, a positive or negative immunoreaction is not always identical with presence or absence of mutations within the corresponding gene. In order to overcome these shortcomings, simple nonradioactive PCR techniques have been developed which allow a rapid determination, e.g., of LOH of tumor-suppressor genes by use of microsatellite markers. In addition, this technique facilitates the detection of instabilities in the length of simple genomic repeats which are caused by mutations within mismatch repair genes. Demonstration of such mutations in DNA from normal tissue or blood forms the molecular basis of HNPCC, which is currently the most frequent cancer predisposition syndrome.

Thus, analysis of gastrointestinal tumors by immunohistological and molecular biological techniques not only allows an improved assessment of the tumor's biological aggressiveness; it also opens a new field in cancer prevention by delineation of cancer predisposition families.

References

Aaltonen LA, Peltomäki P, Leach FS, Sistonen P, Pylkkänen L, Mecklin JP, Järvinen H, Powell SM, Jen J, Hamilton SR, Peterson GM, Kinzler KW, Vogelstein B, de la Chapelle A (1993) Clues of the pathogenesis of familial colorectal cancer. Science 260:812–816

Aaltonen LA, Peltomäki P, Mecklin JP, Järvinen H, Jass JR, Green JS, Lynch HT, Watson P, Tallqvist G, Juhola M, Sistonen P, Hamilton SR, Kinzler KW, Vogelstein B, de la Chapelle A (1994) Replication errors in benign and malignant tumors from hereditary nonpolyposis colorectal cancer patients. Cancer Res 54:1645–1648

Al-Sheneber I, Shibata H, Sampalis J, Jothy S (1993) Prognostic significance of proliferating cell nuclear antigen expression in colorectal cancer. Cancer 71:1954–1959

Baak JPA (1990) Mitosis counting in tumors. Hum Pathol 21:683–685

Baas I, Mulder J-W, Offerhaus G, Vogelstein B, Hamilton S (1994) An evaluation of six antibodies for immunohistochemistry of mutant p53 gene product in archival colorectal neoplasms. J Pathol 172:5–12

Benhattar J, Losi L, Chaubert P, Givel JC, Costa J (1993) Prognostic significance of k-ras mutations in colorectal carcinoma. Gastroenterology 104:1044–1048

Bravo R, Frank R, Blundell PA, McDonald-Bravo H (1987) Cyclin/PCNA is the auxiliary protein of DNA polymerase alpha. Nature 236:515–520

Brooks RF (1992) Regulation of the eukaryotic cell cycle. In: Hall PA, Levison DA, Wright NA (eds) Assessment of cell proliferation in clinical practice. Springer, Berlin Heidelberg New York, pp 1–26

Burkart Ċ (1994) Das Tumorsuppressorprotein p53. Dtsch Arztebl 91:679–684
Correa P, Shiao Y (1994) Phenotypic and genotypic events in gastric carcinogenesis. Cancer Res [Suppl] 54:1941s–1943s
Crocker J, Nar P (1987) Nucleolar organizer regions in lymphomas. J Pathol 151:111–118
Fearon E, Vogelstein B (1990) A genetic model for colorectal tumorigenesis. Cell 61:759–767
Fielding LP, Fenoglio-Preisser CM, Freedman LS (1992) The future of prognostic factors in outcome prediction of patients with cancer. Cancer 70:2367–2377
Finkelstein SD, Sayegh R, Christensen S, Swalsky PA (1993) Genotypic classification of colorectal adenocarcinoma. Cancer 71:3827–3838
Fishel R, Lescoe MK, Rao MRS, Copeland NG, Jenkins NA, Garber J, Kane M, Kolodner R (1993) The human mutator gene homologue MSH2 and its association with hereditary nonpolyposis colon cancer. Cell 75:1027–1038
Friedl W (1994) Familiäre adenomatöse Polyposis. Dtsch Arztebl 91(C):92–94
Graham D, Appelman H (1990) Crohn's-like lymphoid reaction and colorectal carcinoma: a potential histologic prognosticator. Mod Pathol 3:332–335
Greenson JK, Isenhart CE, Rice R, Mojzisik C, Houchens D, Martin EW (1994) Identification of occult micrometastases in pericolic lymph nodes of Duke's B colorectal cancer patients using monoclonal antibodies against cytokeratin and cc49. Correlation with long-term survival. Cancer 73:563–569
Griffiths A (1989) Silver-stained structures (AgNORs), their dependence on tissue fixation and absence of prognostic relevance in rectal adenocarcinoma. J Pathol 159:121–127
Hall PA, McKee PH, Menage HD, Dover R, Lane DP (1993) High levels of p53 protein in UV-irradiated normal skin. Oncogene 8:203–207
Hamelin R, Laurent-Puig P, Olschwang S, Jego N, Asselain B, Remvikos Y, Girodet J, Salmon RJ, Thomas G (1994) Association of p53 mutations with short survival in colorectal cancer. Gastroenterology 106:42–48
Hemming A, Davis N, Kluftinger A, Robinson B, Quenville N, Liseman B, LeRiche J (1992) Prognostic markers of colorectal cancer: an evaluation of DNA content, epidermal growth factor receptor and Ki-67. J Surg Oncol 51:147–152
Hermanek P, Guggenmoos-Holzmann I, Gall F (1989) Prognostic factors in rectal carcinoma. Dis Colon Rectum 32:593–599
Hollywood DP, Lemoine NR (1992) Growth factors, oncogenes and tumour suppressor genes. In: Hall PA, Levison DA, Wright NA (eds) Assessment of cell proliferation in clinical practice. Springer, Berlin Heidelberg New York, pp 27–43
Iino H, Fukayama M, Maeda Y, Koike M, Mori T, Takahashi T, Kikuchi-Yanoshita R, Miyaki M, Mizuno S, Watanabe S (1994) Molecular genetics for clinical management of colorectal carcinoma. Cancer 73:1324–1331
Itoh F, Hinoda Y, Ohe M, Ohe Y, Ban T, Endo T, Imai K, Yachi A (1993) Decreased expression of DCC mRNA in human colorectal cancers. Int J Cancer 53:260–263
Jass JR, Love SB, Northover JMA (1987) A new prognostic classification of rectal cancer. Lancet 6:1303–1306
Jen J, Kim H, Piatadosi S, Liu Z, Levitt R, Sistonen P, Kinzler K, Vogelstein B, Hamilton S (1994) Allelic loss of chromosome 18q and prognosis in colorectal cancer. N Engl J Med 331:213–221
Jino H, Fukayama M, Maeda Y, Koike M, Mori T, Takahashi T, Kikuchi-Yanoshita R, Miyaki M, Mizuno S, Watanabe S (1994) Molecular genetics for clinical management of colorectal carcinoma. 17p, 18q and 22q loss of heterozygosity and decreased DCC expression are correlated with the metastatic potential. Cancer 73:1324–1331
Joyce W (1992) The prognostic value of nucleolar organiser regions in colorectal cancer. Ann R Coll Surg 74:172-6–176-7

Key G, Becker M, Baron B, Duchrow M, Schlüter C, Flad H, Gerdes J (1993) New Ki-67-equivalent murine monoclonal antibodies (MIB 1-3) generated against bacterially expressed parts of the Ki-67 cDNA containing three 62 base pair repetitive elements encoding for the Ki-67 epitope. Lab Invest 68:629–636
Knudson AG (1985) Hereditary cancer, oncogenes, and antioncogenes. Cancer Res 45:1437–1443
Kreipe H, Parwaresch R (1993) A closer look at the cell cycle. Virch Arch [A] 422:341–343
Kreipe H, Wacker H, Heidebrecht J, Haas K, Hauberg M, Tiemann M, Parwaresch R (1993) Determination of the growth fraction in non-Hodgkin's lymphomas by monoclonal antibody Ki-S5 directed against a formalin-resistant epitope of the Ki-67 antigen. Am J Pathol 142:1689–1694
Kubota Y, Petras R, Easley K, Bauer T, Tubbs R, Fasio V (1992) Ki-67-determined growth fraction versus standard staging an grading parameters in colorectal carcinoma. Cancer 70:2602–2609
Kunkel TA (1993) Slippery DNA and diseases. Nature 365:207–208
Laurent-Puig P, Olschwang S, Delattre O, Remvikos Y, Asselain B, Melot T, Validire P, Muleris M, Girodet J, Salmon R, Thomas G (1992) Survival and acquired genetic alternations in colorectal cancer. Cancer 102:1136–1141
Linden M, Ma C, Kubus J, Brown R, Zarbo R (1993) Ki-67 and proliferating cell nuclear antigen tumor proliferative indices in DNA diploid colorectal adenocarcinoma. Am J Clin Pathol 100:206–212
Lynch HT, Smyrk TC, Watson P, Lanspa SJ, Lynch JF, Lynch PM, Cavalieri RJ, Boland CR (1993) Genetics, natural history, tumor spectrum, and pathology of hereditary nonpolyposis colorectal cancer: an updated review. Gastroenterology 104:1535–1549
Marshall CJ (1991) Tumor suppressor genes. Cell 64:313–326
Marx J (1993) New colon cancer gene discovered. Science 260:751–752
Mayer A, Takimoto M, Fritz E, Schellander G, Kofier K, Ludwig H (1993) The prognostic significance of proliferating cell nuclear antigen, epidermal growth factor receptor and mdr gene expression in colorectal cancer. Cancer 71:2454–2460
Miyahara M, Saito T, Kaketani K, Sato K, Kuwahara A, Shimoda K, Kobayashi M (1991) Clinical significance of ras p21 overexpression for patients with an advanced colorectal cancer. Dis Colon Rectum 34:1097–1102
Miyake S, Nagai K, Yosthino K, Oto M, Endo M, Yuasa Y (1994) Point mutations and allelic deletion of tumor suppressor gene DCC in human esophageal squamous cell carcinomas and their relation to metastasis. Cancer Res 54:3007–3010
Motojima K, Urano T, Nagata Y, Shiku H, Tsunoda T, Kanematsu T (1991) Mutations in the Kirsten-ras oncogene are common but lack correlation with prognosis and tumour stage in human pancreatic carcinoma. Am J Gastroenterol 86:1784–1788
Nicolaides NC, Papadopoulos N, Liu B, Wei YF, Carter KC, Ruben SM, Rosen CA, Haseltine WA, Fleischmann RD, Fraser CM, Adams MD, Venter JC, Dunlop MG, Hamilton SR, Peterson GM, de la Chapelle A, Vogelstein B, Kinzler KW (1994) Mutations of two PMS homologues in heredetary nonpolyposis colon cancer. Nature 371:75–80
Öfner D (1990) Silver-stained nucleolar organizer region proteins (Ag-NORs) as a predictor of prognosis in colonic cancer. J Pathol 162:43–49
Öfner D, Bankfalvi A, Riehemann K, Bier B, Schmid KW (1994) Wet autoclave pretreatment improves the visualisation of silver-stained nucleolar organizer regions associated proteins (AgNORs) in routinely formalin-fixed and paraffin-embedded tissues. Mod Pathol 7:946–951
Papadopoulos N, Nicolaides NC, Wei YF, Ruben SM, Carter KC, Rosen CA, Haseltine WA, Fleischmann RD, Fraser CM, Adams MD, Venter JC, Hamilton SR, Peterson GM, Watson P, Lynch HT, Peltomäki P, Mecklin JP, de la Chapelle A,

Kinzler KW, Vogelstein B (1994) Mutation of a mutL homolog in hereditary colon cancer. Science 263:1625–1629

Peltomäki P, Aaltonen LA, Sistonen P, Pylkkänen L, Mecklin JP, Järvinen H, Green JS, Jass JR, Weber JL, Leach FS, Petersen GM, Hamilton SR, de la Chapelle A, Vogelstein B (1993) Genetic mapping of a locus predisposing to human colorectal cancer. Science 260:810–812

Ponz de Leon M, Sant M, Micheli A, Sacchetti C, Di Gregorio C, Fante R (1992) Clinical and pathologic prognostic indicators in colorectal cancer. Cancer 69:626–635

Rayter Z, Surtees P, Tildsley G, Corbishley C (1992) The prognostic value of argyrophil nuclear organiser regions (AgNORs) in colorectal cancer. Eur J Surg Oncol 18:37–40

Rhyu M-G, Park W-S, Jung Y-J, Choi S-W, Meltzer S (1994) Allelic deletions of MCC/APC an p53 are frequent late events in human gastric carcinogenesis. Gastroenterology 106:1584–1588

Rüschoff J (1992) Nucleolar organizer regions (NORs) in diagnostic tumor pathology. Fischer, Stuttgart

Rüschoff J, Plate K, Contractor H, Kern H, Zimmermann R, Thomas C (1990) Evaluation of nucleolar organizer regions (NORs) by automatic image analysis: a contribution to standardization. J Pathol 161:113–118

Schlegel J, Bocker T, Zirngibl H, Hofstädter F, Rüschoff J (1995) Detection of microsatellite instability in human colorectal carcinomas using a non-radioactive PCR-based screening method. Virch Arch 426:223–227

Schlimok G, Funke I, Bock B, Schweiberer B, Witte J, Riethmüller G (1990) Epithelial tumor cells in bone marrow of patients with colorectal cancer: immunocytochemical detection, phenotypic characterization and prognostic significance. J Clin Oncol 8:831–837

Schlimok G, Funke I, Pantel K, Strobel F, Lindemann F, Witte J, Riethmuller G (1991) Micrometastatic aspects of detection and prognostic significance. Eur J Cancer 27:1461–1465

Scott N, Sagar P, Stewart J, Blair GE, Dixon MF, Quirke P (1991) p53 in colorectal cancer: clinicopathological correlation and prognostic significance. Br J Cancer 63:317–319

Simon B, Weinel R, Höhne M, Watz J, Schmidt J, Körtner G, Arnold R (1994) Frequent alterations of the tumor suppressor genes p53 and DCC in human pancreatic carcinoma. Gastroenterology 106:1645–1651

Soussi T, Legros Y, Lubin R, Ory K, Schlichtholz B (1994) Multifactorial analysis of p53 alteration in human cancer: a review. Int J Cancer 57:1–9

Starzynska T, Bromley M, Ghosh A, Stern PL (1992) Prognostic significance of p53 overexpression in gastric and colorectal carcinoma. Br J Cancer 66:558–562

Strand M, Prolla TA, Liskay RM, Petes TD (1993) Destabilization of tracts of simple repetitive DNA in yeast by mutations affecting DNA mismatch repair. Nature 365:274–276

Suchy B, Zietz Ch, Rabes HM (1992) K-ras point mutations in human colorectal carcinomas: relation to aneuploidy and metastasis. Int J Cancer 52:30–33

Taylor C, Shi S-R, Chaiwun B, Young L, Iman A, Cote R (1994) Strategies for improving the immunohistochemical staining of various intranuclear prognostic markers in formalin-paraffin sections: androgen receptor, estrogen receptor, progesterone receptor, p53 protein, proliferating cell nuclear antigen, and Ki-67 antigen revealed by antigen retrieval techniques. Hum Pathol 25:263–270

Thibodeau SN, Bren G, Schaid D (1993) Microsatellite instability in cancer of the proximal colon. Science 260:816–819

Union Internationale Contre le Cancer (UICC) (1993) TNM Atlas, 3rd edn. Springer, Berlin Heidelberg New York

Vasen HFA, Mecklin JP, Meera Khan P, Lynch HT (1991) Hereditary non-polyposis colorectal cancer. Lancet 338:877

Vogel P, Rüschoff J, Kümmel S, Zirngibl H, Hofstädter F, Hohenberger W (1995) Microscopic peritoneal seeding of gastrointestinal malignancies — first results of a prospective study. GUT 37 [Suppl 2]: A101

Yamaguchi A, Nakagawara G, Kuroska Y, Nishimura G, Yonemura Y, Miyazaki J (1993) p53 immunoreaction in endoscopic biopsy specimens of colorectal cancer, and its prognostic significance. Br J Cancer 68:399–402

Molecular Mechanisms and Possibilities of Overcoming Drug Resistance in Gastrointestinal Tumors

M. Dietel

Institut für Pathologie der Charité, Humboldt Universität zu Berlin,
Schumannstr. 20-21, 10117 Berlin, Germany

Abstract

Primary and aquired resistance of tumor cells to antineoplastic drugs is a major cause of the limited efficiency of chemotherapy. Gastrointestinal (GI) tumors have proven to express cytostatic drug resistance at an unusually high rate. One major reason for this is the multidrug resistant (MDR) phenotype which is often found in carcinomas of the stomach, bile duct, pancreas, liver, and colon. MDR is due to the overexpression of a membrane-bound glycoprotein, the so called P-glycoprotein. However, this is not the only resistance mechanisms of GI tumor cells, but the intracellular compartmentalization of drugs with subsequent release to the microenvironment represents an additional potent mechanism of drug resistance. This is independent of P-glycoprotein and as yet cannot be reversed. Alterations of glutathione-*S*-transferase (GST) and topoisomerase I and II may be involved either. Analyses of cell lines for cross resistance against a battery of cytostatic drugs suggest even more mechanisms which may contribute to the marked resistance of gastrointestinal cancer. Only a detailed investigation of all different types of drug insensitivity, if ever possible, might offer a chance to fully understand this multifactorial orchestra of events and to develop complex strategies for overcoming drug resistance.

Introduction

Gastrointestinal (GI) tumors are known to be relatively insensitive to single-agent or combination chemotherapy (Mac Donald et al. 1982) and to exhibit a primary or intrinsic resistance for many different types of cytostatic drugs. There are different mechanisms by which malignant tumor cells are able to overcome the toxic attack of the drugs: (a) overexpression of membrane-bound efflux pumps, such as P-170-glycoprotein or the multidrug resistance

Recent Results in Cancer Research, Vol. 142

(MDR)-associated protein (MRP), (b) intracellular compartmentalization of the cytostatic substances, (c) reduced expression of topoisomerase II, and (d) activation of certain detoxifying or converting enzymes, such as glutathione-*S*-transferase and glutathioneperoxidase. The current paper will focus on the first two pathways, which appear to play the major role in gastrointestinal malignancies.

P-Glycoprotein and Detection of Multidrug Resistance

The MDR phenotype is associated with the overexpression of P-glycoprotein, an integral membrane-bound energy-dependent efflux pump. This channel-forming molecule is capable of removing structurally and functionally unrelated cytostatic drugs, the so-called MDR drugs such as anthracyclins, epidophyllotoxins, alkylating agents, and vinca alkaloids, from inside the tumor cells to the extracellular environment. This decreases the intracellular concentration, resulting in a noneffectiveness of the chemotherapeutic agents. P-glycoprotein was found to be the product of the mdr1 gene (Gros et al. 1986) located on chromosome 7q21.1 (Callen et al. 1987). Sequence analyses of the mdr1 gene support the concept that P-glycoprotein belongs to the ATP-binding casette (ABC) superfamily of transport proteins (Juranka et al. 1989).

A major problem with the clinical value of P-glycoprotein detection is the difficulty of introducing standardized and reproducible assays. A P-glycoprotein assay should be equally applicable to small biopsies, e.g., needle biopsy, and to organ specimens obtained by surgery; it should allow quantitation or at least semiquantitation; and it should work on routinely processed formalin-fixed paraffin-embedded material. Although there are several limitations, the method of choice is immunocytochemistry (IC). To standardize IC (and other approaches) an MDR-Detection Workshop was held in Memphis in 1994 (Beck et al. 1995). Agreement was obtained on the following points:

1. Prior to the application of IC, the systems must be "calibrated" using P-glycoprotein-positive cell lines with different factors of resistance. For solid tumors the KB series and for hematological malignancies the myeloma cell line 8226 (Dalton et al. 1989) was chosen. A positive detection must be possible in the low level P-glycoprotein 8226DOX6 cell line and the KB V-I cell line as control for IC sensitivity of the laboratory. The cell lines were prepared to simulate solid tumors by producing cell pellets or "collodion bags" (Table 1).

   Another possibility for proper control of P-glycoprotein IC staining is to initiate P-glycoprotein-positive tumors in nude mice, e.g., a F4-6ADR solid tumor mouse model (Dietel et al. 1995), to process this tissue routinely and to prepare several paraffin blocks which can deliver series of sections, all covered with identical P-glycoprotein-positive tumor tissue.
2. All clinical specimens should be investigated with at least two antibodies, e.g., C-219, JSB-1, HYB-241, HYB-612, or UIC-2. Preferably, P-glycopro-

Table 1. Semiquantitative IC for the MDR-associated P-glycoprotein, performed at Institute of Pathology, Charité, Berlin

- Reference and control: 8226DOX6 cells,[a] KB V-I cells or F4–6RADR nude mice tumor
- Prepared as "tissue pellet" or "collodion bag"
- Routine fixation and processing of control cell pellet as well as tumor probe
- Covering on one slide
- Routine IH staining procedure
- Quantitative color image analysis of 100 tumor cells (optional)
- Comparison of control cells and tumor cells to be evaluated

[a] Sixfold resistance for doxorubicin

tein IC should be performed on serial sections, and both antibodies should produce a clear signal in the same cells.
3. Immunostaining should clearly be limited to the tumor cells, leaving the stroma cells almost completely unstained.
4. IC allows only semiquantification on a cellular basis, determining the percentage of positive cells and the intensity of staining. This can be supported by a quantitative color image analysis system. The approach is comparable to the IC detection of estrogen receptors in histological sections. However, for P-glycoprotein it is often difficult to evaluate intensity, so agreement was reached that at least 10% of the tumor cells should be stained to define a tumor as P-glycoprotein positive.

When all four prerequisites are fulfilled and there is a clear signal the tumor can be regarded as multidrug resistant. At present, the information can be delivered to the clinician only with the limitation that this is still an experimental approach.

Details of the IC technique are described elswhere (Dietel et al. 1990, 1994). In brief, cells and tumor tissue were processed routinely for paraffin sections. Formalin fixation was not longer than 4–6h. For paraffin sections a microwave pretreatment is necessary for antigen retrieval, using a 10-min application of 600W energy. Subsequently, they were processed by covering with the anti-P-glycoprotein mouse mAbs C219 and JSB-1, applied as a purified IgG preparation in a final concentration of 10mg/ml. The first step was followed by an IgG (final concentration 1mg/ml) directed against mouse IgG and the detection system alkaline phosphatase anti-alkaline phosphatase. Controls were performed (a) by replacing the specific antibody with normal mouse serum or mouse IgG, (b) by replacing the anti-mouse IgG with normal serum or phosphate-buffered saline, or (c) by omitting separately each step of detection.

A difficulty of P-gp IC remains, in that there is no mAb for the easy detection of P-glycoprotein on paraffin sections. In our experience C-219 is the most consistently staining mAb, followed by JSB-1. However, for whatever reason, variations in staining intensity are often observed. The problem of P-glycoprotein mAb specificity, e.g., C-219, was addressed by several authors

(Georges et al. 1990; Schinkel et al. 1991) and is still a matter of discussion. All these notions underline the necessity of proper controls.

If fresh material is available, quantitative reverse transcriptase-polymerase chain reaction (RT-PCR) is recommended as an additional detection system. In our lab (Dietel et al. 1994) RT-PCR for P-glycoprotein is performed using primers designed for cDNA from human mdr1-RNA (Hoof et al. 1991). The primers were provided by Dr. Kullmann (University of Hamburg). In an excellent study comparing different methods of P-glycoprotein analysis (Herzog et al. 1992), RT-PCR was described as the most sensitive and as the best approach for quantification. This may have special implications for clinical specimens, since they often contain only low levels of mdr1 mRNA. Other techniques for detecting P-glycoprotein on the protein (Western blot) or RNA levels (Northern blot) have been used in several studies; however, they have not found general acceptance in diagnostic work.

Multidrug Resistance in Cancer of the Small Bowel, Large Bowel, and Bile Tract

The MDR-associated P-glycoprotein can be found in many adenocarcinomas of the intestinal tract and the bile tract even when there has been no previous chemotherapy. The possible explanation for this observation may be the clearly detectable expression of P-glycoprotein in most normal epithelia of the intestinal mucosa, suggesting a role in the vectorial transport across GI biomembranes. By applying P-glycoprotein-specific IC, we and others (Thiebaut et al. 1987; Cordon-Cardo et al. 1990) demonstrated P-glycoprotein positivity in unaltered epithelia. As exemplified for intrahepatic canaliculi (Fig. 1), P-glycoprotein expression is sharply limited to the apical border of the lining hepatocytes. There is almost no immunostaining in the lateral or basal portion of the cell membrane or in the cytoplasm. A similar distribution pattern is given in normal colon cells. This polarized localization should be considered as an internal control for P-glycoprotein IC and a differing staining pattern should be met with caution. In addition, it must be kept in mind that P-glycoprotein expression shows considerable individual variability in the gastrointestinal tract (Bellamy and Weinstein 1994), which might have an influence on the interpretation of the IC results.

In our own series of 60 immunocytochemically investigated colon cancers and bile tract cancers, P-glycoprotein was found in more than 70% of the cases (Fig. 2). In this study we followed the instructions proposed by the St. Jude MDR-Detection Workshop 1994 (Beck et al. 1996). In a series of eight colon cancer specimens reported by Yamauchi et al. (1992) seven were found to express P-glycoprotein, detected by C-219 immunohistochemistry. Fojo et al. (1987) found high levels of mdr1 mRNA in the majority of colon cancer specimens. In general, the results correlate with the biological behavior of the tumors, since in the clinic it is a well-known fact that in the majority of cases

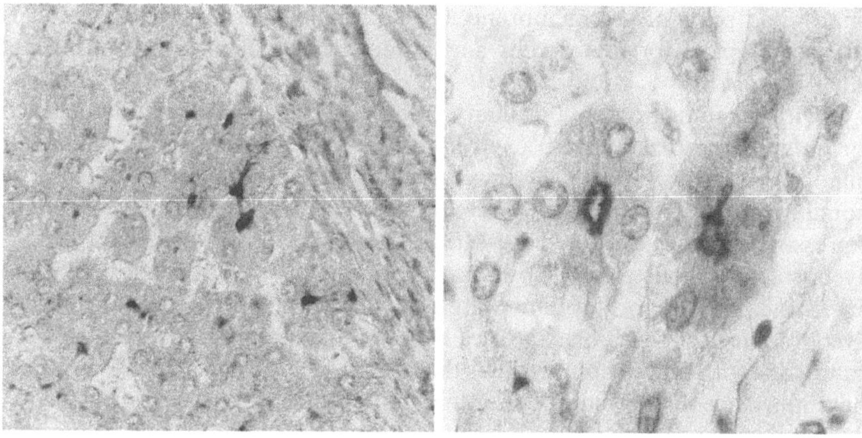

Fig. 1. Immunocytochemistry for P-glycoprotein in normal intrahepatic bile ducts (canaliculi). Clear immunostaining of the apical border of hepatocytes indicating involvement of P-glycoprotein in transmembrane release of bile or other hepatocyte-born substances. MoAb C-219; *left*: ×200, *right*: ×1000

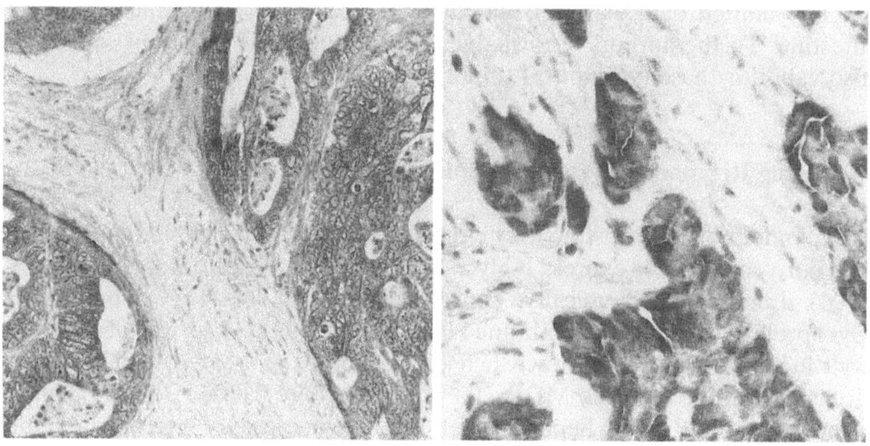

Fig. 2. Invasively growing colon cancer with intensive expression of P-glycoprotein. Loss of polar differentiation with immunostaining of the complete cell surface and even of the cytoplasm. *Left*: well-differentiated part of the tumor; *right*: low-differentiated part. MoAb C-219, *left*: ×200, *right*: ×630

MDR drugs are more or less ineffective in the treatment of GI cancer. In a number of selected cases, clinical follow-up showed resistance to doxorubicin when P-glycoprotein was expressed and sensitivity when P-glycoprotein was not found (Yamauchi 1992).

In the majority of tumors the proportion of positive cells does not exceed 30% and most often is about 15%. Within a given tumor there always is some heteogeneity in local distribution, with groups or "clones" of positive cells among larger areas of nonstained cells. Cytologically, P-glycoprotein is found in all parts of the membrane and additionally in the cytoplasm. This pattern is typical for tumor cells and differs from that observed in normal tissue.

In vitro examination of 20 primary colon cancer cell lines exhibited a high percentage (approximately 80%) of P-glycoprotein positivity detected by immunocytochemistry and PCR (own unpublished data). When tested in the monolayer proliferation assay (Dietel et al. 1994), almost all P-glycoprotein-expressing cell lines exhibited the MDR phenotype. If colon cell lines lack P-glycoprotein, they at least showed a slight sensitivity for doxorubicin and vincristine. In a report by Duensing and Slate (1994), the existence of P-glycoprotein-positive colon cancer cell lines with high sensitivity for doxorubicin was stated. This result underlines the need for functional assays to evaluate the importance of P-glycoprotein in mediating MDR.

Drug resistance may not be the only function of P-glycoprotein. Weinstein et al. (1991) reported an association of P-glycoprotein in colon carcinomas with local aggressiveness. In a subset of tumors a predominance at the invading front is obvious. Whether this suggests some potency of P-glycoprotein in this process or whether it is a sign of dedifferentiation is not clear.

Only limited data exist for malignant tumors of the bile tract and small intestine. To the author's knowledge the data outlined for colon cancer are also valid for these types of GI tumors.

Multidrug Resistance in Hepatocellular Carcinoma

Independent of a preexisting liver cirrhosis, hepatocellular carcinomas (HCC) and derived cell lines express P-glycoprotein to a high percentage (Park et al. 1994). Immunocytochemically, approximately 65% of HCC expressed P-glycoprotein on the cell membrane (Itsubo et al. 1994). This was observed as well in tumors and cell lines which had never been treated with cytostatic drugs, indicating intrinsic MDR (Fardel et al. 1994). Other reports demonstrate that not all MDR hepatoma cell lines must express P-glycoprotein, but that there are other mechanisms mediating drug resistance (Oudard et al. 1991; Shen et al. 1991).

Multidrug Resistance in Gastric Cancer

In our experience, in nontumoral and nondysplastic gastric mucosa P-glycoprotein can hardly be detected by IC. This has also been reported by Pastan and Gottesman (1987) and Vollrath et al. (1991). Other studies, however, found P-glycoprotein in the normal gastric epithelia (Robey-Cafferty et al. 1990), a discrepancy that needs to be clarified. In precursor lesions with increased risk of developing gastric cancer, such as colonic metaplasia or dysplasia, P-glycoprotein positivity was described (Vollrath et al. 1991).

Whether this observation can be interpreted as one step towards malignancy is an interesting question, not yet solved.

Similar to colon cancer, in gastric carcinoma specimens and cell lines a positivity of between 40% and 90% was described (Park et al. 1990; Vollrath et al. 1991; Wallner et al. 1993) when dot-blot techniques or immunocytochemistry were applied. The unfavorable prognosis of gastric cancer in response to chemotherapy, e.g., using doxorubicin, can be interpreted as a clinical equivalent to this observation.

Additional Drug Resistance Mechanisms Observed in Gastrointestinal Cancer

In a P-glycoprotein-negative gastric carcinoma cell line a further mechanism of resistance was disclosed, first by a morphological approach (Dietel et al. 1990). In an ongoing series of functional experiments using electron microscopy, confocal laser microscopy, cell culture assays, and drug transport assays, intracellular drug compartmentalization in vesicular structures was observed. The resistant tumor cells were found to be able to create membrane vesicles which are born in close vicinity to the nucleus. After drug loading they move from the perinuclear region to the peripheral plasma membrane, and there they release the content to the extracellular space via exocytosis. This active transport is performed with the help of the cytoskeleton protein tubulin and the motor protein kinesin, which are both involved in the vectorial transport of the drug-filled vesicles (Seidel et al. 1995). Transport studies using the oil filtration method (Reymann et al. 1989) disclosed that the vesicle-associated transport contributes considerably to reducing intracellular drug concentration in the resistant P-glycoprotein-negative cell line. This oberservation was repeated in cancer lines derived from colon, pancrease, bile duct, ovary, and breast (Seidel et al. 1992; our own unpublished results), as well as in several others (Wilingham 1986; Mujai'c 1991; Schuurhuis 1993; Gervasoni et al. 1991).

The role of overexpressed glutathione-S-tranferase (GST) and its isozymes alpha, mu, and pi in GI tumors is still under debate. Analyses of colon cancer cell lines with intrinsic MDR revealed elevated GST-pi levels, indicating an active role in the resistance mechanism (Chao 1992). In contrast, there are many cell lines, e.g., the human gastric carcinoma cell line EPG85-257NOV and the mouse erythroleukemia cell line F4-6RADR (Dietel et al. 1990, 1994), which are drug resistant and do not show alterations in the GST content. Thus, several authors suggest (Boiocchi et al. 1992) that GST may be only a cofactor in the process of anthracycline resistance. The same assumption appears to be true for topoisomerase. Altered topoisomerase II has been proposed to be a major factor in drug resistance (Beck 1993), but this is certainly not a general mechanism similar to P-glycoprotein overexpression.

Overcoming MDR

The possibility of reversing MDR exists at the protein or the mRNA level, i.e., with (a) agents which interfere with the pumping potency of P-glycoprotein, (b) drug-labeled or nonlabeled mAbs, (c) liposome-encapsulated drugs, or (d) antisense ribozymes to eliminate mdr1 mRNA.

Several membrane-active agents are known to modulate MDR by enhancing cytoplasmic concentration of the anticancer compounds. The reversing drugs are biochemically completely different from each other and include drug analogues (N-acetyl daunomycin), calcium channel blockers (e.g., verapamil, quinidine, diltiazem), calcium antagonists (e.g., azidopine), calmodulin modulators (e.g., trifluoperazine), tubulin inhibitors (e.g., cytochalasin A and B, nacodazole), lysosomotropic agents (chloroquine), tamoxifen, and cyclosporins A/H (for review see Endicott and Ling 1989). The common features are lipid solubility at physiological pH, binding to hydrophobic domains of P-glycoprotein, cationic charge, and binding capacity for P-glycoprotein (Zamora et al. 1988). One of the most potent drugs to reverse MDR is cyclosporin A (CsA) (Twentyman et al. 1987), which has been shown to be a P-glycoprotein-binding protein. In our own experiments it was shown that at therapeutically achievable levels ($1–5 \times 10^{-6} M$) CsA considerably enhances the cytotoxic potency of adriamycin in several MDR gastric and colon cancer cell lines (for an example, see Fig. 3). Nonimmunosuppressive

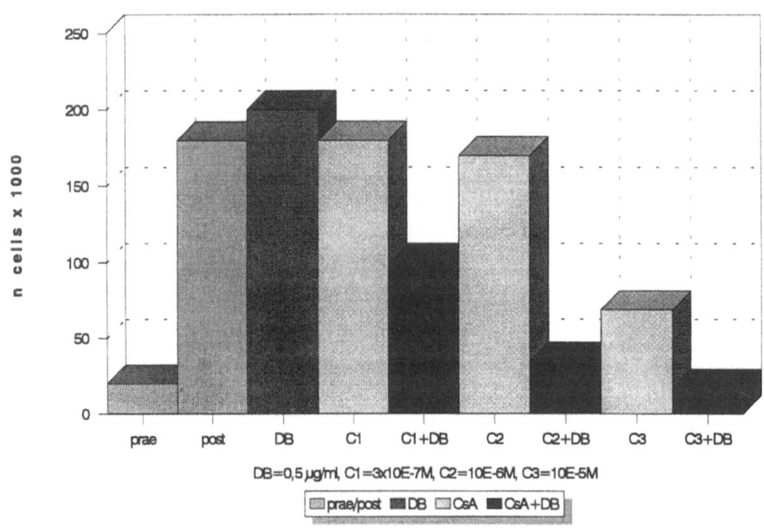

Fig. 3. P-glycoprotein-positive human pancreatic carcinoma cell line EPP85-181RDB (Holm et al. 1994) resistant to daunorubicin (*DB*). Reversal of multidrug resistance by combined application of daunorubicin and cyclosporin A (*CsA*). *prae*, Number of cells at the beginning of the experiment; *post*, number of cells at the end of the experiment; *DB*, daunorubicin; *C1*, *2*, *3*, concentration of cyclosporin A; *CsA*, cyclosporin A

analogues such as CsH and SDZ PSC833 are under investigation to determine which drug has the strongest chemosensitizing potential and the least side effects. First results are promising.

The calcium channel inhibitor dexniguldipine, a compound of low systemic toxicity, was evaluated with respect to its MDR-reversing potency. Several studies exhibited a considerable modulating activity at concentrations achievable in vivo (Reyman et al. 1993; Dietel et al. 1994). Among other tumor types, this was shown for gastrointestinal tumors.

In a nude mouse model the possibility of specific targeting using the anti-P-glycoprotein mAb MRK16 was demonstrated (Pearson et al. 1991; Iwahashi et al. 1993). The administration of MRK16 alone resulted in a limited decrease of the tumor burden, while the combination with doxorubicin led to a considerable antitumor activity and suppression of tumor growth.

To overcome P-glycoprotein activity, liposome-encapsulated doxorubicin was tested in colon cancer cells. The experiments revealed enhanced toxicity of liposome doxorubicin, diminishing the MDR phenotype (Oudard et al. 1991). Whether this might have clinical implications has to be shown.

To reverse MDR in cell cultures, a new antisense strategy was introduced by our group, (Holm et al. 1994) applying a specific hammerhead ribozyme directed against the mdr1 mRNA of a human pancreatic carcinoma cell line expressing the MDR phenotype. It was constructed to possess catalytic activity and to cleave the 880-codon sequence GUC in exon 21 of the mdr1 mRNA. We demonstrated that the ribozyme was able to cleave to the substrate mdr1 mRNA at the GUC position under physiological conditions in a cell-free system. A DNA ribozyme gene was then incorporated into a mammalian expression vector (pHβAPr-1-neo) and transfected into the MDR pancreatic carcinoma cell line EPP86-181DAU. The ribozyme decreased levels of detectable mdr1 mRNA, inhibited expression of P-glycoprotein, and reversed the resistance against daunoblastin. These results show that ribozymes are useful in reversing MDR and may well be a new class of resistance-reversing agents.

An exact understanding of the mechanisms of resistance and the action of reversibility may be helpful in designing MDR modulators, while also opening new possibilities for circumvention of drug resistance. With regard to overcoming drug compartmentalization, many compounds and other strategies have been tested in P-glycoprotein-negative MDR cells with intensive vesicle-forming activity. However, there are no convincing reports on possibilities of specifically reversing this form of resistance. Further experiments are underway.

Clinical Relevance

Many studies on the clinical relevance of P-glycoprotein detection have been published during the past 10 years. The results are controversial; some described a strong correlation between P-glycoprotein expression and chemoresistance as well as poor prognosis (Chan et al. 1991), while others reported no importance of P-glycoprotein for the prediction of chemotherapy, the likelihood of response to chemotherapy, or the possibility of predicting prognosis (Niehans et al. 1992). "Why haven't we cured multidrug-resistant tumors?" is the title of an excellent overview written by Murren and Hait (1992). The authors discussed many factors and arguments which might explain the unsatisfactory situation concerning the possibility of reversing drug resistance in patients.

A major point of explanation is the fact that cancer cells use a variety of unrelated mechanisms to achieve chemoresistance and to circumvent toxic effects of cytostatic drugs. Characterization of a single parameter, such as P-glycoprotein content or vesicular compartmentalization, appears not to be sufficient to adequately determine drug resistance in order to provide a rational basis for the selection of certain drugs for a "specific" treatment of a given tumor. Tumor heterogeneity is an additional factor complicating the MDR story.

Conclusions

The MDR phenotype is often expressed by malignant tumors of the stomach, bile ducts, pancreas, liver, and colon; it appears to play an important role in primary and presumably also in acquired chemoresistance. However, in P-glycoprotein-positive and -negative GI tumor cells intracellular compartmentalization of the drug with subsequent release to the microenvironment represents an additional potent mechanism of drug resistance which up to now cannot be reversed. Alterations of GST and topoisomerase II may be involved as well. Cytostatic drug analyses of cell lines for cross-resistance against a battery of cytostatic drugs suggests that even more mechanisms contribute to the overall resistance of gastrointestinal cancer. Only a detailed analysis of all different types of drug insensitivity might make it possible to fully understand this extraordinarily complex mechanism.

References

Beck WT, Danks MK, Wolverton JS, Ryungsa K, Mei C (1993) Drug resistance associated with altered DNA topoisomerase II. Adv Enzyme Regul 33:113–127

Beck WT, Grogan T, Willman C, Cordon-Cardo C, Raham D, Kuttesch J, Andreeff M, Bates S, Boyet J, Brophy N, Broxterman H, Chan H, Dalton W, Dietel M, Fojo A, Head D, Houghton P, Srivastava K, Paietta E, Pavelic Z, Rimzsa L, Roninson I, Sikic B, Twentyman P, Warnke R, Weinstein R (1996) St. Jude workshop on methods to detect P-gp-associated MDR (accepted for Cancer Res)

Bellamy W, Weinstein RS (1994) Functional diversity in the multidrug resistance gene family. Lab Invest 71:617–620

Boiocchi M, Tumiotto L, Giannini F, Viel A, Biscontin G, Sartor F, Toffoli G (1992) P-glycoprotein but not topoisomerase II and glutathione-S-transferase-pi accounts for enhanced intracellular drug resistance in LoVo MDR human cell lines. Tumori 78:159–166

Callen DF, Baker E, Simmers RN, Seshadri R, Roninson IB (1987) Localization of the human multiple drug resistance gene, MDR1, to 7q21.1. Hum Genet 77:122–126

Chan HSL, Haddad G, Thorner PS, DeBoer G, Lin YP, Ondrusek N, Yeger H, Ling V (1991) P-glycoprotein expression as a predictor of the outcome of therapy for neuroblastoma. N Engl J Med 325:1608–1614

Chao CC, Huang YT, Ma CM, Chou WY, Lin-Chao S (1992) Overexpression of glutathione S-transferase and elevation of thiol pools in a multidrug-resistant human colon cancer cell line. Mol Pharmacol 41:69–75

Cordon-Cardo C, O'Brien JP, Boccia J, Casals D, Bertino JR, Melamed MR (1990) Expression of the multidrug resistance gene product (P-glycoprotein) in human normal and tumor tissues. J Histochem Cytochem 30:1277–1287

Dalton WS, Grogan TM, Rybski JA, Scheper RJ, Richter L, Kailey J, Broxterman HJ, Pinedo HM, Salmon SE (1989) Immunohistochemical detection and quantitation of P-glycoprotein in multiple drug-resistant human myeloma cells: association with level of drug resistance and drug accumulation. Blood 73:747–752

Dietel M, Arps H, Lage H, Niendorf A (1990) Membrane vesicle formation due to acquired mitoxantrone resistance in gastric carcinoma cell line EPG85-257. Cancer Res 50:6100–6106

Dietel M, Bals U, Schaefer B, Herzig I, Arps H, Zabel M (1993) In vitro prediction of cytostatic drug resistance in primary cell cultures of solid malignant tumours. Eur J Cancer 29A:416–420

Dietel M, Herzig I, Brandt I, Schaefer B, Bunge A, Reymann A, Heidebrecht H-J, Seidel A (1994) Secondary combined resistance to the multidrug reversing activity of cyclosporin A in the cell line F4-6ADR-CsA. J Cancer Res Clin Oncol 120:263–271

Dietel M, Boss H, Reymann A, Pest S, Seidel A (1995) In vivo reversibility of multidrug resistance by the MDR modulator dexniguldipine (niguldipine derivative B859-35) and by verapamil. J Exp Ther Oncol

Duensing TD, Slate DL (1994) Intracellular expression of P-glycoprotein in a human colon tumor cell line. Anticancer Res 14:13–9

Endicott JA, Ling V (1989) The biochemistry of P-glycoprotein-mediated multidrug resistance. Annu Rev Biochem 58:137–171

Fardel O, Loyer P, Lecureur V, Glaise D, Guillouzo A (1994) Constitutive expression of functional P-glycoprotein in rat hepatoma cells. Eur J Biochem 219:512–518

Fojo AT, Ueda K, Salmon DJ, Poplacl DG, Gottesmann MM, Pastan I (1987) Expression of a multidrug-resistance gene in human tumors and tissues. Proc Natl Acad Sci U S A 84:265–269

Foxwell BMJ, Mackie A, Ling V, Ryffel B (1989) Identification of the multidrug resistance-related P-glycoprotein as a cyclosporine-binding protein. Mol Pharmacol 36:543–546

Georges E, Bradley G, Gariepy J, Ling V (1990) Detection of P-glycoprotein isoforms by gene-specific monoclonal antibodies. Proc Natl Acad Sci U S A 87:152–156

Gervasoni jr. JE, Fields SZ, Krishna S, Baker MA, Rosado MA, Thuraisamy K, Hindenburg AA, Taub RN (1991) Subcelluar distribution of daunorubicin in P-glycoprotein positive and negative drug-resistant cell lines using laser-assisted confocal microscopy. Cancer Res 51:4955–4963

Gros P, Ben NY, Housman DE (1986) Isolation and expression of a complementary DNA that confers multidrug resistance. Nature 323:728–731

Herzog CE, Trepel JB, Mickley LA, Fojo AT (1992) Various methods of analyses of mdr1/P-glycoprotein in human colon cancer cell lines. J Natl Cancer Inst 84:711–716

Holm PS, Dietel M, Scanlon K (1994) Reversion of multidrug resistance in the P-glycoprotein-positive human pancreatic cell line (EPP85-181RDB) by introduction of a hammerhead ribozyme. Br J Cancer 70:239–243

Hoof T, Riordan JR, Timmler B (1991) Quantitation of mRNA by the kinetic polymerase chain reaction assay – a tool for monitoring P-glycoprotein gene expression. Analyt Biochem 196:162–169

Itsubo M, Ishikawa T, Toda G, Tanaka M (1994) Immunohistochemical study of expression and cellular localization of the multidrug resistance gene product P-glycoprotein in primary liver carcinoma. Cancer 73:298–303

Iwahashi T, Okochi E, Ariyoshi K, Watabe H, Amann E, Mori S, Tsuruo T, Ono K (1993) Specific targeting and killing activities of anti-P-glycoprotein monoclonal antibody MRK16 directed against intrinsically multidrug-resistant human colorectal carcinoma cell lines in the nude mouse model. Cancer Res 53:5475–5482

Juranka PF, Zastawny RL, Ling V (1989) P-glycoprotein: Multidrug-resistance and a superfamily of membrane-associated transport proteins. FASEB J 3:2583–2592

Mac Donald J, Gurderson L, Cohn I (1982) Cancer of stomach. In: De Vita VT, Hellman JS, Rosemberg ST (eds) Cancer of stomach. Lippincott, Philadelphia, pp 534–558

Mujai'c H, Mujai'c Z (1991) Detection of pleiotropic drug resistance by the rapid immunofluorescence assay of drug effects on the cytoskeleton. Oncology 48:202–209

Murren JR, Hait WN (1992) Why haven't we cured multidrug-resistant tumors? Oncol Res 4:1–6

Niehans G, Jaszcz W, Brunetto V, Perri R, Gajl-Peczalska K, Wick M, Tsuruo T, Bloomfield C (1992) Immunohistochemical identification of P-glycoprotein in previously untreated, diffuse large cell and immunoblastic lymphomas. Cancer Res 52:3768–3775

Oudard S, Thierry A, Jorgensen TJ, Rahman A (1991) Sensitization of multidrug-resistant colon cancer cells to doxorubicin encapsulated in liposomes. Cancer Chemother Pharmacol 28:259–265

Park J, Kramer B, Lai S, Goldstein L, Gazdar A (1990) Chemosensitivity patterns and expression of human multidrug resistance-associated MDR1 gene by human gastric and colorectal carcinoma cell lines. J Natl Cancer Inst 82:193–198

Park JG, Lee SK, Hong IG, Kim HS, Lim KH, Choe KJ, Kim WH, Kim YI, Tsuruo T, Gottesman MM (1994) MDR1 gene expression: its effect on drug resistance to doxorubicin in human hepatocellular carcinoma cell lines. J Natl Cancer Inst 86:700–705

Pastan I, Gottesman M (1987) Multiple-drug resistance in human cancer. N Engl J Med 316:1388–1393

Pearson JW, Fogler WE, Volker K, Usui N, Goldenberg SK, Gruys E, Riggs CW, Komschlies K, Wiltrout RH, Tsuruo T et al (1991) Reversal of drug resistance in a human colon cancer xenograft expressing MDR1 complementary DNA by in vivo administration of MRK-16 monoclonal antibody. J Natl Cancer Inst 83:1386–1391

Reyman A, Looft G, Woermann C, Dietel M, Erttmann R (1993) Reversal of multidrug resistance in Friend leukemia cells by dexniguldipine-HCl. Cancer Chemother Pharmacol 32:25–30

Robey-Cafferty SS, Rutledge ML, Bruner JM (1990) Expression of a multidrug resistant gene in esophageal adenocarcinoma. Correlation with response to chemotherapy and comparison with gastric adenocarcinoma. Am J Clin Pathol 93:1–7

Shen DW, Lu YG, Chin KV, Pastan I, Gottesman MM (1991) Human hepatocellular carcinoma cell lines exhibit multidrug resistance unrelated to MRD1 gene expression. J Cell Sci 98:317–322

Schinkel AH, Roelofs EM, Borst P (1991) Characterization of the human MDR3 P-glycoprotein and its recognition by P-glycoprotein-specific monoclonal antibodies. Cancer Res 51:2628–2635

Schuurhuis GJ, van Heiningen THM, Cervantes A, Pinedo HM, de Lange JHM, Keizer HG, Broxtermann HJ, Baak JPA, Lankelma J (1993) Changes in subcellular doxorubicin distribution and cellular accumulation alone can largely account for doxorubicin resistance in SW-1573 lung cancer multidrug-resistant tumor cells. Br J Cancer 68:898–908

Seidel A, Nickelsen M, Dietel M (1992) Mechanisms of resistance in a human gastric carcinoma cell line resistant against daunoblastin. In: Klapdor R (ed) Tumor-associated antigens, oncogenes, receptors, cytokines – tumor diagnosis and therapy in the beginning of the 90th. Zuckschwert, München pp 554–558

Seidel A, Hasmann M, Löser R, Bunge A, Schaefer B, Herzig I, Steidtmann K, Dietel M (1995) Intracellular localization, vesiclular accumulation and kinetics of daunorubicin in sensitive and multidrug-resistant gastric carcinoma EPG85-257 cells. Virchows Arch

Thiebaut F, Tsuruo T, Hamada H, Gottesman MM, Pastan I, Willingham MC (1987) Cellular localization of the multidrug-resistance gene product P-glycoprotein in normal human tissues. Proc Natl Acad Sci U S A 84:7735–7738

Twentyman PR, Fox NE, White DJG (1987) Cyclosporin A and its analogues as modifiers of adriamycin and vincristin resistance in a multidrug resistant human lung cancer cell line. Br J Cancer 56:55–57

Vollrath V, Chiaanale J, Gonzalez S, Duarte I, Andrade L, Ibanez L (1991) Multidrug resistance gene and P-glycoprotein in gastric adenocarcinoma and precursor lesions. Virchows Archiv [B] 60:133–138

Wallner J, Depisch D, Gsur A, Gotzl M, Haider K, Pirker R (1993) MDR1 gene expression and its clinical relevance in primary gastric carcinomas. Cancer 71:667–671

Weinstein RS, Jakate SM, Dominguez JM, Lebovitz MD, Koukoulis GK, Kuszak JR, Klusens LF, Grogan TM, Saclarides TJ, Roninson IB et al (1991) Relationship of the expression of the multidrug resistance gene product (P-glycoprotein) in human colon carcinoma to local tumor aggressiveness and lymph node metastasis. Cancer Res 51:2720–2726

Wilingham MC, Cornwell MM, Cardarelli CO, Gottesman MM, Pastan I (1986) Single cell analysis of daunomycin uptake and efflux in multidrug-resistant and sensitive KB cells: effects of verapamil and other drugs. Cancer Res 46:5941–5946

Yamauchi M, Kumazawa H, Satta T, Sugawara I, Isobe K, Kodera Y, Ito K, Watanabe T, Takagi H (1992) Prediction of doxorubicin resistance in gastrointestinal cancer by P-glycoprotein staining. Eur J Cancer 28A:1422–1427

Zamora JM, Pearce HL, Beck WT (1988) Physical-chemical properties shared by compounds that modulate multidrug resistance in human leukemic cells. Mol Pharmacol 33:454–462

Radiological Modalities in the Staging of Colorectal Tumors: New Perspectives for Increasing Accuracy

T.J. Vogl[1], W. Pegios[1], M.G. Mack[1], M. Rausch[1], H. Hintze[2], M. Hünerbein[3], R. Hammerstingl[1], H. Lobbeck[4], and R. Felix[1]

[1] Department of Radiology, [2] Department of Internal Medicine, [3] Department of Surgery, [4] Department of Pathology, University of Berlin, Rudolf Virchow Clinic, Augustenburger Platz 21, 13353 Berlin, Germany

Abstract

The purpose of this study was to evaluate the diagnostic accuracy of contrast-enhanced endorectal MRI for the staging of rectal adenoma versus rectal carcinoma in correlation to findings from biopsy and histopathology.

Ten volunteers and 20 patients underwent body-coil and endorectal MRI (1.5 T supraconducting unit) using plain, T1-weighted (w) T2-w SE and TSE-w sequences, a dynamic Gd-DTPA enhanced protocol (turboFLASH), and postcontrast T1-w-SE sequences. Histopathological correlation via biopsy ($n = 10$) and surgical resection ($n = 19$) were conducted for all patients. An independent, two-observer, reader evaluation was performed and qualitative and quantitative data calculated.

In volunteers and all patients endorectal MRI reliably delineatel normal wall layers. Rectal adenomas ($n = 7$) were identified by a visualization of an intact muscularis mucosae, a homogeneous inner structure, and a significant contrast enhancement. T1 carcinomas ($n = 4$) were best identified in dynamic turboFLASH sequences by delineation of an intact muscularis propria. The visualization of contrast-enhancing tumor tissue was indicative of a T2 carcinoma ($n = 4$). All T3 ($n = 3$) and T4 ($n = 2$) carcinomas were correctly staged on dynamic and static MRI. The endorectal MRI stage agreed with the staging results from pathological study in 16 of 20 (80%) patients.

Endorectal surface coil MRI provides reliable data for the preoperative staging and evaluation of rectal lesions.

Introduction

According to estimates produced by the American Cancer Society, over 45 000 new cases of rectal carcinoma were expected to be diagnosed in the United

Recent Results in Cancer Research, Vol. 142

States in 1991: 7500 deaths were caused by rectal carcinoma (Boring et al. 1991) Dietary factors, family history, a variety of polyposis sndromes, and long-standing inflammatory bowel disease are risk factors for the development of colorectal carcinoma.

Because specific treatment options will vary with tumor location, the preoperative evaluation of rectal carcinoma is important for therapy planning and the assessment of the prognosis. So far, there are several limitations to determining the infiltration of the wall layers in rectal tumors (adenoma and carcinoma) in width and depth by the usually applied endoscopic and X-ray procedures (barium enema examination, computed tomography), endosconography, and conventional MR imaging.

During the past few years, the indication for barium enema examinations decreased by 20%–30% due to the improvement of other imaging modalities.

Endoscopy is helpful only for the evaluation of macroscopic aspects, localization of the lesion, and morphology, including tactile and visual criteria. The advantages of endoscopy are the possibility of biopsy and the decision about the final treatment modality.

Staging with computed tomography (CT) is accurate in the range of 48%–74% (Moss 1989). Early studies using magnetic resonance imaging (MRI) showed no increased accuracy over CT (Butch et al. 1986). In particular, initial studies demonstrated that the depiction of tumor infiltration was difficult and unreliable on MR images.

Transrectal ultrasound is now an established imaging modality for evaluation of the integrity of the wall layers in the surrounding of colorectal lesions (Rifkin and Marks 1985). Overstaging seems the most frequent error, both in staging of rectal cancer (Tio et al. 1991) and screening of adenomas for infiltrating malignancy (Hulsmans et al. 1992).

MR imaging is helpful for tumor staging and the detection of tumor recurrence, particularly in clarifying questions remaining after endoscopic diagnosis. It is necessary to minimize the movement of the patient in order to improve image quality. Rapid scanning techniques, endoluminal surface coils, and paramagnetic contrast agents in particular are expanding the applications of MRI in the evaluation of rectal and perirectal disease.

We report on our experience using high-resolution endorectal surface-coil MR imaging to evaluate rectal carcinomas and rectal adenomas in a variety of clinical applications. In a propsective study we compared the results of high-resolution MR imaging versus transrectal ultrasound and histopathology.

Material and Methods

During a period of 10 months we performed MR imaging of the rectum with an endorectal surface coil as well as a body coil in ten healthy volunteers (five men and five women) and 20 patients (seven men and 13 women, ages ranging from 36 to 80 years). The ten healthy volunteers were evaluated to study the normal anatomy of the rectum with its different layers and the adjacent tissues. All patients underwent an extensive clinical examination protocol and a barium enema study before MRI. Histopathology was obtained via biopsy ($n = 13$) and operative resection ($n = 7$).

Four patients with rectal carcinoma stages pT4 and pT3 were included in this study in the course of a hyperthermic treatment protocol. In two of these patients (pT4) the indication for the examination was a suspected infiltration of the prostate. Two different types of endorectal surface coils (Medrad, Pittsburgh, PA, USA) were used. In 15 patients a prostate endorectal surface coil and in five patients a colon endorectal surface coil were applied.

MR imaging was performed with a 1.5-T unit (Magnetom SP 63, Siemens, Erlangen). At the beginning of the examination T2-weighted images (TR/TE = 2500/22–90, field of view 350 mm, imaging matrix 160 × 512, slice thickness 4 mm, no gap, acquisition time 6 min) were obtained using the body coil.

Before placement of the endorectal surface coil, a digital examination of the rectum was performed to make sure that there were no obstructions within the lumen. The distance from the rectal lesion to the anus had been determined previously at barium enema examination and endoscopy. The center of the coil was positioned over the center of the lesion. Thereafter, the coil balloon was filled with 60 cm^3 of air. In case of the colon endorectal coil no filling of the balloon was necessary.

The position of the coil was controlled with the patient in the supine position using a sagittal localizer. All endorectal surface coil images were obtained with a 180-mm field of view, 4-mm slice thickness, and an imaging matrix of 180 × 512 in order to get an optimal spatial resolution.

In all patients T2-(TR/TE = 2500/22-90) and T1-weighted (TR/TE = 700/15) precontrast images were acquired. For comparative evaluation, 11 patients received an additional turbospin-echo sequence TSE (TR/TE = 3700/90). Therafter, dynamic MRI at the slice position with the largest tumor extension using a turboFLASH sequence (TR/TE = 7/3, flip angle = 15°) during the application of 0.1 mmol/kg body wt. Gd-DTPA (Schering, Berlin) was performed, followed by static axial and sagittal T1-weighted and fat-saturated sequences. Total examination time including placement of the coil was between 60 and 90 min.

All images were evaluated separately by a panel of three radiologists who used a 4-point rating scale (1 = excellently distinguishable, 2 = well distinguishable, 3 = poorly distinguishable, 4 = not distinguishable) for evaluating the layers of the rectal wall and the perirectal tissue. The lesions were staged according to the TNM staging system (WHO) (Table 1). The radiologists read the images with knowledge of the clinical information but without knowledge of the results of other examinations (endoscopy, CT, endosonography).

The preoperatively posted staging of the lesions was compared with the results of intraoperative inspection and histology after resection or electrolaser resection in all cases (rectal carcinoma $n = 13$, rectal adenoma $n = 7$).

Table 1. TNM staging for cancer of the colon and rectum (from American Joint Committee on Cancer 1992)

Stage	Level of involvement
Tumor	
Tx	Tumor cannot be assessed
To	No evidence of tumor
Tis	Carcinoma in situ[a]
T1	Tumor invades the submucosa
T2	Tumor invades the muscularis propria
T3	Tumor invades trough the muscularis propria into the subserosa or into nonperitonealized pericolic or perirectal tissues
T4	Tumor invades other organs or structures
Nodes	
Nx	Regional lymph nodes cannot be assessed
No	No involved lymph nodes
N1	Fewer than four regional nodes positive for tumor
N2	More than four regional nodes positive for tumor
N3	Central nodes positive for tumor
Metastasis	
Mx	Presence of distant metastasis cannot be assessed
Mo	No distant metastasis
M1	Distant metastasis

[a] Cancer cells within basement membrane or lamina propria with no extension through the muscularis propria into the submucosa

In four patients with large tubulovillous adenomas, of the rectum the endorectal surface coil was used before and after endoscopic electrolaser resection for the follow-up evaluation.

Results

Normal Findings

The barium enema examination is a standard radiological modality for the evaluation of pathologies of the rectum. It gives first information on localization and size of pathological processes. However, it does not allow the identification of different wall layers.

CT does not allow the differentiation of the different rectal wall layers due to the limited spatial resolution and reduced soft-tissue contrast. Often, it is helpful to opacify the rectal lumen with contrast medium to avoid mistaking nonopacified large bowels in order to increase the diagnostic value of the CT. However, CT is inferior to transrectal US for differentiation of the normal layers of the rectal wall.

Transrectal ultrasound allows the identification of the rectal wall composed of five alternating hyper- and hypoechoic layers, including a border layer, mucosa, submucosa, muscularis propria, and, at the outermost extent, the combination of serosa, subserosa, and perirectal fat.

Endoscopy allows the inspection of the rectal mucosa, biopsy, and endoscopic polypectomy or laser photocoagulation. Nevertheless, the exact staging of the infiltration of the lesion is not possible.

Plain MRI using the body coil demonstrates a high soft-tissue contrast of adjacent structures and allows the differentiation of the mucosa as a band with high signal intensity in the T2-weighted sequence surrounded by a layer of low signal intensity related to the muscularis propria. A further differentiation of other rectal layers is uncertain (Fig. 1b).

Plain and contrast-enhanced MRI with the endorectal surface coil using T2- and T1-weighted sequences allows the identification of all layers of the circumference of the rectal wall (Fig. 2). These layers consist of an inner layer of medium signal intensity (the mucus and fluid between the coil and the rectal wall), a layer of low signal intensity (mucosa and muscularis mucosa), a middle layer of medium-high signal intensity (the submucosa), a second layer of low signal intensity (the muscularis propria), and an outer layer of high signal intensity (the perirectal fat) in the T1-weighted sequence. On T2-weighted SE images the inner layer (mucus and fluid between the coil and the rectal wall) and the middle layer (the submucosa) appear with a high signal intensity. All layers of the rectal wall were visualizable in all patients ($n = 20$).

Pathologic Findings

Rectal carcinomas are generally detected by digital evaluation and endoscopy. Because specific treatment options will vary with tumor location, and because prognosis is affected by tumor size, local extent, and presence or absence of metastases, a variety of imaging procedures are employed for tumor staging.

Obstructions or filling defects using the barium enema for the evaluation of rectal lesions are often the first pointer to pathological findings of the rectum. However, this technique does not allow the staging of a lesion or the judgement of the depth of transmural invasion (Fig. 1a).

CT images generally demonstrate carcinoma of the colon as an irregularly marginated but roughly spherical soft-tissue mass. Large tumors may show a central necrosis. Lesions of the rectum are seen as asymmetrical or circumferential thickening of the bowel wall, with deformation and narrowing of the lumen. Other findings may include extension of tumor into perirectal fat, invasion of adjacent structures, lymphadenopathy, adrenal or liver metastases, and masses in the abdominal wall, omentum, or mesentery.

Transrectal US has also been performed for local staging of rectal carcinoma. Rectal carcinomas are seen as hypoechoic masses; tumor extension is indicated as disruption of these layers. However, transrectal sonography does not provide reliable contrast between the tumor and the muscularis propria.

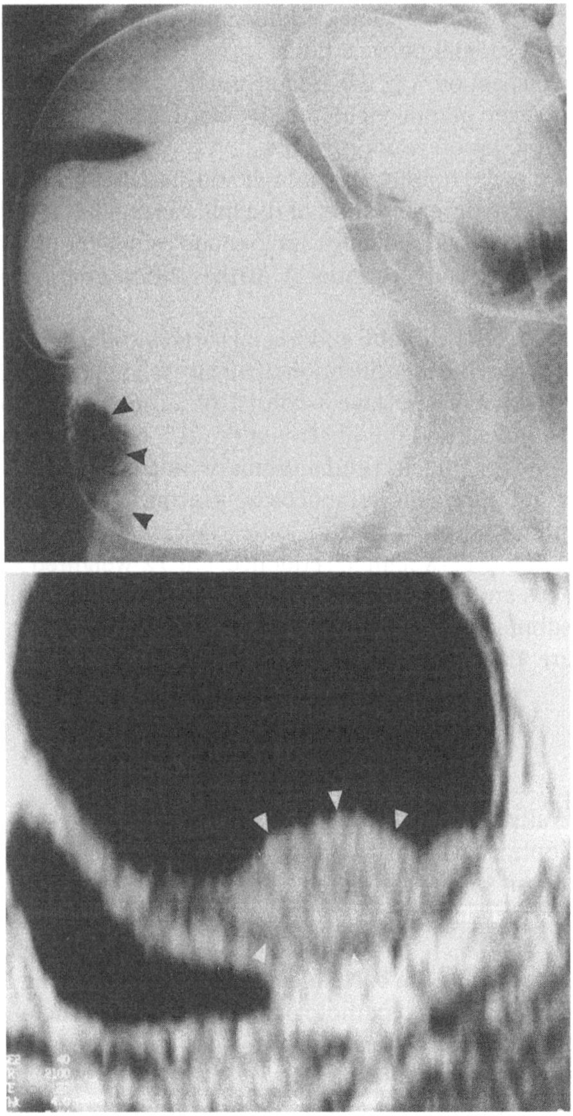

a

b

Fig. 1a,b. Adenoma. **a** Barium enema examination demonstrates a penduculated polypoid lesion approximately 8cm from the anus as a "filling defect" (*black arrowheads*) in the barium enema. **b** Axial T2-weighted SE image (TR/TE = 2100/22) with conventional MR demonstrates an in exact differentiation of a polypoid lesion of the rectum with a low-signal-intensity (*white arrowheads*)

Thus, once the submucosa is breached, it is often difficult to determine the depth of muscle invasion and to detect early perirectal fat invasion.

Using the body coil for MR imaging, rectal carcinomas are demonstrated with high signal intensity in the T2-weighted sequence and are therefore more conspicuous than in T1-weighted images. Infiltration of the bowel wall is best

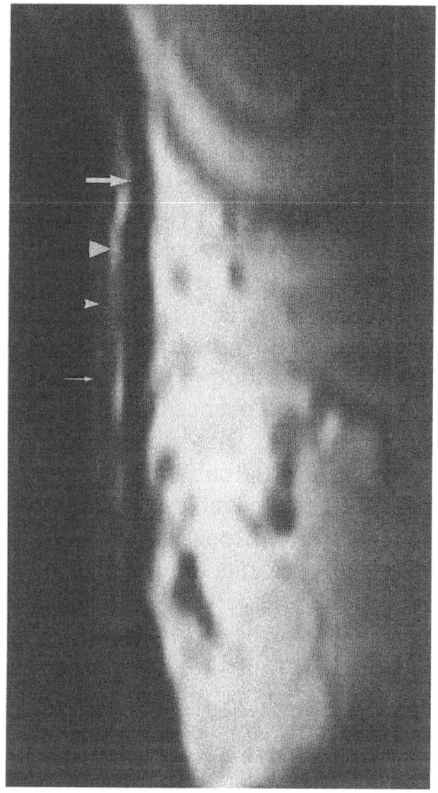

Fig. 2. Sagittal T1-weighted SE image (700/15) of the norml rectal wall. Note the multiple layers visualized: high-signal-intensity mucus within the rectal lumen (*large white arrow*), low-signal-intensity mucosal layer (mucosa and muscularis mucosa) (*small white arrowhead*), high-signal-intensity submucosal layer (*large white arrowhead*), low-signal-intensity muscularis propria (*small white arrow*), and high-signal-intensity perirectal fat (*large black arrow*)

demonstrated in T2-weighted scans, because these images optimally show normal zonal anatomy of the wall and because the contrast between high signal intensity of tumors and low signal intensity of muscle tissue will be maximized. The evaluation of perirectal fat and soft-tissue infiltration by tumor will be most conspicuous in T1-weighted images. Generally, images in transverse slice orientation are the most useful in evaluating rectal wall invasion and perirectal tumor extension.

All patients tolerated endorectal MR imaging well without complications. Endorectal MR imaging enabled correct identification of all layers of the rectal wall and differentiation between the tumor stages. The presence of mucosal thickening with preservation of the submucosal layer is indicative of a stage-T_1 lesion. The extension into, but not through, the muscularis propria with high signal intensity in the T2-weighted images in a band of low signal intensity, with the associated visualization of a partially intact muscularis propria and contrast enhancement, in the T1-weighted images appear to represent valid criteria for diagnosing a stage-T_2 lesion. The complete disruption of the muscularis propria and an unsharp border to the perirectal fat tissue are criteria for a T_3 lesion. A T_4 lesion presents with infiltration of adjacent structures (Fig. 3a,b).

The rectal lesions were different in shape and size. Lesion size ranged from 2.5 to 6.5 cm and the distance between the lesion and the external sphincter varied from 4 to 10 cm.

One patient with the MR diagnosis of a rectal carcinoma stage T_3 was histopathologically staged as a T_2. This was due to the irregularity of the border between the muscularis propria and the perirectal fat tissue in the T1-weighted sequence. However, retrospective evaluation of the dynamic turboFLASH sequence (Fig. 4a–d) and the turbospin-echo T2-weighted sequence demonstrated a clear demarcation of the muscularis propria without infiltration into the perirectal fat tissue. Criteria for the diagnosis of an adenoma are the visualization of the intact muscularis mucosa, a clear demarcation of the submuscosa, sharp borders of the lesion, and a high homogeneous contrast enhancement of the lesion in the dynamic and the T1-weighted sequences.

So far, a differentiation between the carcinoma in situ and a carcinoma stage T_1 is not possible. Two patients with the MR diagnosis of a carcinoma stage T_1 were histopathologically staged as an adenoma with severe cell dysplasia. It was generally possible to differentiate adenomas from carcinomas owing to the higher contrast enhancement and the sharper borders in the T1-weighted sequences (Fig. 5a–c).

The follow-up evaluation of four patients with large tubulovillous adenomas demonstrated the total removal of the tumor after endoscopic electrolaser resection. After therapy, MR imaging with the endorectal surface coil demonstrated the resection of the mucosa and parts of the submucosa (Fig. 6a,b). Again, a clear visualization of the different rectal layers was possible. Only T2-weighted images showed a slight increase of signal intensity and an edematous infiltration of the submucosa at the former localization of the adenoma due to the ongoing repair mechanism.

On the T1-weighted images, the rectal wall was homogeneous and had low to intermediate signal intensity. These images provided good contrast between the perirectal fat and the bowel wall and were helpful for identifying perirectal vessels and lymph nodes (Fig. 7).

In seven patients, histopathology revealed a tubulovillous adenoma; four patients presented with a rectal carcinoma stage pT_1, four patients with stage pT_2, three patients with stage pT_3, and two patients were staged as pT_4. The correlation between the pathologic stage and MR imaging stage is summarized in Table 2A,B. The MR imaging stage agreed with the staging results from pathology in 16 of 20 (80%) patients. The extent of invasion was overestimated in four cases with MR imaging (2 tubulovillous adenomas, 1 T_1 lesion and 1 T_2 lesion were overstaged).

Discussion

Accurate preoperative staging has a definite impact on the surgical management of rectal carcinoma. The standard surgical therapy for rectal cancer is

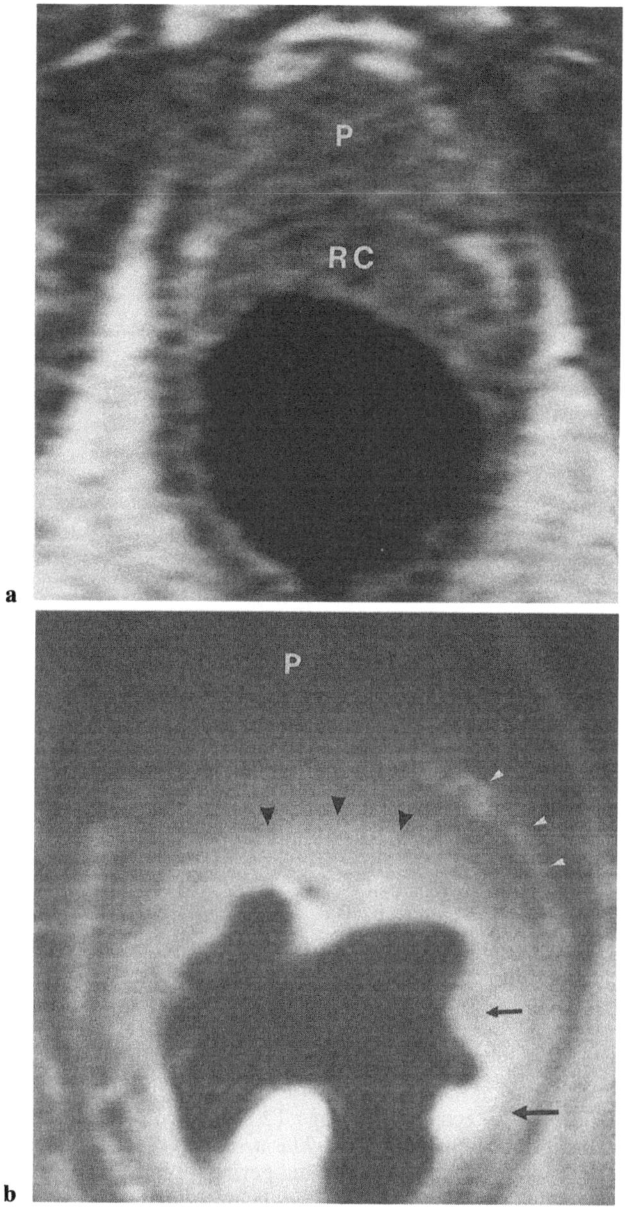

Fig. 3a,b. Rectal cancer stage T4. **a** Axial T2-weighted SE image (2500/22-90) with conventional MR imaging. *RC*, Rectal cancer; *P* prostate. **b** Axial T1-weighted SE image (700/15) with endorectal surface coil post contrast (0.1 mmol/kg body wt. Gd-DTPA) demonstrates rectal cancer with infiltration of submucosa, muscularis propria, perirectal fat, and prostate (indicating a stage-T4 lesion). Visualization of thickened mucosa (*black arrowheads*), as well as normal parts of submucosa (*short black arrow*), muscularis propria (*long black arrow*), perirectal fat (*white arrowheads*), and the prostate (*P*)

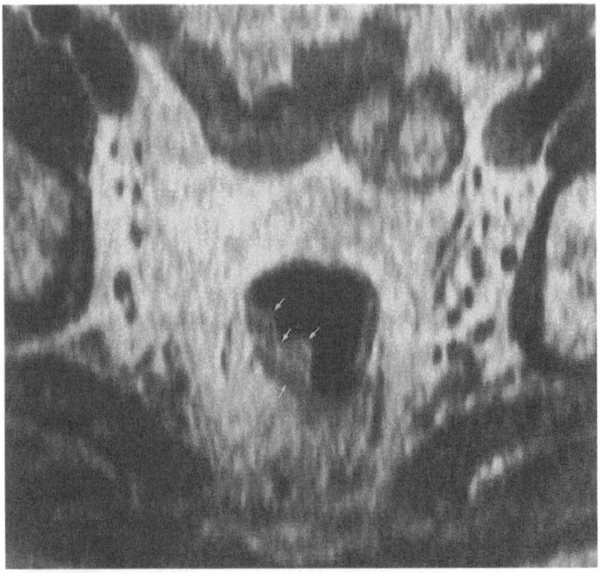

a

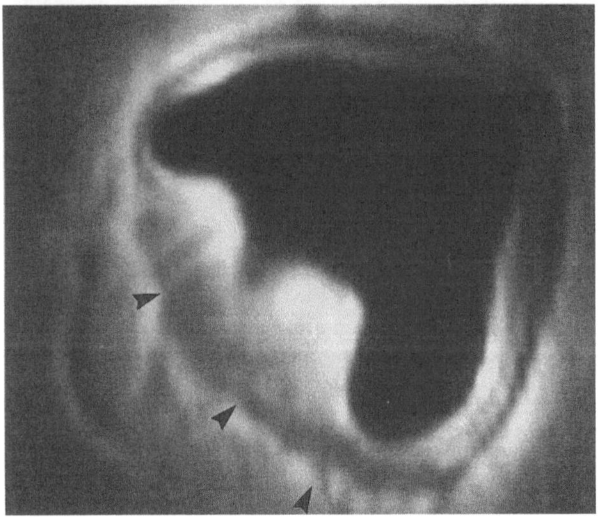

b

Fig. 4a–d. Rectal cancer stage T2. **a** Axial T2-weighted SE image (TR/TE = 2500/22) shows a polypoid lesion (*white arrows*) of the rectum with inexact differentiation between muscularis propria and perirectal fat. This limitation is a result of inadequate spatial resolution. **b** Axial T1-weighted SE image (TR/TE = 700/15) with endorectal surface coil of rectal tumor demonstrates a suspicious irregularity extending into the perirectal fat, which was mistakenly interpreted as invasion into the perirectal fat (*black arrowheads*) (stage T3). **c** Dynamic turboFLASH sequence (TR/TE = 7.5/3) obtained in the same patient as in **b** demonstrates a depressed lesion with complete disruption of the submucosa (*small white arrows*); the muscularis propria (*white arrowheads*) has not been disrupted (stage T2). **d** Histopathology results with hematoxylin-eosin demonstrate tumor invading into but not through the muscularis (*black arrowheads*)

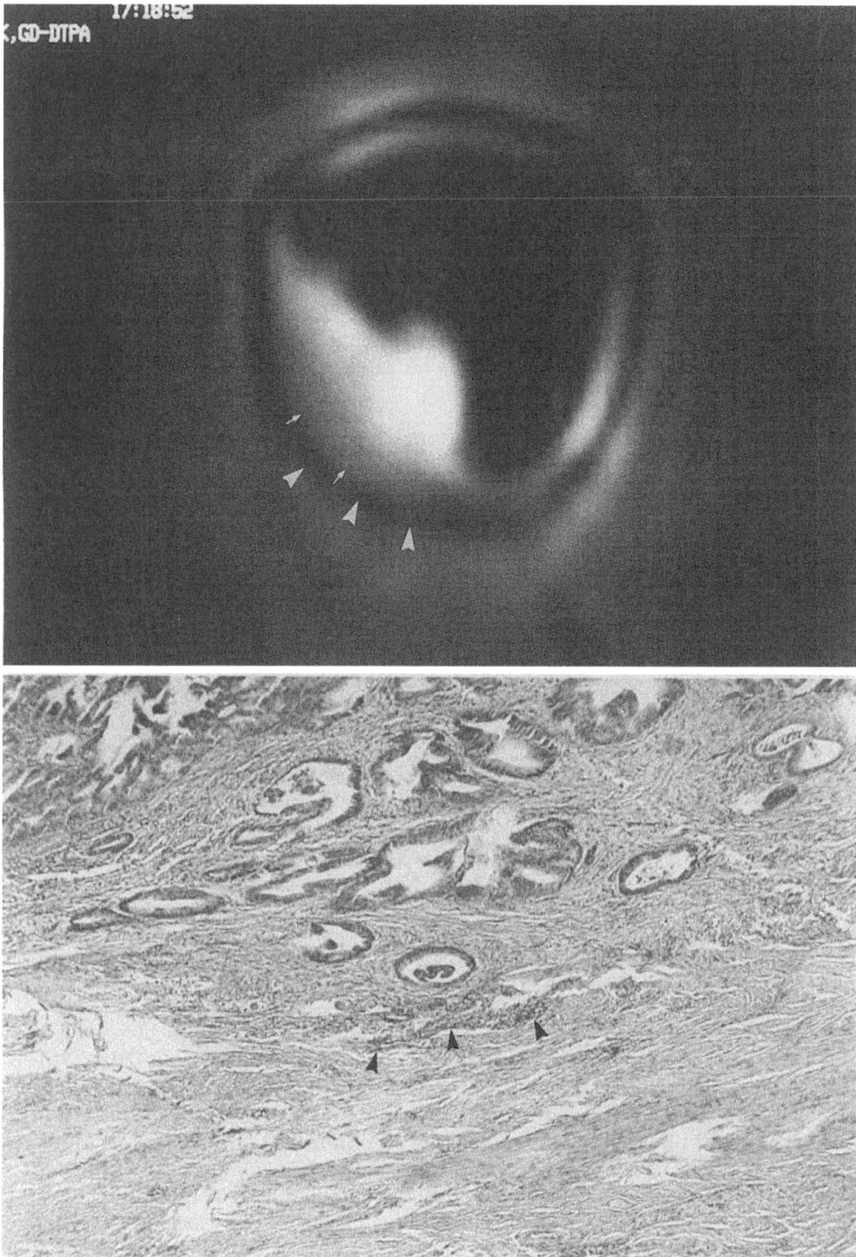

c

d

Fig. 4c,d

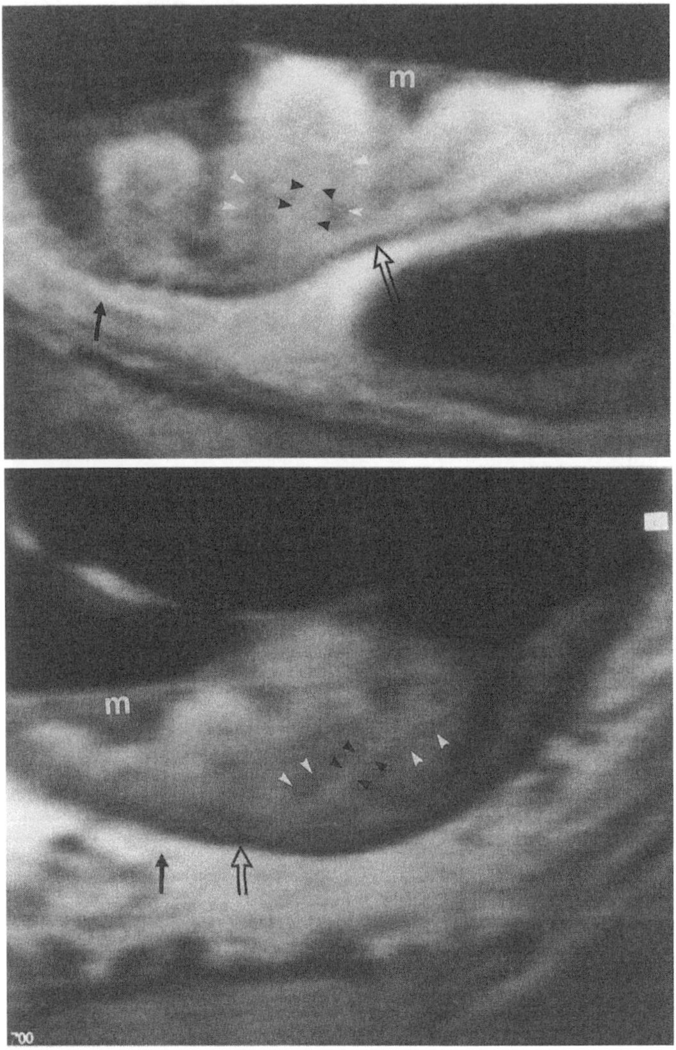

a

b

Fig. 5a–c. Tubulovillous adenoma of the rectum. **a** Axial T1-weighted SE image (700/15). **b** T1-weighted SE image (700/15) post contrast (0.1 mmol/kg body wt., Gd-DTPA) demonstrates a tubulovillous adenoma of the rectum. The different layers of the rectal wall can be identified. Fom lateral to medial, the high signal intensity of the perirectal fatty tissue (*black arrow*), followed by the low signal intensity of the muscularis propria (*open arrow*), followed by a layer of high signal intensity representing the submucosal core (*back arrowheads*) and the low signal intensity of the thickened mucosal layer (contains mucosa and muscularis mucosa; *white arrowheads*). Note the high signalintensity of the mucus within the rectal lumen (*m*). **c** Histologic section demonstrates the normal muscularis mucosa (*white arrowheads*) and the thickened mucosa with typical dysplasia grade III (*black arrowheads*). Vessels within the submucosal layer can also be identified (*black arrows*) c 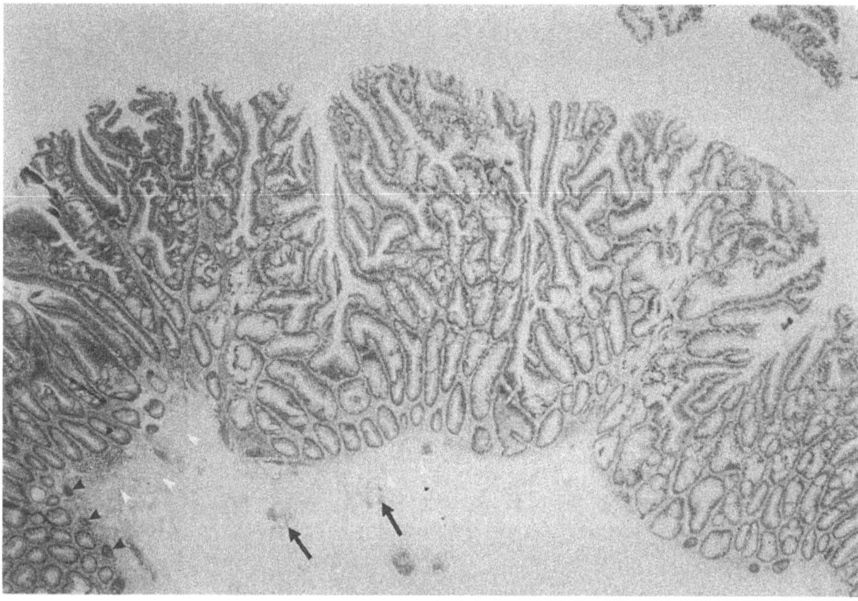

Fig. 5c

Table 2. Camparison of tumor stage at MR imaging and pathologic examination

A: MR imaging

Staging	Adenomas (*n*)	T1 (*n*)	T2 (*n*)	T3 (*n*)	T4 (*n*)
Adenomas	5	0	0	0	0
T1	2	3	0	0	0
T2	0	1	3	0	0
T3	0	0	1	3	0
T4	0	0	0	0	2

B: Pathologic examination of adenomas

n = 3	Tubulovillous (epithelial dysplasia grade II)
n = 2	Tubulovillous (epithelial dysplasia grade II–III)
n = 2	Tubulovillous (epithelial dysplasia grade III with beginning carcinoma in situ

abdominoperineal resection (Curley et al. 1989). Because of the morbidity associated with this procedure, the most notable being the social and physical problems of a permanent colostomy, a number of alternative surgical approaches have been proposed. These include anus-sparing radical resections, such as low anterior resection (Rothenberger and Wong 1985) and local

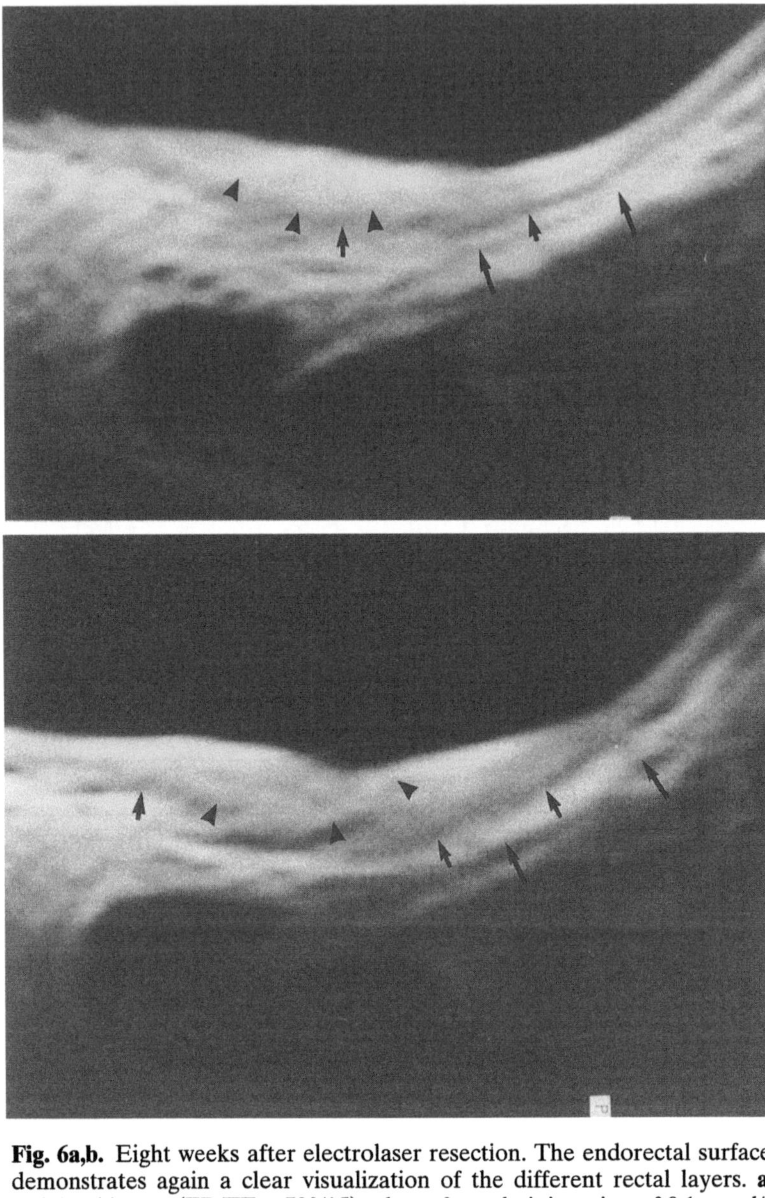

a

b

Fig. 6a,b. Eight weeks after electrolaser resection. The endorectal surface coil image demonstrates again a clear visualization of the different rectal layers. **a,b** The T1-weighted image (TR/TE = 700/15) taken after administration of 0.1 mmol/kg body wt. Gd-DTPA shows a slight increase of signal intensity and an edematous infiltration of the parts of the submucosa (*black arrowheads*). Muscularis propria (*short black arrows*), perirectal fat (*long black arrows*)

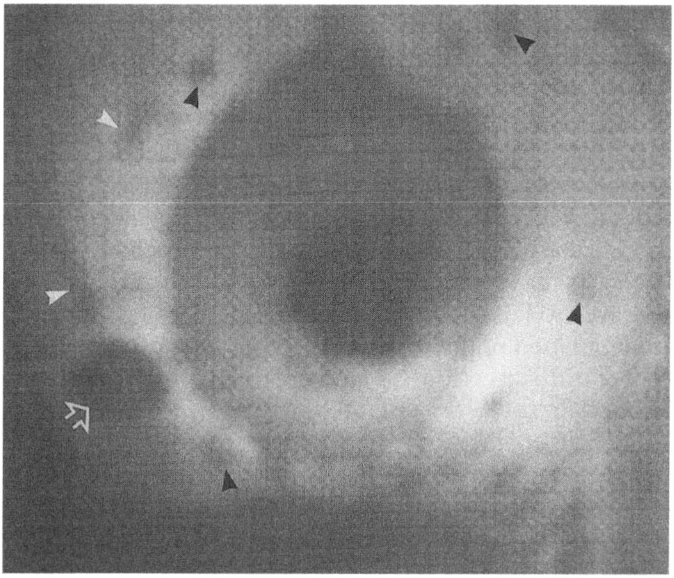

Fig. 7. Axial T1-weighted SE image (TR/TE = 700/15) of the rectum of a patient with stage-T4 rectal cancer. Four small perirectal lymph nodes, 3 and 2 mm in diameter (*black arrowheads*), are detected in the fatty tissue. In addition, one large perirectal lymph node >1 cm in diameter (*open white arrow*) is demonstrated (stage N2); *white arrowheads* indicate vessels

excision (Hager et al. 1983), and nonsurgical approaches such as low-kilovoltage endorectal irradiation, electrocautery, and transanal fulguration.

Patient selection is considered essential for obtaining a good outcome in the treatment of early rectal cancer. Carlson et al. (1985) reported that the prognosis of patients treated for cure with conservative local therapy depends on the extent of the lesion. Consequently, the exact staging of the local extent of rectal cancer is important to the sucessful enforcement of any conservative treatment regimen. The preoperative staging is important as well in selecting patients for planning adjuvant preoperative radiation therapy, chemotherapy, and hyperthermia therapy.

O'Connell et al. (1988) reported that preoperative radiation therapy resulted in a better outcome than postoperative radiation therapy in patients with invasive disease.

The hyperthermia therapy systems based on radiowave irradiation have been commercially available for regional hyperthermia of the pelvis since the mid 1980s. This technology makes it possible to perform sufficiently tolerable and effective regional hyperthermia on rectal carcinomas. Used as a part of curative preoperative and postoperative multimodal therapeutic strategies, hyperthermia can lead to improvement in local control.

For years, the mainstay of local staging of ractal cancer has been the digital rectal examination. The accuracy of the digital rectal examination in correctly staging rectal cancer has been reported to be approximately 70–75% (Hildebrandt and Feifel 1985).

Radiological modalities that have been used in the staging of rectal carcinoma include CT, transrectal US, and MR imaging. The accuracy of staging with CT was reported to be as high as 92% initially (Thoeni et al. 1981). Later published articles showed that CT studies have limited usefulness for accurate staging of local disease or depth of wall invasion (Hodgman et al. 1986). However, CT does not permit evaluation of less extensive tumors because differentiation of the normal layers of the intestinal wall is impossible due to poor soft-tissue contrast. Tumors located low in the rectum were particularly difficult to stage because of the paucity of perirectal fat in this region (Hodgman et al. 1986).

Transrectal ultrasound is now an established imaging modality for evaluation of the integrity of the wall layers underneath the colorectal lesion (Rifkin and Marks 1985). Some articles reported that transrectal US is 77% accurate in demonstrating invasion of carcinoma into the perirectal fat and 50% accurate in demonstrating perirectal lymph node involvement (Rifkin et al. 1989) New articles report a 75–83% accuracy for staging rectal cancer with transrectal US (Milsom and Graffner 1990). However, transrectal US does not provide reliable contrast between the tumor and the muscularis propria. Thus, once the submucosa is breached, it is often diffucult to determine the depth of muscle invasion and to detect early perirectal fat invasion.

Complete removal of adenomatous polyps is the most important measure in prophylaxis of colorectal adenocarcinomas (Shinya and Wolff 1979). Laser photocoagulation is often used in broad-based villous adenomas in patients with a poor surgical or medical condition Mathus-Vliegen and Tytgat (1986).

Few articles have been published about the use of MR imaging with a body coil to stage rectal carcinoma (Butch et al. 1986; Hodgman et al. 1986). The depth of bowel wall invasion cannot be determined, and the accuracy of staging with conventional MR imaging has been reported as not than higher 60% (Hodgman et al. 1986). The limitation of conventional MR imaging in the initial studies was the result of inadequate resolution. de Lange et al. (1990) described results with an external surface coil for MR imaging of rectal cancer; they were able to decrease the voxel volume to 5.7 mm^3 and reported a high accuracy for identifying lesions invading perirectal fat (89%). This technique is disadvantageous in obese patients because the sensitive volume of the surface coil configuration is limited to approximately one radius.

Several authors have reported on the use of a high-resolution endorectal surface coil (Chan et al. 1991). Schanll et al. (1994) reported an accuracy of 81% in staging the extent of the primary lesion in rectal carcinoma. In addition, they reported a specifity of 72% for N1 disease in demonstrating perirectal adenopathy.

However, there are still some problems with using the endorectal surface coil. It is presumed that the pressure from the balloon compressing the low signal intensity mucosa and muscularis propria together makes the layers difficult to be identified. This phenomenon is especially seen with the prostata coil; with the rectal coil these artifacts could be reduced.

Our results demonstrate that endorectal MR imaging can be useful for staging rectal tumors. The layers of the rectal wall are visualizable in all cases. It is important that none of the cases were understaged, because this could prevent patients with highly invasive disease from being adequately treated.

The accuracy of 82% in staging the extent of a primary lesion with MR imaging is better than that reported for CT and body coil MR imaging and similar to that claimed for endorectal sonography.

The follow-up examinations have demonstrated that endorectal surface coil MR imaging probably improves the follow-up studies after electrolaser resection in comparison to transrectal US. This is due to the misinterpretation of inflammatory changes using transrectal US. However, high-resolution endorectal MR imaging was excellent for depicting perirectal nodes.

Clearly, more work and further studies are required to establish criteria for interpreting endorectal MR images.

References

American Joint Committee on Cancer (1992) Manual for staging of cancer, 4th edn. Lippincott, Philadelphia

Boring CC, Squires TS, Tong T (1991) Cancer statistics 1991. Cancer 41:119–151

Butch RJ, Stark DD, Wittenberg J (1986) Staging rectal cancers by MR and CT. AJR 146:1155–1160

Carlson CA, Fabris G, Arslan-Pagnini C et al (1985) Prognostic correlations of operable carcinoma of the retum. Dis Colon Rectum 28:47–50

Chan TW, Kressel HY, Milestone B et al (1991) Rectal carcinoma: staging at MR imaging with endorectal surface coil – work in progress. Radiology 181:461–467

Curley SA, Roh MS, Rich TA (1989) Surgical therapy of early rectal carcinoma. Hematol Oncol Clin North Am 3:87–101

de Lange EE, Fechner RE, Edge SB, Spaulding CA (1990) Preoperative staging of rectal carcinoma with MR imaging: surgical and histopathologic correlation. Radiology 176:623–628

Hager TH, Gall FP, Hermanek P (1983) Local excision of cancer of the rectum. Dis Colon Rectum. 26:149–151

Hildebrandt U, Feifel G (1985) Preoperative staging of rectal cancers by intrarectal ultrasound. Dis Colon Rectum 28;42–46

Hodgman CG, MacCarty RL, Wolf BG et al (1986) Preoperative staging of rectal carcinoma by computed tomography and 0.15 T magnetic resonance imaging. D is Colon Rectum 29:446–450

Hulsmans FJH, Tio TL, Mathus-Vliegen EMH, Bosma A, Tytgat GNJ (1992) Colorectal villous adenoma: transrectal US in screening for invasive malignancy. Radiology 185:193–196

Mathus-Vliegen EMH, Tytgat GNJ (1986) Nd: YAG laser photocoagulation in colorectal adenomas: evaluation of its safety, usefulness and efficacy. Gastroenterology 90:1865–1873

Milsom JW, Graffner H (1990) Intrarectal ultrasonography in rectal cancer staging and in the evaluation of pelvic disease: clinical uses of intrarectal ultrasound. Ann Surg 212:602–606
Moss AA (1989) Imaging of colorectal carcinoma. Radilogy 170:308–310
O'Connell MJ, Gunderson LL, Fleming TR (1988) Adjuvant therapy of rectal cancer. Semin Oncol 15:138–145
Rifkin MD, Marks GJ (1985) Transrectal US as an adjunct in the diagnosis of rectal and extrarectal tumors. Radiology 157:499–502
Rifkin MD, Ehrlich SM, Marks G (1989) Staging of rectal carcinoma: prospective comparison of endorectal US and CT. Radiology 170:319–322
Rothenberger DA, Wong WD (1985) Rectal cancer: adequacy of surgical management. Ann Surg 17:309–312
Shinya H, Wolff W (1979) Morphology, anatomic distribution and cancer potential of colonic polyps: an analysis of 7000 polyps endoscopically removed. Ann Surg 190:679–683
Thoeni R, Moss AA, Schnyder P, Margulis AR (1981) Detection and staging of primary rectal and rectosigmoid cancer by computed tomography. Radiology 141:135–138
Tio TL, Coene PPLO, van Delden OM, Tytgat GNJ (1991) Colorectal carcinoma: preoperative TNM classification with endosonography. Radiology 179:165–170

Immunological and Molecular Classification of Mucosa-Associated Lymphoid Tissue Lymphoma

A. Schmitt-Gräff

Institut für Pathologie, Albert Ludwig Universität Freiburg, Albertstr. 19, 79104 Freiburg, Germany

Abstract

Malignant B-cell lymphoma of mucosa-associated lymphoid tissue (MALT) type is now considered to be a tumor of marginal zone cells of native or, more frequently, acquired MALT. The relationship of MALT lymphoma to the normal counterpart population is acknowledged by the revised European-American classification of lymphoid neoplasms (R.E.A.L.). It fits into the extranodal subtype of marginal zone lymphoma listed as a distinct entity in this recent classification scheme. A typical feature of this lymphoma type is a close lymphocyte–epithelium interaction as reflected by lymphoepithelial lesions. The immunophenotype is characterized by the expression of Sig and B-cell-associated antigens and by the lack of CD5 and CD10. Frequent occurrence of trisomy 3 has been reported.

There is now overwhelming evidence that low-grade MALT lymphomas are subject to immunologic drive. In the stomach, the presence of *Helicobacter pylori* and locally activated T cells appears to be critical for the growth of neoplastic cells. This finding is of clinical significance since the eradication of *H. pylori* has been shown to reverse low-grade MALT lymphoma.

Introduction

Malignant lymphoma presents with significant frequency in the gastrointestinal tract. This site may either be involved in nodal disease or be the origin of primary extranodal lymphoma. In Western countries, most gastrointestinal lymphomas develop in the stomach, while in the Middle East, more than half of the cases are observed in the small bowel. Primary lymphomas arising in the esophagus, colon, and rectum are rare (Domizio et al. 1993; Isaacson 1994b). A variety of lymphoma entities such as Burkitt's lymphoma or mantle cell

Recent Results in Cancer Research, Vol. 142

lymphoma may initially be confined to the gastrointestinal tract. The equivalent of mantle cell lymphoma arising in the mucosa has been designated as lymphomatous polyposis and may manifest as multifocal colorectal polyps (Harris et al. 1994; O'Brien et al. 1989). However, there is overwhelming evidence that characteristic entities, which are significantly different from nodal lymphoma, are closely related to the normal immune system of the gut. Thus, intestinal T-cell lymphoma (ITCL), also designated as enteropathy-associated T-cell lymphoma (O'Farrelly et al. 1986), which was first thought to be of histiocytic origin, is a tumor of intraepithelial T cells (Isaacson et al. 1985; Spencer et al. 1988). Coeliac disease is considered to be a predisposing factor for the development of this neoplasm. ITCL which occurs in the jejunum and/or with multifocal gastrointestinal manifestations has previously been included in the category of mucosa-associated lymphoid tissue (MALT) lymphoma (Isaacson and Spencer 1987). However, the term MALT lymphoma is now generally confined to a specific type of extranodal lymphoma of the B-cell type and is the most common extranodal lymphoid neoplasm (Isaacson 1994b). Here, we delineate pathological, immunophenotypical, and genetic features defining this disease with special emphasis on gastrointestinal manifestations.

Classification of B-Cell Lymphoma of MALT Type and Its Relationship to Marginal Zone Cells

The collective term "MALT lymphoma" was proposed to designate a distinct type of B-cell lymphoma arising in a variety of extranodal sites (Isaacson and Spencer 1987; Isaacson and Wright 1983). The observation that the histology of certain low-grade B-cell lymphomas of the stomach and the small intestine was unlike that of comparable nodal lymphomas but recapitulated features of MALT, led to the concept of this distinct clinicopathological entity (Isaacson and Wright 1983). Primary low-grade MALT lymphoma most frequently occurs in the gastrointestinal tract. A variety of extranodal lymphoid neoplasms arising in other mucosal or nonmucosal sites such as the small intestine (Domizio et al. 1993; Li et al. 1994), salivary glands (Diss et al. 1995; Hyiek et al. 1988), conjunctiva (Wotherspoon et al. 1993b), lung (Li et al. 1990; Schmitt-Gräff et al. 1995), breast (Mattia et al. 1993), thyroid (Hyiek and Isaacson 1988), thymus (Isaacson et al. 1990), urogenital tract (Parveen et al. 1993), and liver (Isaacson et al. 1995) share properties of MALT lymphoma. The majority of lesions previously diagnosed as pseudolymphoma are actually low-grade B-cell lymphoma of MALT type (Isaacson and Spencer 1987).

Gut-associated lymphoid tissue consists of B cells and T cells arranged in organized lymphoid nodules (Peyer's patches) and follicles distributed throughout the lamina propria. The B-cell compartment of Peyer's patches is composed of a follicle surrounded by a mantle and a marginal zone. The dome epithelium is selectively infiltrated by B cells. This lymphoepithelium suggests a close lymphocyte—epithelial interaction (Spencer et al. 1985a, b). In the non-neoplastic MALT, lymphocytes mature into monocytoid B cells and plasma cells upon contact with antigens traversing the epithelium. When they enter the circulation, homing back is mediated by receptors which interact with organ-specific ligands present on high endothelial venules (McDermott and Bienenstock 1979).

The prevailing view is that the marginal zone B cell of MALT is the normal counterpart of the neoplastic cell of B cell lymphoma of MALT type (Harris et al. 1994; Spencer et al. 1990). This relationship is reflected in the behavior of low-grade B-cell lymphoma of MALT which tends to remain confined to the site of origin in stages I and II of extranodal disease. This may be cured by local treatment (Cogliatti et al. 1991). When dissemination occurs, other extranodal sites may be involved, while spreading to the bone marrow is a rare event (Cogliatti et al. 1991; Isaacson 1994b). A follow-up study suggested that the prognosis of high-grade MALT lymphomas may also be more favorable than that of nodal tumors of similar grade (Cogliatti et al. 1991).

MALT type lymphomas are not mentioned in most classifications of malignant lymphomas. A group within the European Association for Haematopathology (J. Diebold, P.G. Isaacson, A.G. Stansfeld, D.H. Wright, and A.C. Feller) proposed that gastrointestinal lymphomas be included in the updated Kiel classification (Stansfeld et al. 1988). Recently, MALT lymphomas have been included in the R.E.A.L. classification (Harris et al. 1994). This classification recognizes the marginal zone B-cell lymphoma as a separate entity. In view of the morphologic and immunophenotypical overlap between nodal monocytoid B-cell lymphoma and extranodal low-grade B-cell lymphoma of MALT, both lymphoma types are listed as subtypes of marginal B-cell lymphoma. Therefore, the term "extranodal marginal zone B-cell lymphoma" was proposed for tumors previously referred to as MALT lymphoma, thus underlining the relationship of this tumor to marginal zone cells (Harris et al. 1994).

Pathological Features of Gastrointestinal B-Cell Lymphoma of MALT

Gastric Low-Grade Lymphoma

In typical low-grade MALT lymphoma the predominant cell is small- to medium-sized with a dense nucleus of irregular shape and a moderately abundant, often pale-staining cytoplasm (Fig. 1). This marginal zone cell resembles follicular center centrocytes and has been designated as centrocyte-like (CCL). There may be an admixture of small lymphocytes, monocytoid B cells, plasma cells, and some larger centroblast- or immunoblast-like cells resulting in cytologic heterogeneity. Plasma-cell differentiation usually predominates beneath the surface epithelium.

In early lesions, neoplastic cells infiltrate the marginal zone and expand into the interfollicular areas arround non-neoplastic follicles. Moreover, coloniza-

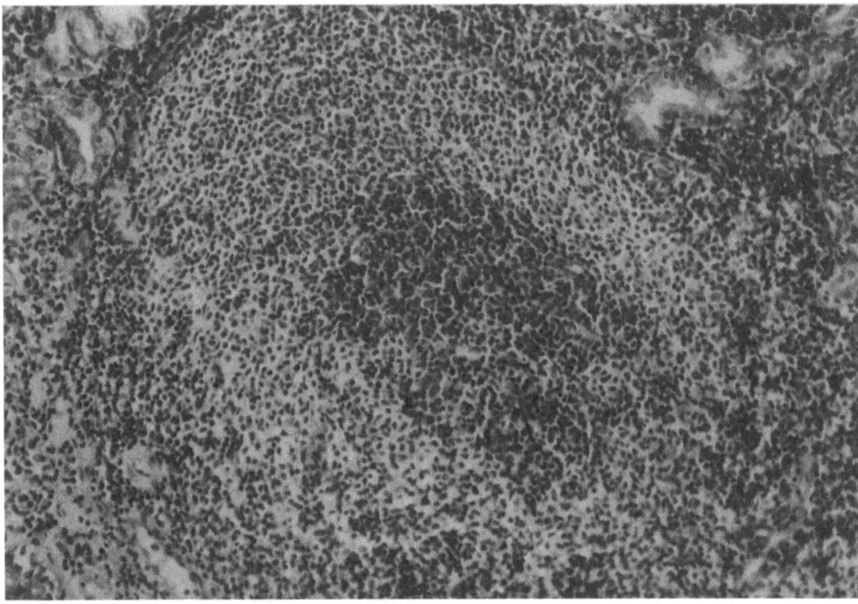

1

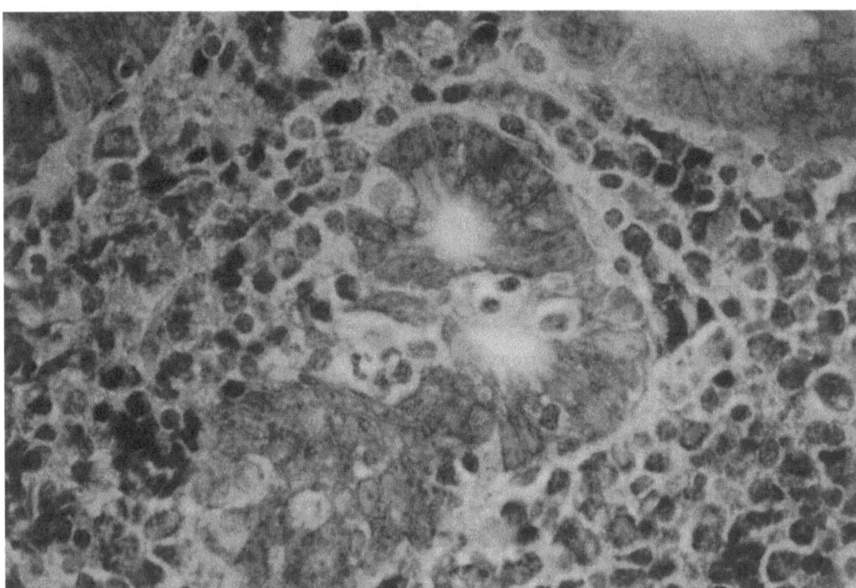

2

Fig. 1. Low-grade B-cell lymphoma of mucosa-associated lymphoid tissue. Centrocyte-like cells are spreading around reactive lymphoid aggregate forming a pale-staining perifollicular area (Giemsa, ×25)

Fig. 2. Low-grade mucosa-associated lymphoid tissue B-cell lymphoma of stomach showing typical lymphoepithelial lesions formed by clusters of tumor cells infiltrating glandular epithelium (Giemsa, ×125) tion of lymphoid follicles by neoplastic cells is frequently encountered. According to Isaacson et al. (1991b) three patterns may occur: (a) CCL cells infiltrate the follicle center while the non-neoplastic mantle zone remains intact; (b) lymphoid follicles are completely replaced by CCL cells; and (c) the intrafollicular cells undergo plasma-cell differentiation. Extensive infiltration of follicles by tumor cells may produce a pattern which resembles follicular center-cell lymphoma. Meshworks of follicular dendritic cells are reminiscent of the original follicles. The hallmark of MALT lymphomas is the presence of lymphoepithelial lesions formed by clusters of CCL cells which invade and destroy the overlying epithelium (Fig. 2). The characteristic infiltration of the glandular epithelium was first recognized in 1979 in cases of immunoproliferative small intestinal disease (IPSID; Isaacson 1979). The infiltration of the epithelium by CCL cells, with close contacts between the membrane of each cell, results in marked ultrastructural changes of the epithelium (Papadaki et al. 1992). It has been suggested that lymphoepithelial lesions may be mediated by membrane-bound signals (Wotherspoon and Isaacson 1995). Multifocal manifestations of low-grade MALT lymphoma are frequently present, especially in the stomach (Wotherspoon et al. 1992). When lymphoid nodes are infiltrated by low-grade MALT lymphoma, tumor cells are predominantly observed in the sinuses and interfollicular areas.

Gastric High-Grade MALT Lymphoma

A low-grade MALT lymphoma may undergo transformation to a high-grade large cell tumor. An important diagnostic feature of high-grade transformation is the presence of confluent clusters of transformed cells outside of colonized follicles (Fig. 3). Large blast cells may display varied cytological appearances and resemble centroblasts or immunoblasts and plasmoblasts with a basophilic cytoplasm. In the high-grade component, glandular invasion with typical lymphoepithelial lesions is a rare event (Chan and Isaacson 1990). When a coexistence of low- and high-grade elements is observed, it may be assumed that both components are related to MALT. However, there are no histological or cytological features whereby high-grade MALT lymphomas lacking a low-grade component can be reliably differentiated from other high-grade B-cell lymphomas (Isaacson 1994b). This is especially the case when reactive follicles and lymphoepithelial lesions are completely absent. However, it cannot be excluded that high-grade types may arise de novo without a low-grade precursor lesion (Cogliatti et al. 1991).

Intestinal B-Cell Lymphoma of MALT

Most intestinal low-grade B-cell lymphomas of the small intestine show features of MALT (Domizio et al. 1993). In a series of 119 cases of primary small

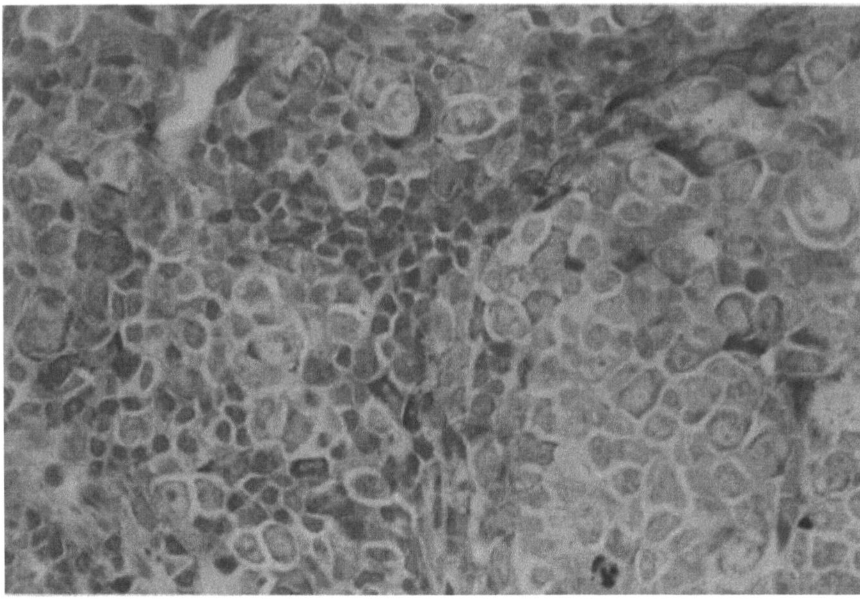

Fig. 3. High-grade mucosa-associated lymphoid tissue B-cell lymphoma of stomach composed of sheets of large-sized blast cells with basophilic cytoplasm (Giemsa, ×150)

bowel lymphoma (Domizio et al. 1993), 20 were classified as low-grade B-cell tumors, among which 15 were of the MALT type. Immunoproliferative small intestinal disease (IPSID) in the Middle East differs from the so-called Western type occurring throughout the world. The Western type is predominantly composed of CCL cells which surround and colonize reactive follicles and form lymphoepithelial lesions (Isaacson 1994b). Tumors may exhibit a combination of low- and high-grade components (Domizio et al. 1993). The morphologic features of IPSID resemble that of low-grade B-cell lymphoma of MALT type but show a more prominent plasma cell component (Isaacson 1979). Three stages of IPSID have been described: in stage A, the mucosa and the mesenteric lymph nodes are involved; in stage B, infiltration spreads beyond the muscularis mucosae; and in stage C, bulky lesions and transformation into a high-grade tumor occur (Isaacson 1994a).

Immunophenotypical and Genetic Features of MALT Lymphoma

Tumor cells of MALT lymphoma are characteristically CD19+, CD20+, CD 22+, CD 79a+ and CD43–/+. Lack of CD5 expression is useful in distinguishing MALT lymphoma from mantle-cell lymphoma and chronic lymphocytic leukemia. Tumor cells express sIg (M > G or A) but not IgD; in about 40%, cytoplasmic Ig (usually IgM) with light chain restriction is observed (Harris et al. 1994; Isaacson 1994b). The absence of CD10 can help to distinguish it from follicular center-cell lymphoma. In IPSID, tumor cells are characterized by the synthesis of alpha heavy chain without a light chain (Isaacson 1979). In the majority of cases, IgA is of subtype IgA1.

In cytokeratin studies, epithelium is labeled by anti-cytokeratin antibodies while lymphocytes are not-thus lymphoepithelial lesions are highlighted (Fig. 4). Staining for T-cell-associated antigens generally shows a high content of reactive T cells intermingled with tumor cells. The growth fraction assessed by using the MiB1 antibody to the Ki-67 antigen is low (generally ≤5%) in low-grade tumors (Fig. 5). High Ki-67 counts (≥70%) are obtained in high-grade tumors.

Heterogeneity of bcl-2 expression in MALT lymphoma has been reported recently (Ashton-Key et al. 1995). Bcl-2 protein, which is implicated in B-cell survival by preventing apoptosis, is expressed in small lymphocytes in the peripheral blood and lymph nodes but disappears from B cells entering the germinal centers. Bcl-2 is present in most follicular lymphomas while it is absent from reactive follicles (Pezzella et al. 1990). Low-grade MALT lymphomas are generally positive for bcl-2, but may have small populations of bcl-negative cells (Isaacson et al. 1991a). Non-neoplastic follicles which are surrounded by tumor cells do not stain for bcl-2 (Fig. 6). When reactive follicles are colonized by CCL cells, bcl-2 staining is generally observed (Fig. 7). However, colonization by blast cells displaying a high growth fraction may be accompanied by loss of bcl-2 (Isaacson 1994b). In high-grade tumors the majority of neoplastic cells is bcl-2 negative (Ashton-Key et al. 1995). It has been speculated that the good prognosis of MALT lymphomas may be related to a normal pattern of bcl-2 expression (Ashton-Key et al. 1995). Genetic analysis failed to demonstrate rearrangements of the bcl-2 gene (t[14;18] translocation) or the bcl-1 gene (t[11;14] translocation) in MALT lymphoma (Finn et al. 1993; Wotherspoon et al. 1994). B-cell monoclonality of MALT lymphomas has been shown indirectly by immunohistochemical demonstration of light chain restriction and by immunoglobulin gene rearrangement studies using Southern blot analysis and the polymerase chain reaction (PCR) (Diss et al. 1993; Norton and Isaacson 1987; Teruya-Feldstein et al. 1995). PCR amplification of immunoglobulin heavy chain (IgH) regions can determine the clonal relationship between lesions removed from different sites or at different times during the course of a disease. Diss et al. (1993) detected a single neoplastic clone in sequential biopsy specimens from a patient with primary gastric MALT lymphoma and Sjögren's syndrome. These authors (Diss et al. 1995) studied the emergence of monoclonal B-cell populations in the context of myoepithelial sialoadenitis. Sheets of CCL cells around lymphoepithelial islands accompanied by B-cell monoclonality signaled the onset of lymphoma. PCR analysis demonstrated identical clonal IgH rearrangements in a low-grade gastric MALT lymphoma progressing into a high-grade tumor (Montalbán et al. 1995). This finding further confirms that low- and high-grade types which have previously been shown to have identical immunoglobulin restriction (Chan and Isaacson 1990) form part of the spectrum of the same

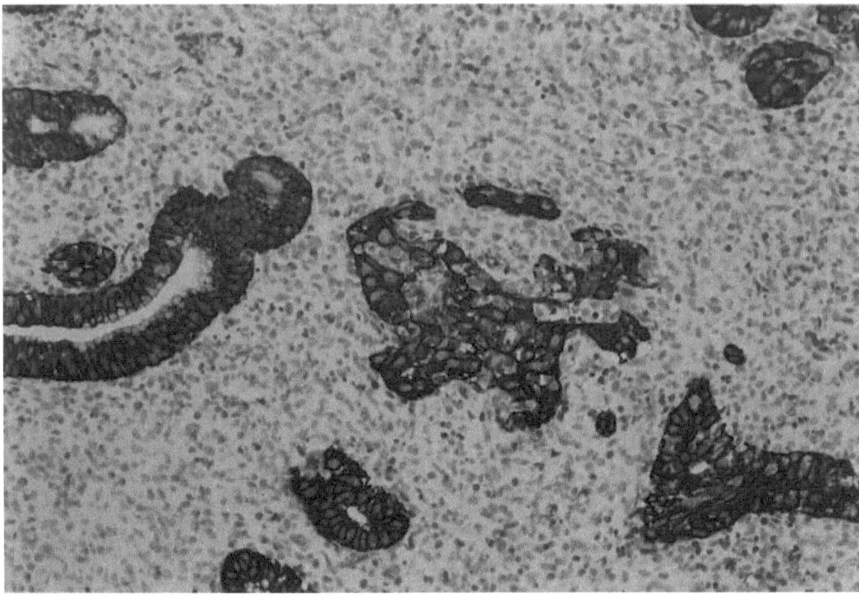

4

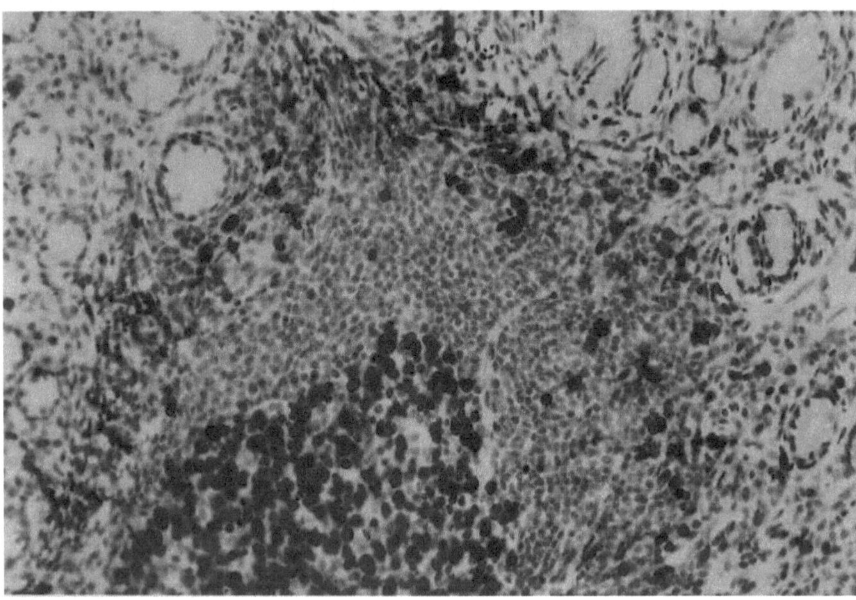

5

Fig. 4. Low-grade mucosa-associated lymphoid tissue B-cell lymphoma of stomach. Staining of epithelium with a broad-spectrum cytokeratin antibody highlights lymphoepithelial lesions (Giemsa, ×40)

Fig. 5. Staining for the Ki-67 antigen (antibody MiB1) shows a high growth fraction in the reactive follicle; scarce tumor cells in the marginal zone are labeled, indicating a small growth fraction of low-grade B-cell lymphoma of stomach (APAAP, ×60)

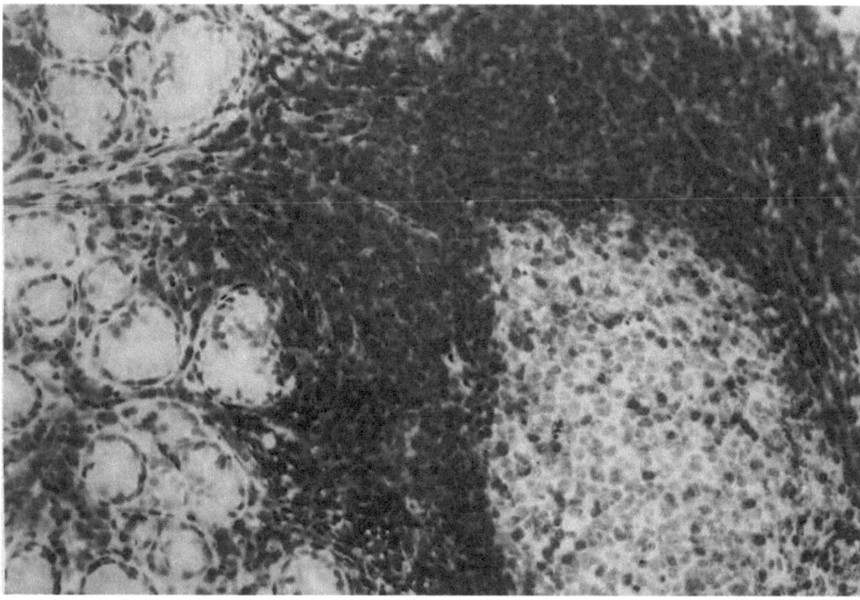

6

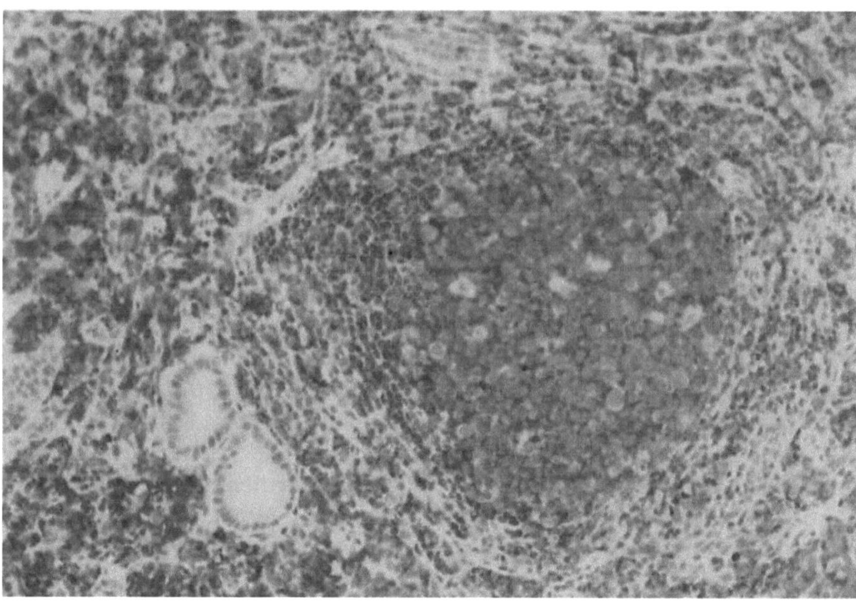

7

Fig. 6. Low-grade B-cell lymphoma of stomach. Bcl-2 protein is expressed by tumor cells surrounding the non-neoplastic germinal center which does not express bcl-2 protein (APAAP, ×60)

Fig. 7. Low-grade B-cell lymphoma of mucosa-associated lymphoid tissue. Colonization of follicle centers by tumor cells expressing high levels of bcl-2 protein (APAAP, ×40) disease. Both types have a trisomy 3 as the most common cytogenetic abnormality (Finn et al. 1993; Wotherspoon et al. 1994). In situ hybridization with chromosome-specific alpha-satellite probes showed trisomy of chromosome 3 in over 50% of MALT lymphomas. It was suggested that this abnormality may be important in its genesis (Finn et al. 1993). In addition, numerical abnormalities of chromosome 7 were reported. Additional genetic alterations may occur during high-grade transformation; *c-myc* rearrangements may be a distinguishing feature of high-grade MALT lymphoma (Raghoebier et al. 1991).

Pathogenetic Aspects of MALT Lymphoma

In mucosal organs and in some histogenetically related sites, organized lymphoid follicles with features of MALT typified by Peyer's patches accumulate as a consequence of chronic inflammation often associated with autoimmune diseases. Example include the stomach in *Helicobacter pylori* infection (Genta et al. 1994; Stolte and Eidt 1989), salivary glands in myoepithelial sialoadenitis usually associated with Sjögren's syndrome (Fig. 8) (Hyiek et al. 1988), and the thyroid in Hashimoto's thyroiditis (Fig. 9) (Hyjek and Isaacson 1988). Paradoxically, the large majority of MALT lymphomas arises from this so-called acquired and not from the indigenous MALT. Several studies have suggested a causal association between gastric colonization by the gram-negative spiral bacterium *H. pylori* and the development of gastric adenocarcinoma (Correa 1991), as well as MALT lymphoma (Eidt et al. 1994; Parsonnet et al. 1994; Wotherspoon et al. 1991). Recently, nine cases of gastric adenocarcinoma occurring simultaneously with low-grade B-cell MALT lymphoma were reported (Wotherspoon and Isaacson 1995). Epidemiologic studies in the Veneto region of Italy have documented an increased frequency of gastric lymphoma. In this region the incidence of *H. pylori* infection and an associated, strikingly severe follicular gastritis is unusually high (Doglioni et al. 1992). Wotherspoon et al. (1991) identified *H. pylori* in over 90% of gastric MALT lymphomas. Parsonnet et al. (1994) attributed 66% of gastric lymphoma to *H. pylori* infection; this case-control study provided evidence that the infection precedes the onset of disease. The demonstration of *H. pylori* in high-grade lymphoma shown in study further substantiates a close relationship between low- and high-grade tumors. While the normal gastric mucosa lacks organized lymphoid tissue *H. pylori* infection induces the acquisition of MALT which may harbor the precursor cell population of MALT lymphoma (Eidt et al. 1994; Genta et al. 1994; Wotherspoon et al. 1991). The induction of a chronic local immune reaction may initiate or promote the development of a lymphoma. By using an anti-idiotypic antibody highly specific for the IgA-MALT lymphoma idiotype, Greiner et al. (1994) showed that B cells with the lymphoma idiotype were generated during *H. pylori* infection. It has been speculated that antigenic stimulation by *H. pylori* may trigger the growth of a lymphoma with anti-self immunoreactivity. According to the

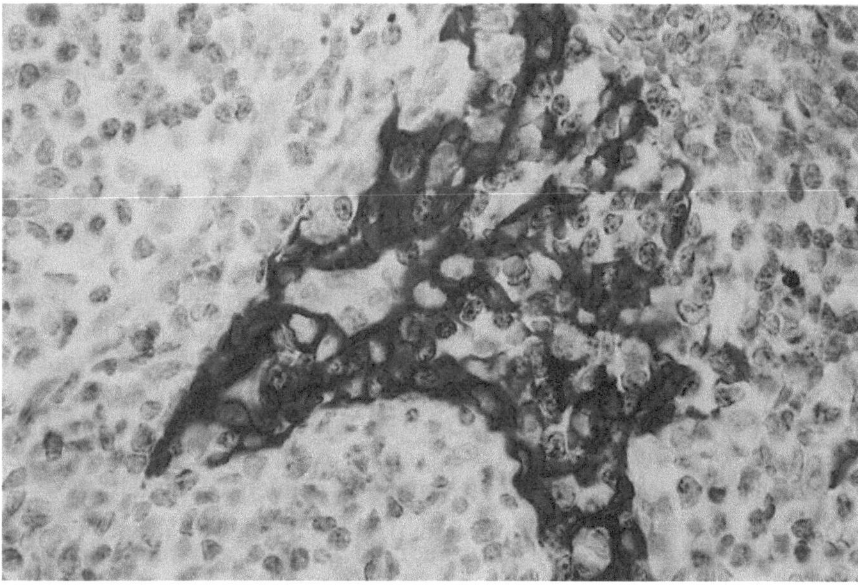

8

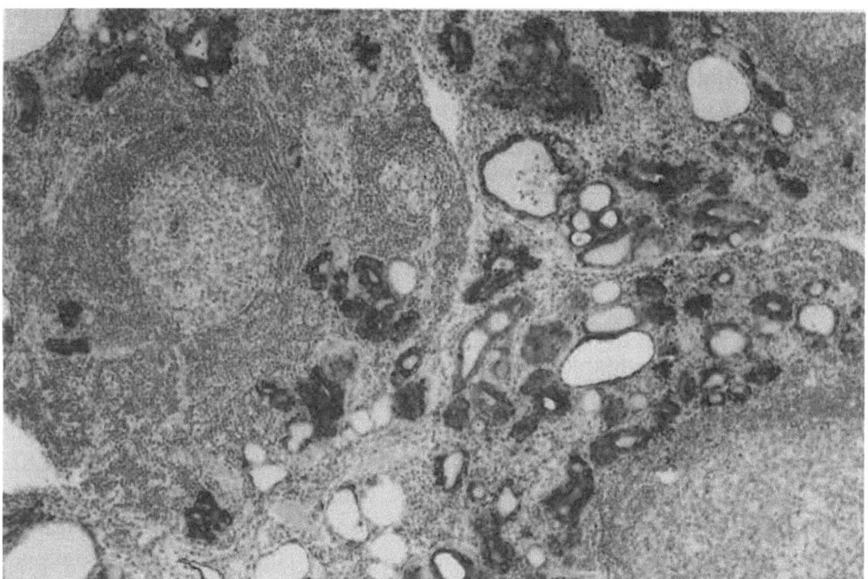

9

Fig. 8. Low-grade mucosa-associated lymphoid tissue-B lymphoma of salivary gland in Sjögren's syndrome. Epithelium labeled by anti-cytokeratin antibodies is surrounded and infiltrated by centrocyte-like cells (APAAP, ×125)

Fig. 9. Low-grade mucosa-associated lymphoid tissue B-cell lymphoma of the thyroid developing in Hashimoto's thyroiditis. Note the presence of reactive lymph follicles. Epithelium is highly labeled by anti-cytokeratin antibodies (APAAP, ×25) results presented by Hussell et al. (1993b), tumor-derived immunoglobulin fails to recognize *H. pylori* antigens but instead recognizes a variety of tissue autoantigens. Hussel et al. (1993a) provided evidence that the growth of low-grade MALT lymphoma cells may be modulated by *H. pylori* and T cells. Co-culturing specific strains of cells from low-grade MALT lymphoma with *H. pylori* resulted in the proliferation of neoplastic B cells and non-neoplastic T cells, an increase in Il-2 receptor expression, and an increase in tumor Ig and Il-2 in the supernatant. Removal of tumor-associated T-cells abrogated these responses.

These data provide evidence that low-grade MALT-lymphomas proliferate in response to *H. pylori* and that the response is strain specific and mediated by H. pylori-specific T cells (Hussell et al. 1993a). Clinical data further indicate that low-grade MALT B-cell lymphoma is sensitive to cytokines produced by *H. pylori*-responsive T cells (Isaacson 1994a). It is well documented that eradication of *H. pylori* leads to the regression of low-grade MALT lymphoma by eliminating the stimulus for T cells and T-cell-dependent help for B-cell proliferation (Wotherspoon et al. 1993a). Long-term follow-up studies are needed to determine whether recurrence of lymphoma and transformation to high-grade tumor is a problem.

In line with the observation that a high incidence of *H. pylori* infection is associated with a low incidence of gastric tumors in some regions (Holcombe 1992) is the suggestion that the effect of *H. pylori* infection depends on environmental, socioeconomic, and genetic factors. Carcinogenesis may also be related to specific strains of *H. pylori*. There is evidence that *H. pylori* strains with the *cagA* gene are associated with an enhanced acute inflammation and an increased risk for gastric cancer (Blaser et al. 1995). The presence of the *cagA* gene may also be related to the development of gastric MALT lymphoma. Since *H. pylori* is not present in all cases of MALT lymphoma, other as yet undefined risk factors may be involved in the development of MALT lymphoma. The development of IPSID and its progression to high-grade lymphoma is problably triggered by recurrent parasitic and bacterial infections and is reversible upon antibiotic treatment (Ben-Ayed et al. 1989). Nevertheless, despite antibiotic therapy, high-grade transformation disseminating from the abdomen may evolve in some patients.

Chronic antigenic stimulation may trigger the development of MALT lymphoma at other sites. In the salivary glands, this lymphoma arises in a background of myoepithelial sialoadenitis associated with Sjögren's syndrome (Diss et al. 1993; Hyiek et al. 1988). Since Epstein-Barrvirus (EBV) sequences can only be detected in a minority of cases, EBV is apparently not associated with the pathogenesis of this lymphoma type (Diss et al. 1993). In the lung, chronically recurrent infections leading to hyperplasia of bronchus-associated lymphoid tissue may be the prerequisite for the development of MALT lymphoma. Single cases of gastrointestinal and pulmonary low-grade MALT lymphoma were reported in HIV-antibody positive patients (Coker et al. 1992; Teruya-Feldstein et al. 1995). It was speculated that MALT lymphoma may represent a new category of HIV-related disease (Teruya-Feldstein et al. 1995). However, the association between HIV and MALT lymphomas seems to be extremly rare. Further work is required to elucidate the mechanisms of antigenic stimulation triggering the development of MALT lymphoma in various organs.

Conclusion

MALT is a native constituent of mucosal organs and may accumulate in response to various stimuli even in nonmucosal sites. Both the indigenous and acquired MALT contain reactive lymphoid follicles. Their marginal zone cells are now considered to be the normal counterpart of tumor cells of low-grade MALT lymphoma. The characteristic cell type of MALT lymphoma, also designated as a CCL cell, retains biological properties of non-neoplastic counterparts, i.e., the formation of lymphoepithelial lesions and the propensity to home to the tissue of origin. This phenomenon is reflected by the biological behavior characterized by a remarkably favorable clinical outcome. The prognosis of high-grade tumors of MALT still seems to be better than that of high-grade nodal lymphomas. The most common type of MALT lymphomas in the Western world occurs in the stomach, where it is generally associated with *H. pylori* infection. There is increasing evidence indicating that both morphological and clinical remission may be induced by eradication of *H. pylori*. In vitro studies have shown that the growth of MALT lymphoma-derived B cells is controlled by tumor-infiltrating T cells. This response is restricted to those T cells at the site of *H. pylori* infection. It may be speculated that growth of other neoplasms with a high content of non-neoplastic T cells may also be modulated by immunologic mechanisms.

References

Ashton-Key M, Biddolph SC, Stein H, Gatter KC, Mason DY (1995) Heterogeneity of bcl-2 expression in MALT lymphoma. Histopathology 26:75–78

Ben-Ayed F, Halphen M, Najjar T et al (1989) Treatment of alpha chain disease – results of a prospective study in 21 Tunisian patients by the Tunisian-French Intestinal Lymphoma Study Group. Cancer 63:1251–1256

Blaser MJ, Perez-Perez GI, Kleanthous H, Cover TL, Peek RM, Chyou PH, Stemmermann GN, Normura A (1995) Infection with Helicobacter pylori strains possessing cagA is associated with an increased risk of developing adenocarcinoma of the stomach. Cancer Res 55:2111–2115

Chan JKC, Isaacson PG (1990) Relationship between high-grade lymphoma and low-grade B-cell mucosa-associated lymphoid tissue lymphoma (MALToma) of the stomach. Am J Pathol 136:1153–1164

Cogliatti SB, Schmid U, Schumacher U et al (1991) Primary B-cell gastric lymphoma: a clinicopathological study of 145 patients. Gastroenterology 101:1159–1170

Coker RJ, Lau R, Isaacson PG, Kelly SA, Price P, Weber J (1992) Mucosa-associated gastric lymphoma occurring in an HIV-antibody-positive patient. AIDS 6:336–337
Correa P (1991) Is gastric carcinoma an infectious disease? N Engl J Med 325:1170–1171
Diss TC, Peng H, Wotherspoon AC, Panb L, Speight PM, Isaacson PG (1993) A single neoplastic clone in sequential biopsy specimens from a patient with primary gastric-mucosa-associated-lymphoid tissue lymphoma and Sjögren's syndrome. N Engl J Med 329:172–175
Diss TC, Wotherspoon AC, Speight P, Langxing P, Isaacson PG (1995) B-cell monoclonality, Epstein Barr virus and t(14;18) in myoepithelial sialadenitis and low-grade B-cell MALT lymphoma of the parotid gland. Am J Surg Pathol 19:531–536
Doglioni C, Wotherspoon AC, Moschini A, de Boni M, Isaacson PG (1992) High incidence of primary gastric lymphoma in northeastern Italy. Lancet 339:834–835
Domizio P, Owen Ra, Shepherd NA, Talbot IC, Norton AJ (1993) Primary lymphoma of the small intestine. A clinicopathological study of 119 cases. Am J Surg Pathol 17:429–442
Eidt S, Stolte M, Fischer R (1994) Helicobacter pylori gastritis and primary gastric non-Hodgkin's lymphomas. J Clin Pathol 47:436–439
Finn T, Isaacson PG, Wotherspoon AC (1993) Numerical abnormalities of chromosomes 3, 7, 12, and 18 in low grade lymphomas of MALT-type and splenic marginal zone cell lymphomas detected by interphase cytogenetics on paraffin embedded tissue. J Pathol 170:335A
Genta RM, Huberman RM, Graham DY (1994) The gastric cardia in Helicobacter pylori infection. Hum Pathol 25:915–919
Greiner A, Marx A, Heesemann J, Leebmann J, Schmaußer B, Müller-Hermelink HK (1994) Idiotype identity in a MALT-type lymphoma and B cells in Helicobacter pylori associated chronic gastritis. Lab Invest 70:572–577
Harris NL, Jaffe ES, Stein H, Banks PM, Chan JKC, Cleary ML, Delsol G, De Wolf-Peeters C, Falini B, Gatter KC, Grogan TM, Isaacson PG, Knowles DM, Mason DY, Muller-Hermelink HK, Pileri SA, Piris MA, Ralfkiaer E, Warnke RA (1994) A revised European-American classification of lymphoid neoplasms: a proposal from the international lymphoma study group. Blood 84:1361–1392
Holcombe C (1992) Helicobacter pylori: the African enigma. Gut 33:429–431
Hussell T, Isaacson PG, Crabtree JE, Spencer J (1993a) The response of cells from low-grade B-cell gastric lymphomas of mucosa-associated lymphoid tissue to Helicobacter pylori. Lancet 342:571–574
Hussell T, Isaacson PG, Crabtree JE, Dogan A, Spencer J (1993b) Immunoglobulin specificity of low grade-B-cell gastro-intestinal lymphoma. Am J Pathol 142:285–292
Hussell T, Isaacson PG, Spencer J (1995) Tumour infiltrating T-cells in gastric lymphoma (editorial). Virchows Arch 426:1–2
Hyjek E, Isaacson PG (1988) Primary B-cell lymphoma of the thyroid and its relationship to Hashimoto's thyroiditis. Hum Pathol 19:1315–1326
Hyiek E, Smith WJ, Isaacson PG (1988) Primary B-cell lymphoma of the salivary gland and its relationship to myoepithelial sialadenitis. Hum Pathol 19:766–776
Isaacson PG (1979) Middle east lymphoma and alpha-chain disease. An immunohistochemical study. Am J Pathol 3:431–441
Isaacson PG (1994a) Gastric lymphoma and Helicobacter pylori (editorial). N Engl J Med 330:1310–1311
Isaacson PG (1994b) Gastrointestinal lymphoma. Hum Pathol 25:1020–1029
Isaacson PG, Spencer J (1987) Malignant lymphoma of mucosa-associated lymphoid tissue. Histopathology 11:445–462
Isaacson PG, Wright DH (1983) Malignant lymphoma of mucosa-associated lymphoid tissue. Cancer 52:1410–1416

Isaacson PG, Spencer J, Connolly C, Pollock D, Stein H, O'Connor N, Bevan D, Kirham N, Wainscoat J, Mason D (1985) Malignant histiocytosis of the intestine: a T-cell lymphoma. Lancet 2:688–699
Isaacson PG, Chan JKC, Tang C, Addis B (1990) Low-grade B-cell lymphoma of mucosa-associated lymphoid tissue arising in the thymus. A thymic lymphoma mimicking myoepithelial sialadenitis. Am J Surg Pathol 14:342–351
Isaacson PG, Wotherspoon AC, Diss TC, Pan LX (1991a) Bcl-2 expression in lymphomas (letter; comment). Lancet 337:175–176
Isaacson PG, Wotherspoon AC, Diss TC et al (1991b) Follicular colonization in B cell lymphoma of mucosa associated lymphoid tissue. Am J Surg Pathol 15:819–828
Isaacson PG, Banks PM, Best PV, McLure SP, Muller-Hermelink K, Wyatt SI (1995) Primary low-grade hepatic B-cell lymphoma of mucosa-associated lymphoid tissue (MALT) type. Am J Surg Pathol 19:571–575
Li G, Hansmann ML, Zwingers T, Lennert K (1990) Primary lymphomas of the lung: morphological, immunohistochemical and clinical features. Histopathology 16:519–531
Li G, Ouyang Q, Liu K, Wang Y, Yang X (1994) Primary non-Hodgkin's lymphoma of the intestine: a morphological, immunohistochemical and clinical study of 31 Chinese cases. Histopathology 25:113–121
Mattia AR, Ferry JA, Harris NL (1993) Breast lymphoma. A B-cell spectrum including the low-grade B-cell lymphoma of mucosa-associated lymphoid tissue. Am J Surg Pathol 96:738–745
McDermott MR, Bienenstock J (1979) Evidence for a common mucosal immunologic system. I. Migration of B immunoblasts into intestinal, respiratory and genital tissues. J Immunol 122:1892–1898
Montalbán C, Manzanal A, Castrillo JM, Escribano L, Bellas C (1995) Low grade gastric B-cell MALT lymphoma progressing into high grade lymphoma. Clonal identity of the two stages of the tumor, unusual bone involvement and leukaemic dissemination. Histopathology 27:89–91
Norton AJ, Isaacson PG (1987) Detailed phenotypic analysis of B-cell lymphoma using a panel of antibodies reactive in routinely fixed wax-embedded tissue. Am J Pathol 128:225–240
O'Brian D, Kennedy M, Daly P, O'Brian A, Tanner W, Rogers P, Lawlor E (1989) Multiple lymphomatous polyposis of the gastro-intestinal tract: a clinicopathologically distinctive form of non-Hodgkin's lymphoma of centrocytic type. Am J Surg Pathol 13:691–699
O'Farrelly C, Feighery C, O'Brien DS et al (1986) Humoral response to wheat protein in patients with coeliac disease and enteropathy associated T-cell lymphomas. Br Med J 293:908–910
Papadaki L, Wotherspoon AC, Isaacson PG (1992) The lymphoepithelial lesion of gastric low-grade B-cell lymphoma of mucosa-associated lymphoid tissue (MALT): an ultrastructural study. Histopathology 21:415–421
Parsonnet J, Hansen S, Rodriguez L, Gelb AB, Warnke RA, Jellum E, Orentreich N, Vogelman JH, Friedman GD (1994) Helicobacter pylori infection and gastric lymphoma. N Engl J Med 330:1267–1271
Parveen T, Navarro-Roman L, Medeiros LJ, Raffeld M, Jaffe ES (1993) Low-grade B-cell lymphoma of mucosa-associated lymphoid tissue arising in the kidney. Arch Pathol Lab Med 117:780–783
Pezzella F, Tse AG, Cordell JL, Pulford KA, Gatter KC, Mason DY (1990) Expression of the bcl-2 oncogene protein is not specific for the 14;18 chromosomal translocation. Am J Pathol 137:225–232
Raghoebier S, Kramer MHH, van Krieken JHJM et al (1991) Essential differences in oncogene involvement between primary nodal and extranodal large cell lymphoma. Blood 78:2680–2685

Schmitt-Gräff A, Raff T, Rahn W, Stein H (1995) Primäre pulmonale B-Zell-Lymphome vom MALT-Type Primary pulmonary B-cell lymphoma of the MALT-type. Pathologe 16:328–335

Spencer J, Finn T, Isaacson PG (1985a) Gut associated lymphoid tissue: a morphological and immunocytochemical study of the human appendix. Gut 26:672–679

Spencer J, Finn T, Pulford KAF et al (1985b) The human gut contains a novel population of B lymphocytes which resemble marginal zone cells. Clin Exp Immunol 62:607–612

Spencer J, Cerf-Bensussan N, Jarry A, Guy-Grand D, Brousse N, Krajewski M, Isaacson P (1988) Enteropathy-associated T-cell lymphoma is recognized by a monoclonal antibody (HML-1) that defines a membrane molecule on human mucosal lymphocytes. Am J Pathol 132:1–5

Spencer J, Diss T, Isaacson P (1990) A study of the properties of a low-grade mucosal B-cell lymphoma using a monoclonal antibody specific for the tumour immunoglobulin. J Pathol 160:231

Stansfeld A, Diebold J, Kapanci Y, Kelenyi G, Lennert K, Mioduszewska O, Noel H, Rilke F, Sudstrom C, van Unni J, Wright D (1988) Updated Kiel classification for lymphomas. Lancet 1:292

Stolte M, Eidt S (1989) Lymphoid follicles in antral mucosa: immune response to Campylobacter pylori? J Clin Pathol 42:1269–1271

Teruya-Feldstein J, Temeck BK, Sloas MM, Kingma DW, Raffeld M, Pass HI, Mueller B, Jaffe ES (1995) Pulmonary malignant lymphoma of mucosa-associated lymphoid tissue (MALT) arising in a pediatric HIV-positive patient. Am J Surg Pathol 19:357–363

Wotherspoon AC, Isaacson PG (1995) Synchronous adenocarcinoma and low-grade B-cell lymphoma of mucosa associated lymphoid tissue (MALT) of the stomach. Histopathology 27:235–331

Wothersppon AC, Ortiz-Hidalgo C, Falzon MR, Isaacson PG (1991) Helicobacter pylori-associated gastritis and primary B-cell gastric lymphoma Lancet 338:1175–1176

Wotherspoon AC, Doglioni C, Isaacson PG (1992) Low-grade gastric B-cell lymphoma of mucosa-associated lymphoid tissue (MALT): a multifocal disease. Histopathology 20:29–34

Wotherspoon AC, Doglioni C, Diss TC, Pan L, Moschini A, de Boni M, Isaacson PG (1993a) Regression of primary low-grade B-cell gastric lymphoma of mucosa-associated lymphoid tissue type after eradication of Helicobacter pylori. Lancet 342:575–577

Wotherspoon AC, Diss TC, Pan LX et al (1993b) Low grade B-cell lymphoma of the conjunctiva: a mucosa associated lymphoid tissue (MALT) type lymphoma. Histopathology 23:417–424

Wotherspoon AC, Finn T, Isaacson PG (1994) Numerical abnormalities of chromosomes 3 and 7 in lymphomas of mucosa associated lymphoid tissue and the splenic marginal zone. Lab Invest 70:124A

Somatostatin Receptor Scintigraphy in the Diagnosis of Neuroendocrine Gastroenteropancreatic Tumors

M. Bäder and K. Koppenhagen

Department of Radiology and Nuclear Medicine, University Medical Center Benjamin Franklin, Free University of Berlin, Hindenburgdamm 30, 12200 Berlin, Germany

Abstract

Somatostatin receptor scintigraphy is a new, very sensitive procedure for detecting receptor-positive neuroendocrine tumors. Radiolabeled somatostatin analogues are selectively taken up after intravenous administration by tissue carrying somatostatin receptors and, as with the skeletal scintiscan, permit a whole-body visualization of receptor-positive tumors and metastases. Somatostatin receptor scintigraphy shows an overall sensitivity of about 84% for neuroendocrine gastroenteropancreatic tumors. This kind of scintigraphy should be applied in primary tumor localization, staging, and course control in a confirmed or highly probable neuroendocrine gastroenteropancreatic tumor. Furthermore, the use of a gamma probe for intraoperative tumor localization is demonstrated. Therapy with radioactively marked somatostatin analogues should be possible because of the highly selective tumor uptake. The development of an optimal tracer is the subject of current research.

Introduction

Somatostatin is a cyclic peptide hormone consisting of 14 amino acids which occurs in mammals as somatostatin-14 and as somatostatin-28. It is well known that somatostatin inhibits the secretion of numerous hormones (e.g., growth hormone, insulin, gastrin, glucagon), gastric juice, and pancreatic enzymes (Reichlin 1983). Somatostatin analogues inhibit in vitro the growth of neuroendocrine tumors (literature survey in Weckbecker et al. 1994). Receptor-mediated activation of phosphotyrosine phosphatase and the inhibition of adenylate cyclase in receptor-positive tumors are considered as direct mechanisms. Moreover, an indirect mechanism can also be observed for receptor-negative tumors. The indirect mechanism consists in the down-regulation of

Recent Results in Cancer Research, Vol. 142

growth-stimulating factors such as hormones and growth factors (Patel et al. 1990; Weckbecker et al. 1994). Since natural somatostatin has a half-life of only 1–2 min, a somatostatin analogue with a longer half-life was developed for therapeutic purposes; the octapeptide octreotide proved to be successful with a half-life of approximately 80–100 min (SMS 201-995, Sandostatin) (Bauer et al. 1982).

Biomechanical methods (Reichlin 1983) and receptor autoradiography (Reubi and Maurer 1985) were applied to study the distribution of somatostatin and somatostatin receptors in normal human and animal tumor tissue (Reubi et al. 1987a,b). Most of the neuroendocrine gastroenteropancreatic (NEGEP) tumors carry, in contrast to the surrounding tissue, highly affinitive binding sites for somatostatin (Reubi et al. 1987a,b, 1990b). The first in vivo visualization of somatostatin receptor-positive tumor tissue, reported by Krenning et al. (1989), used [^{123}I-Tyr^3] octreotide, an iodine-123-marked somatostatin analogue. Compared with somatostatin, this gamma-emitting somatostatin analogue has the same biological activity and almost the same affinity to the SRIF receptor (Bakker et al. 1990). Parallel application of in vivo receptor scintigraphy and in vitro autoradiography confirmed that [I-123-Tyr^3] octreotide scintigraphy does in fact correspond to the accumulation of radiopharmacons in specific functional somatostatin receptors (Lamberts et al. 1990b).

Despite its successful visualization of different receptor-carrying tissues (Bakker et al. 1990, 1991b; Krenning et al. 1992b), scintigraphy with [I-123-Tyr^3] octreotide has some disadvantages. These are a complicated marking technique, the high costs of cyclotrone-manufactured I-123, the relatively short half-life of the radiopharmacon in combination with a rapid blood reduction rate that makes imaging more difficult after 24 h, and the high abdominal background activity due to primarily hepatobiliary excretion (Bakker et al. 1990).

To overcome these problems, another somatostatin analogue which could be radiolabeled was looked for. Bakker et al. (1991b) introduced [In-111-DTPA-D-Phe^1] octreotide (pentetreotide, Octreoscan 111, Mallinckrodt, Holland). Here, In-111 is complexly bound by the functional groups of diethylenetriaminepenta acetic acid (Fig. 1). Apart from a somewhat lower receptor affinity (Bakker et al. 1991b), In-111 pentetreotide exhibited the following advantages over [I-123-Tyr^3] octreotide: Labeling is very easy; it is done by simply adding activity to the lyophylized pentetreotide, and further purification steps are unnecessary. The labeling yield is more than 95%; in our own investigations it was 98% with a standard deviation of 0.3%. Images can be obtained without problems after 24 h or even after several days owing to the long half-life (2.8 days) of Indium 111. A major advantage is the predominantly renal clearance. With In-111 pentetreotide, it is possible to obtain images with little background activity in the abdominal region that is of special interest.

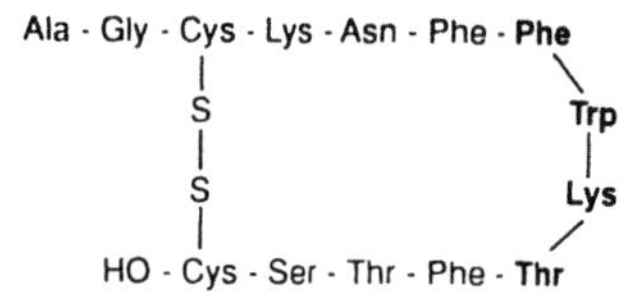

somatostatin

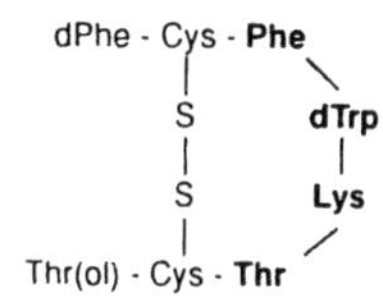

octreotide

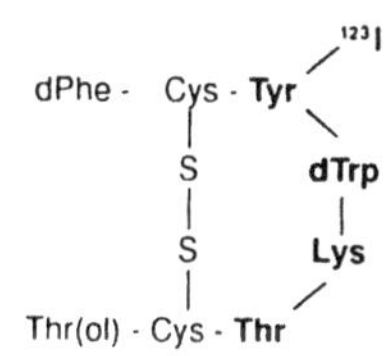

^{123}I-Tyr^{3}-octreotide

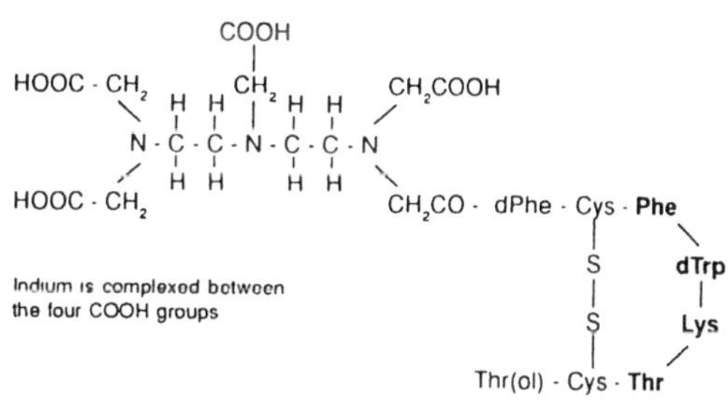

[111 In-DTPA-D-Phe^{1}] -octreotide
pentetreotide

Fig. 1. Structural formulas of native somatostatin, octreotide (Sandostatin), (^{123}I-labeled-Tyr^{3}) octreotide and (^{111}In-labeled-DTPA-D-Phe^{1}) octreotide (^{111}In-labeled pentetreotide). The bioactive aminoacid structure is printed fat

Somatostatin Receptors

Distribution in Normal Tissue

Somatostatin receptors were initially detected in pituitary cells (Schönbrunn and Tashjian 1978), then also in other somatostatin target organs: the anterior pituitary lobe (Enjalbert et al. 1982); the brain (Reubi et al. 1981; Srikant and Patel 1981); and the gastrointestinal tract, for example, in the endocrine and exocrine pancreas (Srikant and Patel 1986; Viguerie et al. 1988, Amherdt et al. 1987); as well as in the thyroid C cells (Van Noorden et al. 1977; Yamada et al. 1977) and the lymphocytes (Sreedharan et al. 1989).

Distribution in Tumor Tissue

Most of the tumors originating from somatostatin target organs preserve their capacity to express somatostatin receptors. Highly affinitive somatostatin receptors in high density were described for the first time in cases of acromegaly in the anterior pituitary lobe (Reubi 1984). The survey study by Lamberts et al. (1991) includes an overview of the somatostatin receptor prevalence in human tumor tissue (Table 1).

Somatostatin Receptor Subtypes

The existence of receptor subtypes was suspected because of the observation that effector cells are differently influenced by natural somatostatin 14 and somatostatin 28 (Srikant and Patel 1987; Wang et al. 1989). Also, normal rat and human brains showed different affinities to somatostatin analogues (Reubi 1984; Reubi et al. 1987b; Heimann et al. 1987; Markstein et al. 1989) in some areas like the cortex, hippocampus, substantia nigra, and pituitary gland (Reubi 1984; Reubi et al. 1987; Heimann et al. 1987; Markstein et al. 1989).

Following the first somatostatin receptor subtypes (Yamada et al. 1992a), another five receptor subtypes were cloned that were named SSTR1–5 in the order of their discovery (Yamada et al. 1992a,b; Rohrer et al. 1993; Kluxen et al. 1992; O'Caroll et al. 1992). Somatostatin 14 and somatostatin 28 have a high affinity to all receptor subtypes, whereas octreotide has a high affinity to SSTR2 and SSTR5 ($IC_{50} = 0.3\,nM$ and $IC_{50} = 0.2\,nM$) but only a very low affinity to SSTR1 and SSTR4 ($IC_{50} > 1000\,nM$) and only a moderate affinity to SSTR3 ($IC_{50} = 30\,nM$) (Weckbecker et al. 1993). The binding characteristics of other known short somatostatin analogues (RC-160, BIM 2314, MK 678) are similar to those of octreotide. They are selective ligands for SSTR2 and SSTR5. SSTR2 is apparently the dominating subtype in somatostatin receptor-positive tumors (Weckbecker et al. 1993).

Table 1. Incidence of somatostatin receptors in human tumors (Lamberts et al. 1991)

	Observed incidence[a]	
	In vitro Autoradiography (%)	In vivo Scintigraphy (%)
Pituitary adenoma		
GH	42/43 (98)	4/4 (100)
TSH	2/2	2/2
Inactive	6/15 (40)	6/8 (75)
Endocrine pancreatic tumors	31/35 (89)	18/21 (86)
Carcinoids	54/62 (87)	37/39 (95)
Paragangliomas	11/12 (92)	29/31 (94)
Pheochromocytomas	38/52 (73)	2/5 (40)
Medullary thyroid carcinomas	10/26 (38)	7/12 (58)
Bronchial carcinomas		
Small cell	4/7 (57)	5/8 (63)
Non-small cell	0/17 (0)	3/4 (75)
Neuroblastomas	15/23 (65)	5/5 (100)
Meningiomas	54/55 (98)	11/11 (100)
Gliomas		
Astrocytomas	14/17 (82)	4/4 (100)
Glioblastomas	1/45 (2)	0/2
Merkel-cell tumors		4/5 (80)
Mamma carcinomas		
Total	72/356 (20)	
Large tumors	33/72 (46)	39/52 (75)
Adenocarcinomas		
Unknown origin		5/9 (56)
Pancreas	0/12 (0)	0/20 (0)
Ovary	3/57 (5)	
Colorectal	3/26 (11)	
Lymphomas	27/31 (87)	10/10 (100)

[a] The tumors of 50 patients in this table were studied in vivo and in vitro. The results concurred in 47 cases

In the future, there might be the possibility of a differentiated therapy with somatostatin analogues that selectively bind receptor subtypes (Weckbecker et al. 1993), or of selective demonstration of tumors with certain subtypes and also characteristic properties.

Scintigraphic Examination Technique

A prerequisite for scintigraphic examination, from the point of view of equipment, is a wide-angle gamma camera with a medium-energy or Indium-111-optimized collimator. The energy windows are centered on 173 and 247 keV with a 20% window width. The imaging times of 4 and 24 h post injection (p.i.)

are usually chosen after injection of 110–220 MBq In-111-pentetreotide. For plane images, at least 300000 impulses are registered for 4 h p.i. on the head and neck – if necessary, also on the extremities. Thorax and abdomen are recorded with 500000 counts. At 24 h p.i., imaging is terminated after reaching the same number of impulses or after 10–15 min; 500000 counts are rarely obtained here. For the abdomen, especially in the region of the liver, spleen, and kidneys, single-photon emission computed tomography (SPECT) is performed with an imaging time of approximately 1 h. SPECT enables superimposition-free visualization, so that some pathological uptake can be differentiated from uptake in other organs like the kidney only by this procedure (Fig. 2). In cases of unclear abdominal findings, additional plane imaging with an imaging time of up to 20 min should be applied between days 2 and 5 p.i. (Fig. 3). Intestinal activity is usually not detectable here; thus, it is easier to

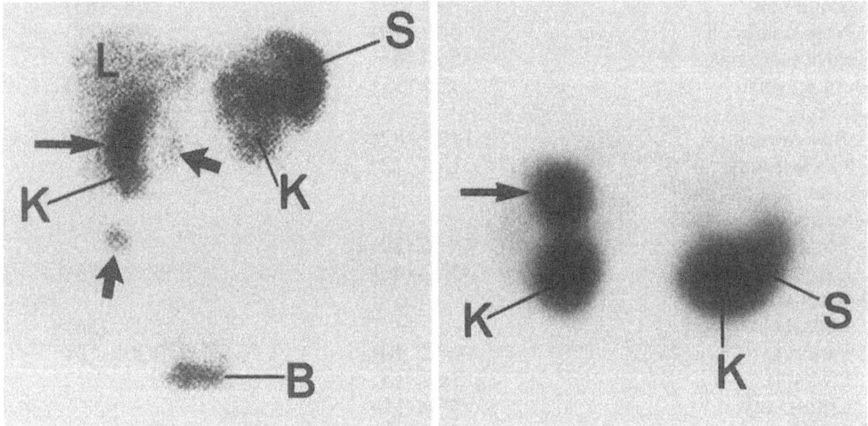

a b

Fig. 2a,b. Anterior somatostatin receptor scintigraphic view of a midgut carcinoid (**a**) shows primary tumor (*short arrow*) and a questionable area in projection to the right kidney (*long arrow*). The transversal slices of single photon emission computed tomography (**b**) clearly show a liver metastasis (*long arrow*) in front of the right kidney. *L*, liver; *S*, spleen; *K*, kidney; *B*, bladder

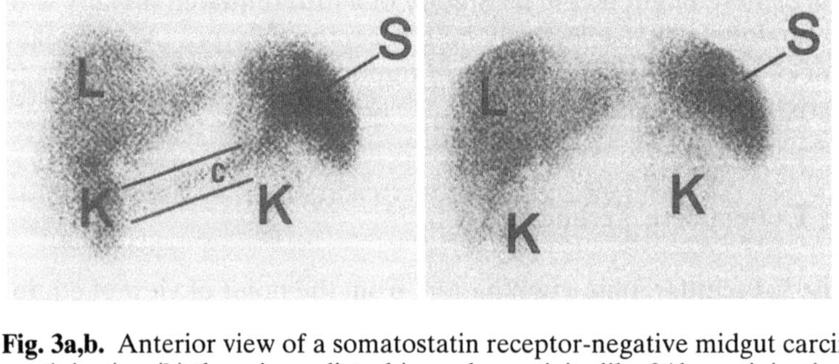

a b

Fig. 3a,b. Anterior view of a somatostatin receptor-negative midgut carcinoid. At 72 h postinjection (**b**) there is no disturbing colon activity like 24 h postinjection (**a**) *L*, liver; *S*, spleen; *K*, kidney; *C*, colon differentiate between physiological and pathological intestinal accumulation. To avoid colon activity, the use of laxatives is highly recommended.

Biokinetics

Blood activity in humans usually drops to 33% of the applied dose 10min after injection. Less than 2% is eliminated via the feces within 72h. There is rapid renal clearance; 25% of the applied activity is eliminated via the kidneys after 3h, 50% after 6h, 85% after 24h, and more than 90% after 48h (Krenning et al. 1992a). The effective equivalent dose is 0.08mSv/MBq. At 0.45mGy/MBq, the effective renal dose is the largest for any organ (Table 2, Krenning et al. 1992a).

Our evaluation of the first 40 patients examined yielded long half-lives for the liver, spleen, kidneys, and tumor tissue, while the pulmonary and abdominal background decreased comparatively fast with a half-life of 11–17h (see

Table 2. Dose estimates after intravenous administration of In-111-DTPA-D-Phe-1-octreotide in man on the basis of gamma camera measurements ($n = 24$), urinary excretion measurements ($n = 10$), and fecal excretion measurements ($n = 4$)[a] (Krenning et al. 1992a)

Target organ	Absorbed dose (mGy/MBq)	Range (mGy/Mbq)
Kidneys	0.45[MD]	0.19–0.80
Liver	0.07[MD]	0.04–0.15
Spleen	0.32[MD]	0.1–0.66
Gonads	0.019[MD]	0.015–0.026
Red marrow	0.020[MD]	0.016–0.026
Urinary bladder wall	0.18[MN]	n.a.
GI tract		
Small intestinal wall	0.03[MN,b]	n.a.
ULI wall	0.04[MN,b]	n.a.
LLI wall	0.06[MN,b]	n.a.
Thyroid gland	0.04[MX]	
Pituitary	0.11[MX]	
Median effective dose equivalent (mSv/MBq)		Range (mSv/MBq)
0.08		0.05–0.12

MD, median; *MN*, mean; *MX*, calculations for maximum uptake; *n.a.* not applicable due to the model

[a] The input to the small intestines is taken to be the same as the fecal excretion during 72h ($n = 4$), namely 1.7%. For the thyroid and the pituitary ($n = 6$), the radiation dose corresponds to the maximum organ uptake measured in these patients

[b] ICRP30 GI model used

Table 3). Since tumor tissue has a particularly long half-life, images can be obtained after 24 h with good tumor/nontumor quotients. If necessary, images can also be obtained after 2, 3, or 4 days, and although they take longer because of a decrease in the number of impulses, they are occasionally used by us to clarify questionable abdominal foci.

Side Effects

Side effects in the form of clinical complaints or changes in hematological or clinical and chemical laboratory parameters were observed neither in the course of our investigations nor in the European multicenter study (Dop 1994). The biological effect of octreotide is ten times stronger than that of [In-111-DTPA-D-Phe[1]] octreotide (Bakker et al. 1991a). For the usual dose of 110–220 MBq, the substance amount of the applied radiopharmacon is 10–20 μg (the contents of one or two kits), while a low-dose octreotide therapy requires a daily subcutaneous application of $3 \times 100\,\mu$g.

Side effects are also not to be expected after a single dose of [In-111-DTPA-D-Phe[1]] octreotide because of the low effective strength of In-111 pentetreotide and the small amount of substance applied, and in view of the small number of side effects found with octreotide.

Accumulations in the Scintigram

In normal individuals, an intensive accumulation in the liver, spleen, and kidneys is observed with In-111-pentetreotide in the somatostatin receptor scintigram. The bladder is intensely visualized 4 h p.i. and also parts of the upper and lower urinary tract; 24 h p.i. the bladder is barely visible. Far weaker

Table 3. Biological half-life of In-111-pentetreotide determined in intervals between 4 h and 24 h p.i. in 40 patients with NEGEP tumors. Calculation from planar gamma camera images

Organ	Biological half-life in hours
Liver	56.9
Spleen	99.2
Kidneys	44.7
Liver without metastases	32.2
Liver with metastases	63.7
Liver metastases	138.5
Background lungs	12.2
Background abdomen	16.9

accumulations are observed in the pituitary (Fig. 4), in the thyroid, and in some cases in the mammae. Visualization of the gallbladder and the colon is inconsistent after 24 h p.i. It occurs very frequently in fasting patients or in patients with disturbed bile flow, as for example sludge. Colon visualization can be reduced but not completely prevented by giving laxatives.

Frequently, there is a weak demonstration of the articular joints (4 h p.i.), and the heart is regularly seen 4 h p.i. Since fresh surgical scars are often demonstrated, assessment in the surgical area is restricted to 3–6 months postoperatively (Fig. 5).

The imaging sequences after 4 and 24 h are reliable, in our opinion. Whereas a more favorable tumor/nontumor ratio is usually found on the 24-h image, assessment is rendered more difficult by colon visualization, less frequently also by visualization of other intestinal segments as well as the gallbladder. The disadvantages of intestinal activity and gallbladder demon-

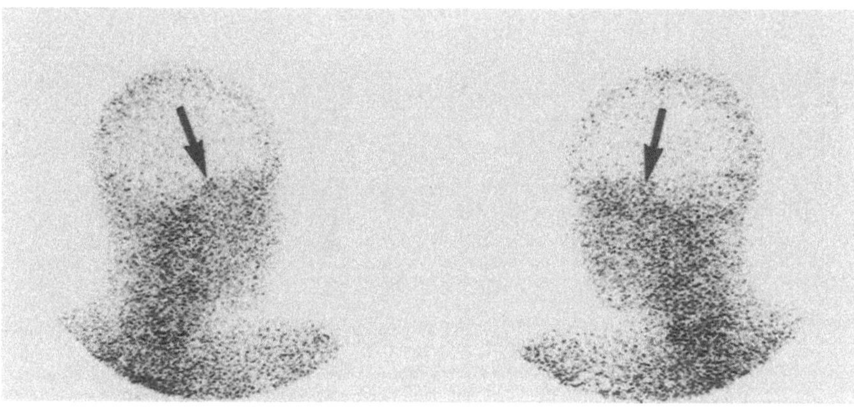

Fig. 4. Normal pituitary. Lateral views of head and neck at 4 h postinjection show a slight tracer uptake in pituitary (*arrow*)

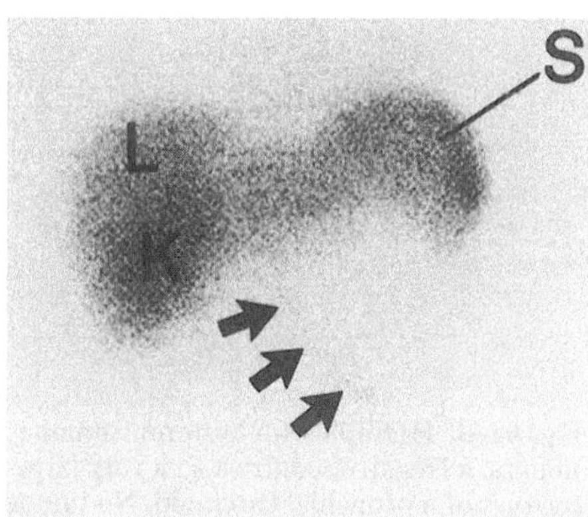

Fig. 5. Example of visualization of a scar. Anterior view of a patient with neuroendocrine tumor 2 weeks after nephrectomie. *L*, liver; *S*, spleen; *K*, right kidney

stration are hardly encountered in the 4-h image, which should result in optimal sensitivity and specificity, especially when imaging sequences are compared.

Problems in Assessing Scintigrams

Although assessability of scintigrams is very often unproblematic because of intensive accumulations, delineation problems may indeed occur with less intensive uptake (Fig. 6). The more difficult assessability in cases of colon and gallbladder visualization has already been discussed and can be largely eliminated by SPECT and a comparison of imaging sequences.

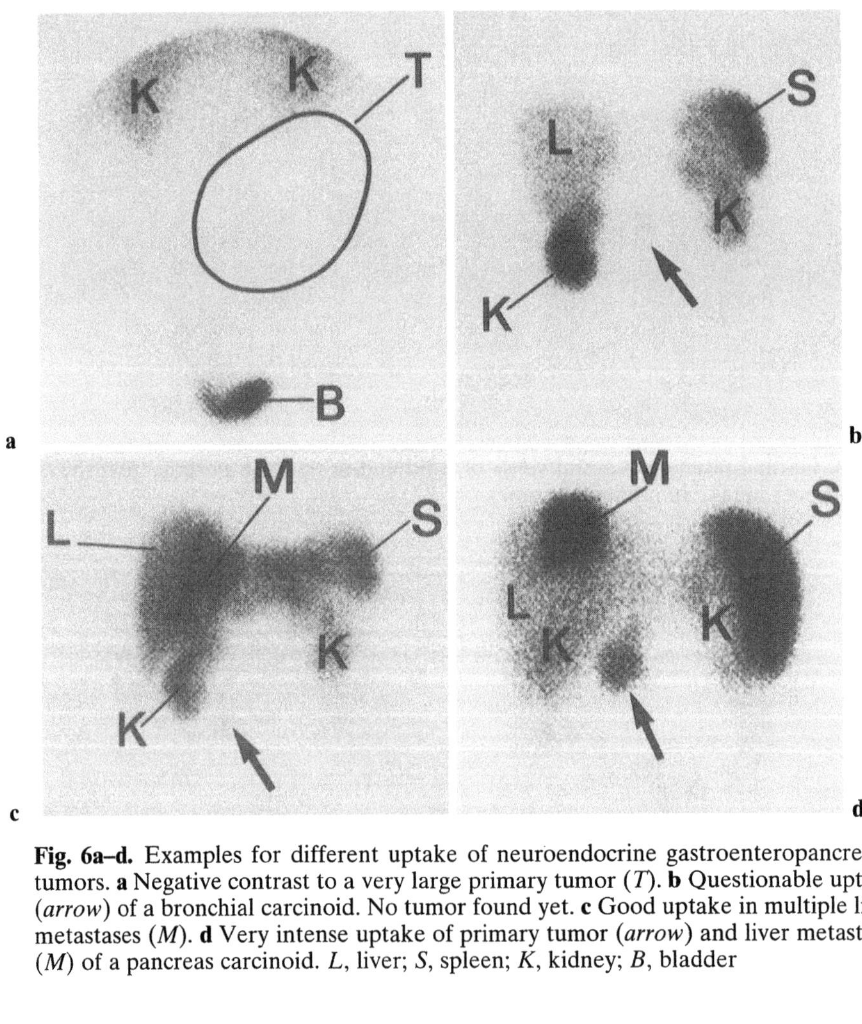

Fig. 6a–d. Examples for different uptake of neuroendocrine gastroenteropancreatic tumors. **a** Negative contrast to a very large primary tumor (*T*). **b** Questionable uptake (*arrow*) of a bronchial carcinoid. No tumor found yet. **c** Good uptake in multiple liver metastases (*M*). **d** Very intense uptake of primary tumor (*arrow*) and liver metastasis (*M*) of a pancreas carcinoid. *L*, liver; *S*, spleen; *K*, kidney; *B*, bladder

As a rule, somatostatin receptor scintigraphy allows only a statement on whether nonphysiological accumulation can be visualized with the present radiopharmacon. Nonphysiological accumulation may, however, be due to receptor binding of the tumor, another condition (see Table 1), or a disease with activated lymphocytes like sarcoidosis or tuberculosis (Lamberts et al. 1991). Enlarged lymph nodes in the common cold are apparently not visualized (Lamberts et al. 1991). Furthermore, postoperative demonstration of scars is also possible.

No pathological accumulation in the scintigram may indicate that there is no tumor, or a tumor that either has no somatostatin receptors or expresses the wrong somatostatin receptor subtype, as for example with insulinomas in 57% of the cases (Krenning et al. 1993; Lamberts et al. 1991).

The aforementioned reasons, in connection with a positive and negative somatostatin receptor scintigram, do not allow its application as a screening method. However, in a correspondingly selected patient group, false-positive findings, in the sense that another disease with positive somatostatin receptor status is detected instead of the targeted tumor, are very rare.

Neuroendocrine Gastroenteropancreatic Tumors

NEGEP tumors can be embryologically classified into foregut, midgut, and hindgut carcinoids (see Table 4), midgut carcinoids having a more favorable prognosis than the other two (Wiedenmann and Gregor 1991). Foregut carcinoids, a heterogeneous group, mainly of the pancreas, are classically subdivided according to their hormone secretion into insulinomas, gastrinomas, vipomas, glucagonomas, and somatostinomas, as well as functional nonactive tumors (Arnold et al. 1992).

Depending on the size, not more than 40–60% of hormone-active tumors are preoperatively diagnosed by sonography, CT, angiography, or MRI (Zimmer et al. 1994). With the exception of insulinomas, NEGEP tumors are usually malignant and have already metastasized at the time of diagnosis (Stefanini et al. 1974). Since localization of the primary tumor and its metastases is of decisive importance for curative or palliative surgical treatment, it is very desirable to use an imaging procedure with a high degree of sensitivity.

Table 4. Localization and classification of the carcinoids (Heitz and Klöppel 1987)

	Foregut carcinoid	Midgut carcinoid	Hindgut carcinoid
Localization	Bronchial system, thymus, esophagus, stomach, duodenum, pancreas	Jejunum, ileum, appendix, colon ascendens	Colon transversum, colon descendens, sigmoid, rectum, ovary

Results of Somatostatin Receptor Scintigraphy with In-111 Pentetreotide in NEGEP Tumors

In our own study of 74 patients with an immunohistologically confirmed NEGEP tumor, a sensitivity of 81.1% (60/74) was obtained with In-111 pentetreotide scintigraphy. Sensitivity is somewhat lower in foregut carcinoids at 65.5% best in the midgut region at 96.6% (28/29), and lies between the two for hindgut tumors in 80.0% (4/5). Scintigraphy was positive in 82% (9/11) of cases with a metastatic spread and an unknown primary tumor. Similar results were obtained by other study groups (Dörr et al. 1993; Höring et al. 1994; Joseph et al. 1993; Krenning et al. 1993, Scherübl et al. 1993). For a comparison, the results of the European multicenter study are given in Table 5.

Comparison of Somatostatin Receptor Scintigraphy and Other Imaging Procedures

Somatostatin receptor scintigraphy (SRS) was compared with the usual imaging procedures like sonography, computed tomography (CT), magnetic resonance imaging (MRI), and with endosonography in the foregut. Table 7 shows that SRS is the most sensitive procedure in the foregut after endosonography, and that none of the other procedures were superior to SRS in other primary tumor localizations, as can be seen in Table 6.

Table 5. Results of the European multicenter study (Dop 1994)

Diagnosis	*n*	Positive scintigraphy (%)
Carcinoid	182	87
Nonsecreting	60	82
Gastrinoma	67	73
Insulinoma	24	46
Others	14	93
Total	347	84

Table 6. Sensitivity of imaging technique depending on the primary tumor

Tumor	*n*	SRS	Sono	CT	MRI
Total	54	83.3	68.5	75.9	66.6
Foregut	23	65.2	47.8	52.2	52.2
Midgut	19	89.5	73.7	89.5	77.8
Hindgut	2	100	100	100	50
Unknown	10	100	100	100	90

The heterogeneous group of foregut carcinoids was separately evaluated in our study (Zimmer et al. 1994). The excellent sensitivity of endosonography in detecting even the smallest primary tumors (see Table 7) should be emphasized here, as well as the higher sensitivity of SRS compared with the conventional imaging procedures like sonography, CT, and MRI (Table 8).

Table 7. Comparison of sensitivities of various imaging procedures in detecting primary tumor lesions of neuroendocrine tumors depending on size and location (Zimmer et al. 1994)

Sensitivity [*n* (%)]	EUS	US	CT	MRI	SRS
Total	22/25 (88)	8/25 (32)	9/25 (36)	6/25 (24)	13/25 (52)
<2 cm	15/17 (88)	1/17 (6)	2/17 (12)	0/17 (0)	6/17 (35)
>2 cm	7/8 (87)	7/8 (87)	7/8 (87)	6/8 (75)	7/8 (87)
Pancreas	16/17 (94)	7/17 (41)	8/17 (47)	5/17 (29)	8/17 (47)
Extrapancreatic	6/8 (75)	1/8 (12)	1/8 (12)	1/8 (12)	5/8 (62)

EUS, Endoscopic ultrasound; *US*, ultrasound; *CT*, computed tomography; *MRI*, magnetic resonance imaging; *SRS*, somatostatin receptor scintigraphy

Table 8. Comparison of sensitivities of various imaging procedures in detecting primary tumor lesions of neuroendocrine tumors depending on functional state (Zimmer et al. 1994)

Sensitivity [*n* (%)]	EUS	US	CT	MRI	SRS
Total	22/25 (88)	8/25 (32)	9/25 (36)	6/25 (24)	13/25 (52)
Gastrinomas	4/5 (80)	3/5 (60)	3/5 (60)	3/5 (60)	5/5 (100)
Insulinomas	7/8 (87)	0/8 (0)	1/8 (12)	0/8 (0)	1/8 (12)
Carcinoids	1/1 (100)	1/1 (100)	1/1 (100)	1/1 (100)	1/1 (100)
Non-functional tumors	10/11 (91)	4/11 (36)	4/11 (36)	2/11 (18)	6/11 (54)

EUS, Endoscopic ultrasound; *US*, ultrasound; *CT*, computed tomography; *MRI*, magnetic resonance imaging; *SRS*, somatostatin receptor scintigraphy

New Findings

SRS enables the localization of tumors that cannot be demonstrated with any other procedure (Fig. 7). In this connection, the situation may occasionally arise that a positive finding in the SRS cannot be confirmed for a while by any other imaging technique, despite an intensive search. Thus, a separate evaluation of somatostatin receptor-positive findings in 19 of 61 patients showed no correlation in transabdominal ultrasound, CT, and MRI. However, when these patients were followed up at regular intervals, six of 19 examined at intervals of up to 24 months showed a correlated focal finding intraoperatively or in the conventional procedure (Faiss et al. 1994). In our study as well as in others, new tumor localizations were found in 30–40% of cases (Kwekkeboom et al. 1993; Joseph et al. 1993; Dörr et al. 1993; Pauwels et al. 1992).

False-negative Findings

In our own investigations, SRS yielded 20% false-negative findings compared with sonography, CT, and MRI (Scherübl et al. 1993). Other investigators found false-negative scintigrams in 10–20% of cases (Joseph et al. 1993; Dop 1994). Somatostatin receptors are detected by receptor autoradiography with

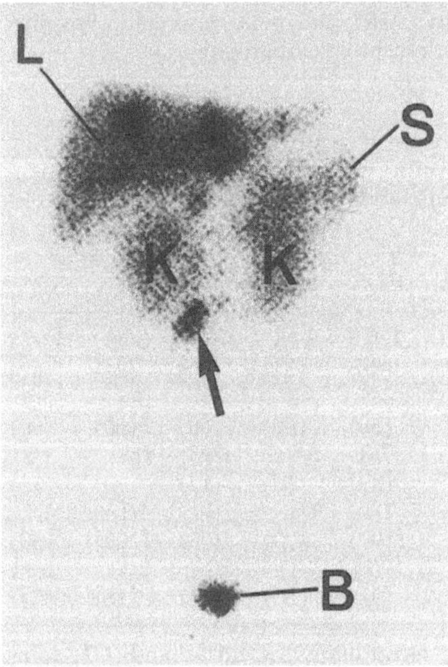

Fig. 7. Multiple liver metastases in gastrinoma of the duodenum (*arrow*). Anterior view 4h p.i.. Liver metastases had been missed by conventional ultrasonography, computed tomography, and magnetic resonance imaging. *L*, liver with multiple metastases; *S*, spleen; *K*, kidney; *B*, bladder

Tyr[3]-octreotide in 88% of pancreatic tumors (Reubi et al. 1987a) and in 87% of carcinoids. Because of the close correlation between receptor autoradiography with Tyr[3] octreotide and SRS (Lamberts et al. 1990b), it may be assumed that the false-positive findings in SRS are composed mainly of a larger portion of actual receptor-negative findings and to a smaller extent of findings that are either too small for visualization or whose receptor intensity is not strong enough compared with the surrounding area.

The Value of SRS in Whole-body Examinations

SRS differs considerably from other conventional imaging procedures by way of its whole-body character. Thus, SRS differs clearly not only from endosonography, which is methodologically limited to the areas of the abdomen, duodenum, pancreas, and surrounding lymph nodes, but also from other imaging procedures in the detection of all tumor localizations (Fig. 8).

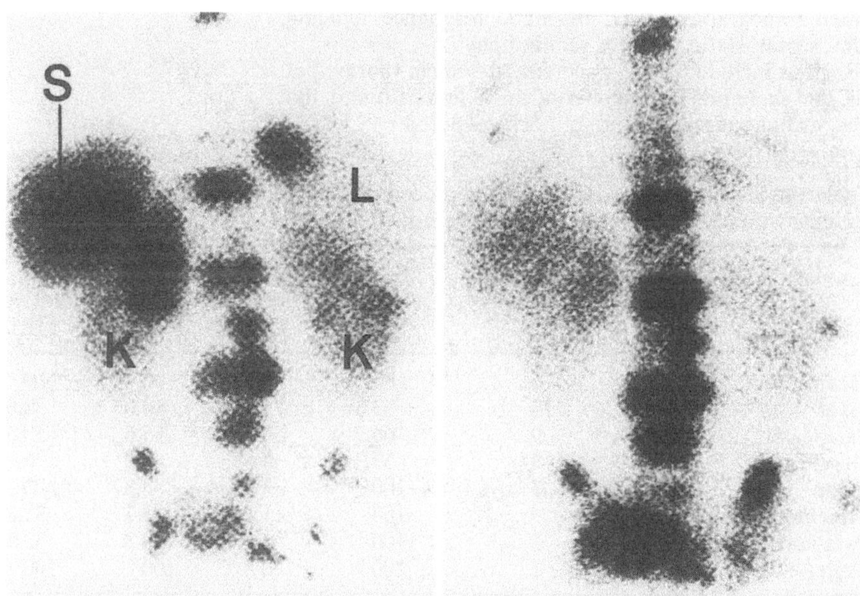

a b

Fig. 8a,b. Dual isotope scintigraphy in patient with pancreas carcinoid. **a** Posterior view of somatostatin receptor scintigraphy shows multiple bony metastases and other metastases in liver and tail of pancreas. **b** Bone scan that is done at the same time using a ^{99m}Tc-labeled diphosphonate. In **b** there are multiple bony metastases in spine, ribs, and pelvis. Note the slight visualization of spleen and liver caused by the ^{111}In-labeled pentetreotide, which is uncommon on bone scans

Evaluation of Tumor Regions

The value of SRS as a whole-body examination becomes obvious in an evaluation according to tumor regions. In this connection, tumor manifestations in 92 regions were detected in the first 56 patients examined by us. These regions included the liver, pancreas, abdomen, thorax, pelvis, and skeleton. The number of single lesions, as in liver and bone metastases, were not included here. Under these conditions, SRS proves to be clearly superior to all other procedures, with a sensitivity of 79% for all tumor regions (sonography 45%, CT 58%, MRI 45%, endosonography 30%) (Table 9). As shown in Table 10, SRS

Table 9. Sensitivity of various imaging procedures in whole-body diagnostics; evaluation of 92 tumor localizations in 56 patients[a]

	EUS	US	CT	MRI	SRS
Sensitivity (%)	30	45	58	45	79

EUS, Endoscopic ultrasound; *US*, ultrasound; *CT*, computed tomography; *MRI*, magnetic resonance imaging; *SRS*, somatostatin receptor scintigraphy
[a] Regions included: liver, pancreas, abdomen, thorax, pelvis, und skeleton. The number of single lesions found, like liver or bone metastases, were not considered

Table 10. Sensitivity of various imaging procedures for detection of tumor sites in 40 patients with 63 tumor localizations (Scherübl et al. 1993)

Localization of tumor	No. of patients	Sensitivity (%)			
		SRS	US[a]	CT	MRI
Mediastinum	5	80.0	ND	100[b]	ND
Liver	30	93.3	73.3	80.0	78.6[c]
Pancreas[d]	9	66.7	55.6	55.6	55.6
Duodenum[e]	3	33.3	0	0	0
Ileum	3	100	33.3	33.3	ND
Mesenteric lymph nodes	9	100	11.1	33.3	33.3
Para-aortic lymph nodes	3	100	0	33.3	33.3
Skeleton[f]	1	100	ND	100	100

ND, Not done
[a] Transabdominal ultrasonography
[b] In one patient CT was not performed because of noncompliance
[c] In two patients MRI was not possible because of claustrophobia
[d] In three patients the tumor was detectable only by endosonography
[e] In two patients the tumor was detectable only by endosonography
[f] The bony metastases (spine, pelvis, and femora) were first detected by SRS, and those in the spine were consecutively confirmed by CT and MRI

also had the highest sensitivity in the liver region (more than 90%), with the most frequent localization of metastases compared with other imaging procedures.

Hormone Status

An evaluation of 56 patients regarding scintigraphic detectability with respect to the hormone status yielded no significant difference between hormone-forming (79.3%) and functionally inactive (70.4%) GEP tumors. There was nevertheless a certain tendency favoring the visualization of functionally active tumors that could also be observed in conventional imaging procedures (Table 11).

Remarkable is the poor sensitivity of SRS in insulinomas (12.5% in our study group, 57% in the study by Krenning et al. 1992b), which has also been described by other study groups and agrees with the observation that insulinomas frequently express a receptor subtype which cannot be marked with short-chain somatostatin analogues (Lamberts et al. 1991).

Dependence on Size

In our prospective study of 18 patients with a total of 25 lesions and a primary epigastric tumor, the dependence of the imaging procedures on size was analyzed. In this context, endosonography was independent of size and hormone status (Table 7) and allowed tumor identification in 88% below and in 87% above a size of 2 cm. SRS, on the other hand, exhibited a clear size dependence with sensitivities of 35% and 87%, respectively. CT and MRI were of little value with tumors smaller than 2 cm and exhibited sensitivities of 12% and 0%, respectively. For visualization on the scintigram, the size of the lesion is less important than the intensity of the receptor density. Thus, it is possible to visualize tumor foci as small as approximately 0.5 cm with sufficiently intensive receptor density (Gadiot et al. 1993); other sources give a lower limit of 1 cm (Joseph et al. 1993).

Table 11. Dependence of various imaging procedures on the functional activity of NEGEP tumors in 56 patients

Method	Hormone-producing (%)	Functionally inactive (%)
SRS	23/29 (79.3)	19/27 (70.4)
Sonography	22/29 (75.8)	15/27 (55.6)
CT	23/29 (79.3)	18/27 (66.7)
MRI	23/29 (79.3)	12/25 (48)[a]

[a] In two patients with functionally inactive tumors, MRI was not possible because of claustrophobia

Intraoperative Tumor Localization with a Gamma Probe

Multiple metastases are frequently found with NEGEP tumors. The SRS is very well suited as a whole-body examination for detecting hitherto unknown tumor localizations, especially cervical, mediastinal, or abdominal lymph nodes. The intraoperative localization of smaller tumors may be very problematic, for example, when it is necessary to differentiate between metastasized and normal lymph nodes. This clinical problem, as well as the frequently intensive somatostatin receptor accumulation on neuroendocrine tumors, makes it desirable to use a gamma probe for intraoperative differentiation between tumor and normal tissue.

Selverstone et al. (1949) were the first to report on the intraoperative application of radioactivity-measuring probes for the detection of brain tumors. Survey studies by Woolfenden and Barber (1989) and Perkins (1993) discuss the development, possible area of application, presently available industrially produced gamma probes, and the requirements made on the radiopharmaceutical used and the gamma probe.

The most likely area in which gamma probes are now applied was described by Colton and Hardy (1983) in connection with the osteid osteoma. The gamma probe permits exact intraoperative localization of the nidus and thus complete tumor removal with the least loss of bone mass (Kirchner et al. 1993). Moreover, the method is applied with radioactively marked antibodies against tumor cells and is called here radioimmunoguided surgery (RIGS) (Sardi et al. 1989).

We report in this paper on the intraoperative application of a gamma probe in a patient with a metastasized gastrinoma. Figure 9 shows SRS in a 37-year-old patient with a large neuroendocrine, gastrin-producing pancreatic-head tumor. Two small dorsal and ventral accumulations in the liver were visualized additionally. Remarkable is the gallbladder visualization 27 h p.i. in the parenterally fed patient which caused no more interference 56 h p.i. Further imaging (ultrasound, CT, MRI) did not confirm the suspicion of liver metastases. Both intraoperative liver sonography and palpation carried out in connection with the partial pancreatic resection yielded no sign of liver metastases. The histological examination of the resected pancreas tumor confirmed the diagnosis of a gastrinoma. Follow-up examinations with conventional imaging techniques in the first postoperative year yielded no results. Two years postoperatively, another complete staging was carried out in connection with a persistently pathological secretin test. The CT with and without contrast application provided no evidence of liver metastases. An MRI was initially also without findings. Only a spiral CT performed subsequently with contrasting of the hepatic arteries via an indwelling angiographic catheter revealed a focus in the right caudal dorsal liver lobe (Fig. 10b). This localization corresponds exactly to the increased accumulation described 2 years earlier with SRS. The scintigraphic course control revealed constant foci that were also well correlated to the CT by emission computed tomography (Fig.

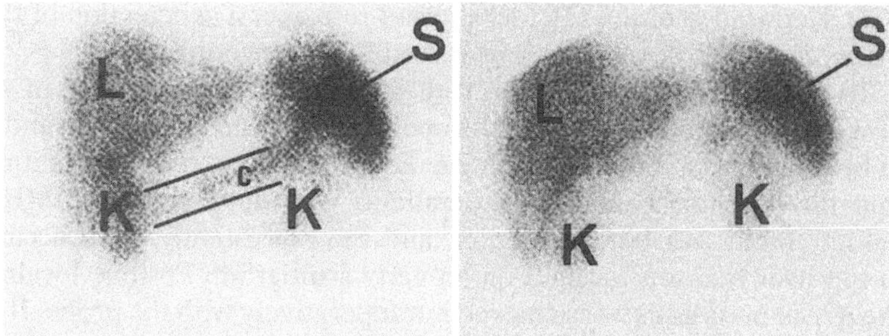

a b

Fig. 9a,b. Anterior view 27h p.i. **a** A great primary tumor of gastrinoma and tracer accumulation of the gallbladder. The gallbladder can not be seen 56h p.i. **b** A small ventral metastasis is still visible. Pronounced gallbladder visualization is caused by intravenous nutrition

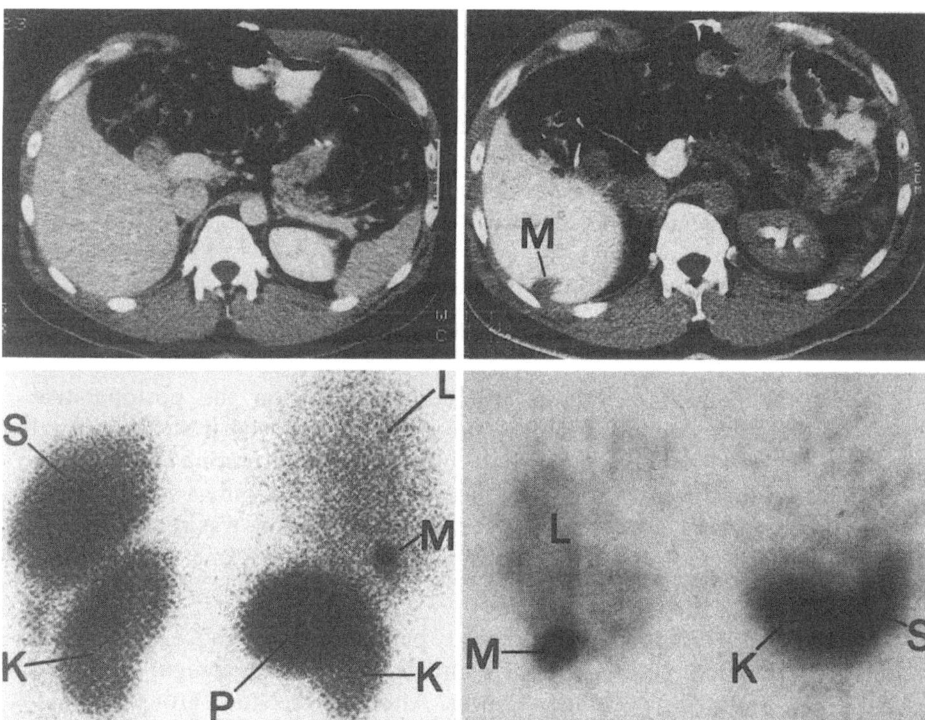

a b c d

Fig. 10a–d. Metastasis (*M*) of a gastrinoma can be clearly seen (**c**) in the dorsal right caudal liver lobe. *L*, liver; *S*, spleen; *K*, kidney; *P*, primary tumor. This metastasis could also be localized only when 24 months later a spiral computed tomography (CT) was performed (*M* in **b**). The CT at time of first scintigraphy was negative (**a**): **d** Corresponding transversel slice on single photon emission computed tomography which shows metastasis (*M*) exact at the same localization as spiral CT (**b**)

10d). Knowledge of the CT foci allowed retrospective detection of the dorsal foci in the MRI. A ventral focus was still not detectable.

In this situation, reoperation with intraoperative application of a gamma probe was planned. The aim of the operation was the localization and removal of both accumulations detectable on the somatostatin receptor scintigram and thus the potential healing of the patient. We administered 220 MBq In-111 pentetreotide 24 h before surgery, and the consistently good accumulation in the liver foci was verified on an early scintigram. Positive localization of the dorsal metastasis was achieved intraoperatively with the probe. It revealed 800 counts per second compared with 300 counts per second (tumor to nontumor ratio: 2.7/1) in the area of the surrounding liver tissue. This focus was also localized by palpation and by intraoperative ultrasound. The ventral focus could not be localized by the probe. The intraoperative ultrasound examination revealed no further focus. Considering the scintigram, a ventral palpation finding right above the former gallbladder bed was also questionable in the presence of a condition after cholecystectomy. However, palpation was rendered more difficult due to scarring in the former gallbladder bed. The histological examination yielded neuroendocrine tumor cells in this case as well.

Somatostatin receptor scintigraphy was performed 2 days postoperatively as a control. The dorsal focus was no longer detectable (Fig. 11b,d). However, demonstration of the ventral focus was practically unchanged (Fig. 11a,c). Ex vivo compared with in vivo measurements yielded a considerably higher tumor to nontumor ratio (dorsal focus to normal liver = 24:1, ventral tissue removal to normal liver = 5:1).

The following conclusions can be drawn:

1. The dorsal focus was exactly localized with the intraoperative gamma probe.
2. Since the ventral focus was still demonstrable on the postoperative scintigram, and tumor tissue was nevertheless removed from the ventral area, it may be concluded that either a somatostatin-receptor-poor metastasis of the gastrin-forming tumor was found, or only a small portion of the metastasis, appearing as a ventral accumulation, was removed.
3. Somatostatin receptor scintigraphy is suitable for postoperative therapy control.

Ahlmann et al. (1994) report in a recently published paper about their experience with the intraoperative use of a gamma probe in five foregut carcinoids and in two endocrine pancreatic tumors. Although the study group also successfully localized liver metastases, Ahlmann et al. describe probe-guided localizations in the abdomen as particularly difficult, due to the very high background activity of the liver, spleen, and kidneys. A less difficult localization was achieved in the pelvis, especially in cervical lymph nodes. Intraoperative measurements underestimated the tumor to nontumor ratio in smaller tumors. The operations were carried out 24 h, 48 h, or 120 h after the injection of In-111 pentetreotide. A reliable statement on the optimal time

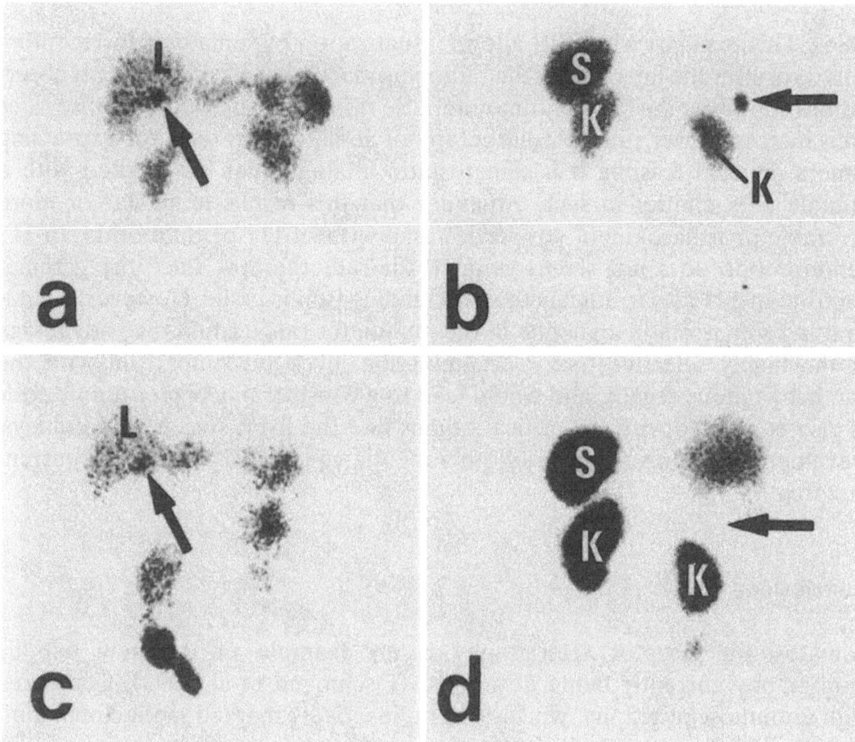

Fig. 11a–d. Anterior (**a**) and posterior (**b**) scintigraphic view before operation. *Arrow* shows ventral metastasis in (**a**) and dorsal metastasis in (**b**). *L*, liver. **c** Anterior view postoperatively still shows ventral metastasis (*arrow*). **d** Posterior view after operation no longer shows uptake where metastasis was removed (*arrow*)

interval could not be made; the relation between tumor activity and surroundings was not significantly changed.

Further experience is necessary for a better assessment of the value, the special areas of indication, and the effort required for the intraoperative use of the gamma probe in cases of NEGEP tumors. The following questions are still unanswered: Can very small tumors that were not even detected with the most sensitive scintigraphy be localized intraoperatively with the gamma probe? If so, how often does this happen, and does it justify application of the probe in specific constellations? Is it possible to deduce a quantitative criterion from the preoperative scintigram which can predict the probability of intraoperative probe localization?

Therapy with Radioactively Marked Somatostatin Analogues

It has been shown in animal experiments that somatostatin is introduced in the cell via the somatostatin membrane receptors (Draznin et al. 1985; Morel et al.

1986). This explains why SRS allows visualization of somatostatin receptors cells days after the injection of the radiopharmaceutical agent. Our own observations show that the ratio of tumor impulse rates to background impulse rates even increases over time. Radiotherapy of somatostatin receptor-expressing tumors appears feasible if a somatostatin analogue can be marked with a suitable beta emitter in such a manner that this results in similar or more favorable pharmacokinetic properties than with In-111 pentetreotide. In-111 pentetreotide does not seems suitable for radiotherapy, since the gamma-emitting In-111 also irradiates the surrounding tumor tissue. However, a beta-emitting somatostatin analogue in the millimeter range could take advantage of the highly selective tumor accumulation, even in comparison with the parenchymatous organs, and would lead to a considerably higher tumor dosis as also compared with the critical organs like the liver, spleen, and kidneys. Development of this type of radiotherapeutic agents is the subject of current research.

Conclusions

Somatostatin receptor scintigraphy is an example of the new peptide scintigraphy currently being developed (Fischmann et al. 1993). Compared with immunoscintigraphy, which uses radioactively marked monoclonal antibodies and fragments, the great advantage of peptide scintigraphy is a considerably smaller molecule size. This smaller molecule size results in a markedly shorter half-life in the blood vessels and thus in relatively little background activity.

Somatostatin receptor scintigraphy with In-111 pentetreotide is a highly sensitive imaging technique for the diagnosis of NEGEP tumors. It is suitable for primary tumor localization, staging, and course control. A prerequisite for visualization is the expression of somatostatin receptors with a high affinity for short-chain somatostatin analogues. In NEGEP tumors, this high in vitro affinity is given in about 88% of the cases. Correspondingly, a sensitivity of 84% is being reported in studies with a greater number of cases.

In whole-body examinations, SRS is particularly important for dissemination diagnostics. Current experience shows that the metastases of receptor-positive primary tumors are also receptor positive. SRS cannot be applied as the only procedure because of the possibility of receptor-negative tumors. When necessary, it is complemented by other imaging techniques such as sonography, CT, and MRI. However, it should be applied relatively early after the diagnosis of a neuroendocrine gastroenteropancreatic tumor, since the complementary examination procedures can then be specifically applied. Endosonography is the most sensitive procedure for localizing primary tumors, but not their metastases, in the abdomen, pancreas, and duodenum.

Identification of a positive somatostatin receptor status can possibly predict the therapeutic success with octreotide in inhibiting tumor hormone production (Lamberts et al. 1990a). Although an antiproliferative effect in NEGEP tumors has been confirmed, the results obtained thus far in a small patient group speak against the predictive value of SRS with respect to an antiproliferative effect in human beings (Joseph et al. 1993).

The following may be regarded as an indication for somatostatin receptor scintigraphy: Localization of a primary tumor and metastases in connection with whole-body scintigraphy, as well as therapy and course control in a confirmed or highly probable neuroendocrine gastroenteropancreatic tumor. The clinical value of, as well as the special indications for, intraoperative tumor localization with a radioisotope-guided gamma probe have to be confirmed in studies with a greater number of cases.

Because of highly selective tumor accumulation, radiotherapy with a beta emitter-marked somatostatin analogue appears possible. However, such a substance does not exist at the present time.

References

Ahlman H, Wängberg B, Tisell LE, Nilsson O, Fjälling M, Forssell-Aronsson E (1994) Clinical efficacy of octreotide scintigraphy in patients with midgut carcinoid tumors and evaluation of intraoperative scintillation detection. Br J Surg 81:1144–1149

Amherdt M, Patel YC, Orci L (1987) Selective binding of somatostatin-14 and somatostatin-28 to islet cells revealed by quantitative electron microscopic autoradiography. J Clin Invest 80:1455–1458

Arnold R, Neuhaus C, Trautmann ME (1992) Therapie endokriner gastroenteropankreatischer Tumoren mit dem Somatostatin-Analogon Octreotid. Dtsch Med Wochenschr 117:1067–1071

Bakker WH, Albert R, Bruns C, Breeman WAP, Hofland LJ, Marbach P, Pless J, Pralet D, Stolz B, Koper JW, Lamberts SWJ, Visser TJ, Krenning EP (1991a) [In-111-DTPA-D-Phe[1]]-Octreotide, a potential radiopharmaceutical for imaging of somatostatin receptor-positive tumors: synthesis, radiolabeling and in vitro validation. Life Sci 49:1583–1591

Bakker WH, Krenning EP, Breeman WAP, Kooij PPM, Reubi JC, Koper JW, de Jong M, Lameris JS, Visser TJ, Lamberts SWJ (1991b) In vivo use of a radioiodinated somatostatin analogue: dynamics, metabolism and binding to somatostatin receptor-positive tumors in man. J Nucl Med 32:1184–1189

Bakker WH, Krenning EP, Breeman WAP, Koper JW, Kooij PPM, Reubi JC, Klijn JGM, Visser TJ, Docter R, Lamberts SWJ (1990) Receptor scintigraphy with a radioiodinated somatostatin analogue: radiolabeling, purification, biological activity and in vivo applications in animals. J Nucl Med 31:1501–1509

Bauer W, Briner U, Doepfner W, Haller R, Huguenin R, Marbach P, Peteher TJ, Pless J (1982) SMS 201-995: a very potent and selective octapeptide analogue of somatostatin with prolonged action. Life Sci 31:1133–1140

Colton CL, Hardy JG (1983) Evaluation of a sterilizable radiation probe as an aid to the surgical treatment of osteoid-osteoma. J Bone Joint Surg (BR) 65:1019–1022

Dop F-J (1994) The European multicentre clinical trial group on GEP neuroendocrine tumors. J Nucl Med 35:96P

Dörr U, Räth U, Schürmann G, Höring E, Bach D, Wurm K, Scholz M, Adrian HJ, Bihl H (1993) Somatostatin-Rezeptor-Szintigraphie. Ein neues bildgebendes Verfahren zum spezifischen Nachweis von Dünndarmkarzinoiden. Fortschr Röntgenstr 158:67–73

Draznin B, Sherman N, Sussman KE, Dahl R, Vatter R (1985) Internalization and cellular processing of somatostatin in primary culture of rat anterior pituitary cells. Endocrinology 117:960

Enjalbert A, Tapia-Arancibia L, Rieutort M et al (1982) Somatostatin receptors on rat anterior pituitary membranes. Endocrinology 110:1634–1640

Faiss S, Scherübl H, Bäder M, Fett U, Koppenhagen K, Wiedenmann B, Riecken EO (1994) Bedeutung falsch-positiver Befunde in der Diagnostik neuroendokriner Tumoren des gastroenteropankreatischen Systems. Z Gastroenterol 32:243–246

Fischmann AJ, Babick JW, Strauss HW (1993) A ticket to ride: peptide radiopharmaceuticals. J Nucl Med 34:2253–2263

Gadiot G, de Kerviler E, Le Guludec D, Camhaji B, Sobhani I, Ruszniewski P, Mignon M (1993) In patients with the Zollinger-Ellison syndrome (ZES) the main interest of somatostatin receptor scintigraphy (SRS) is to detect previously unknown metastases. Gastroenterology 104:A298

Heiman ML, Murphy WA, Coy DH (1987) Differential binding of somatostatin agonists to somatostatin receptors in brain and adenohypophysis. Neuroendocrinology 45:429

Heitz P, Klöppel G (1987) Endokrine Tumoren des Pankreas und des Duodenum. Verh Dtsch Ges Pathol 71:202–221

Höring E, Räth U, Rücker S, von Gaisberg U, Meincke J, Walendzik J, Dörr U, Bihl H (1994) Somatostatinrezeptor-Szintigraphie in der Primärdiagnostik und Nachsorge bei Gastrinomen. Dtsch Med Wochenschr 119:367–374

Joseph K, Stapp J, Reinecke J, Skamel HJ, Höffken H, Neuhaus C, Lenze H, Trautmann ME, Arnold R (1993) Receptor scintigraphy with ^{111}In-pentetreotide for endocrine gastroenteropancreatic tumors. Hormone Metab Res 27 [Suppl]:28–35

Kirchner B, Hillman A, Lottes G, Sciuk J, Bartenstein P, Winkelmann W, Schober O (1993) Intraoperative, probe-guided curettage of osteid osteoma. Eur J Nucl Med 20:609–613

Kluxen F, Bruns C, Lübbert H (1992) Expression cloning of a rat brain somatostatin receptor cDNA. Proc Natl Acad Sci U S A 89:4618–4622

Krenning EP, Bakker WH, Breeman WAP, Koper JW, Kooij PPM, Ausema L, Lameris JS, Lamberts SWJ (1989) Localization of endocrine related tumors with radioiodinated analogue of somatostatin. Lancet 1:242–245

Krenning EP, Bakker WH, Kooij PPM, Breeman WAP, Oei HY, de Jong M, Reubi J-C, Visser TJ, Bruns C, Kwekkeboom DJ, Reijs AEM, van Hagen PM, Koper JW, Lamberts SWJ (1992a) Somatostatin receptor scintigraphy with Indium-111-DTPA-D-Phe-1-octreotide in man: metabolism, dosimetry and comparison with Iodine-123-Tyr-3-octreotide. J Nucl Med 33:652–658

Krenning EP, Kwekkeboom DJ, Oei HY, Reubi JC, van Hagen PM, Kooij PPM, Reijs AEM, Lamberts SWJ (1992b) Somatostatin receptor imaging of endocrine gastrointestinal tumors. Schweiz Med Wochenschr 122:634–637

Krenning EP, Kwekkeboom DJ, Reubi J-C, van Hagen PM, van Eijck CHJ, Oei HY, Lambers SWJ (1993) ^{111}In-Octreotide scintigraphy in oncology. Digestion 54 [Suppl 1]:84–87

Kwekkeboom DJ, Krenning EP, Bakker WH. Oei HY, Kooij PPM, Lamberts SWJ (1993) Somatostatin analogue scintigraphy in carcinoid tumours. Eur J Nucl Med 20:283–292

Lamberts SWJ, Bakker WH, Reubi J-C, Krenning EP (1990a) Somatostatin-receptor imaging in the localization of endocrine tumors. N Engl J Med 232:1246

Lamberts SWJ, Hofland LJ, van Koetsveld PM, Reubi J-C, Bruining HA, Bakker WH, Krenning EP (1990b) Parallel in vivo and in vitro detection of functional somatostatin receptors in human endocrine pancreatic tumors: consequences with regard to diagnosis, localization and therapy. J Clin Endocrinol Metab 71:566

Lamberts SWJ, Krenning EP, Reubi J-C (1991) The role of somatostatin and its analogs in the diagnosis and treatment of tumors. Endocr Rev 12:450–482
Markstein R, Stoeckli KA, Reubi J-C (1989) Differential effects of somatostatin on adenylate cyclase as functional correlates for different brain somatostatin receptor subpopulations. Neurosci Lett 104:13
Morel G, Pelletier G, Heisler S (1986) Internalization and subcellular distribution of radiolabeled somatostatin-28 in mouse anterior pituitary tumor cells. Endocrinology 119:1972
O'Caroll AM, Lolait SJ, König M, Mahan LC (1992) Molecular cloning and expression of a pituitary somatostatin receptor with preferential affinity for somatostatin-28. Mol Pharmacol 42:939–946
Patel YC, Murthy KK, Escher EE, Banville D, Spiess J, Srikant CB (1990) Mechanism of action of somatostatin: an overview of receptor function and studies of the molecular characterization and purification of somatostatin receptor proteins. Metabolism 39:63–69
Pauwels S, Jamar F, Leners N, Fiasse R (1992) Efficacy of ^{111}In-pentetreotide scintigraphy in endocrine gastroentero-pancreatic (GEP) tumors. Gastroenterology 102:A387
Perkins A (1993) Perioperative nuclear medicine. Editorial. Eur J Nucl Med 20:573–575
Reichlin, S (1983) Somatostatin. N Engl J Med 309:1495–1501, 1556–1563
Reubi J-C (1984) Evidence of two somatostatin-14 receptor types in rat brain cortex. Neurosci Lett 49:259
Reubi J-C, Landolt AM (1984) High density of somatostatin receptors in pituitary tumors from acromegalic patients. J Clin Endocrinol Metab 59:1148–1151
Reubi J-C, Maurer R (1985) Antoradiographic mapping of somatostatin receptors in the rat central nervous system and pituitary. Neuroscience 15:1183–1193
Reubi J-C, Perrin M, Rivier J et al (1981) High affinity binding sites for a somatostatin-28 analog in rat brain. Life Sci 28:2191–2198
Reubi J-C, Häcki WH, Lamberts SWJ (1987a) Hormone-producing gastrointestinal tumors contain a high density of somatostatin receptors. J Clin Endocrinol Metab 65:1127–1134
Reubi J-C, Probst A, Cortes R, Palacios JM (1987b) Distinct topographical localisation of two somatostatin receptor subpopulations in the human cortex. Brain Res 406:391
Reubi J-C, Krenning E, Lamberts SWJ, Kvols L (1990a) Somatostatin receptors in malignant tissues. J Steroid Biochem Mol Biol 37:1073–1077
Reubi J-C, Kvols L, Krenning E, Lamberts SWJ (1990b) Distribution of somatostatin receptors in normal and tumor tissue. Metabolism 39 [Suppl 2]:78–81
Reubi J-C, Kvols LK, Waser B, Nagorney DM, Heitz PU, Charboneau JW, Reading CC, Moertel CG (1990c) Detection of somatostatin receptors in surgical and percutaneous needle biopsy samples of carcinoids and islet cell carcinomas. Cancer Res 50:5960
Reubi J-C, Maurer R, von Werder K, Torhorst J, Klijn JGM, Lamberts SWJ (1990d) Somatostatin receptors in human endocrine tumors. Cancer Res 47:551–558
Rohrer L, Raulf F, Bruns C, Buettner R, Hofstaedter F, Schüle R (1993) Cloning and characterization of a fourth human somatostatin receptor. Proc Natl Acad Sci U S A 90:4196–4200
Sardi A, Workman M, Mojzisik C, Hinkle G, Nieroda C, Martin EW (1989) Intraabdominal recurrence of colorectal cancer detected by radioimmunoguided surgery (RIGS system). Arch Surg 124:55–59
Scherübl H, Bäder M, Fett U, Hamm B, Schmidt-Gayk R, Koppenhagen K, Dop F-J, Riecken EO, Wiedenmann B (1993) Somatostatin-receptor imaging of neuroendo-

crine gastroenteropancreatic tumors. A new, diagnostically relevant procedure. Gastroenterology 105:1705–1709
Schönbrunn A, Tashjian A (1978) Characterization of functional receptors for somatostatin in rat pituitary cells in culture. J Biol Chem 253:6483
Selverstone B, Sweet WH, Robinson CV (1949) The clinical use of radioactive phosphorous in the surgery of brain tumors. Ann Surg 130:643–651
Sreedharan SP, Kodama KT, Peterson KE, Goetzl EJ (1989) Distinct subsets of somatostatin receptors on cultured human lymphocytes. J Biol Chem 264:949–953
Srikant CB, Patel YC (1981) Receptor binding of somatostatin-28 is tissue specific. Nature 294:259–260
Srikant CB, Patel YC (1986) Somatostatin receptors on rat pancreatic acinar cells. Pharmacological and structural characterization and demonstration of down regulation in streptozotocin diabetes. J Biol Chem 261:7690–7696
Srikant CB, Patel YC (1987) Somatostatin receptor: evidence for structural and functional heterogeneity. In: Reichlin S (ed) Somatostatin, basic and clinical aspects. Plenum, New York, pp 89–102
Stefanini P, Carboni M, Patrassi N, Basoli A (1974) Beta-islet tumors of the pancreas: results of a study on 1067 cases. Surgery 75:597
Van Noorden S, Polak JM, Pearse AGE (1977) Single cellular origin of somatostatin and calcitonin in the rat thyroid gland. Histochemistry 53:243–247
Viguerie N, Tahiri-Jouti N, Esteve JP et al (1988) Fuctional somatostatin receptors on a rat pancreatic acinar cell line. Am J Physiol 255:G113–G120
Wang HL, Bogen C, Reisine T, Dichter M (1989) Somatostatin-14 and somatostatin-28 induce opposite effects on potassium currents in rat neocortical neurons. Proc Natl Acad Sci U S A 86:16
Weckbecker G, Raulf F, Stolz B, Bruns C (1993) Somatostatin analogs for diagnosis and treatment of cancer. Pharmacol Ther 60:245–264
Wiedenmann B, Gregor M (1991) Empfehlungen zur Diagnostik und Therapie von Karzinoiden (Neuroendokrinen epithelialen Tumoren) im Raum Berlin. Berl Arztebl 104:182–183
Woolfenden JM, Barber BH (1989) Radiation detector probes for tumor localization using tumor-seeking radioactive tracers. Am J Roentgenol 153:35–39
Yamada Y, Ito S, Matsubara Y, Kobayashi S (1977) Immunohistochemical demonstration of somatostatin-containing cells in the human, dog and rat thyroids. Tohoku J Exp Med 122:87–92
Yamada Y, Post SR, Wang K, Tager HS, Bell GI, Seino S (1992a) Cloning and functional characterization of a family of human and mouse somatostatin receptors expressed in brain, gastrointestinal tract and kidney. Proc Natl Acad Sci U S A 89:251–255
Yamada Y, Reisine T, Law SF, Ihara Y, Kubota A, Kagimoto S, Seino M, Seino Y, Bell GI, Seino S (1992b) Somatostatin receptors, an expanding gene family: cloning and functional characterization of human SSTR3, a protein coupled to adenylyl cyclase. Mol Endocrinol 6:2136–2142
Zimmer T, Ziegler K, Bäder M, Fett U, Hamm B, Riecken E-O, Wiedenmann B (1994) Localisation of neuroendocrine tumors of the upper gastrointestinal tract. Gut 35:471–475

III. Therapeutic Approaches

Basis and Consequences of Primary and Secondary Prevention of Gastrointestinal Tumors

P. Goldin-Lang[1], E-D. Kreuser[2], and H.J.F. Zunft[1]

1 Department of Epidemiology and Nutritional Behavior, German Institute of Human Nutrition, Arthur-Scheunert-Allee 114-116, 14558 Bergholz-Rehbruecke, Germany
2 Department of Hematology and Oncology, Klinikum Benjamin Franklin, Free University of Berlin, Hindenburgdamm 30, 12200 Berlin, Germany

Abstract

Carcinomas of the gastrointestinal tract (GI) are among the most common malignancies with regard to their incidence and mortality. Nutritional factors play an important role in the tumor development. The strength of their influence varies with the localization in the GI tract. Epidemiological studies focusing on GI cancer incidence or mortality as an endpoint necessitate large numbers of subjects to achieve significant results. Generally, a low energy and fat intake and a high intake of antioxidative vitamins (vitamin C, E, β-carotene) and secondary plant metabolites (especially polyphenols) appear to be protective in GI carcinogenesis. Moderate drinking of alcohol and increased consumption of whole grain products, as opposed to highly refined carbohydrates, may help to reduce the risk of colon cancer. The recommended type of diet is low in fat, especially in saturated fatty acids, includes monounsaturated fatty acids, and includes moderate amounts of polyunsaturated fatty acids (no more than 10% of calories). Moderate consumption of salt and of highly salted, smoked, and barbecued foods should be encouraged. Obesity should be avoided by trying to match energy intake with expenditure while increasing physical activity levels. The mechanisms by which nutritional factors act especially on molecular events still remain to be examined. The use of molecular biomarkers will help us better understand cancer development as well as the role and significance of nutritional factors in this process.

Introduction

Gastrointestinal cancer, especially colorectal cancer (CRC), is one of the most common malignancies worldwide (Shike et al. 1990). Nutrition is widely ac-

Recent Results in Cancer Research, Vol. 142

cepted to be among the most important exogenous factors influencing carcinogenesis in gastrointestinal organs (oral cavity, pharynx, esophagus, stomach, colon, rectum) (Cheah 1990; Weisburger 1991; Nair and Mayberry 1994).

The incidence of cancers shows a marked geographic variation. The rates of CRC, for example, are as much as ten times higher in industrialized countries than in developing nations. This fact is suggested to reflect environmental differences, including nutritional factors (Stemmermann 1989). Moreover, the tumor rate changes with alterations in lifestyle. This is obvious from the increasing westernization of Japan after World War II and the migration of Japanese to Hawaii. Both these events have resulted in substantial dietary, social, and economic changes. The changes in dietary practice are an increased consumption of fat and protein and a decreased consumption of complex carbohydrates.

Based of various kinds of studies, it has been suggested that several food components are involved in the process of gastrointestinal carcinogenesis, having either a procarcinogenic (dietary fat, red meat, and alcohol) or a protective (calcium, vitamin D, fruits, and vegetables) effect. However, carcinogenesis is a multifactorial event, and numerous etiologic factors act together to produce the final outcome. Some factors may be causative, others enhancing and promoting or protective. To estimate the role of these causative and modifying factors and their relationship, a multidisciplinary approach is essential to acquire a complete data base using investigations in man, in animal models, and in relevant laboratory studies.

First, information is obtained with epidemiological studies investigating geographic pathology, special populations, and time trends. Second, results are obtained from laboratory studies comparing the epidemiological with metabolic and biochemical data on high- and low-risk populations, followed by comparative studies in animal models and/or cell and organ cultures. Third, there is a need to develop hypotheses and to define mechanisms, based both on established risk factors and their mode of action and on suspected risk factors and their possible role. Finally, intervention programs have to be designed and applied to control promoting or enhancing agents and to use protective or inhibiting factors.

Epidemiological Evidence on Food Components, Exposition Factors, and Gastrointestinal Cancer

Epidemiological studies have revealed that there are several environmental factors influencing the cancer risk at different locations in the intestinal tract. The results of more recent studies are summarized in Table 1. General trends are supported by several studies.

Table 1. Epidemiological studies (1990–1995) of nutrient and non-nutrient exposure and risk of GI cancer

Exposure	Study design	Association between exposure and outcome	Target organ	References
Total energy intake	Case-control	Positive	Colon, rectum	Peters et al. 1992
Total (animal) fat	Case-control	Posistive	Esophagus, stomach	Kabat et al. 1993
	Case-control	Positive	Stomach	Gonzalez et al. 1994
	Case-control	No association	Stomach	Tuyns et al. 1992
Bread, sweets, salted and cured meat, smoked and fried food, fermented beans	Case-control	Positive	Stomach	Lee et al. 1990
	Case-control	Positive	Stomach	Boeing et al. 1991
	Case-control	Positive	Colon, rectum	Peters et al. 1992
Lean meat	Case-control	Negative	Stomach	Tuyns et al. 1992
Cholesterol	Case-control	Positive	Stomach	Gonzalez et al. 1994
	Case-control	Positive	Colon, rectum	Zaridze et al. 1993
Oil with high P/S ratio	Case-control	Negative	Stomach	Tuyns et al. 1992
PUFA	Case-control	Negative	Colon, rectum	Zaridze et al. 1993
Crude fiber	Case-control	Negative	Distal esophagus/cardia	Kabat et al. 1993
	Case-control	Negative	Ascending colon	Peters et al. 1992
Fiber, sucrose	Case-control	No association	Colon, rectum	Peters et al. 1992
Cereal fiber	Case-control	Negative	Colon, rectum	Arbman et al. 1992
Grain, flour products, white bread, sugar	Case-control	Positive	Stomach	Tuyns et al. 1992
	Case-control	Negative	Stomach	Lee et al. 1990
	Case-control	Negative	Colon, rectum	Zaridze et al. 1993
Whole meal bread	Case-control	Negative	Stomach	Boeing et al. 1991
Calcium	Case-control	Negative	Colon	Arbman et al. 1992
	Case-control	Negative	Colon, rectum	Peters et al. 1992
Cheese	Case-control	Negative	Stomach	Boeing et al. 1991
Yogurt	Case-control	Negative	Colon, rectum	Peters et al. 1992
Vegetables	Case-control	Negative	Stomach	Kneller et al. 1992
	Case-control	Negative	Stomach	Peters et al. 1992
	Case-control	Negative	Stomach	Gonzalez et al. 1994
	Case-control	Negative	Colon	Steinmetz et al. 1994
	Case-control	Negative	Colon, rectum	Zaridze et al. 1993

Table 1. *Continued*

Exposure	Study design	Association between exposure and outcome	Target organ	References
	Case-control	Negative	Colon, rectum	Tuyns et al. 1988
	Case-control	No association	Colon, rectum	Tuyns et al. 1992
Fruit	Case-control	Negative	Stomach	Gonzalez et al. 1994
	Case-control	Negative	Stomach	Boeing et al. 1991
	Case-control	Negative	Colon	Steinmetz et al. 1994
Fruit, vegetables	Case-control	Negative	Stomach	Gridley et al. 1990
	Case-control	Negative	Stomach	LaVecchia et al. 1994
	Case-control	Negative	Stomach	Oreggia et al. 1991
	Case-control	Negative	Stomach	Graham et al. 1990
	Case-control	Negative	Stomach	DeStefani et al. 1990
	Cohort	Negative	Stomach	Chyou et al. 1990
	Case-control	Negative	Stomach	Demirer et al. 1990
	Case-control	Negative	Stomach	Graham et al. 1990
	Case-control	Negative	Stomach	Willett et al. 1990
	Case-control	Negative	Stomach	Forman 1991
	Case-control	Negative	Stomach	Boeing et al. 1991
	Case-control	Negative	Colon	Hu et al. 1992
	Case-control	Negative	Colon, rectum	Zaridze et al. 1993
	Case-control	Negative	Colon, rectum	Wu-Williams et al. 1990
	Case-control	Negative	Colon, rectum	Freudenheim et al. 1990
	Case-control	Negative	Colon, rectum	Kato et al. 1990
Vitamin C	Intervention	Negative	Esophagus, stomach	Dawsey et al. 1994
	Intervention	Negative	Stomach	Wang et al. 1994
	Case-control	Negative	Stomach	La Vecchia et al. 1994
	Case-control	Negative	Stomach	Hansson et al. 1994
	Case-control	Negative	Stomach	Boeing et al. 1991
	Case-control	Negative	Stomach	Buiatti et al. 1990
	Case-control	Negative	Colon, rectum	Zaridze et al. 1993

Vitamin A	Case-control	Positive	Esophagus, stomach	Kabat et al. 1993
β-Carotene	Intervention	Negative	Esophagus, stomach	Taylor et al. 1994
	Case-control	Negative	Stomach	La Vecchia et al. 1994
	Intervention	Negative	Stomach	Hwang et al. 1994
	Case-control	Negative	Stomach	Kneller et al. 1992
	Case-control	No	Colon, rectum	Peters et al. 1992
	Case-control	Negative	Colon, rectum	Zaridze et al. 1993
Lycopene	Case-control	Negative	Oral cavity, pharynx, Esophagus, stomach, Colon, rectum	Franceschi et al. 1994
Vitamin E	Intervention	Negative	Esophagus, stomach	Taylor et al. 1994
	Case-control	Negative	Stomach	Buiatti et al. 1990
Selenium	Intervention	Negative	Esophagus, stomach	Taylor et al. 1994
	Case-control	Negative	Stomach	Kneller et al. 1992
	Cross-sectional	Positive	Stomach	Tsugane et al. 1992
Coffee	Case-control	No association	Stomach	Hansson et al. 1993
	Case-control	No association	Stomach	Memik et al. 1992
	Case-control	No association	Stomach	Agudo et al. 1992
Tea	Case-control	Positive	Stomach, esophagus	Lee et al. 1990
	Case-control	No association	Stomach	Demirer et al. 1990
	Case-control	Negative	Stomach	Yu et al. 1991
	Case-control	No association	Stomach	LaVecchia 1992
	Case-control	No association	Stomach	Agudo et al. 1992
	Case-control	Negative	Colon, rectum	Kato et al. 1990
	Case-control	Negative	Colon, rectum	Kono 1992
	Case-control	Positive	Colon, rectum	LaVecchia et al. 1992
Alcohol	Case-control	Positive	Esophagus, stomach	Kabat et al. 1993
	Case-control	Positive	Stomach	Lee et al. 1990
	Case-control	Positive	Stomach	Boeing et al. 1991
	Cohort	Positive	Rectum	Arbman et al. 1992
	Case-control	Positive	Rectum	Goldbohm et al. 1994

Table 1. *Continued*

Exposure	Study design	Association between exposure and outcome	Target organ	References
Smoking, tobacco	Case-control	Positive	Esophagus, stomach	Kabat et al. 1993
	Case-control	No association	Stomach	Agudo et al. 1992
	Case-control	Positive	Stomach	Lee et al. 1990
	Case-control	Positive	Stomach	Forman 1991
	Case-control	No association	Stomach	Boeing et al. 1991
N-nitroso compounds	Case-control	Positive	Esophagus, stomach	Kumar et al. 1992
	Case-control	Positive	Stomach	Buiatti et al. 1990
	Cross-sectional	Positive	Stomach	Tsugane et al. 1992
	Case-control	Positive	Stomach	Gonzalez et al. 1994
Aspirin	Cohort	Negative	Esophagus, stomach Colon, rectum	Thun et al. 1993
	Cohort	No association	Esophagus, stomach, Colon, rectum	Heath et al. 1994
	Cohort	Negative	Colon, rectum	Paganini-Hill et al. 1989
	Case-control	Negative	Colon, rectum	Rosenberg et al. 1991

Intake of Energy and Macronutrients

Total energy intake is positively correlated with the risk of CRC (Peters et al. 1992). The positive association with total energy intake has important implications for interpreting data on macronutrient influences, because all of them tend to be correlated with total energy intake (Willett 1994). There is, however, evidence that the intake of animal fat, meat, or alcohol is associated with an increasing risk of gastrointestinal cancer, independent of the energy intake. Total (animal) fat and cholesterol showed a positive correlation to esophageal, gastric, and colorectal cancer (Tuyns et al. 1992; Kabat et al. 1993; Zaridze et al. 1993; Gonzalez et al. 1994).

Polyunsaturated fatty acids (PUFA) were shown to be protective against CRC (Zaridze et al. 1993) and against stomach cancer, as determined in a case-control study by Tuyns et al. (1992).

Red meat (salted, cured, fried) and poultry are positively correlated with an increased risk of stomach cancer and CRC (Lee et al. 1990; Boeing et al. 1991; Peters et al. 1992), whereas lean meat shows a negative association with stomach cancer risk (Tuyns et al. 1992). Dietary nitrate, frequently used as a meal preservative, does not appear per se to be a risk factor for cancer, but the excessive consumption of salt-preserved foods may lead to mucosal changes which predispose individuals to increased nitrosation and ultimately further mucosal damage (Correa 1992).

Carbohydrate-rich foods are reported to a lesser extent to be involved in carcinogenesis. Flour products, refined grains, white bread, sucrose, and sugar seem to be positively associated with gastric cancer (Tuyns et al. 1992), whereas whole-grain bread shows a protective function against stomach cancer (Boeing et al. 1991).

Dietary Fiber

Dietary fiber, sometimes measured as cereal fiber or crude fiber, is a group of food constituents consisting mainly of nonstarch polysaccharides (NSP). The intake of dietary fiber is negatively associated with CRC (Peters et al. 1992; Arbman et al. 1992), especially crude fiber with tumors of the distal esophagus/cardia and ascending colon (Peters et al. 1992; Kabat et al. 1993). On a worldwide basis, estimated intakes of dietary fiber tend to be higher in countries where the risk of CRC is low, but when fat and meat consumption are controlled for, this inverse association is reduced substantially. The case-control studies carried out since 1969 have been reviewed by Bingham (1990). Eleven of 22 studies reported that individuals with cancer consumed less fiber than controls; no significant differences were reported in nine studies, and in two studies the cancer patients reported eating more fiber. Principally, epidemiological studies are difficult to interpret because they usually report only the total amount of dietary fiber eaten. Intervention studies indicate that wheat bran dietary fiber may be protective (Harris and Ferguson 1993). Obviously, any inhibitory effect on colorectal carcinogenesis depends on the type of fiber, but wheat bran and cellulose are more consistent in this respect. Cellulose was found to be protective against CRC (Zaridze et al. 1993). On the other hand, pectin apparently either enhanced tumor development or showed no effect. In all studies examining the sources of fiber separately, grain fiber or cereal intake was either unrelated or positively associated with risk of colon cancer, whereas intake of fiber from fruits and vegetables was protective (LaVecchia et al. 1988). High intake of fruits and vegetables has been consistently related to lower risk of colon cancer, but consumption of cereal products has not. On the other hand, the reported favorable effect may be caused by dietary fiber, because fruits and vegetables are an important source of NSP in Western diets. It may also reflect the influence of other bioactive components: antioxidant vitamins, minerals, and phytochemicals.

Antioxidants (β-Carotene, Vitamin E, Selenium, Vitamin A, Vitamin C, Lycopene)

Vegetables and fruits were found to be protective against esophageal, gastric, and colorectal cancer in 25 case-control studies (Gridley et al. 1990; Graham et al. 1990; DeStefani et al. 1990; Demirer et al. 1990; Chyou et al. 1990; Wu-Williams et al. 1990; Freudenheim et al. 1990; Kato et al. 1990; Willett et al. 1990; Steinmetz and Potter 1991; Oreggia et al. 1991; Forman 1991; Hu et al. 1992; Zaridze et al. 1993). Overall, these studies tend to show a reduction in bowel cancer risk, and vegetables and fruits therefore appear to be protective. Besides NSP, other nonnutrient ingredients (phytochemicals) such as polyphenols and glucosinolates may be responsible for the protective effect. Protective effects are reported from specific substances such as β-carotene (Kneller et al. 1992; Peters et al. 1992; Zaridze et al. 1993; LaVecchia et al. 1994; Hwang et al. 1994; Taylor et al. 1994), vitamin E (Buiatti et al. 1990; Taylor et al. 1994), and selenium (Buiatti et al. 1990; Taylor et al. 1994). With regard to vitamin C (Buiatti et al. 1990; Boeing et al. 1991; Zaridze et al. 1993; LaVecchia et al. 1994; Dawsey et al. 1994; Wang et al. 1994; Hansson et al. 1994), both the epidemiological evidence and mechanistic studies suggest a protective role (Willett 1994). Vitamin A causes an increased risk of esophageal and gastric cancer (Kabat et al. 1993). In one analysis no association was found between the intake of vegetables and CRC (Peters et al. 1992). In several studies the intake of cruciferous vegetables was positively correlated to CRC (Tuyns et al. 1992).

In a case-control study for lycopene, Franceschi et al. (1994) showed protection for all sites, most notably for gastrointestinal neoplasms (oral cavity, pharynx, esophagus, stomach, colon, rectum), and one cross-sectional study showed a positive association to stomach cancer risk (Tsugane et al. 1992).

Other Vitamins and Methyl Group Transferring Agents

Folate, methionine, and alcohol influence the methyl group availability, and a methyl-deficient diet may be linked to early stages of colorectal neoplasia. A dietary pattern that increases methyl availability could reduce incidence of colorectal cancer, as shown by the Health Professionals Follow-up Study (Giovannucci et al. 1993). Alcohol intake is positively associated with cancers of the upper aerodigestive and digestive tract (oral cavity, pharynx, larynx, esophagus, stomach, and colon) (Kabat et al. 1993; Lee et al. 1990), and beer intake is positively correlated with rectal carcinomas (Arbman et al. 1992; Goldbohm et al. 1994).

Minerals (Calcium)

Case-control studies showed that low calcium intake has been associated with risk of CRC (Peters et al. 1992; Arbman et al. 1992), but the evidence has not been consistent (Bostick et al. 1993). It has been hypothesized that increased dietary calcium intake reduces the hyperproliferative and cancer-promoting effect of the dietary fat intake characteristic for Western-style diets. Calcium may also be responsible for the uniformly negative association between dairy products (milk, yogurt, cheese) and both stomach cancer and CRC (Lee et al. 1990; Boeing et al. 1991; Peters et al. 1992; Zaridze et al. 1993; Kampman et al. 1994).

Phenolic Compounds as Ingredients of Coffee and Tea

Case-control studies about the correlation of coffee intake and stomach cancer show an overall nonsignificant outcome (Agudo et al. 1992; Memik et al. 1992; Hansson et al. 1993). About tea consumption and gastrointestinal tumors there are contradictory results. Three studies show no association (LaVecchia et al. 1992; Demirer et al. 1990; Agudo et al. 1992), one study a positive (Lee et al. 1990), and three other studies a negative association (Kato et al. 1990; Kono 1991; Yu and Hsieh 1991). Previous research has suggested that coffee may be rather protective against colon cancer, whereas investigation regarding tea has yielded inconsistent results (Yang and Wang 1993; Baron et al. 1994). Overall, coffee consumption appears to be protective against colon cancer, and tea against rectal tumors (Rosenberg 1990).

Other Factors of Exposure

Aspirin as a putative chemopreventive non-nutrient factor was found to reduce the risk of gastrointestinal cancer in four of five studies (Paganini-Hill et al. 1989; Rosenberg et al. 1991; Thun et al. 1993). Heath et al. (1994), however, proposed a rather positive correlation to the risk of CRC.

Smoking and the intake of N-nitroso compounds is unequivocally associated with tumors of the esophagus and stomach. In only two of eight studies is there no correlation to stomach cancer (Boeing et al. 1991; Agudo et al. 1992), whereas the other six show a positive association to esophageal and gastric cancer (Buiatti et al. 1990; Lee et al. 1990; Forman et al. 1991; Kumar et al. 1992; Tsugane et al. 1992; Kabat et al. 1993; Gonzalez et al. 1994).

General Effects of Food or Food Components in Gastrointestinal Carcinogenesis

From model investigations using laboratory animals or human cell cultures, several mechanisms have been derived for the pro- and anticarcinogenic action of nutrients and nonnutrients (Table 2).

There is no suggested mechanism for the effect of total energy intake. It may act via the intake of macronutrients, mainly fat. Dietary fat, especially of animal origin, may develop its procarcinogenic effect by stimulation of bile secretion, causing an increase in the luminal concentration of secondary bile acids with a proliferative and suggested mutagenic and cocarcinogenic activity (Weisburger 1991). Furthermore, it changes the protein kinase C (PKC) isozyme expression and influences PKC activity that is correlated with cell proliferation (Chapkin et al. 1993; Davidson et al. 1995). Thus, red meat may be procarcinogenic, acting as a cocarcinogen with accompanying fat, but also with ammonia produced by intestinal bacteria or the strongly carcinogenic heterocyclic amines (2-amino-1-methyl-6-phenylimidazo[4,5-b]-pyridine [PHIP], 2-amino-3-methylimidazo[4,5-f] quinoline [IQ]) formed during food processing (Willett et al. 1990). The concentration of these latter substances depends both on the type of food and on the cooking method used. Grilling and frying generate more heterocyclic amines because of the higher surface temperatures involved. They have been shown to be carcinogenic in animals in various organs, particularly the gastrointestinal tract, a fact that may be of significance in man.

For the protective action of dietary fiber (bran, cellulose) several different mechanisms are described. Nutrients with a dietary fiber-like action (e.g., resistant starch) and fruits and vegetables usually rich in dietary fiber, act mainly protectively in the colon and rectum by binding luminal water, diluting the content of the large bowel lumen, reducing the time that putative carcinogens are in contact with the large bowel mucosa, and increasing the fecal weight (Bingham 1990; Willett et al. 1990; Steinmetz and Potter 1991; Weisburger et al. 1993). To decide which of these proposed mechanisms predominates in man the use of better-defined dietary fibers is necessary. Both cellulose and wheat bran reduced fecal mutagenicity and secondary bile acid secretion compared with control diet periods, but oat bran did not affect either

Table 2. Effects of foods and nutrients on GI carcinogenesis (Observations from E-epidemiological studies A-animal experiments H-investigations with human beings and human cell cultures)

Food or food component	Observed effect	Suggested mechanism of action	References
Red meat	Procarcinogenic (A, E, H)	Colon: cocarcinogenic action of accompanying fat, of heterocyclic amines formed during food processing, or of ammonia produced by intestinal bacteria	Bingham 1990; Willett et al. 1990
Dietary fiber: bran cellulose	Anticarcinogenic (A)	Colon and rectum: increase in fecal weight, reduced transit time, diluted contents of the large bowel lumen, reduced time for putative carcinogens to be in contact with the large bowel mucosa	Bingham et al. 1990; Willett et al. 1990; Steinmetz and Potter 1991
Fruits and vegetables	Anticarcinogenic (A, E, H)	Colon and rectum: increase in fecal weight, reduced transit time, diluted contents of the large bowel lumen, reduced time for putative carcinogens to be in contact with the large bowel mucosa	Weisburger et al. 1993
Calcium	Anticarcinogenic (A, E)	Colon: binding of the potentially carcinogenic bile acids to unsoluble soaps	Reshef et al. 1990; Newmark 1992
	Anticarcinogenic (A, E)	Stomach: decrease in norepinephrine in the gastric wall and consequent stimulation of proliferation of antral epithelial cells	Tatsuta et al. 1993
	Anticarcinogenic (A, E)	Colon: precipitates luminal surfactants and thus inhibits cytolytic activity, epithelial cell damage, and colonic proliferation	Govers et al. 1994
Vitamin C	Anticarcinogenic (A, E, H)	Stomach: lowers the body burden of intragastrically formed N-nitroso compounds; may scavenge and reduce nitrite, thus reducing the substrate for the reaction with secondary amines to form nitrosoamines; antioxidant; hydroxylation of lysine and proline in the synthesis of connective tissue proteins (e.g., collagen)	Steinmetz and Potter 1991; Byers et al. 1992; Bartsch 1991
Carotenoids	Anticarcinogenic (A, E, H)	General: deactivate excited oxygen molecules generated as by-products of normal metabolic processes and trap free radicals	Steinmetz and Potter 1991; Byers and Perry 1992; Hill et

Table 2. *Continued*

Food or food component	Observed effect	Suggested mechanism of action	References
			al. 1992
		Stomach: decrease the constitution-dependent enzymatic activation in the gastric mucosal membrane and inhibition of focus formation with abnormally high activity of ornithine decarboxylase	Draudin-Krylenko et al. 1992
Vitamin E		General: intracellular antioxidant protecting unsaturated fatty acids in cell membranes from oxidative damage; keeps selenium in the reduced state; reduces the expression of *c-myc* and *H-ras*	Steinmetz and Potter 1991; Prasad et al. 1990; Byers and Perry 1992
Selenium	Anticarcinogenic (A)	General: protects oxidative tissue damage as cofactor of glutathione peroxidase; suppresses cell proliferation	Steinmetz and Potter 1991;
Folic acid	Anticarcinogenic (A)	General: decreases micronuclei formation and chromosomal damage	Steinmetz and Potter 1991
Polyphenols	Anticarcinogenic (A, E, H)	Stomach: lowers the body burden of intragastrically formed N-nitroso compounds, suppresses activation of carcinogens, traps genotoxic agents	Bartsch 1991; Yang et al. 1993
Coffee	Anticarcinogenic (A, E, H)	Colon: decreases the stool concentrations of cholesterol and bile acids	Ekbom et al. 1993
Tea	Anticarcinogenic (A, E, H)	Colon, rectum: decreases the stool concentrations of cholesterol and bile acids; inhibition of metabolic activation and carcinogen-DNA binding; induction of antioxidant and phase-II enzyme activities	Chen 1992; Yamane et al. 1991; Wang et al. 1992; Takahashi 1991
Sulfur-containing compounds (dithiolthiones, oxazolidinthiones, glucosinolates	Anticarcinogenic (A, H)	General: induction of phase-II enzymes	Prestera et al. 1993
Alcohol	Procarcinogenic (E)	Rectum: action of accompanying nitrosamines in alcoholic beverages	Longnecker et al. 1990

E, Epidemiological studies; *A*, animal experiments; *H*, investigations with human beings and human cell cultures of these parameters. Another hypothesis has developed from the realization that fermentation by colonic bacteria is of considerable importance in large bowel physiology and therefore may also be involved in protection against cancer. Carbohydrate entering the large bowel undergoes anaerobic fementation producing short chain fatty acids (SCFA), particularly acetate, propionate, and butyrate, and gas (carbon dioxide, hydrogen, and methane), and consequently increasing microbial cell mass. This in itself increases stool bulk, but there is also evidence that SCFA, especially butyrate, have an antiproliferative activity in epithelial cells of the colon (Bingham 1990; Freudenheim et al. 1990; Scheppach et al. 1992).

Epidemiological data suggest that increased risk of colon cancer is correlated with a higher facal pH and increase of ionization and solubilization of fecal long-chain free fatty acids and unconjugated free bile acids in colon chyme. At a high pH most of the bile acids are in solution. The lower the pH, the greater their portion forming insoluble calcium salts. Consequently, their contact with the colonic mucosa and their potential for damaging epithelial cells is reduced. However, the exact mechanism of bile acid action in the colon is uncertain. A proliferating effect via increased ornithine decarboxylase activity or PKC activity and expression is suggested (Chapkin et al. 1993; Davidson et al. 1994). Promoters, however, include the secondary bile acids, particularly deoxycholic acid and lithocholic acid, concentrations of which are influenced also by the level of dietary fat (Reddy et al. 1992).

Calcium exerts its anticarcinogenic effect in the stomach by decreasing norepinephrine in the gastric wall and subsequently stimulating proliferation of antral epithelial cells (Tatsuta et al. 1993). In animal studies, it was demonstrated that orally administered calcium supplements suppressed the action of bile acids and fatty acids on the colon epithelium, presumably by precipitating their anions as insoluble calcium soaps in the lumen. This binding of the potentially carcinogenic bile acids and precipitating luminal surfactants may inhibit cytolytic activity, epithelial cell damage, and colonic proliferation (Reshef et al. 1990; Newmark and Lupton 1990; Govers et al. 1994). The similar efficacy of calcium carbonate, calcium phosphate, and other milk minerals indicates that the antiproliferative effect of milk is mediated by its calcium content and is not inhibited by phosphate (Govers et al. 1994). Data from intervention studies in patients at high risk for colon cancer and in normal volunteers suggest that dietary calcium is able to diminish the risk of colon cancer by reducing proliferation of colonic epithelial cells, probably by influencing secondary bile acids in the colonic lumen. The exact mechanism, however, is yet to be established (Lapré and Van der Meer 1992).

The nutrients which act in a variety of ways to counteract oxidative and free radical damage are frequently referred to as antioxidants. They include vitamin A and its precursors, the carotenoids, vitamin C, vitamin E, and certain trace minerals, notably selenium. It is well documented that retinol and other retinoids, referred to collectively as vitamin A, can influence carcinogenesis, notably by influencing cellular differentiation, especially in epithelial cells, intercellular communication, and the immune response. Carotenoids play a protective role by trapping free radicals and deactivating excited oxygen molecules generated as by-products of normal metabolic processes (Steinmetz and Potter 1991; Byers and Perry 1992; Hill and Grubbs 1992). β-Carotene could be important in protecting body fat and lipid membranes against oxidation. In the gastric mucosal membrane constitution-dependent enzymes were activated, and focus formation with abnormally high activity of ornithine decarboxylase is inhibited (Draudin-Krylenko et al. 1992). Furthermore, carotenoids arrest transformation of carcinogen-initiated cells and enhance gap-junctional cell-cell communication (Wolf 1992).

Vitamin C (ascorbic acid) may scavenge and reduce nitrite, thus eliminating the substrate for the reaction with secondary amines to form nitrosamines; it plays a role as an antioxidant and in the hydroxylation of lysine and proline in the synthesis of connective tissue proteins such as collagen (Steinmetz and Potter 1991; Byers and Perry 1992). Its protective function, especially in the stomach, is to lower the body burden of intragastrically formed N-nitroso compounds (Bartsch 1991). It is also believed that the strong associations between low vitamin C status and gastric and esophageal cancer may be explained by the role of vitamin C in preventing the formation of potentially carcinogenic nitrosamines. There is evidence that vitamin C inhibits the formation of fecal mutagens and protects the colonic mucosa (Shike et al. 1990). Vitamin E (tocopherol) functions as an intracellular antioxidant protecting unsaturated fatty acids in cell membranes from oxidative damage. Thus, it may prevent carcinogenesis by neutralizing the damaging effects of free radicals, particularly those resulting from the metabolism of fat (Shike et al. 1990). Furthermore vitamin E keeps selenium in its reduced state and reduces the expression of c-myc and H-ras (Prasad and Edwards-Prasad 1990; Steinmetz and Potter 1991; Byers and Perry 1992). Vitamin E has also been shown to enhance the body's immune response. In addition, vitamin E operates together with vitamin C to inhibit the formation of nitrosamines from nitrites in the stomach. In tumorigenesis, vitamin E has been shown to inhibit oral carcinogenesis and to influence colon carcinogenesis in different directions. These variable effects may be due to interactions with other dietary components such as fat and selenium. Thus, before definite conclusions can be drawn about the possible protective effect of vitamin E in gastrointestinal cancer, further data from ongoing prospective and intervention trials have to be assessed.

Selenium is essential for destroying lipid hydroperoxides. As a cofactor of glutathione peroxidase it protects several tissues from damage and suppresses cell proliferation (Steinmetz and Potter 1991). It has been proposed that high levels of selenium may be toxic to rapidly proliferating cancer cells, or that the mineral might enhance the activity of the liver microsomal enzymes involved in carcinogen metabolism. Other vitamins and methyl group transferring agents (folic acid, methionine) decrease micronuclei formation and chromosomal damage (Steinmetz and Potter 1991). They interact in methylation reactions with other nutrients: choline, vitamin B_{12}. These reactions are crucial to the synthesis of DNA and membranes and to lipid metabolism. DNA methylation plays a role in the regulation of gene activity. Reduced methylation of DNA, occurring when one or more of these factors are deficient in the diet, is believed to lead to deranged replication of cells and loss of normal growth control. Low dietary folate and methionine and high intake of alcohol may reduce levels of S-adenosylmethionine, which is required for DNA methylation. Alcohol was shown to be procarcinogenic in rectal cancer due to accompanying nitrosamines in alcoholic beverages (Longnecker et al. 1990), but the exact mechanism by which alcohol exerts its carcinogenic effects is uncertain. Its metabolite, acetaldehyde, is a potent carcinogen, but it may also act via an alteration in hormonal balance, by a direct toxic effect, or as a promoting factor in initiated cells (Lancet Editorial 1990).

Polyphenols, especially flavonoids as a subgroup of secondary plant metabolites, play a role as anticarcinogens as regards their antioxidative activity, induction of phase-I and phase-II enzymes, and nucleophilic binding of carcinogenic electrophiles, thus reducing their bioavailability during the gastrointestinal passage (Huang and Ferraro 1992; Newmark 1992; Yang and Wang 1993). The flavonoids biochanin A and genistein inhibit cell growth in vitro in stomach cancer cell lines through activation of a signal transduction pathway for apoptosis (Yanagihara et al. 1993); in human gastric and colon cancer cells isoflavones block cell progression from the G1 to the S phase and inhibit cell growth (Yoshida et al. 1990). The flavonoid quercetin decreases the colon tumor rate induced by azoxymethane (AOM) in mice by 75% and inhibits procarcinogen-activating enzymes (Hosokawa et al. 1990; Deschner et al. 1993). A similar potective effect (63% decrease in AOM-induced colon tumor yield) is observed with rutin (Deschner et al. 1993; Dragsted et al. 1993).

Coffee, particularly unfiltered or boiled, is protective against colon cancer, decreasing the stool concentrations of cholesterol and bile acids and thereby probably increasing serum cholesterol (Ahola et al. 1991). The mechanism of the protective effect of tea against esophageal cancer and CRC involves an inhibition of metabolic activation and carcinogen-DNA binding and subsequent induction of antioxidant and phase-II enzyme activities, as well as a decrease of the stool concentrations of cholesterol and bile acids (Yamane et al. 1991; Chen 1992; Katiyar et al. 1993). Sulphur-containing compounds (dithiolthiones, oxazolidinthiones, glucosinolates) are also potent anticarcinogens inducing phase-II enzymes (Prestera et al. 1993).

Possible Non-nutritive Causes of Gastrointestinal Cancer

Although the impact of dietary factors on the development of gastrointestinal cancers is high, there are several non-nutritive factors relevant to this process (Table 3). The complexity of the diet/gastrointestinal cancer problem lies in nutritional interactions and in the individual response to dietary factors, which

Table 3. Possible non-nutrient- or nutrition-mediated causes of GI cancer

Causes of GI cancer	Target organ	Observed effect	Suggested mechanism of action	References
Genetic susceptibility	Gastrointestinal organs (esophagus, stomach, colon, rectum)	Genetic alterations related to carcinogenesis	Gene amplification, deletion, mutation, overexpression	Yasui and Tahara 1994; Risio 1992; Stemmermann et al. 1994
Number of children and age at first birth	Colon, rectum	Protection by increasing parity and decreasing age at birth of the first child	Role of female sex hormones whittled away as suggested mechanism	Kune 1995
Physical activity	Colon, rectum	Protective	Increase in motility and mixing of the contents of the colon	Kune et al. 1990
Exercise	Colon	Protective	Increase in prostacyclin, decrease in platelet aggregation, possible decrease of the platelet-derived growth factor	Simopoulos 1990
Personality type	Colon, rectum	Depression increases risk	Psychological variables may influence both the neuro-endocrine and immune systems of the body in such a way that the proliferation of cancer cells is promoted	Kune et al. 1992
Stress	Stomach, colon, rectum	Procarcinogenic	Immunodepression and subsequent cancer growth	Kune et al. 1992
pH and bile acids	Colon, rectum	Procarcinogenic (A, E, H)	Mechanism uncertain; proliferation via increased ornithine decarboxylase activity or protein kinase C activity and expression	Chapkin et al. 1993; Davidson et al. 1995; Newmark and Lupton 1990
Meal frequency	Intestinal mucosa	Protective (E)	Gallbladder contracts and releases bile acids; influence on the enterohepatic circulation and the exposure time of intestinal mucosa to bile acids	Franceschi et al. 1992

Fecapentaenes	Colon	Procarcinogenic (A, H)	Fecapentaenes are direct-acting genotoxins, which may react with DNA through free radical mechanisms, and/or aldehyde formation	Povey et al. 1991
Tobacco	Esophagus, stomach, colon, rectum	Procarcinogenic (E)	Endogenous synthesis of N-nitroso compounds	Forman 1991
Aspirin	Colon, rectum	Protective	Inhibition of cyclooxigenase and thereby blocking of the prostaglandin production that is involved in increased cellular proliferation	Baron and Greenberg 1991

E, Epidemiological studies; *A*, animal experiments; *H*, investigations with human beings and human cell cultures in turn are determined by genetic, physiological, and lifestyle factors. Genetic alterations (gene amplification, deletion, mutation, overexpression) related to gastrointestinal carcinogenesis and paired with the family history are a useful marker for screening and early detection of this cancer. Multiple genetic alterations affecting both cellular proto-oncogenes and tumor suppressor genes are involved during the development and progression of both esophageal and gastric cancers. While very exciting for molecular biologists and geneticists, as these findings enhance the understanding of colorectal carcinogenesis, this research track is unlikely to offer an increased understanding of CRC etiology, unless it is combined with epidemiological studies performed in the same set of respondents (Kune et al. 1989; Risio 1992; Stemmermann et al. 1994; Yasui et al. 1994).

The number of children and the age at first birth also play a critical role in the etiology of CRC. Nulliparity and increasing age at birth of the first child increase the risk, whereas increasing parity is protective against CRC. However, the suggested role of female sex hormones in gastrointestinal carcinogenesis is being whittled away (Kune 1995).

There is an inverse correlation between physical activity and CRC. Exercise increases motility and mixing of contents of the colon, increases prostacyclin, decreases platelet aggregation, and possibly decreases platelet-derived growth factor (PDGF) (Kune et al. 1990; Simopoulos 1990). Depression and psychological variables may influence both the neuroendocrine and immune systems of the body in such a way that the proliferation of cancer cells is promoted. Therefore, personality type seems to be a further risk for CRC (Kune et al. 1992; Kinlen 1992). Immunodepression evoked by stress is related to an increased risk for gastric and colorectal cancer (Kune et al. 1992). Self-reported "perceived" religiousness, as practiced by Mormons and Seventh-Day Adventists, is shown to have a statistically significant protection against CRC, whereas Jews of European origin have an increased risk for CRC (Kune et al. 1993).

Constipation, diarrhea, and laxative use are shown not to be risk factors for CRC, although anthraquinone laxatives possess mutagenic activity under experimental conditions (Kune et al. 1988a). Nevertheless, reduced constipation is a clear benefit of higher fiber intake. Cholecystectomy and asbestos exposure were not risk factors for colorectal tumors (Soltero et al. 1990; Garabrant et al. 1992; Ekbom et al. 1993; Kune 1995). Two meals per day or fewer reduce the risk of CRC. A role of meal frequency in the etiology of colorectal cancer is biologically plausible, because after meal ingestion the gallbladder contracts and releases bile acids. Thus, eating patterns can influence the enterohepatic circulation and, consequently, the exposure time of intestinal mucosa to bile acids (Franceschi et al. 1992).

Fecapentaenes possess a procarcinogenic effect, although patients with CRC excrete fewer fecapentaenes than patients without (Povey et al. 1991). The suggested mechanism in the colon is that fecapentaenes are direct-acting genotoxins which may react with DNA through free radical mechanisms and/or aldehyde formation.

The use of aspirin seems to be protective against CRC, because aspirin inhibits cyclooxigenase and thereby blocks the production of prostaglandins that are involved in increased cellular proliferation (Baron and Greenberg 1991).

Generalized Mechanisms of Action: Events on the Cellular Level

Process of Carcinogenesis in the Stomach

The human model of gastric carcinogenesis comprises the following sequential stages: chronic gastritis, atrophy, intestinal metaplasia, and dysplasia (Stemmermann et al. 1994). p53 abnormalities occur frequently in tumors arising in the stomach, and they can be observed in precancerous lesions as well as in overt cancer. Subsequent abnormalities affecting other genes, e.g., epidermal growth factor receptors (EGFRs), potentially enhance the growth potential of tumors. The initial stages of gastritis and atrophy have been linked to excessive salt intake and to infection with Helicobacter pylori. The intermediate stages have been associated with the ingestion of ascorbic acid and nitrate, determinants of intragastric nitrosation. The final stages have been linked with the supply of β-carotene and with excessive salt intake. Nitrosating agents are candidate carcinogens and could originate in the gastric cavity or in the inflammatory infiltrate (Correa 1992).

Molecular Events in Colorectal Carcinogenesis

The progression from adenoma to carcinoma can be followed on the molecular level, and a sequence of allelic losses on the chromosomes 5q, 12p, 18q, and 17p has been described (Fearon and Vogelstein 1990). Presumably, a developing cancer is the consequence of both an activation of oncogenes and an inactivation of tumor suppressor genes. The best-studied oncogenes in colon carcinogenesis are the K-ras oncogenes. This oncogene is altered by point mutations in 9% of small adenomas, in 58% of adenomas greater than 1 cm, and in 47% of colon cancers (Bos 1989). Allelic deletions in the locus of the p53 tumor suppressor gene are rare in adenomas and most common in carcinomas of the colorectal region (Baker et al. 1990).

It is generally accepted that most, if not all, colon cancers have their origin in previously benign adenomas (Itzkowitz and Kim 1993). This is based not only on epidemiological studies indicating that the prevalence of adenomas parallels the prevalence of colon cancer, but also on clinical and pathological investigations. Not all polyps develop to malignant tumors (Potter 1992).

Furthermore, the transforming growth factor β receptor (TGFβR) potentially enhances the growth of tumors (Markowitz et al. 1995).

Role of Bile as a Carcinogen

Xenobiotics processed by the cellular detoxifying phase-I and phase-II enzymes are partially excreted via bile. This is another source of carcinogenic potential in bile, besides the direct tumor-promoting potency of secondary bile acids described above. A direct reaction of bile constituents with DNA of epithelial cells may be assumed, too, from data of patients with familial adenomatous polyposis. By using the ^{32}P-postlabeling method, both an excess of DNA adducts in the duodenum and a higher level of directly acting genotoxic compounds in the bile of these patients compared with healthy individuals have been found (Scates et al. 1993). A direct adduct-forming capacity of bile acids or their metabolites incubated with DNA in vitro, however, could not be detected (Scates et al. 1994).

Role of the Intestinal Flora in Colon Carcinogenesis

Many of the hypotheses existing to explain colon carcinogenesis include a role of the intestinal microflora in the process. Composition and metabolic activity of the gut flora are influenced by a combination of numerous dietary and endogenous factors. The relative importance of these factors is unknown and may depend on individual characteristics, e.g., of hormonal regulation, age, and gender. This is reflected by gender-dependent differences in frequency and localization of colon cancer, with a female excess of right-sided colon cancers and a male excess of left-sided cancers. The activity of enzymes such as β-glucuronidase and β-glucosidase produced by the anaerobic species Bacteroides and Clostridia provide a measure of the ability of intestinal microorganisms to stimulate carcinogenic processes. They liberate aglycones which have been bound in the cells of liver and gut mucosa by detoxifying phase-II enzymes to solubilizing groups such as glucuronide and sulfate residues and then excreting them. The activity of these enzymes is influenced by nutritional factors such as dietary fiber.

Primary Prevention

Primary prevention is defined as the identification of etiologic factors in the environment that are related to carcinogenesis and the subsequent correction or elimination of them. Principally, it has been shown that a diet high in vegetables, fruit, cellulose, vitamins, and PUFA is associated with a low risk of gastrointestinal cancer, and that a diet high in proteins and saturated fatty acids relative to the more beneficial dietary components is associated with high risk. The chemopreventive aspects of specific vitamins or combinations of vitamins and minerals may also prove to be important in individuals or populations at particular risk for certain cancers (Vargas and Alberts 1992). Data from an intervention trial in Linxian, China, a region with one of the world's highest rates of cancer of the esophagus and gastric cardia, has been published recently (Dawsey et al. 1994). In this region the variety and amount of food available are limited, the intake of many micronutrients is consistently low, and marginal nutritional deficiencies are common.

Chemoprevention of gastrointestinal cancer, especially colorectal cancer, by aspirin is evident from different research disciplines. However, future epidemiological and basic research of a pharmacologic and clinical nature should examine all digestive tract cancers in considering the chemopreventive or therapeutic potential of nonsteroidal anti-inflammatory drugs.

Secondary Prevention

With regard to secondary prevention, which is defined as the identification and eradication of the earliest premalignant stage of disease before lethal consequences can develop, screening for adenomatous polyps and colorectal cancer is now advised for both average and high-risk patients. The average-risk group includes patients in the asymptomatic general population who are 50 years of age or older. Although an annual digital rectal examination is recommended for average-risk patients, the more proximal localization of colorectal cancer means that fewer than 10% of cancers are detected by this method. Adenomas may be detected by fecal occult blood testing, barium enema, sigmoidoscopy, colonoscopy, and ultrasound diagnostics. As screening methods, the fecal occult blood test (FOBT) and sigmoidoscopy are in use. Beginning at the age of 50, patients should undergo a FOBT annually. It involves the use of guaiac slide tests or an immunochemical test that is specific for human hemoglobin. A positive result in a hemoccult test can be found in 1–3% of asymptomatic adults over the age of 40, but only polyps above 1 cm in size usually bleed. Therefore, fewer than 40% of patients with adenomas show a positive hemoccult test. Beginning at the age of 50, asymptomatic individuals should also be encouraged to undergo flexible sigmoidoscopy every 3–5 years (Winawer et al. 1993). However, screening by sigmoidoscopy every 10 years may be nearly as efficacious as more frequent screening (Selby and Friedman 1989). Polyps are detected by sigmoidoscopy in 10–15% of asymptomatic people over the age of 40.

Colonoscopy is usually recommended for patients whose FOBT is positive or in whom results of a biopsy by sigmoidoscopy indicate the presence of an adenomatous polyp (Rex et al. 1991). Laser-induced fluorescence spectroscopy during colonoscopy is a technique that is able to differentiate adenomas from normal colonic mucosa and hyperplastic polyps in 97% of the specimens studied (Cothren et al. 1990).

Polyps above 1 cm in size can be detected in the colon by a transcutaneous ultrasound technique. Endoscopic ultrasound reveals the depth of tumor penetration and gives an assessment of lymph node involvement, thereby helping to determine the stage of cancer (Winawer et al. 1993).

Conclusion

From existing evidence, it is obvious that a variety of dietary components, as well as the level of dietary energy intake, can influence the risk of cancer in various regions of the gastrointestinal tract. For colon cancer, there is evidence for a sequence of pathological events beginning with hyperproliferation and involving specific genetic mutations. It can be concluded that there is a possible role for dietary components in promoting (fat and/or energy) and inhibiting (NSP, calcium, and antioxidant nutrients) colon carcinogenesis.

Although various cancers, including gastrointestinal cancer, have been linked to either total energy or type of fat consumption, there is no clear evidence suggesting that the relationship is causal (LaVecchia 1992). It is difficult to separate the influence of fat from the influence of the total energy content of the diet. A clear protective effect of NSP or their constitutive fractions has not been demonstrated consistently. It must be concluded that NSP are probably important in the etiology of CRC and that more information is required on the influence of butyrate in particular on colonic cell proliferation in human beings.

The strongest and most consistent evidence for cancer-protective effects comes from epidemiological studies which have examined the consumption of vegetables and fruit, especially those rich in carotenes (yellow/green/orange vegetables and fruit). The evidence is consistent for cancers of the mouth, pharynx, esophagus, stomach, colon, and rectum. It is believed that much of this apparent protective effect might be accounted for by the presence of antioxidants, both nutrients (carotenoids, ascorbic acid, tocopherol, selenium) and non-nutrients (polyphenols), in plant foods.

Predisposing factors such as genetic susceptibility are proven; smoking, number of children and age at first birth, physical activity, and personality type play a possible role, while constipation, diarrhea, laxative use, cholecystectomy, asbestos, and female sex hormones play unimportant roles in gastrointestinal cancer etiology. However, the precipitating factor stress and the perception of strees possibly increase the CRC risk (Kune et al. 1991).

In some epidemiological studies tobacco has been shown to play a procarcinogenic role because of the endogenous synthesis of N-nitroso compounds (Forman 1991); with regard to smoking, other studies reveal only a possible risk for CRC (Kune 1995).

Future Outlook

A long-term increase in vegetable and fruit intake is expected to reduce the risk of gastrointestinal cancer, including esophageal cancer, even with exposure to specific carcinogenic compounds (e.g., those from cigarette smoke). Although the epidemiological data on gastrointestinal cancer provide solid support for recommendations to consume an abundance of vegetables and fruits, more studies are needed for precise recommendations about the types and amounts of these foods. Further testing of the relevant compounds in vitro and in vivo will provide more evidence regarding the specific compounds and their sites and modes of action. These nutrients and non-nutrient compounds in fruit and vegetables interact in modifying cancer risk and may augment each other's effect. Moreover it is still unclear precisely which components of the foods are most protective. Therefore, it seems to be better to increase consumption by eating more fruits and vegetables, rather than by taking supplements. Only for individuals at specific risk, e.g., populations at high risk for esophageal or stomach cancer due to nutrient deficiencies, the intake of vitamin supplements is to be recommended.

Moderate drinking of alcohol and increased consumption of whole grain products, as opposed to highly refined carbohydrates, may help to reduce the risk of colon cancer, although this has been difficult to demonstrate epidemiologically. On the basis of current data, it can be concluded that a moderate consumption of coffee (5 cups of instant coffee per day) does not contribute to an increased risk of gastrointestinal cancer. Overall, the diet should be varied and based on foods which are rich in essential nutrients. The recommended type of dietary pattern is low in fat, especially in saturated fatty acids, includes monounsaturated fatty acids, and has moderate amounts of PUFA (no more than 10% of calories). Moderate consumption of salt and of highly salted, smoked, and barbecued foods should be encouraged. Obesity should be avoided by trying to match energy intake with expenditure while increasing physical activity levels.

There are a number of naturally occurring carcinogens present in food, as well as those formed during cooking and those present as microbial and environmental contaminants. There is a plethora of convincing data, however, pointing to the fact that current average levels of consumption contribute no measurable risk in terms of cancer. Some studies focus on gastrointestinal cancer incidence or mortality as an end point, but this clearly necessitates very large numbers of subjects to achieve statistically significant results. Increasingly, biomarkers of earlier events are used. These are parameters which are believed to bear specific relevance to the cancer in question and include the assessment of premalignant lesions such as dysplasia. The identification and measurement of molecular biomarkers in individuals will certainly increase the number and type of epidemiological studies that can be conducted by better identifying exposed individuals. Furthermore, molecular biomarkers that are related to disease end points can be used to identify individuals who may be at higher risk because of inherent genetic factors or lifestyles.

References

Agudo A, Gonzalez CA, Marcos G, Sanz M, Saigi E, Verge J, Boleda M, Ortego J (1992) Consumption of alcohol, coffee, and tabacco, and gastric cancer in Spain. Cancer Causes Control 3:137–143

Ahola I, Jauhiainen M, Aro A (1991) The hypercholesterolaemic factor in boiled coffee is retained by a paper filter. J Intern Med 230:293–297

Arbman G, Axelson O, Ericsson-Begodzki AB, Fredriksson M, Nilsson E, Sjodahl R (1992) Cereal fiber, calcium, and colorectal cancer. Cancer 69:2042–2048

Baker JS, Preisinger AC, Jessup JM et al (1990) p53 gene mutations occur in combination with 17p allelic deletions as late events in colorectal tumorigenesis. Cancer Res 50:717–722

Baron JA, Greenberg ER (1991) Could aspirin really prevent colon cancer? N Engl J Med 325:1644–1645

Baron JA, Gerhardsson de Verdier M, Ekbom A (1994) Coffee, tea, tabacco, and cancer of the large bowel. Cancer Epidemiol Biomarkers Prev 3:565–570

Bartsch H (1991) N-nitroso compounds and human cancer: where do we stand? IARC Sci Publ 105:1–10

Bingham SA (1990) Mechanisms and experimental and epidemiological evidence relating dietary fibre (non-starch polysaccharides) and starch to protection against large bowel cancer. Proc Nutr Soc 49:153–171

Bingham SA (1993) Plant cell wall material and cancer protection. In: Waldron KW et al (eds) Food and cancer prevention. Royal Society of Chemistry, Cambridge, pp 339–347

Boeing H, Frentzel-Beyme R, Berger M, Berndt V, Gores W, Korner M, Lohmeier R, Menarcher A, Mannl HF, Meinhardt M et al (1991) Case-control study on stomach cancer in Germany. Int J Cancer 47:858–864

Bos JL (1989) Ras oncogenes in human cancer: a review. Cancer Res 49:4682–4689

Bostick RM, Potter JD, Fosdick L, Grambsch P, Lampe JW, Wood JR, Louis TA, Ganz R, Grandits G (1993) Calcium and colorectal epithelial cell proliferation: a preliminary randomized, double-blinded, placebo-controlled clinical trial. J Natl Cancer Inst 85:132–141

Buiatti E, Palli D, Decarli A, Amadori D, Avellini C, Bianchi S, Bonaguri C, Cipriani F, Cocco P, Giacosa A et al (1990) A case-control study of gastric cancer and diet in Italy. II. Association with nutrients. Int J Cancer 45:896–901

Byers T, Perry G (1992) Dietary carotenes, vitamin C, and vitamin E as protective antioxidants in human cancers. Annu Rev Nutr 12:139–159

Chapkin RS, Gao J, Lee D-YK, Lupton JR (1993) Dietary fiber and fat alter rat colon protein kinase C activity: correlation to cell proliferation. J Nutr 123, 649–655

Cheah PY (1990) Hypothesis for the etiology of colorectal cancer – an overview. Nutr Cancer 14:5–13

Chen J (1992) The effects of Chinese tea on the occurrence of esophageal tumors induced by N-nitrosomethylbenzylamine in rats. Prev Med 21:385–391

Chyou PH, Nomura AM, Hankin JH, Stemmermann GN (1990) A case-cohort study of diet and stomach cancer. Cancer Res 50:7501–7504

Correa P (1992) Human gastric carcinogenesis: a multistep and multifactorial process – first American Cancer Society Award Lecture on cancer epidemiology and prevention. Cancer Res 52:6735–6740

Cothren RM, Richards-Kortum R, Sivak MV et al (1990) Gastrointestinal tissue diagnosis by laser-induced fluorescence spectroscopy at endoscopy. Gastrointest Endosc 36:105–111
Davidson LA, Lupton JR, Jiang Y-H, Chang W-J, Aukema HM, Chapkin RS (1995) Dietary fat and fiber alter rat protein kinase C isozyme expression. J Nutr 125, 49–56
Dawsey SM, Wang GQ, Taylor PR, Li JY, Blot WJ, Li B, Lewin KJ, Liu FS, Weinstein WM, Wiggett S et al (1994) Effects of vitamin/mineral supplementation on the prevalence of histological dysplasia and early cancer of the esophagus and stomach: results from the dysplasia trial in Linxian, China. Cancer Epidemiol Biomarkers Prev 3:167–172
Demirer T, Icli F, Uzunalimoglu O, Kucuk O (1990) Diet and stomach cancer incidence. A case-control study in Turkey. Cancer 65:2344–2348
Deschner EE, Ruperto JF, Wong GY, Newmark HL (1993) The effect of dietary quercetin and rutin on AOM-induced acute colonic epithelial abnormalities in mice fed a high-fat diet. Nutr Cancer 20:199–204
DeStefani E, Munoz N, Esteve J, Vasallo A, Victora CG, Teuchmann S (1990) Mate drinking, alcohol, tobacco, diet, and esophageal cancer in Uruguay. Cancer Res 50:426–431
Dragsted LO, Strube M, Larsen JC (1993) Cancer-protective factors in fruits and vegetables: biochemical and biological background. Pharmacol Toxicol 72:116–135
Draudin-Krylenko VA, Bukin IuV, Levchuk AA, Davei F (1992) Potential cancer-protective effect of beta-carotene in experimental stomach carcinogenesis. Vopr Med Khim 38:36–39
Editorial (1990) Alcohol and cancer. Lancet 335:634–635
Ekbom A, Yuen J, Adami H, McLaughlin J, Chow W, Persson I, Fraumeni J (1993) Cholecystectomy and colorectal cancer. Gastroenterology 105:142–147
Fearon ER, Vogelstein B (1990) A genetic model for colorectal tumorigenesis. Cell 61:759–767
Forman D (1991) The etiology of gastric cancer. IARC Sci Publ 105:22–32
Franceschi S, Bidoli E, LaVecchia C, Talamini R, D'Avanzo B, Negri E (1994) Tomatoes and risk of digestive-tract cancers. Int J Cancer 59:181–184
Franceschi S, LaVecchia C, Bidoli E, Negri E, Talamini R (1992) Meal frequency and risk of colorectal cancer. Cancer Res 52:3589–3592
Freudenheim JL, Graham S, Horvath PJ, Marshall JR, Haughey BP, Wilkinson G (1990) Risks associated with source of fiber and fiber components in cancer of the colon and rectum. Cancer Res 50:3295–3300
Garabrant DH, Peters RK, Homa DM (1992) Asbestos and colon cancer: lack of association in a large case-control study. Am J Epidemiol 135:843–853
Giovannucci E, Stampfer MJ, Colditz GA, Rimm EB, Trichopoulos D, Rosner BA, Speizer FE Willett WC (1993) Folate, methionine, and alcohol intake and risk of colorectal adenoma. J Natl Cancer Inst 85:875–884
Goldbohm RA, Van den Brandt PA, Vant't Veer P, Dorant E, Sturmans F, Hermus RJ (1994) Prospective study on alcohol consumption and the risk of cancer of the colon and rectum in the Netherlands. Cancer Causes Control 5:95–104
Gonzalez CA, Riboli E, Badosa J, Batiste E, Cardona T, Pita S, Sanz JM, Torrent M, Agudo A (1994) Nutritional factors and gastric cancer in Spain. Am J Epidemiol 139:466–473
Govers MJ, Termont DS, Van der Meer R (1994) Mechanism of the antiproliferative effect of milk mineral and other calcium supplements on colonic epithelium. Cancer Res 54:95–100
Graham S, Haughey B, Marshall J, Brasure J, Zielezny M, Freudenheim J, West D, Nolan J, Wilkinson G (1990) Diet in the epidemiology of gastric cancer. Nutr Cancer 13:19–34

Gridley G, McLaughlin JK, Block G, Blot WJ, Winn DM, Greenberg RS, Schoenberg JB, Preston-Martin S, Austin DF, Fraumeni JF Jr (1990) Diet and oral and pharyngeal cancer among blacks. Nutr Cancer 14:219–225
Hansson LE, Nyren O, Bergstrom R, Wolk A, Lindgren A, Baron J, Adami HO (1993) Nutrients and gastric cancer risk. A population-based case-control study in Sweden. Int J Cancer 55:181–189
Hansson LE, Nyren O, Bergstrom R, Wolk A, Lindgren A, Baron J, Adami HO (1994) Nutrients and gastric cancer risk. A population-based case-control study in Sweden. Int J Cancer 57:638–644
Harris PJ, Ferguson LR (1993) Dietary fiber: its composition and role in protection against colorectal cancer. Mutat Res 290:97–110
Heath CW, Thun MJ, Greenberg ER, Levin B, Marnett LJ (1994) Nonsteroidal antiinflammatory drugs and human cancer. Report of an interdisciplinary research workshop. Cancer 74:2885–2888
Hill DL, Grubbs CJ (1992) Retinoids and cancer prevention. Annu Rev Nutr 12:161–181
Hosokawa N, Hosokawa Y, Sakai T, Yoshida M, Marui N, Nishino H, Kawai K, Aoike A (1990) Inhibitory effect of quercetin on the synthesis of a possibly cell-cycle-related 17-kDa protein in human colon cancer cells. Int J Cancer 45:1119–1124
Hu N, Dawsey SM, Wu M, Bonney GE, He LJ, Han XY, Fu M, Taylor PR (1992) Familial aggregation of oesophageal cancer in Yangcheng Country, Shanxi Province, China. Int J Epidemiol 21:877–882
Huang MT, Ferraro T (1992) Phenolic compounds in food and cancer prevention. In: Huang MT, Ho CT, Lee CY (eds) Phenolic compounds in food and their effects on health, vol II: antioxidants and cancer prevention. ACS Symposium Series 502, Washington DC, pp 8–33
Hwang H, Dwyer J, Russell RM (1994) Diet, *Helicobacter pylori* infection, food preservation and gastric cancer risk: are there new roles for preventative factors? Nutr Rev 52:75–83
Itzkowitz SH, Kim YS (1993) Polyps and benign neoplasms of the colon. In: Sleisenger MH, Fordtran JS (eds) Gastrointestinal disease. pathophysiology, diagnosis, managment, vol 2. Saunders, Philadelphia, pp 1402–1430
Kabat GC, Ng SK, Wynder EL (1993) Tobacco, alcohol intake, and diet in relation to adenocarcinoma of the esophagus and gastric carida. Cancer Causes Control 4:123–132
Kampman E, van't Veer P, Hiddink GJ, van Aken Schneijder P, Kok FJ, Hermus RJ (1994) Fermented dairy products, dietary calcium and colon cancer: a case-control study in the Netherlands. Int J Cancer 59:170–176
Katiyar SK, Agarwal R, Zaim MT, Mukhtar H (1993) Protection against N-nitrosodiethylamine and benzo[a]pyrene-induced forestomach and lung tumorigenesis in A/J mice by green tea.
Kato I, Tominaga S, Ito Y, Kobayashi S, Yoshii Y, Matsuura A, Kameya A, Kano T (1990) A comparative case-control analysis of stomach cancer and atrophic gastritis. Cancer Res 50:6559–6564
Kinlen LJ (1992) Immunosuppression and cancer. IARC Sci Publ 116:237–253
Kneller RW, Guo WD, Hsing AW, Chen JS, Blot WJ, Li JY, Forman D, Fraumeni JF Jr (1992) Risk factors for stomach cancer in sixty-five Chinese counties. Cancer Epidemiol Biomarkers Prev 1:113–118
Kono S (1992) Green tea and colon cancer. Jpn J Cancer Res 83:669
Kumar R, Mende P, Wacker CD, Spiegelhalder B, Preussmann R, Siddiqi M (1992) Caffeine-derived N-nitroso compounds. Nitrosable precursors from caffeine and their potential relevance in the etiology of oesophageal and gastric cancers in Kashmir, India. Carcinogenesis 13:2179–2182
Kune GA (1995) The causes of colorectal cancer. GI Cancer 1:25–31

Kune GA, Kune S, Field B, Watson LF (1988a) The role of chronic constipation, diarrhea, and laxative use in the etiology of large bowel cancer. Data from the Melbourne colorectal cancer study. Dis Colon Rectum 31:507–512

Kune GA, Kune S, Watson LF (1988b) Colorectal cancer risk, chronic illnesses, operations, and medications: case control results from the Melbourne Colorectal Cancer Study. Cancer Res 48:4399–4404

Kune GA, Kune S, Watson LF (1989) The role of heredity in the etiology of large bowel cancer: data from the Melbourne colorectal cancer study. World J Surg 13:124–131

Kune G, Kune S, Field B, Watson L (1990) The nutritional causes of large bowel cancer. In: Prasad KN, Meyskens FL (eds) Nutrients and cancer prevention. Humana, Clifton, NJ, pp 241–259

Kune GA, Kune S, Watson LF, Bahnson CB (1991) Personality as a risk factor in large bowel cancer. Data from the Melbourne colorectal cancer study. Psychol Med 321:29–41

Kune GA, Bannerman S, Watson LF (1992) Attributable risk for diet, alcohol, and family history in the Melbourne colorectal cancer study. Nutr Cancer 18:231–235

Kune GA, Kune S, Watson LF (1993) Perceived religiousness is protective for colorectal cancer. Data from the Melbourne colorectal cancer study. J R Soc Med 86:645–647

Lan Editorial (1990) Alcohol and cancer. Lancet 335:634–635

Lapré JA, Van der Meer R (1992) Dietary modulation of colon cancer risk: the roles of fat, fiber and calcium. Trends Food Sci Tech 3:320–324

LaVecchia C (1992) Cancers associated with high-fat diets. J Natl Cancer Inst Monographs 12:79–85

LaVecchia C, Harris RE, Wynder EL (1988) Comparative epidemiology of cancer between the United States and Italy. Cancer Res 48:7285–7293

LaVecchia C, Ferraroni M, D'Avanzo B, Decarli A, Franceschi S (1994) Selected micronutrient intake and the risk of gastric cancer. Cancer Epidemiol Biomarkers Prev 3:393–398

Lee HH, Wu HY, Chuang YC, Chang AS, Chao HH, Chen KY, Chen HK, Lai GM, Huang HH, Chen CJ (1990) Epidemiologic characteristics and multiple risk factors of stomach cancer in Taiwan. Anticancer Res 10:875–881

Longnecker MP, Orza MJ, Adams ME, Vioque J, Chalmers TC (1990). A metaanalysis of alcoholic beverage consumption in relation to risk of colorectal cancer. Cancer Causes Control 1:59–68

Markowitz S, Wang J, Myeroff L, Parsons R, Sun L, Lutterbaugh J, Fan RS, Zborowska E, Kinzler KW, Vogelstein B, Brattain M, Willson JKV (1995) Inactivation of the type II TGF-β receptor in colon cancer cells with microsatellite instability. Science 268:1336–1338

Memik F, Nak SG, Gulten M, Ozturk M (1992) Gastric carcinoma in northwestern Turkey: epidemiologic characteristics. J Environ Pathol Toxical Oncol 11:335–338

Nair P, Mayberry JF (1994) Vegetarianism, dietary fibre and gastro-intestinal disease. Dig Dis 12:177–185

Newmark HL (1992) Plant phenolic compounds as inhibitors of mutagenesis and carcinogenesis. In: Huang MT, Lee CY, Ho CT (eds) Phenolic compounds in food and their effects on health, vol II. Antioxidants and cancer prevention. ACS Symposium Series 502, Washington DC, pp 48–52

Newmark HL, Lupton JR (1990) Determinants and consequences of colonic luminal pH: implications for colon cancer. Nutr Cancer 14:161–173

Oreggia F, De Stefani E, Correa P, Fierro L (1991) Risk factors for cancer of the tongue in Uruguay. Cancer 67:180–183

Paganini-Hill A, Chao A, Ross RK, Henderson BE (1989) Aspirin use and chronic disease: a cohort study of elderly. BMJ 299:1247–1250

Peters RK, Pike MC, Garabrant D, Mack TM (1992) Diet and colon cancer in Los Angeles county, California. Cancer Causes Control 3:457–473
Potter JD (1992) Reconciling the epidemiology, physiology, and molecular biology of colon cancer. JAMA 268:1573–1577
Povey AC, Schiffman M, Taffe BG, Harris CC (1991) Laboratory and epidemiologic studies of fecapentaenes. Mutat Res 259:387–397
Prasad KN, Edwards-Prasad J (1990) Expressions of some molecular cancer risk factors and their modification by vitamins. J Am Coll Nutr 9:28–34
Prestera T, Holtzclaw WD, Zhang Y, Talalay P (1993) Chemical and molecular regulation of enzymes that detoxify carcinogens. Proc Natl Acad Sci U S A 90:1965–1969
Reddy BS, Engle A, Simi B, Goldman M (1992) Effect of dietary fiber on colonic bacterial enzymes and bile acids in relation to colon cancer. Gastroenterology 102:1475–82
Reshef R, Rozen P, Fireman Z, Fine N, Barzilai N, Shasha SM, Shkolnik T (1990) Effect of a calcium-enriched diet on the colonic epithelial hyperproliferation induced by N-methyl-N-nitro-N-nitrosoguanidine in rats on a low calcium and fat diet. Cancer Res. 50:1764–67
Rex DK, Lehman GA, Hawes RH, Ulbright TM, Smith JJ (1991) Screening colonoscopy in asymptomatic average-risk persons with engative fecal occult blood tests. Gastroenterology 100:64–67
Risio M (1992) Histology, histochemistry, tumor and serum markers in gastrointestinal tract cancer. Curr Opin Oncol 4:714–727
Rosenberg L (1990) Coffee and tea consumption in relation to the risk of large bowel cancer: a review of epidemiologic studies. Cancer Lett 52:163–171
Rosenberg L, Palmer JR, Zauber AG, Warshauer ME, Stolley PD, Shapiro S (1991) A hypothesis: nonsteroidal anti-inflammatory drugs reduce the incidence of large-bowel cancer. J Natl Cancer Inst 83:355–358
Scates DK, Spigelman AD, Nugent KP, Phillips RKS, Venitt S (1993) DNA adducts, detected by ^{32}P-postlabelling, in DNA treated in vitro with bile from patients with familial adenomatous polyposis and from unaffected controls. Carcinogenesis 14:1107–1110
Scates DK, Spigelman AD, Venitt S (1994) Bile acids do not form adducts when incubated with DNA in vitro. Carcinogenesis 15:2945–2948
Scheppach W, Bartram P, Richter A, Richter F, Liepold H, Dusel G, Hofstetter G, Rüthlein J, Kasper H (1992) Effect of short-chain fatty acids on the human colonic mucosa in vitro. J Parent Ent Nutr 16:43–48
Selby JV, Friedman GD (1989) Sigmoidoscopy in the periodic health examination of asymptomatic adults. JAMA 261:594–601
Shike M, Winawer SJ, Greenwald PH, Bloch A, Hill MJ, Swaroop SV (1990). Colorectal cancer. The WHO Collaborating Centre for the Prevention of Colorectal Cancer. Bull World Health Organ 68:377–385
Simopoulos AP (1990) Energy imbalance and cancer of the breast, colon and prostate. Med Oncol Tumor Pharmacother 7:109–120
Soltero E, Cruz NI, Lopez RE, Alonso A (1990) Cholecystectomy and right colon cancer in Puerto Rico. Cancer 66:2249–2252
Steinmetz KA, Potter JD (1991). Vegetables, fruit, and cancer. I. Epidemiology. Cancer Causes Control 2:325–357
Steinmetz KA, Kushi LH, Bostick RM, Folsom AR, Potter JD (1994) Vegetables, fruit, and colon cancer in the lowa Women's Health Study. Am J Epidemiol 139:1–15
Stemmermann GN (1989) Geographic epidemiology of colorectal cancer: the role of dietary fat: In: Seitz HK, Simanowski UA, Wright N (eds) Colorectal cancer. From pathogenesis to prevention? Springer, Berlin Heidelling New York, pp 3–23
Stemmermann G, Heffelfinger SC, Noffsinger A, Hui YZ, Miller MA, Fenoglio-Preiser CM (1994) The molecular biology of esophageal and gastric cancer and their precur-

sors: oncogenes, tumor suppressor genes, and growth factors. Hum Pathol 25:968–981
Takahashi T (1991) In hibition of azoxy-methane-induced colon carcinogenesis in rat by green tea polyphenol fraction. Jpn J Cancer Res 82:1336–1339
Tatsuta M, Iishi H, Baba M, Uehara H, Nakaizumi A, Taniguchi H (1993) Enhancing effects of calcium-deficient diet on gastric carcinogenesis by N-methyl-N′-nitro-N-nitrosoguanidine in Wistar rats. Jpn J Cancer Res 84:945–950
Taylor PR, Li B, Dawsey SM, Li JY, Yang CS, Guo W, Blot WJ (1994) Prevention of esophageal cancer: the nutrition intervention trials in Linxian, China. Linxian Nutrition Intervention Trials study Group. Cancer Res 54:2029s–2031s
Thun MJ, Namboodiri MM, Calle EE, Flanders WD, Heath CW Jr (1993) Aspirin use and risk of fatal cancer. Cancer Res 53:1322–1327
Tsugane S, Tsuda M, Gey F, Watanabe S (1992) Cross-sectional study with multiple measuremets of biological markers for assessing stomach cancer risks at the population level. Environ Health Perspect 98:207–210
Tuyns AJ, Kaaks R, Haelterman M (1988) Colorectal cancer and the consumption of foods: a case-control study in Belgium. Nutr Cancer 11:189–204
Tuyns AJ, Kaaks R, Haelterman M, Riboli E (1992) Diet and gastric cancer. A case-control study in Belgium. Int J Cancer 51:1–6
Vargas PA, Alberts DS (1992) Primary prevention of colorectal cancer through dietary modification. Cancer 70:1229–1235
Wang ZY, Hong JY, Huang MT, Reuhl KR, Conney AH, Yang CS (1992) Inhibition of N-nitrosodiethylamine-and4(methylnitrosamino)-1-(3-pyridyl)-1-butanone-induced tumorigenesis in A/J mice by green tea and black tea. Cancer Res 52:1943–1947
Wang GQ, Dawsey SM, Li JY, Taylor PR, Li B, Blot WJ, Weinstein WM, Liu FS, Lewin KJ, Wang H et al (1994) Effects of vitamin/mineral supplementation on the prevalence of histological dysplasia and early cancer of the esophagus and stomach: results from the General Population Trial in Linxian, China. Cancer Epidemiol Biomarkers Prev 3:161–166
Weisburger JH (1991) Causes, relevant mechanisms, and prevention of large bowel cancer. Semin Oncol 18:316–36
Weisburger JH, Reddy BS, Rose DP, Cohen LA, Kendal ME, Wynder EL (1993) Protective mechanisms of dietary fibers in nutritional carcinogenesis. Basic Life Sci 61:45–63
Willett WC (1994) Diet and health: what should we eat? Science 264:532–537
Willett WC, Stampfer MJ, Colditz GA, Rosner BA, Speizer FE (1990) Relation of meat, fat, and fiber intake to the risk of colon cancer in a prospective study among women. N Engl J Med 323:1664–1672
Winawer SJ, Zauber AG, O'Brien MJ et al (1993) Randomized comparison of surveillance intervals after colonoscopic removal of newly diagnosed adenomatous polyps. N Engl J Med 328:901–906
Wolf G (1992) Retinoids and carotenoids as inhibitors of carcinogenesis and inducers of cell-cell communication. Nutr Rev 50:270–274
Wu-Williams AH, Yu MC, Mack TM (1990) Life-style, workplace, and stomach cancer by subsite in young men of Los Angeles County. Cancer Res 50:2569–2576
Yamane T, Hagiwara N, Tateishi M, Akashi S, Kim M, Okuzumi J, Kitao Y, Inagake M, Kuwata K, Takahashi T (1991) Inhibition of azoxymethane-induced colon carcinogenesis in rat by green tea polyphenol fraction. Jpn J Cancer Res 82:1336-1339
Yanagihara K, Ito A, Toge T, Numoto M (1993) Antiproliferative effects of isoflavones on human cancer cell lines established from gastrointestinal tract. Cancer Res 53:5815–5821
Yang CS, Wang Z-Y (1993) Tea and cancer. J Natl Cancer Inst 85:1038–1049

Yasui W, Tahara E (1994) Molecular diagnosis on gastrointestinal cancers. Rinsho Byori 42:359–363
Yoshida M, Sakai T, Hosokawa N, Marui N, Matsumoto K, Fujioka A, Nishino H, Aoike A (1990) The effect of quercetin on cell cycle progression and growth of human gastric cancer cells. FEBS Lett 260:10–13
Yu GP, Hsieh CC (1991) Risk factors for stomach cancer: a population-based case-control study in Shanghai. Cancer Causes Control 2:169–174
Zaridze D, Filipchenko V, Kustov V, Serdyuk V, Duffy S (1993) Diet and colorectal cancer: results of two case-control studies in Russia. Eur J Cancer 29A:112–115

Drug Therapy in Metastatic Neuroendocrine Tumors of the Gastroenteropancreatic System

S. Faiss, H. Scherübl, E.O. Riecken, and B. Wiedenmann

Department of Internal Medicine and Gastroenterology, Universitätsklinikum Benjamin Franklin, Freie Universität Berlin, Hindenburgdamm 30, 12200 Berlin, Germany

Abstract

Successful treatment of neuroendocrine tumor disease of the gastroenteropancreatic system requires a multimodal approach. Radical tumor surgery is required before other therapies are initiated. So far, only surgery has proven to be curative. If surgical intervention is not possible or a tumor-free state cannot be achieved, biotherapy with the somatostatin analogues octreotide or lanreotide should then be preferably carried out in patients with functional tumors. Interferon-α can alternatively be given. In patients with gastrinoma, therapy with proton pump inhibitors (e.g., omeprazol) is the initial treatment of choice. In patients with nonfunctional tumors, indication for treatment is only given in cases of documented tumor progress.

In case of progressive tumor disease or functionality under the above-mentioned therapies, treatment with somatostatin analogues can be intensified by dose escalation or alternatively by a combination therapy with interferon-α and a somatostatin analogue. On the basis of the less favorable response of neuroendocrine foregut tumors to biotherapy, chemotherapy should be initiated after failure of biotherapy in documented tumor progression. A combination of streptozotocin and 5-fluorouracil, possibly combined with D,L-folinic acid, is the treatment of choice, considering the response and side effect rates. In case of predominantly anaplastic neuroendocrine tumors in advanced stages, good tumor response rates with a chemotherapeutic scheme consisting of cisplatin and etoposide can be achieved. Since the chemotherapy scheme is less effective in patients with midgut or hindgut tumors, chemoembolization of liver metastases should follow biotherapy. The response to chemoembolization may be increased by simultaneous systemic chemotherapy. Attention should always be paid to an adequate analgesic drug administration.

Recent Results in Cancer Research, Vol. 142

Introduction

Neuroendocrine tumors of the gastroenteropancreatic system are characterized by a relatively low incidence (1–2/100000) and normally slow tumor growth. Starting at a certain primary size, these tumors metastasize mainly to the liver. About half of the tumors are functionally active; i.e., via increased release of "tumor-specific" hormones and neurotransmitters they cause a characteristic "hypersecretion syndrome" with considerable restrictions on the patients' quality of life. According to the primary localization of these tumors, one differentiates between foregut tumors (esophagus, stomach, duodenum, pancreas), midgut tumors (jejunum, ileum, appendix, right-sided colon), and hindgut tumors (transverse colon, left-sided colon, sigmoid and rectum). Neuroendocrine tumors are also found outside of the gastroenteropancreatic system in the hepatobiliary and bronchial system, thymus, prostate, in the ovaries, and in other organs.

Neuroendocrine tumors with primary localization in the stomach or the small intestine and secretion of serotonin as well as other neurotransmitters or polypeptides (granins, tachykinines, bradykinines) are also classified as carcinoids. The clinical picture resulting from the release of neurotransmitters leading to flush, diarrhea, bronchoconstriction, and right-heart involvement in the form of endocardiac fibrosis is therefore also classified as carcinoid syndrome. But also in patients with nonfunctional neuroendocrine tumors right-heart involvement can occur (Dingerkus et al. 1994). One third of all patients with a functional neuroendocrine tumor ultimately die, not from the direct consequences of tumor growth but from the consequences of severe cardiac insufficiency, triggered by long-standing specific right-heart alterations. Left untreated, patients with metastasizing serotonin-producing neuroendocrine tumors with primary localization in the small intestine have a 5-year survival rate of merely 20% (Moertel 1987; Norheim et al. 1987).

Other, nonserotonin-producing, functional neuroendocrine tumors are primarily localized in the pancreas as well as the duodenum and are called insulinoma, gastrinoma, glucagonoma, and vipoma, depending on the respective secreted hormone. In contrast to midgut tumors, these tumors have a more heterogeneous tumor biology with variable proliferation characteristics (Öberg 1993). Whereas only 10–15% of all insulin-producing pancreatic tumors exhibit the criteria of malignant growth, tumors producing other hormones can be largely classified as being malignant. Aggressive growth behavior can be observed in neuroendocrine pancreatic tumors without hormone-related clinical syndromes. In contrast to functional pancreatic tumors, nonfunctional tumors produce mostly inactive peptides, but complete peptides like alpha- and beta-HCG or pancreatic polypeptide are also found (Öberg 1993).

Of all patients with a multiple neoplasia type 1 (MEN-1), 30–80% have adenomas of the anterior pituitary as well as of the parathyroids. Neuroendocrine pancreatic tumor disease can be detected in up to 80% of MEN-1 patients. The survival rate of patients with neuroendocrine pancreatic tumors and a simultaneous MEN-1 constellation appears to differ considerably from that for other functional and nonfunctional neuroendocrine pancreatic tumors. Patients with a MEN-1 constellation and a gastrinoma can survive more than 20 years despite liver metastases, whereas patients with nonfunctional sporadic neuroendocrine pancreatic tumors generally die within a few years after diagnosis (Eriksson et al. 1990; Skogseid et al. 1991).

Provided the primary tumor is known and resectable, radical tumor surgery is the treatment of choice for all neuroendocrine tumors of the gastroenteropancreatic system. For inoperable metastasized tumors, several drug therapy approaches are available, their goal being not only the control of clinical symptoms in functional tumors but also a tumor size reduction. Since these tumors are usually slowly growing, tumor debulking also leads to a prolonged survival (Ahlman et al. 1994).

An indication for nonsurgical treatment in neuroendocrine tumors of the gastroenteropancreatic system is given after tumor progression has occurred. Tumor progression should be substantiated not only by conventional imaging techniques (abdomen sonography, computed tomography, MRI) but also by somatostatin receptor scintigraphy and endosonography in the upper and lower gastrointestinal tract. These imaging techniques are complemented by tumor-specific biological parameters. Besides directly assessing the release of hormones and neurotransmitters (serotonin, insulin, gastrin, glucagon, VIP), it is diagnostically important to demonstrate 5-hydroxyindolacetate in urine and increased chromogranin-A levels in serum.

In the following we describe the possibilities of drug treatment for metastasized neuroendocrine tumors of the gastroenteropancreatic system.

Somatostatin Analogues

Somatostatin analogues are long-acting derivatives of human somatostatin. Among many other functions, somatostatin interferes with the release of hormones and neurotransmitters. So far, five different somatostatin receptor subtypes have been identified (Yamada et al. 1992). Recent studies in our laboratory show that somatostatin analogues activate primarily somatostatin receptor subtype 2 and possibly also subtype 5 in vivo (John et al. 1996; Scherübl et al. 1994a). Activation of somatostatin receptors blocks vesicular release of hormones and transmitters. In addition to inhibition of vesicular release, somatostatin appears to directly interfere with gene expression (Todisco et al. 1994), which explains some of the observed antiproliferative effects of somatostatin.

When somatostatin is medically applied, it often results in a disappearance of clinical symptoms in neuroendocrine tumors of the gastroenteropancreatic system. Since native somatostatin has a very short half-life (Frohlich et al. 1978), somatostatin analogues such as octreotide and lanreotide have been developed; they have a half-life of several hours and are therefore administered subcutaneously 2–3 times daily (Kvols et al. 1986). Recently, a slow-release form of lanreotide has also been developed which has to be applied only at 2 weeks intervals (Scherübl et al. 1994b).

Somatostatin analogues have become the drugs of choice for the symptomatic treatment of carcinoid syndrome in particular. They are clinically effective at a dosage ranging from 2–3 times 0.05 mg daily to 2–3 times 0.5 mg daily with a reported 50–96% reduction in the incidence of diarrhea and flush (Kvols 1989; Vinik et al. 1989; Öberg et al. 1991; Arnold et al. 1993). In parallel, a reduced excretion of the serotonin metabolite 5-hydroxyindolicacetic acid (5-HIAA) in urine as well as chromogranin-A in serum is observed. Biochemical response, defined as at least 50% reduction in 5-HIAA urinary excretion, to treatment with 3 × 0.150 mg octreotide was observed in 70% of the cases in a small patient population (Kvols et al. 1986) (cf. Table 1). Side effects leading to termination of treatment are rare and are to only some extent dose dependent. Most side effects are only temporarily observed at the initiation of somatostatin analogues, and generally disappear during the course of treatment. The entire spectrum of side effects of the somatostatin analogues is given in Table 2.

Several studies report tumor regression under treatment with rather low doses of somatostatin analogues in individual cases (Kvols et al. 1986;

Table 1. Biochemical, objective, and symptomatic (subjective) response to different treatments with somatostatin analogues in patients with metastatic neuroendocrine tumors of the gastroenteropancreatic system. Before high-dose lanreotide (3 × 5 mg/day s.c.) therapy started, all patients showed progressive tumor disease under conventional dosages of somatostatin analogues

Response	Octreotide[a] 3 × 0.15 mg/day s.c.	Lanreotide[b] 3 × 5 mg/day s.c.	Lanreotide[c] 1 × 30 mg/14 days i.m.
Biochemical, *n* (%)			
PR	18/25 (72)	14/26 (54)	6/11 (55)
SD	7/25 (28)	12/26 (46)	2/11 (18)
PD	0	0	3/11 (27)
Objective, *n* (%)			
CR	–	1/26 (4)	0
PR	1/25 (4)	1/26 (4)	0
SD	–	12/26 (46)	7/11 (64)
PD	–	7/26 (27)	4/11 (36)
Symptomatic, *n* (%)	22/25 (88)	11/26 (42)	8/11 (73)

CR, Complete remission; *PR*, partial remission; *SD*, stable disease; *PD*, progressive disease

[a] Kvols et al. 1986
[b] S. Faiss et al., unpublished results
[c] Scherübl et al. 1994b

Table 2. Frequency of typical side effects of octreotide and interferon-alpha

Octreotide:	
Malabsorption/diarrhea	17%
Abdominal pain	23%
Cholecystolithiasis	7%
Cholangitis	4%
Allergic reactions	2%
Bradycardia	2%
Interferon-alpha:	
Flu-like symptoms	74%
Fatigue, muscle pain	53%
Anorexia, weight loss	37%
Anemia	30%
Allergic reactions	5%
Autoimmune vasculitis	5%
Hypothyreosis	5%

Wiedenmann et al. 1988; Stöckmann et al. 1988). Since a dose-dependent antiproliferative effect of somatostatin has been reported, studies with high doses (2–3 mg/day) of the somatostatin analogue lanreotide have been started (Anthony et al. 1993). A study of 26 patients with metastatic neuroendocrine tumors of the gastroenteropancreatic system in our center, together with the University of Heidelberg, showed that lanreotide given at a high dosage (3 × 5 mg/day) can even lead to complete or partial remission. Moreover, imaging procedures revealed a cessation of tumor growth in 46% of all patients. The clinical and biochemical response rates were 42% and 54%, respectively (Table 1). These response rates are low compared with other studies using normal doses of octreotide. This is probably due less to the effectiveness of the substance itself than to the composition of the selected patient population. All patients had in fact been clinically progressive under previous therapy with normal doses of somatostatin analogues. Imaging procedures revealed a continuous progression under high-dose therapy with lanreotide in seven patients. The side effects were similar to those under normal-dosed octreotide therapy (Table 2). Consequently, at least in individual cases, an additional antiproliferative action can be obtained with high-dose somatostatin analogue therapy in patients with progressive metastatic neuroendocrine tumors of the gastroenteropancreatic system.

Further advances in somatostatin analogue treatment include the application of long-acting depot forms administered by intramuscular injections at 10- to 14-day intervals (Heron et al. 1993; Scherübl et al. 1994b). Comparable biochemical, radiological, and clinical response rates with conventional octreotide therapy can also be observed with a depot formulation in most patients with functional neuroendocrine tumors (Scherübl et al. 1994). Table 1 gives a survey of the response rates of metastatic neuroendocrine tumors of the gastroenteropancreatic system under therapy with octreotide, high-dose lanreotide (3 × 5 mg), and a lanreotide depot form (30 mg i.m.).

Interferon

Alternatively to somatostatin and its analogues, interferon-alpha is used as a monosubstance in the therapy of metastatic neuroendocrine tumors of the gastroenteropancreatic system. In addition to their known antiviral action, alpha- and beta-interferons also appear to affect cell division. Moreover, they are potent immunomodulators (Balkwill 1989). In some earlier studies it was shown that interferon-alpha has an antiproliferative action in neuroendocrine tumors of the gastroenteropancreatic system and simultaneously reduces the tumor secretion products, and thus can lead to an improvement of symptoms (Öberg et al. 1983, 1986; Smith et al. 1987). Flu-like symptoms, a typical interferon-alpha side effect, can be kept well under control by simultaneous administration of 500 or 1000 mg paracetamol. The common spectrum of typical interferon-alpha side effects is shown in Table 2.

In a meta-analysis of all studies performed with interferon-alpha up to 1993, Öberg obtains a mean tumor response, defined as a reduction in tumor size by at least 50% (PR = partial remission) in 11% of 310 patients, and the biochemical response was positive in 42% (Öberg 1993). However, studies are compared within this meta-analysis with partially different patient populations and varying high dosages of interferon. The dosages range from 5 Mio I.U. interferon-alpha 3×/week to 5 Mio I.U. 8 ×/week up to 2 Mio I.U./m interferon-alpha 12×/week (Hanssen et al. 1989; Bartsch et al. 1990; Öberg et al. 1991). The patient population consists of patients with neuroendocrine tumors at different primary sites and pretreatment with different substances. In one study, an embolization of the hepatic artery is simultaneously performed with interferon therapy (Hanssen et al. 1989). On the whole, an exact statement on the definitive response rates within this meta-analysis is not possible. In one report, Eriksson and Öberg (1993) describe a clinical response to interferon-alpha therapy with 5 Mio I.U. 3×/week in 47% of 57 patients with neuroendocrine pancreatic tumors. There was a reduction in tumor size in 12% of the patients, as demonstrated in imaging procedures, while in 24% of the patients there was a cessation of tumor growth. In this patient population, interferon-alpha therapy was superior to treatment with octreotide (Table 3).

In the largest study with interferon-alpha so far, Öberg et al. describe a biochemical therapeutic response to 5 Mio I.U. interferon-alpha 3×/week of 42% in 111 patients with functional and nonfunctional neuroendocrine tumors of the intestine. Imaging procedures demonstrate a partial tumor remission in 15%. In 66% of all patients there was a cessation of tumor growth; 68% of the patients showed clinical improvement in tumor-related symptoms (Table 4) (Öberg et al. 1991).

Table 3. Biochemical, objective, and symptomatic (subjective) response to octreotide and interferon-alpha therapy in patients with metastatic neuroendocrine tumors of the pancreas (Eriksson and Öberg 1993)

Response	Octreotide *n* (%)	Interferon-alpha *n* (%)
Biochemical	6/19 (31.5)	27/57 (47.4)
Objective		
CR	0	0
PR	0	7/57 (12.3)
SD	6/19 (31.5)	14/57 (24.5)
PD	7/19 (37)	14/57 (24.5)
Symptomatic	6/19 (31.5)	29/57 (51)

CR, Complete remission; *PR*, partial remission; *SD*, stable disease; *PD*, progressive disease

Table 4. Biochemical, objective, and symptomatic (subjective) response to interferon-alpha therapy in patients with metastatic neuroendocrine tumors of the gut (Öberg and Eriksson 1991)

Response	Interferon-alpha *n* (%)
Biochemical	
PR	47/111 (42)
SD	43/111 (39)
PD	21/111 (19)
Objective	
CR	0
PR	16/111 (15)
SD	74/111 (66)
PD	21/111 (19)
Symptomatic	76/111 (68)

CR, Complete remission; *PR*, partial remission; *SD*, stable disease; *PD*, progressive disease

A comparison of these two studies performed on relatively large patient populations shows that interferon-alpha therapy can obtain good response rates with relatively few side effects. Öberg et al. postulate a better response to interferon than to somatostatin in patients with neuroendocrine tumors of the pancreas. In order to enhance the antiproliferative effect of interferon-alpha, it seemed useful to apply a combination with somatostatin analogues, which have, as presented above, an antiproliferative effect, in addition to reducing tumor-related symptoms. While Creutzfeld and co-workers demonstrated that interferon in combination with the somatostatin analogue octreotide has no additional antiproliferative effect (Creutzfeld et al. 1991), more recent studies have shown, at least in individual cases, a synergistic effect of somatostatin analogues combined with interferon-alpha (Joensuu et al. 1992). In a larger study of 20 patients, Tiensuu Janson et al. (1992) reported a growth cessation in 15 of the 20 patients (75%) under a combined therapy of interferon-alpha and octreotide in metastatic neuroendocrine tumors with a primary location in the small and large intestine (Table 5).

There was a significant reduction of initially increased values of 5-hydroxyindolicacetic acid in 24-h urine in 77% of the patients. In comparison, Nold et al. (1994) report on a patient with a partial remission concerning tumor size in a small patient population ($n = 7$) with neuroendocrine pancreatic tumors.

To what extent a combination of somatostatin analogues with interferon-alpha can obtain an increase in efficacy as compared with the respective monotherapies has not yet been examined in a prospective, randomized study. Thus, our study group is presently involved in setting up a three-armed prospective randomized study, which will be performed multicentrically in Germany. In this study, monotherapy with interferon-alpha and lanreotide will be compared with the combined therapy of both substances.

Chemotherapy

In the early 1980s, chemotherapy was considered a mainstay of medical therapy for neuroendocrine tumors of the gastroenteropancreatic system. Based on good response rates to streptozotocin therapy of metastatic, neuroendocrine pancreatic tumors, a variety of combination therapies were tested in clinical studies. The results of the most diverse monotherapies published and the combination therapies developed therefrom led to an objective re-

Table 5. Biochemical and objective response to octreotide therapy combined with interferon-alpha in patients with metastatic neuroendocrine tumors of the gut and pancreas

Response	Neuroendocrine tumor of the gut (Tiensuu Janson et al. 1992)	Neuroendocrine pancreatic tumor (Nold et al. 1994)
Biochemical, n (%)		
PR	17/22 (77)	2/7 (29)
SD	4/22 (18)	–
PD	1/22 (4.5)	–
Objective, n (%)		
CR	0	0
PR	0	1/7 (14)
SD	15/20 (75)	3/7 (43)
PD	5/20 (25)	3/7 (43)

CR, Complete remission; *PR*, partial remission; *SD*, stable disease; *PD*, progressive disease sponse in approximately 30–70% of all patients with neuroendocrine pancreatic tumors (Moertel et al. 1980, 1992). Among intestinal neuroendocrine tumors, on the other hand, the response rate of 0–26% is markedly lower (Engström et al. 1984; Öberg 1993). The period of remission likewise appears to be markedly shorter than in patients with neuroendocrine pancreatic tumors. A survey of the complied results is given in Tables 6 and 7.

Table 6. Objective response and response duration of different chemotherapies in patients with metastatic neuroendocrine tumors of the gut

	Patients (*n*)	Objective response (%)	Response duration (months)
Monotherapy:			
Doxorubicin[a]	81	21	6
5-FU[b]	19	26	3
Dacarbazine[e,b]	18	17	5
Streptozotocin[b]	6	17	2
Combination therapy:			
Streptozotocin + 5-FU[a]	80	22	7.2
Cyclophosphamide + MTX[b]	16	0	–
Cyclophosphamide + streptozotocin[b]	14	0	–

[a] Engström et al. 1984
[b] Öberg et al. 1993

Table 7. Objective response and response duration of different chemotherapies in patients with metastatic neuroendocrine tumors of the pancreas

	Patients (*n*)	Objective response (%)	Response duration (months)
Monotherapy:			
Streptozotocin[a]	17	41	7
Doxorubicin[a]	17	17	4
Chlorozotocin[b]	33	30	16
Combination therapy:			
Streptozotocin			
+5-FU[a]	30	63	19
+5-FU[b]	34	45	16
+5-FU[c]	31	54	26
+Doxorubicin[b]	38	69	27
+Doxorubicin[c]	25	36	22
+5-FU +D,L-folinic acid[d]	12	67	4

[a] Moertel et al. 1980
[b] Moertel et al. 1992
[c] Eriksson et al. 1990
[d] S. Faiss et al., unpublished results

The most comprehensive study published in recent years compared, in a three-armed approach, the efficacy of chemotherapy with streptozotocin plus 5-fluorouracil with that of streptozotocin plus doxorubicin and with a chlorozotocin monotherapy in 105 patients with metastasized neuroendocrine pancreatic tumors (Moertel et al. 1992). The results demonstrate that treatment with streptozotocin plus doxorubicin is superior to streptozotocin plus 5-fluorouracil with regard to the objective response rates (69% and 45%, $p = 0.05$) and remission time (20 and 6.9 months, $p = 0.001$). The former combination therapy shows a significant increase in the survival time of the patients (2.2 and 1.4 years, $p = 0.004$). Response rates around 30% can be reached with chlorozotocin alone and a comparable remission and survival time are obtained with streptozotocin plus 5-fluorouracil. These results largely agree with those published earlier by the Mayo Clinic (Moertel 1987). They differ merely in a low response rate to treatment with streptozotocin plus 5-fluorouracil, which had been reported to be as high as 60% in earlier studies (Moertel et al. 1980, 1992) (cf. Table 7). Possible differences result from a dissimilar composition of the treated patient groups. Thus, due to fewer side effects, we suggest administering primarily a combination therapy with streptozotocin plus 5-fluorouracil instead of streptozotocin plus doxorubicin.

In another study published by Moertel et al. in 1991, a total of 45 patients with metastasizing neuroendocrine tumors were treated with a combination of etoposide and cisplatin. Twenty-seven of these patients had a well-differentiated neuroendocrine tumor with primary localization in the region of the foregut or midgut. Eighteen patients had an anaplastic neuroendocrine tumor of the foregut. Merely two of the patients with well-differentiated tumors (7%) had a reduction in tumor size. One the other hand, the patient group with anaplastic tumors had a response rate of 67%. Even three complete remissions were reported. However, almost all the patients treated exhibited considerable side effects (nausea, leukopenia, anemia, thrombocytopenia, alopecia, and neuropathy). Altogether, considerable response rates can be obtained with these schemes in patients with anaplastic neuroendocrine tumor disease.

A recent study from the Mayo Clinic reports that response rates of up to 80% were obtained in a total of 111 patients with systemic chemotherapy (doxorubicin plus dacarbazine or streptozotocin plue 5-fluorouracil) as a supplement to chemoembolization of liver metastases (Moertel et al. 1994). In the future, this could be a promising therapeutic approach in patients with progressive tumor conditions. A response rate as high as 60% was actually achieved in this study with chemoembolization alone.

The basis for chemoembolization is the fact that liver metastases possess a pronounced blood supply via the branches of the hepatic artery and have practically no connection to the branches of the portal vein. In recent years, a range of improved procedures up to the superselective microembolization have been developed which make it possible to directly treat intrahepatic metastatic foci and embolize with or without the addition of chemotherapeutic agents (Carrasco et al. 1986; Marlink et al. 1990; Moertel et al. 1994). Response rates of up to 80% were obtained in patients with neuroendocrine tumors at various sites (Carrasco et al. 1986). However, a full response was obtained in some patients only after repeated chemoembolization.

Symptomatic Therapy

Symptomatic drug therapy of neuroendocrine tumors of the gastroenteropancreatic system is directed toward the syndromes caused by the tumors. If diarrhea is predominant in carcinoid syndrome and cannot be reduced to a degree acceptable for the patient by somatostatin analogues and interferon-alpha, accompanying antidiarrheal agents (loperamide, opium tincture) can be successfully administered. Therapy of flush symptoms is most successful with somatostatin analogues. In patients with right-heart involvement and consecutive cardiac insufficiency, consistent treatment of cardiac insufficiency is important.

Since the introduction of proton pump inhibitors (e.g., omeprazol), Zollinger-Ellison syndrome can be well controlled. To reduce the need for continuous glucose in patients with advanced insulinoma, treatment with diazoxide is useful. To control excessive diarrhea in VIP-producing neuroendocrine tumors, somatostatin analogues are the mainstay in therapy.

As in other metastatic diseases, pain control by adequate analgesic therapy is ncesseary in all patients with neuroendocrine tumors of the gastroenteropancreatic system. In patients with increasing weight loss, due either to uncontrollable diarrhea or to the progressive tumor condition, a temporary, high-calorie formula feeding together with the administration of steroids or even parenteral hyperalimention in the framework of chemotherapy can contribute to the subjective improvement of the patient's condition.

Conclusion

Successful treatment of neuroendocrine tumor disease of the gastroenteropancreatic system requires a multimodal apporach. Radical tumor surgery is prerequisite before other therapies are initiated. So far, only with surgery is a curative approach possible. If surgical intervention is not possible or a tumor-free state cannot be achieved, a biotherapy with the somatostatin analogues octreotide or lanreotide should then be preferably carried out in patients with functional tumors. Alternatively, interferon-alpha can be applied. In patients with a gastrinoma, therapy with proton pump inhibitors (e.g., omeprazol) is the initial treatment of choice. In patients with nonfunctional tumors, indication for treatment is given only in cases of documented tumor

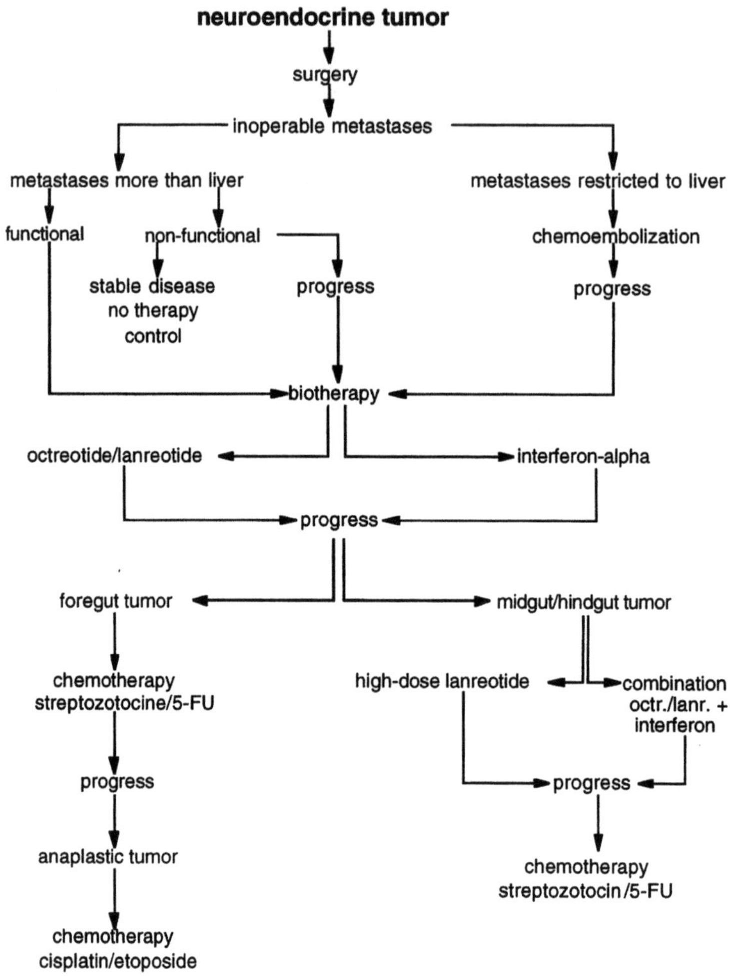

Fig. 1. Alternative methods in the treatment of patients with metastatic neuroendocrine tumors of the gastroenteropancreatic system

progress. In general, response rates (partial and complete remissions) in functional and nonfunctional tumors do not differ.

In case of progressive tumor disease or functionality under the above-mentioned therapies, treatment with somatostatin analogues can be intensified by escalating the dose of the somatostatin analogue lanreotide up to 3 × 5 mg or, alternatively, by a combination therapy with interferon-alpha and a somatostatin analogue (e.g., 3 × 0.5 mg lanreotide). On the basis of the less favorable response of neuroendocrine foregut tumors to biotherapy, chemotherapy should be initiated after failure of biotherapy in documented tumor progress. A combination of streptozotocin and 5-fluorouracil, possibly combined with D,L folinic acid, is the treatment of choice, considering the response and side-effect rates. In case of predominantly anaplastic neuroendocrine tumors at advanced stages, good tumor response rates with a chemotherapeutic protocol consisting of cisplatin and etoposide can be achieved. Since chemotherapy is less effective in patients with midgut or hindgut tumors, chemoembolization of liver metastases should follow biotherapy. The response to chemoembolization may be increased by simultaneous systemic chemotherapy. If the reported positive results of chemoembolization are also confirmed in other studies, applying this therapeutic procedure after biotherapy failure and before beginning systemic chemotherapy will be justified.

In all therapeutic steps, attention should be always be paid to adequate analgesic drug administration. Additional antidiarrheal agents can be used to improve symptoms caused by hormone and neurotransmitter release and various drugs for right-heart involvement.

A survey of the conservative therapeutic possibilities in metastasized neuroendocrine tumors of different origin and function of the gastroenteropancreatic system is given in Fig. 1. Overall, further controlled studies are certainly necessary in order to develop an even better therapeutic concept for all patients with metastasized neuroendocrine tumors of the gastroenteropancreatic system.

References

Ahlman H, Wängberg B, Tisell LE, Nilsson O, Fjälling M, Forsell-Aronsson E (1994) Clinical efficacy of octreotide scintigraphy in patients with midgut carcinoid tumours and evaluation of intraoperative scintillation detection. Br J Surg 81:1144–1149

Anthony L, Johnson D, Hande K (1993) Somatostatin analogue phase I trials in neuroendocrine neoplasms. Acta Oncol 32:217–223

Arnold R, Neuhaus C, Benning R, Schwerk W, Trautmann ME (1993) Somatostatin analog Sandostatin and inhibition of tumor growth in patients with metastatic endocrine gastroenteropancreatic tumors, World J Surg 17:511–519

Balkwill FR (1989) Interferons. Lancet 1:1060–1063

Bartsch HH, Stockman F, Arnold R, Creutzfeldt W (1990) Treatment of patients with metastatic carcinoid tumors by recombinant human interferon-alpha: results from a phase II study. J Cancer Res Clin Oncol 116:305

Carrasco CH, Charnsangavej C, Ajani J, Samaan NA, Richli W, Wallace S (1986) The carcinoid syndrome: palliation by hepatic artery embolization. Am J Rad 147:149–154

Creutzfeld W, Bartsch HH, Jacubaschke K, Stöckmann F (1991) Treatment of gastrointestinal endocrine tumors with alpha-interferon and octreotide. Acta Oncol 30:529–535

Dingerkus H, Völler H, Schröder K, Dißmann R, Henning L, Agrawal R, Linderer T, Wiedenmann B (1994) Endokardfibrose bei neuroendokrinen Tumoren des gastroenteropankreatischen Systems. Dtsch Med Wochenschr 119:647–652

Engström PF, Lawin PT, Moertel CG, Fölsch E, Douglass HO (1984) Streptozocin plus fluorouracil versus doxorubicin therapy for metastatic carcinoid tumors. J Clin Oncol 2:1255–1259

Erikssön B, Skogseid B, Lundqvist G, Wide L, Wilander E, Öberg K (1990) Medical treatment and long-term survival in a prospective study of 84 patients with endocrine pancreatic tumors. Cancer 65:1883–1890
Eriksson B, Öberg K (1993) An update of medical treatment of malignant endocrine pancreatic tumors. Acta Oncol 32:203–208
Frohlich JC, Bloomgarden ZT, Oates JA, McGugan J, Rabinowitz D (1978) The carcinoid flush: provocation by pentagastrin and inhibition by somatostatin. N Engl J Med 299:1055–1057
Hanssen LE, Schrumpf E, Kolbenstvedt AN, Tausjö J, Dolva LO (1989) Treatment of malignant metastatic midgut carcinoid tumours with recombinant human alpha-2b-interferon with or without prior hepatic artery embolization. Scand J Gastroenterol 24:787–795
Heron I, Thomas F, Dero M (1993) Pharmacokinetics and efficacy of a long-acting formulation of the new somatostatin analogue BIM 23014 in patients with acromegaly. J Clin Endocrinol Metab 76:721–727
Joensuu H, Katka K, Kujari H (1992) Dramatic response of a metastatic carcinoid tumor to a combination of interferon and octreotide. Acta Endocrinol (Copenh) 126:184–185
John M, Meyerhof W, Richter D, Waser B, Schaer JC, Boese-Landgraf J, Neuhaus P, Scherübl H, Riecken E-O, Reubi JC, Wiedenmann B (1996) Positive somatostatin receptor scintigraphy correlates with the presence of somatostatin receptor subtype 2. Gut 38 (in press)
Kvols LK, Moertel CG, O'Connell MJ, Schutt AK, Rubin J, Hahn RG (1986) Treatment of the malignant carcinoid syndrome. Evaluation of a long-acting somatostatin analogue. N Engl J Med 315:663–666
Kvols LK (1989) Therapy of malignant carcinoid syndrome. Endocrinol Metabol Clin North Am 18:557–568
Marlink RG, Lokich T, Robins JR, Clouse ME (1990) Hepatic arterial embolization for metastatic hormone-secreting tumor: technique, effectivness, and complications. Cancer 65:2227–2232
Moertel CG (1987) An odyssey in the land of small tumors. J Clin Oncol 5:1502–1522
Moertel CG, Hanley JA, Johnson LA (1980) Streptozocin alone compared with streptozocin plus fluorouracil in the treatment of advanced islet-cell carcinoma. N Engl J Med 303:1189–1194
Moertel CG, Kvols LK, O'Connell MJ, Rubin J (1991) Treatment of neuroendocrine carcinomas with combined etoposide and cisplatin. Cancer 68:227–232
Moertel CG, Lefkopoulo M, Lipsitz S, Hahn RG, Klaassen D (1992) Streptozocin-doxorubicin, streptozocin-fluorouracil, or chlorozotocin in the treatment of advanced islet-cell carcinoma. N Engl J Med 326:519–523
Moertel CG, Johnson CM, McKusick MA, Martin JK, Nagorney DM, Kvols LK, Rubin J, Kunselman S (1994) The management of patients with advanced carcinoid tumors and islet cell carcinomas. Ann Intern Med 120:302–309
Nold R, Frank M, Kajdan U, Trost U, Klose KJ, Arnold R (1994) Kombinierte Behandlung metastasierter neuroendokriner Tumoren des Gastrointestinaltrakts mit Octreotid und Interferon-Alpha. Z Gastroenterol 32:193–197
Norheim I, Öberg K, Theodorsson Norheim, E, Lindgren PG, Lundin I, Lundqvist G, Magnusson A, Wide L, Wilander E (1987) Malignant carcinoid tumors: an analysis of 103 patients with regard to tumor localization, hormone production and survivgal. Ann Surg 206:115–125
Öberg K (1993) Chemotherapy and biotherapy in neuroendocrine tumors. Curr Opin Oncol 5:110–120
Öberg K, Eriksson, B (1991) The role of interferons in the mangement of carcinoid tumors. Acta Oncol 30:519–522

Öberg K, Funa K, Alm G (1983) Effects of leucocyte interferon on clinical symptoms and hormone levels in patients with mid-gut carcinoid tumors and carcinoid syndrome. N Engl J Med 309:129–133
Öberg K, Norheim I, Lind E, Alm G, Lundquist G, Wide L, Jonsdottir B, Magnusson A, Wilander E (1986) Treatment of malignant carcinoid tumors with human leucocyte interferon: long-term results. Cancer Treat Rep 11:1297–1304
Öberg K, Norheim I, Theodorsson E (1991) Treatment of malignant midgut carcinoid tumors with the long-acting somatostatin-analogue, octreotide. Acta Oncol 30:503–507
Scherübl H, Hescheler J, Bychkov R, Cuber JC, John M, Riecken EO, Wiedenmann B (1994a) Elecrical activity and calcium channels in neuroendocrine cells. Ann NY Acad Sci 733:335–339
Scherübl H, Wiedenmann B, Riecken E-O, Faiss S, Thomas F, Kommerell B, Räth U (1994b) Treatment of the carcinoid syndrome with a depot formulation of the somatostatin analogue lanreotide. Eur J Cancer 6:1590–1591
Skogseid B, Eriksson B, Lundqvist G, Lörelius LE, Rastad J, Wide L, Wilander E, Akerström G, Öberg K (1991) Multiple endocrine neoplasia type 1: a ten-year prospective screening study in four kindreds. J Clin Endocrinol Metab 73:281–287
Smith DB, Scarffe JH, Wagstaff J, Johnston RJ (1987) Phase II trial of rDNA alfa 2b interferon in patients with malignant carcinoid tumor. Cancer Treat Rep 7:1265–1268
Stöckmann F, Creutzfeld W (1988) Behandlung gastrointestinaler neuroendockriner Tumoren mit dem Somatostatin-Analog Octreotide (Sandostatin). Z Gastroenterol 26:665
Tiensuu Janson EM, Ahlström H, Andersson T, Öberg K (1992) Octreotide and interferon alfa; a new combination for the treatment of malignant carcinoid tumors. Eur J Cancer 28A:1647–1650
Todisco A, Seva C, Takeuchi Y, Dickinson CJ, Yamada T (1994) Inhibition of AP-1 function via SSTR2 mediates somatostatin inhibition of cell proliferation. Dig Dis Sci 8:1788
Vinik AI, Thompson N, Echkauser F, Mottari AR (1989) Clinical features of carcinoid syndrome and the use of somatostatin analogue and its management. Acta Oncol 28;389–402
Wiedenmann B, Räth U, Rädsch R, Becker F, Kommerell B (1988) Tumor regression of an ileal carcinoid under the treatment with the somatostatin analogue SMS 201–995. Klin Wochenschr 6;75–77
Yamada Y, Reisine T, Law SF, Ihara Y, Kubota A, Kagimoto S, Seino M, Seino Y, Bell GI, Seino S (1992) Somatostatin receptors, an expanding gene family: cloning and functional characterization of human sstr 3, a protein coupled to adenylyl cyclase. Mol Endocrinol 6:2136–2142

Laparoscopic Lymph Node Assessment in Pretherapeutic Staging of Gastric and Esophageal Cancer

B. Rau, M. Hünerbein, B. Reingruber, P. Hohenberger, and P.M. Schlag

Virchow Klinikum, Medical Faculty of the Humboldt University, Robert-Rössle Cancer Hospital, Max Delbrück Center of Molecular Medicine, Lindenberger Weg 80, 13122 Berlin, Germany

Abstract

In gastric cancer lymph node metastases at the hepatoduodenal ligament and in esophageal cancer, metastases at the celiac axis are classified as distant metastases (M1 LYMPH) and implying a poor prognosis. In pretherapeutic staging, imaging procedures such as computed tomography of the abdomen or transcutaneous ultrasonic examination are of limited value in the assessment of enlarged or metastatic lymph nodes. Conversely, laparoscopic staging with subsequent biopsy of suspicious lymph nodes provides essential diagnostic information.

After exclusion of distant metastases (liver, lung, bone) in 73 patients with esophageal- ($n=21$) and gastric cancer ($n=52$), staging laparoscopy, including laparoscopic ultrasound, were performed during an 18-month-period (July/93–December/94). After laparoscopic exclusion of peritoneal seedings, the hepatoduodenal ligament was examined and enlarged lymph nodes were biopsied.

In a total of 73 patients, laparoscopy revealed previously undiagnosed liver metastases in 14 and peritoneal carcinosis in 19 patients. Additionally, in eight (esophageal cancer; $n = 3$, gastric cancer; $n = 5$) of the remaining 40 patients, lymph nodes in the M1-position were regarded suspicious and biopsied. In six of these, malignant spread was observed. Thus, in a further six of 40 patients, surgically incurable situations could be detected.

In esophageal and gastric cancer, staging laparoscopy, including laparoscopic ultrasound and biopsy, is a sensitive technique to assess local tumor spread and distant metastases. The detection of M1- lymph node metastases is facilitated by the use of laparoscopic ultrasound. Tumor spread, which limits surgical curability, can be properly assessed and exploratory laparotomy avoided.

Recent Results in Cancer Research, Vol. 142

Introduction

Curative resection for tumors of the upper gastrointestinal tract yields the best long-term results, but is linked with a high morbidity and mortality rate (Fortner et al. 1994; Vist et al. 1988). Palliative surgical interventions, especially exploratory laparotomy, are also connected with a high morbidity and mortality rate (Böttcher et al. 1994; Viste et al. 1988). Of all the patients with gastric cancer analyzed by the German Gastric Cancer Study Group, 17% underwent an exploratory laparotomy only. The 30-day mortality rate of these patients was 13% (Böttcher et al. 1994). Exact preoperative assessment of locoregional tumor spread is therefore highly desirable.

In addition to excluding liver and lung metastases and peritoneal carcinosis, the recognition of metastatic lymph nodes at the hepatoduodenal ligament and at the celiac axis is essential for the assessment of tumor spread. These lymph nodes are classified as distant metastases (M1 lymph) and indicate that the malignant disease cannot be curatively treated by surgical means alone (Schlag et al. 1989). Enlarged (≥1 cm) or tumor-infested abdominal lymph nodes can be recognized by computed tomography (CT) with an accuracy of 45%–75% (Lehr et al. 1988; Reeders et al. 1993) and by abdominal ultrasound with an accuracy of 37% (Palazzo et al. 1993). Frequently, transcutaneous ultrasound examination is of limited value because of artifacts (ribs or meteorism).

The advantage of diagnostic laparoscopy, in combination with laparoscopic ultrasound, in the detection of distant metastases (nodular peritoneal carcinosis, liver metastases of less than 1 cm in diameter), but also in the detection of M1 lymph nodes within the hepatoduodenal ligament or in the para-aortic position, lies in the fact that it provides a means of direct visual evaluation and histological verification.

Patients and Methods

Between July 1993 and December 1994, 164 patients with carcinoma of the upper gastrointestinal tract (esophageal cancer, n = 41; carcinoma of the esophagocardial junction, n = 37; gastric cancer, n = 86) were admitted to hospital for examination and treatment. In 33 of 164 patients (20%), operative treatment was not an option, as clinical investigations and imaging procedures showed incurable disease or the poor state of the patient caused functional inoperability. Fifty-eight of 164 patients (35%) were gastrectomized (without prior laparoscopy) for endoscopically and endosonographically suspected early cancer or with a primarily palliative intention. Here, further investigative tumor assessment was limited. In 73 of 164 patients (esophageal cancer, n = 21; carcinoma of the esophagocardial junction, n = 30; gastric cancer, n = 22), staging laparoscopy was performed after the presence of distant metastases was excluded by abdominal ultrasound and CT of the abdomen and chest.

Laparoscopy was performed under general anesthesia using standard equipment (Olympus). After inflation of the peritoneum using a Veress needle, a 45° side-angle lens system was introduced via a 10-mm trocar placed para-umbilically. First, careful inspection of the peritoneal cavity was carried out, with special attention paid to liver metastases, peritoneal carcinosis, and ascites. The bursa omentalis was then explored through a dissected gastrocolic ligament. Further trocars were placed if more instruments were required. If the laparoscopic view did not suggest a disseminated tumor (n = 35), laparoscopic ultrasound was subsequently performed. A flexible ultrasonic endoscope (Pentax FG 32 UA) with a 5/7.5-MHz transducer was employed. This instrument has a maximal diameter of 12 mm and can be introduced into the peritoneal cavity using a 15-mm trocar. A systematic examination of the liver and of the relevant intra-abdominal lymph node positions (celiac axis, hepatoduodenal ligament, para-aortic position) was carried out. The examination lasted an average of 20–30 min. Suspected tumors were excised under visual or ultrasonic control, and titanic clips were applied to close dissected lymphatic vessels.

Results

Using staging laparoscopy, infiltration of tumor into neighboring organs was verified in five patients. In one patient with carcinoma of the cardia, a previously undiagnosed wide infiltration into the liver was seen. In four patients, the tumor infiltrated the pancreas.

With laparoscopy, liver metastases were newly discovered in 14 and peritoneal carcinosis in 19 patients. Suspiciously enlarged lymph nodes (n = 8) in the hepatoduodenal ligament were found in esophageal carcinoma (n = 3) and in gastric cancer (n = 5) (Table 1). Excision of these lymph nodes revealed malignancy in six of eight patients. In the other two patients the lymph nodes

Table 1. Additional information provided by staging laparoscopy compared to conventional staging

Added information	Positive results					
	Peritoneal carcinosis (n)	Liver metastases (n)	M1 Lymph nodes (n)	Nonresectable disease (n)	Total patients	
					n	%
Laparoscopy (n = 73)	19	10	2	5	36	49
Subsequent laparoscopic ultrasound (n = 35)	–	4	4	–	8	23

showed inflammatory changes. Thus, in six patients out of 40 (15%) a previously unknown M1 lymph node metastasis was found.

In 25 out of 29 patients, a subsequent laparotomy confirmed the laparoscopic assessment of tumor spread. False-negative results were found in four patients (13%); peritoneal carcinosis within the bursa omentalis ($n = 2$) and peritoneal seedings on the duodenum ($n = 1$) were detected by laparotomy only. In a further patient, an M1 lymph node metastasis in the hepatoduodenal ligament was not recognized.

Alteration of the tumor stage established by conventional means as a result of staging laparoscopy occurred in 44 of 73 patients (60%). This led to a modification of therapeutic procedures in 38 patients (Fig. 1).

In five patients, a palliative surgical procedure was performed for laparoscopically diagnosed disseminated disease (e.g., percutaneous laparoscopic gastrostomy, $n = 4$; jejunal feeding tube, $n = 1$). In six patients, gastrectomy was performed with a primarily palliative intention for resectable, but stenosing gastric cancer. In 33 patients, neoadjuvant radiochemotherapy was initiated.

Complications of staging laparoscopy occurred in three of 73 patients. Two patients required blood tranfusions (two units of packed cells per patient) due to hemorrhage; bleeding from a liver biopsy site in one patient and hemorrhage from the trocar insertion wound in another made laparotomy necessary for hemostasis. In one patient, laparoscopic cholecystectomy was necessary

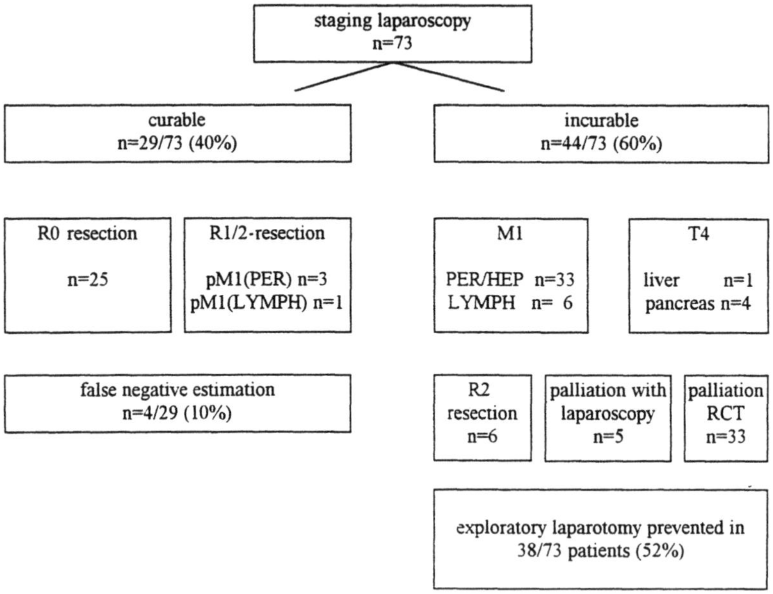

Fig. 1. Therapeutic consequences of staging laparoscopy for esophageal and gastric cancer. *RCT*, radiochemotherapy; *PER*, peritoneal carcinosis; *HEP*, hepatic metastasis

after an injury to the cystic artery, inflicted during the dissection of the hepatoduodenal ligament.

Discussion

In gastric cancer surgery, exploratory laparotomy is performed and the operation terminated without resection of the tumor in 15%–30% of all cases because the extent of the tumor is underestimated preoperatively (Böttcher et al. 1994; Irvin and Bridger 1988). Exploratory laparotomy entails undeniable risks of mortality and morbidity (Hallisscy et al. 1988). Serious complications occur in 10%–20% of all patients (Böttcher et al. 1994; Viste et al. 1988), with a 30-day mortality of 17%–25%. An open procedure should therefore be avoided as far as possible.

With the development of minimally invasive surgical procedures, laparoscopy has gained importance in the diagnosis and treatment of gastrointestinal tumors. Analogous to exploratory laparotomy, the aim of staging laparoscopy is the histopathological verification of local tumor spread and lymph node metastasis and the diagnosis of distant metastases. In contrast to exploratory laparotomy, diagnostic laparoscopy has a complication rate of 1% and a mortality rate of 0.05% (Dagnini et al. 1989). We observed complications in 4% of patient.

Additional invasive diagnostic procedures are necessary due to the limited resolution of the imaging techniques currently available. Sonography, CT, or magnetic resonance imaging (MRI) often fail to provide a clear idea about the extent of local tumor infiltration. The accuracy of these procedures in the detection of lymph node or hepatic metastases is only limited 46%–75% (Lehr et al. 1988; Reeders and Bartelsman 1993), and only 49% for lesions of less than 1 cm in diameter (Wernecke et al. 1991). In a prospective study, lymph node metastases was detected by endoscopic ultrasound in 87%, by transcutaneous ultrasound in 47%, and by CT in 76% of cases (Palazzo et al. 1993).

Laparoscopy combined with laparoscopic ultrasound provides an additional means of evaluating local tumor extent and distant metastasis (Huenerbein et al. 1995). Superficial distant metastases can be proven laparoscopically. In 35%–58% of cases, additional pathological lesions are found on the liver and peritoneum (Feussner et al. 1994; Kriplani and Kapur 1991; Shandall and Johnson 1985; Watt et al. 1989). In patients with carcinoma of the upper gastrointestinal tract, this technique revealed a 60% difference in tumor stage compared to that previously defined by imaging techniques. Hepatic metastases were found in 19% of patients, peritoneal carcinosis in 26%, infiltration by the tumor of neighboring organs in 7%, and M1 lymph node metastases in 8%.

Even though minute tumor seedings can be detected with the optic magnification of the laparoscope, the method is limited to superficial lesions. In three of 29 patients, laparotomy revealed nodular peritoneal carcinosis which had been missed by laparoscopy. This confirms other reports in which rates of false-negative results in the detection of peritoneal carcinosis were 5%–10% (Brady et al. 1991; Dagnini et al. 1989). The reason for this is a limited assessment of the peritoneum due to adhesions and poor visibility in the Douglas and the retrogastric space.

M1 lymph nodes are of special interest in pretherapeutic diagnostics for esophageal and gastric carcinomas because a tumor manifestation at this site would impede a surgical procedure. The evaluation of lymph node metastases by laparoscopy is difficult. Even enlarged lymph nodes cannot be detected by laparoscopy if they are located in the adipose tissue of the hepatoduodenal ligament or in the para-aortic position. Watt and colleagues (1989) report up to 26% of false-negative results in the laparoscopic evaluation of the lymph node status. By employing laparoscopic ultrasound, it has become possible to discover enlarged lymph nodes more easily and to subsequently resect them. The dissection of lymph nodes, however, is time-consuming and not without complications. In our series, one of eight patients with hepatoduodenal ligament dissection had to undergo laparoscopic cholecystectomy after the cystic artery had been injured. Therefore, it seems reasonable to dissect these positions at the end of the staging laparoscopy after already having excluded superificial lesions.

By combining ultrasound with laparoscopy, in two of 21 patients with esophageal carcinoma and in four of 52 patients with gastric cancer, surgical incurability was histologically proven after the presence of liver metastases and peritoneal carcinosis was excluded.

In our opinion, laparoscopic staging of lymph nodes in esophageal and gastric cancer should be limited to the M1 lymph node positions, since therapeutic consequences would only ensue due to involvement of these sites. Furthermore, the dissection of these positions should only be performed after exclusion of pathological lesions of the peritoneum and the liver. With this policy, the cascade of invasive staging of patients with upper gastrointestinal tumors can be further optimized.

References

Böttcher K, Siewert JR, Roder JD, Busch R, Hermanek P, Meyer HJ (GGCS'92) (1994) Risiko der chirurgischen Therapie des Magencarcinoms in Deutschland. Chirurg 65:298–306

Brady PG, Peebles M, Goldschmid S (1991) Role of laparoscopy in the evaluation of patients with suspected hepatic or peritoneal malignancy. Gastrointest Endosc 37:27–30

Dagnini G, Caldironi MW, Marin G, Buzzaccarini O, Tremolada C, Ruol A (1989) Laparoscopy in abdominal staging of esophageal carcinoma. Gastrointest Endosc 32:400–402

Feussner H, Kraemer SJ, Siewert JR (1994) Technik der laparoskopischen Ultraschalluntersuchung bei der diagnostischen Laparoskopie. Langenbecks Arch Chir 379:248–254

Fortner JG, Lauwers GY, Thaler HT, Concepcion R, Friedlander-Klar H, Kher U, Maclean BJ (1994) Nativity, complications, and pathology are determinants of surgical results for gastric cancer. Cancer 73:8–14
Hallissey MT, Allum WH, Roginsky C, Fielding JWL (1988) Palliative surgery for gastric cancer. Cancer 620:440–444
Huenerbein M, Rau B, Schlag PM (1995) Laparoscopy and laparoscopic ultrasound for staging of upper gastrointestinal tumours. Eur J Surg Oncol 21:50–55
Irvin TT, Bridger JE (1988) Gastric cancer: an audit of 122 consecutive cases and the results of R1 gastrectomy. Br J Surg 75:106–109
Kriplani AK, Kapur BM (1991) Laparoscopy for pre-operative staging and assessment of operability in gastric carcinoma. Gastrointest Endosc 37:441–443
Lehr L, Rupp N, Siewert JR (1988) Assessment of resectability of esophageal cancer by computed tomography and magnetic resonance imaging. Surgery 103:344–350
Palazzo L, Roseau G, Gayet B et al (1993) Endoscopic Ultrasonography in the diagnosis and staging of pancreatic adenocarcinoma. Endoscopy 25:143–150
Reeders JWAJ, Bartelsman JFWM (1993) Radiological diagnosis and preoperative staging of oesophageal malignancies. Endoscopy 25:10–27
Schlag P, Buhl K, Schwarz V, Möller P, Herfarth C (1989) Die neue TNM-Klassifizierung und ihre Auswirkung auf die chirurgische Behandlung des Magen-Carcinom. Chirurg 60:8–15
Shandall A, Johnson C (1985) Laparoscopy or scanning in oesophageal and gastric carcinoma? Br J Surg 72:449–451
Valen B, Viste A, Haugstvedt T, Elide GE, Soreido O (1988) Treatment of stomach cancer, a national experience. Br J Surg 75:708–712
Viste A, Haugstvedt T, Eide E, Soreide O (1988) Postoperative complications and mortality after surgery for gastric cancer. Ann Surg 7
Watt I, Stewart I, Anderson D, Bell G, Anderson JR (1989) Laparoscopy, ultrasound and computed tomography in cancer of the oesophagus and gastric cardia: a prospective comparison for detecting intra-abdominal metastases. Br J Surg 76:1036–1039
Wernecke K, Rummeny E, Bongartz G, Vassallo P, Kivelitz D, Wiesmann W, Peters P, Reers B, Reiser M, Pircher W (1991) Detection of hepatic masses in patients with carcinoma: comparative sensitivities of sonography, CT, and MR imaging. AJR 157:731–739

Radiation Therapy Alone or Combined with Chemotherapy in the Treatment of Esophageal Cancer

B.D. Minsky

Department of Radiation Oncology, Memorial Sloan Kettering Cancer Center, 1275 York Ave., New York, NY 10021, USA

Abstract

Radiation therapy has been used in the adjuvant setting or as a primary treatment modality for esophageal cancer. Although there are design flaws in all of the trials of adjuvant radiation therapy for esophageal cancer, there is no clear survival advantage when radiation therapy is delivered in the adjuvant setting (preoperatively or postoperatively). Phase II results of preoperative, combined modality therapy are encouraging; however, the approach remains investigational. When radiation therapy is used as a primary modality, the most favorable results are seen when it is combined with adequate doses of systemic chemotherapy. Phase III intergroup trials are in progress which are examining the effectiveness of higher doses of radiation therapy when combined with chemotherapy.

Introduction

There are a number of approaches to the use of radiation therapy in the treatment of esophageal cancer. These include radiation therapy in the adjuvant setting (preoperatively and/or postoperatively) or as a primary treatment modality (alone or in conjunction with chemotherapy). In general, the results of external-beam radiation therapy alone in the treatment of esophageal cancer have been as discouraging as those with surgery. Depending upon the series, the median survival is generally less than 1 year, and 5-year survival rates range from 2 to 20%.

Although the overall results of surgery and radiation therapy are similar, the patient population selected for treatment with each modality is quite different. First, poor prognostic patients are commonly selected for treatment with radiation therapy. These include patients who are not surgical candidates due to medical contraindications and/or locally advanced or metastatic

Recent Results in Cancer Research, Vol. 142

disease. Second, nonoperative series report results based on clinically staged patients, whereas surgical series report results based on pathologically staged patients. Pathologic staging has the advantage of excluding some patients with metastatic disease. Third, since many patients treated with radiation therapy alone are approached in a palliative rather than potentially curative fashion, the doses and techniques of radiation therapy are commonly suboptimal. Despite these adverse selection factors, the use of radiation therapy does offer a defined cure rate as well as significant impact on the palliation of dysphagia.

Much of this discussion will focus on the results of randomized trials. In the settings where randomized trials are not available, selected nonrandomized trials will be discussed.

Primary Radiation Therapy Alone

External Beam

Many series have reported results of external beam radiation therapy alone for esophageal carcinoma. The majority of these series include patients with unfavorable features such as clinical T4 lesions, positive lymph nodes, and unresectable disease. For example, in the study by De-Ren, 184 of the 678 patients had stage-IV disease (De-Ren 1989).

The use of radiation therapy in the potentially curative setting requires doses of at least 5000 cGy at 180–200 cGy/fraction. Given the large size of many unresectable esophageal cancers, doses in the range of 6000 cGy or greater are probably required. The results of selected series of radiation therapy alone are seen in Table 1 (De-Ren 1989; Newaishy et al. 1982; Okawa et al. 1989). Overall, the 5-year survival for patients with carcinoma of the esophagus treated with radiation therapy alone is approximately 10%.

External Beam Plus Intraluminal Brachytherapy

Intraluminal brachytherapy has been used in a variety of settings for esophageal cancer (Armstrong 1993). It can be delivered by high dose rate or low dose rate (Caspers et al. 1993). Although there are technical differences between the two dose rates, there are no clear therapeutic advantages. Briefly, a radioactive source is placed intraluminally via bronchoscopy or a nasogastric tube.

The major limitation of brachytherapy is the effective treatment distance. The primary isotope is iridium-192, which can effectively treat to a distance of 1 cm from the source. Therefore, if any portion of the tumor is >1 cm it will receive a suboptimal radiation dose.

Table 1. Radiation therapy alone for esophageal cancer: selected series

Reference	Histology	Stage	No. of patients	5-Year survival (%)
Newaishy et al. 1982	Squamous	"Inoperable"	444	9
Okawa et al. 1989	Squamous	I	43	20
		II	130	10
		III	92	3
		IV	23	0
		T1	47	18
		T2	147	10
		T3	94	3
		Total	288	9
De-Ren 1989	Various	II	177	22
		III	501	28
		<5 cm	59	25
		5 cm	115	25
		>5 cm	504	6
		Total[a]	678	8

[a] Includes 184 patients with stage-IV disease

In the curative setting, the best approach is to add brachytherapy as a boost (1000–2000 cGy) following external-beam radiation (5000–6000 cGy). The limited non-randomized data suggest that outcome may be improved when brachytherapy is added to external beam. This approach is being prospectively examined by the Radiation Therapy Oncology Group (RTOG 92-07). In the palliative setting, it is used to improve swallowing. The effectiveness of intraluminal brachytherapy in this setting is controversial.

Adjuvant Radiation Therapy

The rationale of adjuvant therapy in clinically resectable esophageal cancer is based on the patterns of failure following potentially curative surgery. Unfortunately, few surgical series report patterns of failure data. The incidence of local/regional failure in the surgical control arms from the preoperative radiation therapy randomized trials by Mei et al. (1989) and Gignoux et al. (1987) was 12% and 67%, respectively. The local/regional failure rate in the surgical control arm from the postoperative radiation therapy randomized trial by Teniere et al. (1991) was 35% for patients with negative local/regional lymph nodes and 38% for patients with positive local/regional lymph nodes. Therefore, although most patients with esophageal cancer die of distant metastasis, the incidence of local/regional failure following surgery alone in patients with clinically resectable disease is high enough to support the use of adjuvant radiation therapy.

Preoperative Radiation Therapy

Rationale

Theoretical advantages of preoperative radiation therapy in the treatment of esophageal cancer include biological (decreased tumor seeding and increased radiosensitivity due to more oxygenated cells), physical (increased resectability), and dosimetric (patients who undergo a gastric pull-up or intestinal interposition are not limited to the postoperative dose of 4500–5000 cGy).

Results

As seen in Table 2, there have been six randomized trials of preoperative radiation therapy for esophageal cancer (Launois et al. 1981; Arnott et al. 1993; Mei et al. 1989; Gignoux et al. 1987; Nygaard et al. 1992). The series of Launois et al. (1981), Gignoux et al. (1987) and Nygaard et al. (1992) are limited to patients with squamous cell carcinoma. Patients with both squamous cell carcinoma and those with adenocarcinoma are included in the series of Arnott et al. (1993). The reports by Huang et al. (1988) and Mei et al. (1989) do not mention the histology.

Overall, there were no differences in resectability rates between patients who underwent preoperative radiation therapy and those who underwent surgery alone. Local/regional failure rates were reported for only two of the six series. Mei et al. (1989) reported no difference in local/regional failure; however, Gignoux et al. (1987) reported a significant decrease in local/regional failure (46% versus 67%) among patients who received preoperative radiation therapy compared with those who had surgery alone.

Two of the six series showed an improvement in survival with preoperative radiation therapy. The series of Nygaard and associates was a four-arm trial in which patients were randomized preoperatively to chemotherapy (cisplatin/bleomycin × two cycles), radiation therapy, combined modality therapy, or surgery alone (Nygaard et al. 1992). Patients who received preoperative radiation therapy (with or without chemotherapy) had a significant improvement in overall 3-year survival (18% versus 5%, $p = 0.009$). The 48 patients who received preoperative radiation therapy alone had a 20% 3-year survival; however, this did not reach statistical significance. A similar improvement in survival (46% versus 25%) was reported by Huang et al. (1988). However, a statistical analysis was not performed.

There are many criticisms of the preoperative randomized trials. For example, none used conventional doses of radiation therapy. Second, none allowed an adequate radiation therapy–surgery interval (usually 4–5 weeks following the completion of radiation). Because of these unconventional techniques, a meaningful analysis of radiation-related morbidity is precluded.

Table 2. Randomized trials of preoperative radiation therapy for esophageal cancer

Reference	Type	No. of patients	Total dose (cGy)	Fraction size (cGy)	Resectable (%)		Local failure (%)		5-Year survival (%)	
					Surg	RT	Surg	RT	Surg	RT
Arnott et al. 1993	Squamous and adenocarcinoma	176	2000	200	NR	NR	NR	NR	17	9
Gignoux et al. 1987	Squamous	229	3300	330	58	47	67	46*	8	10
Nygaard et al. 1992	Squamous	186	3500[b]	175	NR	NR	NR	NR	5	18 (3-year)*
Launois et al. 1981	Squamous	109	4000	NR	70	76	NR	NR	10	10
Huang et al. 1988	NR	160	4000	200	90	92	NR	NR	25	46[a]
Mei et al. 1989	NR	206	4000	NR	85	93	12	13	30	35

NR, Information not reported in the manuscript; *SURG*, surgery; *RT*, radiation therapy
* $p = 0.009$
[a] Statistical analysis was not performed
[b] With or without chemotherapy

In summary, since only two of the six series have reported local/regional failure rates, it is difficult to draw firm conclusions regarding the influence of preoperative radiation therapy on the incidence of local/regional failure. Regarding the impact on survival, two series showed an improvement (one in which 50% of the patients received chemotherapy). However, four of the six series showed no advantage in overall survival. Yadava et al. (1991) and Sugimachi et al. (1986) also reported no survival benefit in nonrandomized trials. Based on the available randomized – albeit poorly designed – trials, adjuvant preoperative radiation therapy does not appear to improve local/regional control or survival.

Postoperative Radiation Therapy

Rationale

The primary advantage of adjuvant postoperative radiation therapy is more accurate case selection based on pathologic findings. Patients with pathologic stage-T1–2N0M0 disease and those with metastatic disease can be excluded from treatment. The major disadvantage is dosimetric, since patients who undergo a gastric pull-up or intestinal interposition are limited to 4500–5000 cGy.

Results

There are many encouraging nonrandomized reports of postoperative radiation therapy in the treatment of esophageal cancer. For example, Kasai et al. reported an 88% 5-year survival for node-negative patients who received postoperative radiation therapy (Kasai et al. 1978). There have been only two randomized trials (Table 3). The discussion here will be limited to patients treated in the adjuvant setting (complete resection and negative margins with or without positive local/regional lymph nodes).

Teniere and colleagues (Teniere et al. 1991) reported results of 221 patients with squamous cell carcinoma randomized to surgery alone versus postoperative radiation therapy (4500–5500 cGy at 180 cGy/fraction). The minimum follow-up was 3 years. For the total patient group the addition of postoperative radiation therapy had no significant impact on survival.

The series of Fok et al. (1993) included patients with both squamous cell carcinoma and adenocarcinoma. It should be emphasized that both patients with curative and those with palliative resections were included in this series. Although the total dose of radiation therapy was conventional, the dose per fraction (350 cGy/fraction) was unconventional. There was no significant im-

Table 3. Randomized trials of postoperative radiation therapy for esophageal cancer

Reference	No. of patients	Median survival (months)	Survival (%)		Local failure (%)			Distant failure (%)
			DFS	Overall	LN+	LN−	Overall	
Teniene et al. 1991								
Radiation	119		85	19	30	10*		
Surgery	102		70	19	38	35		
Fok et al. 1993								
Radiation	30	15					10	40
Surgery	30	21					13	30

DFS, Disease-free survival; *LN+*, lymph node positive; *LN−*, lymph node negative
* Statistically significant

provement in median survival, local failure, or distant failure with the addition of postoperative radiation therapy.

Postoperative radiation therapy is commonly recommended for patients with positive local/regional lymph nodes. Although the data from Teniere et al. (1991) support the use of postoperative radiation therapy for local/regional control, the benefit was limited to patients with negative lymph nodes. Postoperative radiation therapy decreased local failure from 35% to 10%. There was no significant benefit for patients with positive nodes.

In summary, although adjuvant postoperative radiation therapy may improve local/regional control in node-negative patients, it has no impact on overall survival.

Pre- Plus Postoperative Versus Postoperative Radiation Therapy

An alternative approach to adjuvant therapy is pre- plus postoperative radiation therapy. Iizuka et al. (1988) compared this approach with that in patients who received postoperative radiation therapy alone. There was no surgical control arm. In their trial, 364 patients with a variety of histologies were randomized to pre- plus postoperative radiation therapy (3000cGy followed by surgery followed by postoperative radiation therapy up to 5400cGy) versus postoperative radiation therapy alone (5000cGy). Limiting the analysis to the 207 eligible patients, there was a significant improvement in 4-year survival (33% versus 20%) as well as in median survival (22 months versus 13 months) among patients who received postoperative radiation therapy compared with those who received pre- plus postoperative radiation therapy. The major criticisms of this trial are that only 207 of 364 randomized patients were eligible for analysis, and that a higher percentage of patients who received pre- plus postoperative radiation therapy had primary tumors greater than 7cm in size (56% versus 39%).

Combined Modality Therapy for Esophageal Cancer

Given the limited success of radiation therapy when used as either a single modality or in the adjuvant setting (preoperative or postoperative), a number of investigators have explored the use of systemic chemotherapy in conjunction with radiation therapy. There is a good rationale for combining systemic chemotherapy with radiation therapy for the treatment of esophageal cancer. It is based on the fact that there is an objective response rate of 40–60% in patients with metastatic disease, on the observation that most patients with esophageal cancer die of distant metastasis, and on the fact that many of the active agents in esophageal cancer (i.e., 5-FU, cisplatin, mitomycin C) are radiation sensitizers.

Preoperative Combined-Modality Therapy

In general, there are two approaches to preoperative combined-modality therapy. Patients either have a planned operation (Table 4) or, for a variety of reasons, are selected to undergo an operation (Table 5). It is important to analyze the data from these two approaches separately, since the selection factors for surgery may have an impact on the results.

The results of selected series in which patients undergo planned preoperative combined-modality therapy followed by a planned operation are seen in Table 5. Initial studies by Leichman and colleagues from Wayne State University reported the results of 21 patients with squamous cell carcinoma (Leichman et al. 1984). Patients received 3000 cGy at 200 cGy/fraction with two cycles of concurrent 5-FU and cisplatin. If there was residual tumor in the specimen, patients received an additional 2000 cGy postoperatively. Of the 21, 19 underwent an operation. The pathologic complete response rate was 37% and the median survival was 18 months. The operative mortality was 27%. In addition to the substantial mortality, 48% of patients required hyperalimentation during the preoperative therapy.

Although the morbidity and mortality were high, since the complete response rates were encouraging, this pilot trial was expanded to a Southwest Oncology Group trial (SWOG 80-37). The results were reported by Poplin et al. (1987). A toatl of 113 patients with squamous cell carcinoma underwent the preoperative therapy designed by Leichman. Of the 113, only 71 underwent surgery. The pathologic complete response rate was 16% and the operative mortality was 11%. Despite a 3-year actuarial sruvival rate of 16%, all patients were dead of disease by 4 years.

At the University of Michigan, two separate series were studied. Urba et al. reported the results of 24 patients with adenocarcinoma of the esophagus who underwent preoperative continuous-infusion 5-FU and concurrent radiation therapy, followed by a transhiatal esophagectomy (Urba et al. 1992). It should be noted that transhiatal esophagectomy is a more conservative approach,

Table 4. Planned preoperative combined-modality therapy for esophageal cancer: selected series

Reference	No. of patients	Histology	No. who underwent surgery	CR (%)	Survival (%)	Operative mortality (%)
Le Prise et al. 1994	39	Squamous	35	11	47% 1-year	9
Leichman et al. 1984 (Wayne State)	21	Squamous	19	37	18 months (median)	27
Poplin et al. 1987 (SWOG 8037)	113	Squamous	71	16	12 months (median) 16% 3-year (all DOD at 4 years)	11
Naunheim et al. 1992	47	Squamous and adeno	39	21	23 months (median) 40% 3-year	5
Forastiere et al. 1990, Forastiere 1992 (U Michigan)	43	Squamous and adeno	39	27	29 months (median) 46% 3-year	2
Urba et al. 1992 (U Michigan)	24	Adeno	19	10	11 months (median)	16
Stewart et al. 1993	24	Adeno	23	25	76% 2-year	0

Adeno, Adenocarcinoma; *DOD*, dead of disease; *CR*, pathologic complete response

Table 5. Preoperative combined-modality therapy ± surgery for esophageal cancer: selected nonrandomized series

Reference	No. of patients	Local failure (%)	Distant failure (%)	Median survival (months)		
				Squamous cell	Adenocaroinoma	Both
Gill et al. 1992						
Surgery	46	25	36	36	14	
No surgery	36	17	12	26	15	
Kavanagh et al. 1992[a]						
Surgery	72	24	39			9[b]
No surgery	71	44	38			15[c]

[a] Results limited to the 103 of 143 patients who had no clinical evidence of metastatic disease at the time of preoperative assessment
[b] All dead of disease by 5 years
[c] All dead of disease by 3.5 years

since the thorax is not entered. Patients received 4900 cGy at 350 cGy/fraction. The pathologic complete response rate was 11% and the median survival was only 11 months. The operative mortality was 16%. The large radiation fraction sizes may have contributed to the morbidity and mortality reported in this series.

In the other series from the University of Michigan, Forastiere and colleagues reported a group of 39 patients with both squamous cell cancer and adenocarcinoma who received preoperative 5-FU, vinblastine, cisplatin and concurrent radiation therapy (Forastiere et al. 1990; Forastiere 1992). Radiation therapy was delivered either with large fractions (250 cGy) or with hyperfractionation (150 cGy b.i.d.). Patients received the therapy on an inpatient basis for 21 days. Following the preoperative therapy, a transhiatal esophagectomy was performed. The pathologic complete response rate was 27%, the 3-year actuarial survival rate was 46%, and the operative mortality was only 2%. A randomized trial of this approach is now being performed at the University of Michigan.

It is unclear whether the addition of surgery following combined-modality therapy is of benefit (Table 5). In a nonrandomized trial by Gill et al., patients received two cycles of 5-FU, cisplatin, and radiation therapy (Gill et al. 1992). Patients who either were treated palliatively or were medically inoperable were excluded from surgery. Therefore, the patients with a better prognosis were selected for surgery. Although the differences were not statisticaly significant, the local failure and distant failure rates were higher in the patients who underwent surgery compared with those who did not undergo surgery.

A similar trial was reported by Kavanagh et al. (1992). Patients received 4400–4600 cGy plus chemotherapy with either VP-16, 5-FU, cisplatin, or carboplatin. Following re-evaluation, those who were potentially operable underwent surgery, and if they had positive margins they received postoperative radiation therapy. Patients who were either medically or technically inoperable also received additional radiation therapy, bringing the total dose to 6000–6400 cGy. The patients who underwent surgery had a lower local failure rate (44% versus 24%), but there was no difference in distant failure or median survival. However, regardless of the type of treatment, all patients were dead of disease within 3.5–5 years.

In summary, the phase-II results of preoperative combined-modality therapy are encouraging; however, the approach remains investigational. The randomized trial from the University of Michigan should help to better define the role of this approach in this group of patients.

Radiation Therapy Alone Versus Combined-Modality Therapy

Nonrandomized Trials

There are a number of single-arm trials of combined-modality therapy alone for esophageal cancer (Table 6) (John et al. 1989; Coia et al. 1991; Izquierdo et al. 1993; Seitz et al. 1990; Valerdi et al. 1994). The trial reported by Coia and associates is the only combined-modality therapy trial in which patients with clinically early stage esophageal cancer (stages I and II) were treated and analyzed separately (Coia et al. 1991). Patients received 5-FU and mitomycin C concurrently with 6000 cGy. Combining clinical stages I and II, the local failure rate was 25%, the 5-year actuarial sruvival rate was 30%, and the 5-year actuarial local relapse-free survival rate was 70%.

Table 6. Combined-modality therapy alone for esophageal cancer: selected series

Reference	Clinical stage	No. of patients	Histology	Local failure (%)	Actuarial survival (%)	
					Overall	LRF
Coia et al. 1991	I	13	Both	26	73 (5-year)	100 (5-year)
	II	44	Both	45	20	59
	AII	16	Adenocarcinoma	NR	38	71
	AII	39	Squamous cell	NR	27	58
	Total	57	Both	25	30	70
John et al. 1989	I–III	30	Squamous and adeno	27	29 (2-year)	NR
Seitz et al. 1990	I–III	35	Squamous	NR	21 (2-year)	NR
Izquierdo et al. 1993	"Unresectable"	25	Squamous	NR	8 (4-year) 8 months (median)	NR

NR, Information was not reported in the manuscript; *LRF*, local relapse free

Randomized Trials

Table 7 details four randomized trials comparing radiation therapy alone with combined modality therapy (Araujo et al. 1991; Herskovic et al. 1992; Roussel 1988; Nygaard et al. 1992). Unfortunately, in three of the four trials inadequate doses of systemic chemotherapy were delivered. For example, in the small trial from Araujo and colleagues patients received only one cycle of 5-FU, mitomycin-C, and bleomycin. In the EORTC trial reported by Roussel et al. subcutaneous methotrexate was used. In the Scandinavian trial (Nygaard et al. 1992), patients received inadequate doses of chemotherapy (cisplatin 20 mg/m2 and bleomycin 10 mg/m^2 for a maximum of two cycles).

The only trial which was designed to deliver adequate doses of systemic chemotherapy with concurrent radiation therapy was that of the Radiation Therapy Oncology Group (RTOG 85-01; Herskovic et al. 1992) This is shown in Fig. 1. This intergroup included primarily patients with squamous cell carcinoma. They received four cycles of 5-FU (1000 mg/m^2 × 4 days) and cisplatin (75 mg/m^2, day 1). Radiation therapy (5000 cGy) was given concurrently with chemotherapy, beginning on day 1. Cycles 3 and 4 of chemotherapy were delivered every 3 weeks (weeks 8 and 11) as opposed to every 4 weeks (weeks 9 and 13). This intensification may explain, in part, why only approximately half of the patients finished all four cycles of the chemotherapy. The control arm was radiation therapy alone, albeit a higher dose (6400 cGy).

At 2 years, patients who received combined-modality therapy showed a significant improvement in survival (38% versus 10%) as well as significant

Table 7. Randomized trials of radiation therapy vs. combined-modality therapy for esophageal cancer

Reference	No. of patients	Complete response (%)	Survival (%)	Failure (%)	
				Local	Distant
RTOG (Herskovic et al. 1992)					
Radiation alone	60	NR	0 (3-year)*	65	26
Combined-modality	61	NR	31	44*	12*
NCI Brazil (Araujo et al. 1991)					
Radiation alone	31	58	6 (5-year)	84	23
Combined-modality	28	75	16	61	32
EORTC (Roussel et al. 1988)					
Radiation alone	69	NR	6 (3-year)	NR	NR
Combined-modality	75	NR	12	NR	NR
SCANDINAVIA (Nygaard et al. 1992)					
Radiation alone	51	NR	6 (3-year)	NR	NR
Combined-modality	46	NR	0	NR	NR

NR, Information was not reported in the manuscript
* Statistically significant

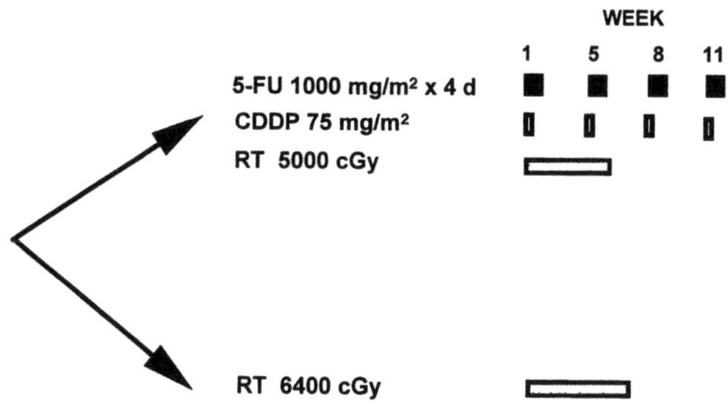

Fig. 1. Phase-III intergroup RTOG 8501 for patients with squamous cell and adenocarcinoma of the esophagus selected for a nonoperative approach. *CDDP*, Cisplatin

decreases in local failure (44% versus 65%) and distant failure (12% versus 26%). With longer follow-up, the 3-year actuarial survival of patients who received combined-modality therapy was 31%. There were no 3-year survivors in the radiation therapy control arm (Al-Sarraf et al. 1993).

A similar randomized trial of radiation therapy alone versus combined-modality therapy (ECOG EST-1282) was performed by the Eastern Cooperative Oncology Group (Sischy et al. 1990). However, since patients had the option of surgery after receiving 4000 cGy, the results are more difficult to interpret. An interim analysis revealed a significant improvement in median survival (14.9 months versus 9 months) for patients who received combined-modality therapy. Final results of this trial are pending.

Toxicity

It should be emphasized that combined-modality therapy is associated with acute toxicity. In a separate toxicity analysis from Coia and associates, an additional 33 patients with stage-III and -IV disease were included (Coia et al. 1991). For the total group of 90 patients, the incidence of grade-III toxicity was 22%, that of grade-IV toxicity 6%. There was no treatment-related mortality. A similar increase in toxicity was noted in the RTOG 85-01 trial. Compared with radiation therapy alone, the use of combined-modality therapy was associated with a higher incidence of grade-III toxicity (44% versus 25%) and grade-IV toxicity (20% versus 3%). Including the one treatment-related death (2%), the incidence of total grade-III+ toxicity was 66%.

Newer Approaches

Based on the positive results from the RTOG 85-01 trial, the conventional nonoperative treatment for esophageal carcinoma in the United States is combined-modality therapy, rather than radiation therapy alone. Although there was a significant improvement in local control and survival with combined-mondality therapy compared with radiation therapy alone, the local/regional failure rate was at least 44% and the 3-year actuarial survival rate was 31%.

Neoadjuvant Chemotherapy

In an attempt to improve these results, the phase-II intergroup trial 0122 (ECOG PE289/RTOG 9012) was designed to intensify the RTOG 85-01 combined-modality arm (Fig. 2). Both the chemotherapy and radiation therapy were modified as follows: (a) the 5-FU continuous infusion (1000 mg/m^2/24 h) was increased from 4 days to 5 days, (b) the total number of cycles of chemotherapy was increased from four cycles to five cycles, (c) three cycles of full-dose neoadjuvant 5-FU/cisplatin were delivered prior to combined-modality therapy, and (d) the radiation dose was increased from 5000 cGy to 6480 cGy. Eligibility was limited to patients with squamous cell carcinoma.

The development of this neoadjuvant trial was based, in part, on the results of a randomized trial from the Memorial Sloan-Kettering Cancer Center. In this trial, 96 patients with potentially resectable squamous cell carcinoma of the esophagus were randomized to preoperative radiation therapy (5500 cGy) or preoperative (neoadjuvant) chemotherapy (Kelsen et al. 1990). There were no significant differences in the resectability rates (65 vs. 58%), overall objective response rates (64% vs. 55%), or the local failure rates (15% vs. 6%) between the two preoperative therapies. Since there was a cross-over postoperatively, it was not possible to compare the survival rates. The overall survival

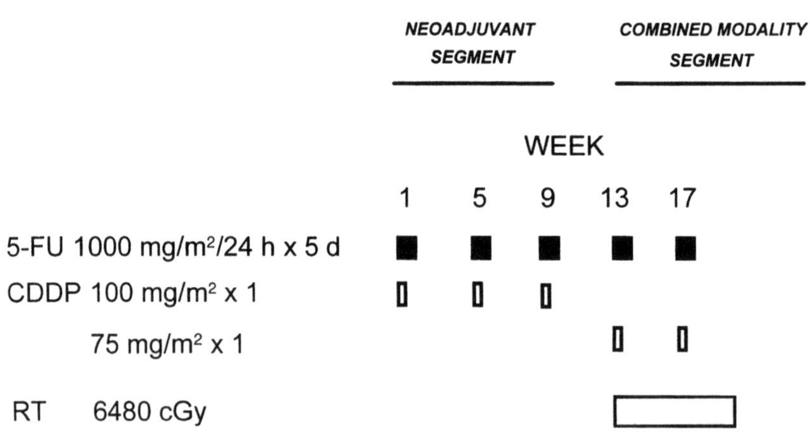

Fig. 2. Phase-II intergroup 0122 (ECOG PE 289, RTOG 90-12) for patients with squamous cell carcinoma of the esophagus selected for a nonoperative approach. *CDDP*, Cisplatin

for both arms was 20% at 5 years, and the median survival was 10–12 months. Therefore, since chemotherapy and radiation therapy offered the same benefits prior to surgery, and chemotherapy has the potential to treat micrometastasis, the neoadjuvant approach was integrated with combined-modality therapy.

The preliminary results of the intergroup trial 0122 have been analyzed (Minsky et al. 1996). Although the incidence of grade-III+ toxicity in trial 0122 was similar to that reported in the RTOG 85-01 combined-modality arm (61–72% vs. 66%, respectively), the treatment-related mortality was 11% compared with 2% in the RTOG 8501 combined-modality arm.

A similar approach with neoadjuvant chemotherapy was reported by Valerdi et al. (1994). In their trial, 40 patients with clinical stage-II and -III squamous cell carcinoma of the esophagus received two cycles of neoadjuvant cisplatin/vindesine/bleomycin (days 1 and 29), followed by 6000 cGy. However, no chemotherapy was delivered with the radiation therapy. Following the completion of radiation, the pathologic complete response rate was 53%. With a median follow-up of 78 months, the median survival was 11 months, and the 3-year and 5-year actuarial survival rates were 20% and 15%, respectively. The local/regional failure rate was 62%. These results are similar to those obtained with the RTOG 85-01 combined-modality arm. However, the incidence of treatment-related deaths was increased to 5%. Based on the increased treatment-related mortality reported in these trials, neoadjuvant chemotherapy should be used with caution in patients with esophageal carcinoma who are selected for a nonoperative approach.

Increased Radiation Dose

There are limited data regarding the tolerance of radiation doses ≥6000 cGy plus concurrent chemotherapy in patients with esophageal cancer. In a separate toxicity analysis from Coia and associates, a total of 90 patients with clinical stages I–IV squamous cell and adenocarcinoma of the esophagus were reported (Coia et al. 1991). The incidence of grade-III toxicity was 22%, that of grade-IV toxicity 6%. There were no treatment-related deaths.

Calais et al. reported the results of 53 patients with unresectable esophageal carcinoma who received 5-FU/cisplatin/mitomycin-C and 6500 cGy (Calais et al. 1994) The full dose of radiation was delivered in 96% of patients. The incidence of WHO grade-III+ toxicity was 30% and the overall 2-year survival was 42%. It should be noted that the chemotherapy in this trial was not delivered at full systemic doses.

The large majority of patients in the intergroup 0122 trial and in the trial of Calais et al. (96% and 94%, respectively) who started radiation were able to complete the full course (6480–6500 cGy). Therefore, this higher dose of radiation is used in the experimental arm of the replacement intergroup esophageal trial (INT 0123, RTOG 94-05). In this replacement trial for RTOG 8501, patients with both squamous cell and adenocarcinoma of the esophagus who are selected for a nonoperative approach will be randomized to a slightly modified RTOG 85-01 combined-modality regimen plus 5040 cGy or to the same chemotherapy plus 6480 cGy (Fig. 3). The trial opened to accrual in late 1994.

Adenocarcinoma Versus Squamous Cell Carcinoma

Given the increasing incidence of adenocarcinoma of the esophagus compared with squamous cell carcinoma, treatment results need to be examined by histology. In the series by Coia et al. (1991) patients with adenocarcinoma had improved survival compared with those with squamous cell carcinoma. In contrast, Gill et al. (1992) and Forastiere and colleagues (Forastiere et al. 1990; Forastiere 1992) reported that patients with squamous cell carcinoma had an improved survival compared with those who had adenocarcinoma. Naunheim and associates reported no survival difference with histology (Naunheim et al. 1992). Until randomized trials are performed where patients are stratified, the impact of histology cannot be adequately assessed.

Toxicity of Radiation Therapy

The morbidity of radiation therapy is a function of dose, technique, and whether the patient received chemotherapy or underwent surgery. There are

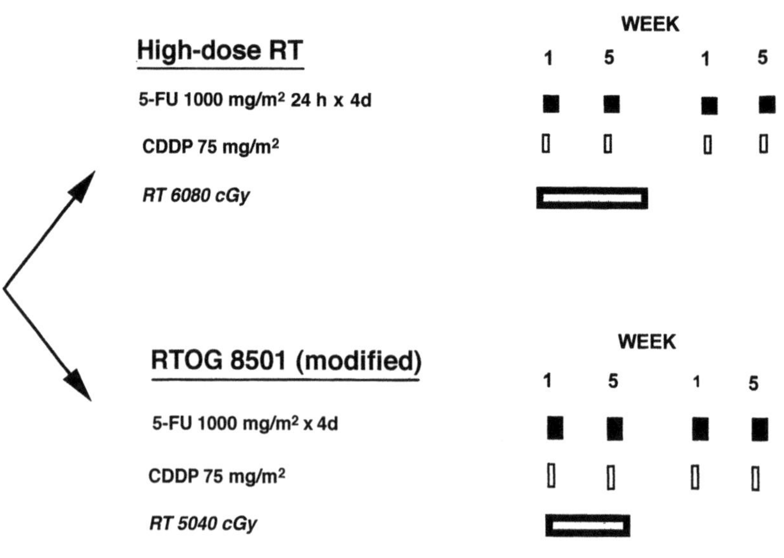

Fig. 3. Phase-III intergroup trial 0123 (RTOG 94-05) for patients with squamous cell and adenocarcinoma of the esophagus selected for a nonoperative approach. *CDDP*, Cisplatin

very limited toxicity data for patients who received radiation therapy in the adjuvant setting. As previously discussed, the preoperative adjuvant radiation therapy trials used unconventional radiation doses and techniques, thereby making the data difficult to interpret.

The best-documented acute radiation-related morbidity data are from the control arm of RTOG 85-01 (Herskovic et al. 1992; Al-Sarraf et al. 1993) In this arm, 60 patients received radiation therapy alone, to a dose of 6400 cGy. The incidence of acute grade-III toxicity was 25%, that of grade-IV toxicity was 3%. There were not treatment-related deaths.

Likewise, there are few reports of long-term radiation-related morbidity. In general, patients who receive radiation therapy alone have a 30–60% incidence of esophageal stricture. However, almost half of the strictures are associated with a local recurrence. The incidence of grade-III+ pneumonitis and/or pericarditis is 5%. If appropriate radiation techniques are used, spinal cord myelitis should not occur.

Conclusions

Due to selection bias, it is difficult to determine what is the best treatment for esophageal cancer. Although there are design flaws in all of the trials of adjuvant radiation therapy for esophageal cancer, there is no clear survival advantage when radiation therapy is delivered in the adjuvant setting (preoperative or postoperative). Pre- plus postoperative radiation therapy does not appear to have an advantage over postoperative radiotehrapy alone. If radiation therapy is used as a primary modality, the most favorable results are seen when it is combined with adeuqate doses of systemic chemotherapy. Phase-III intergroup trials are in progress to examine the effectiveness of higher doses of radiation therapy (INT 0123/RTOG 94-05).

References

Al-Sarraf M, Pajak T, Herskovic A et al (1993) Progress report of combined chemoradiotherapy (CT-RT) vs. radiotherapy (RT) alone in patients with esophageal cancer. An intergroup study. (Abstract) Proc ASCO 12:197

Araujo CMM, Souhami L, Gil RA et al (1991) A randomized trial comparing radiation therapy versus concomitant radiation therapy and chemotherapy in carcinoma of the thoracic esophagus. Cancer 67:2258–2261

Armstrong JG (1993) High dose rate remote afterloading brachytherapy for lung and esophageal cancer. Semin Radiat Oncol 4:270–277

Arnott SJ, Duncan W, Kerr GR et al (1993) Low-dose preoperative radiotherapy for carcinoma of the oesophagus: results of a randomized clinical trial. Radiother Oncol 24:108–113

Calais G, Jadavil E, Chapet C et al (1994) High dose radiotherapy (RT) and concomitant chemotherapy (CT) for nonresectable esophageal cancer. Results of a phase-II study. Proc ASCO 13:197

Caspers RJL, Zwinderman AH, Griffioen G et al (1993) Combined external-beam and low dose rate intraluminal radiotherapy in oesophageal cancer. Radiother Oncol 27:7–12
Coia LR, Engstrom PF, Paul AR et al (1991) Long-term results of infusional 5-FU, mitomycin-C, and radiation as primary management of esophageal cancer. Int J Radiat Oncol Biol Phys 20:29–36
De-Ren S (1989) Ten-year follow-up of esophageal cancer treated by radical radiation therapy: analysis of 869 patients. Int J Radiation Oncol Biol Phys 16:329–334
Fok M, Sham JST, Choy D et al (1993) Postoperative radiotherapy for carcinoma of the esophagus: a prospective, randomized controlled trial. Surg 113:138–147
Forastiere A, Orringer MB, Perez-Tamayo C et al (1990) Concurrent chemotherapy and radiation therapy followed by transhiatal esophagectomy for local-regional cancer of the esophagus. J Clin Oncol 8:119–127
Forastiere A (1992) Treatment of local-regional esophageal cancer. Semin Oncol 19:57–63
Gignoux M, Roussel A, Paillot B et al (1987) The value of preoperative radiotherapy in esophageal cancer: results of a study of the EORTC. World J Surg 11:426–432
Gill PG, Denham JW, Jamieson GG et al (1992) Patterns of treatment failure and prognostic factors associated with the treatment of esophageal carcinoma with chemotherapy and radiotherapy either as sole treatment or followed by surgery. J Clin Oncol 10:1037–1043
Herskovic A, Martz L, Al-Sarraf M et al (1992) Combined chemotherapy and radiotherapy compared with radiotherapy alone in patients with cancer of the esophagus. N Engl J Med 326:1593–1598
Huang GJ, Gu XZ, Wang LJ et al (1988) Combined preoperative irradiation and surgery for esophageal carcinoma. In: Delarue NC (ed) International trends in general theracic surgery. Mosby, St. Louis, pp 315–318
Iizuka T, Ide H, Kakegawa T et al (1988) Preoperative radioactive therapy for esophageal carcinoma: randomized evaluation trial in eight institutions. Chest 93:1054–1058
Izquierdo MA, Marcuello E, Gomez de Segura G et al (1993) Unresectable nonmetastatic squamous cell carcinoma of the esophagus managed by sequential chemotherapy (cisplatin and bleomycin) and radiation therapy. Cancer 71:287–292
John MJ, Flam M, Ager Mowry PA et al (1989) Radiotherapy alone and chemoradiation for nonmetastatic esophageal carcinoma. Cancer 63:2397–2403
Kasai M, Mori S, Watanabe T (1978) Follow-up results after resection of thoracic esophageal carcinoma. World J Surg 2:543–551
Kavanagh B, Anscher M, Leopold K et al (1992) Patterns of failure following combined modality therapy for esophageal cancer, 1984–1990. Int J Radiat Oncol Biol Phys 24:633–642
Kelsen DP, Minsky BD, Smith M et al (1990) Preoperative therapy for esophageal cancer: a randomized comparison of chemotherapy vs. radiation therapy. J Clin Oncol 8:1352–1361
Launois B, Delarue D, Campion JP et al (1981) Preoperative radiotherapy for carcinoma of the esophagus. Surg Gynecol Obstet 153:690–692
Le Prise E, Etienne PL, Meunier B et al (1994) A randomized study of chemotherapy, radiation therapy, and surgery versus surgery for localized squamous cell carcinoma of the esophagus. Cancer 73:1779–1784
Leichman L, Steiger Z, Seydel HG et al (1984) Preoperative chemotherapy and radiation therapy for patients with cancer of the esophagus: a potentially curative approach. J Clin Oncol 2:75–79
Mei W, Xian-Zhi G, Weibo Y et al (1989) Randomized clinical trial on the combination of preoperative irradiation and surgery in the treatment of esophageal carcinoma: report on 206 patients. Int J Radiat Oncol Biol Phys 16:325–327

Minsky BD, Neuberg D, Kelsen D, Pisansky TM, Ginsberg R, Benson AI (1996) Neoadjuvant chemotherapy plus concurrent chemotherapy and high dose radiation for squamous cell carcinoma of the esophagus – a preliminary analysis of the Phase II intergroup trial 0122. J Clin Oncol 14:149–155

Naunheim KS, Petruska PJ, Roy TS et al (1992) Preoperative chemotherapy and radiotherapy for esophageal carcinoma. J Thorac Cardiovasc Surg 5:887–895

Newaishy GA, Read GA, Duncan W et al (1982) Results of radical radiotherapy of squamous cell carcinoma of the esophagus. Clin Radiol 33:347–352

Nygaard K, Hagen S, Hansen HS et al (1992) Pre-operative radiotherapy prolongs survival in operable esophageal carcinoma: a randomized, multicenter study of preoperative radiotherapy and chemotherapy. The second Scandinavian trial in esophageal cancer. World J Surg 16:1104–1110

Okawa T, Kita M, Tanaka M et al (1989) Results of radiotherapy for inoperable locally advanced esophageal cancer. Int J Radiat Oncol Biol Phys 17:49–54

Poplin E, Fleming T, Leichman L et al (1987) Combined therapies for squamous-cell carcinoma of the esophagus, a Southwest Oncology Group Study (SWOG-8037). J Clin Oncol 5:622–628

Roussel A, Jacob JH, Jung GM et al (1988) Controlled clinical trial for the treatment of patients with inoperable esophageal carcinoma: a study of the EORTC Gastrointestinal Tract Cancer Cooperative Group. Recent Results Cancer Res 2:21–30

Seitz JF, Giovannini M, Padaut-Cesana J et al (1990) Inoperable nonmetastatic squamous cell carcinoma of the esophagus managed by concomitant chemotherapy (5-fluorouracil and cisplatin) and radiation therapy. Cancer 66:214–219

Sischy B, Ryan L, Haller D et al (1990) Interim report of EST 1282 phase-III protocol for the evaluation of combined modalities in the treatment of patients with carcinoma of the esophagus. (Abstract) Proc ASCO 9:105

Stewart JR, Hoff SJ, Johnson DH et al (1993) Improved survival with neoadjuvant therapy and resection for adenocarcinoma of the esophagus. Ann Surg 218:571–578

Sugimachi K, Matsufuji H, Kai H et al (1986) Preoperative irradiation for carcinoma of the esophagus. Surg Gynecol Obstet 162:174–176

Teniere P, Hay J, Fingerhut A et al (1991) Postoperative radiation therapy does not increase survival after curative resection for squamous cell carcinoma of the middle and lower esophagus as shown by a multicenter controlled trial. Surg Gynecol Obstet 173:123–130

Urba SG, Orringer MB, Perez-Tamayo C et al (1992) Concurrent preoperative chemotherapy and radiation therapy in localized esophageal adenocarcinoma. Cancer 69:285–291

Valerdi JJ, Tejedor M, Illarramendi JJ et al (1994) Neoadjuvant chemotherapy and radiotherapy in locally advanced esophagues carcinoma: long-term results. Int J Radiat Oncol Biol Phys 27:843–847

Yadava OP, Hodge AJ, Matz LR et al (1991) Esophageal malignancies: is preoperative radiotherapy the way to go? Ann Thorac Surg 51:189–193

Preoperative Chemotherapy in Gastric Cancer

H. Wilke[1], H.J. Meyer[2], and U. Fink[3]

[1] Department of Internal Medicine (Cancer Research), Essen University Medical School, Hufelandstr. 55, 45122 Essen, Germany
[2] Department of Surgery, Hanover University Medical School, 30625 Hanover, Germany
[3] Department of Surgery, Technical University of Munich, Klinikum rechts der Isar, 81675 Munich, Germany

Abstract

Even with extended surgery, including systematic lymphadenectomy of the lymph node compartment II, only half of the patients with locally advanced gastric cancer (LAGC) – which comprises stages IIIA, IIIB, and IV – undergo macroscopic and microscopic tumor-free resection (i.e., R0 resection, according to UICC 1987/AICC 1988). An improvement in this situation is best accomplished by preoperative treatment modalities to increase the R0 resection rate and by preoperative and postoperative treatment to reduce local recurrences and distant metastases. For LAGC, which includes approximately two thirds of patients with locoregionally confined tumors, preoperative chemotherapy (CTx) represents a promising approach. Among a group of patients with surgically or clinically staged unresectable LAGC, approximately half underwent R0 resection after downstaging induced by active CTx. The long-term survival of these patients seems to be improved. Even in patients who had primarily unresectable tumors as defined by explorative laparotomy, the long-term survival was about 20% after preoperative CTx and subsequent surgery. Based on these experiences, randomized trials investigating preoperative CTx versus surgery alone are clearly needed to define whether such an approach has an impact on R0 resection rates and survival of patients with LAGC. Preconditions for such trials are clinical staging procedures, including endoscopic ultrasonography (T category) and surgical laparoscopy plus lavage (excluding peritoneal carcinomatosis), and a standardized surgical procedure.

Introduction

Surgery is the cornerstone of treatment of locoregionally confined gastric cancer with curative intention. Especially in the early stages of this disease,

Recent Results in Cancer Research, Vol. 142

surgery may cure up to 80% of patients with stage I and 50%–(70%) of patients with stage II disease. In locally advanced stages (stage IIIA, IIIB, localized stage IV) the prognosis remains poor. Also after R0 resection (macroscopically and microscopically tumor-free resection margins) the 5-year survival rates usually do not exceed 20%, with the best results in stage IIIA (Roder et al. 1993; Meyer et al. 1991) and the worst results in localized stage IV (<5%). However, only 40%–50% of patients with locally advanced gastric cancer (LAGC) can undergo a R0 resection. Taking this into account, only 10% of patients with LAGC can be cured by surgery alone. The main reasons for this poor outcome are primarily unresectable tumors and a high incidence of locoregional and distant recurrences even after "curative" resection. Perioperative irradiation (pre-, intra-, postoperative) did not lead to better results (Caudrey 1992). This clearly indicates spread of disease beyond those borders which can be reached by local treatment alone. It also indicates that an improvement of these results can only be expected by combining local and systemic treatment.

As part of such a multimodal treatment approach, chemotherapy (CTx) has been predominantly used as a postoperative (adjuvant) measure. However, up to now, postoperative CTx has failed to show a clinically relevant survival benefit compared to surgery alone (Schein 1992).

More promising appears to be preoperative CTx which has attracted increasing interest during the past 8–10 years. Preoperative CTx has been investigated in patients with clinically staged, potentially resectable tumors and in patients with locally advanced disease (LAGC).

The trials which are being done with preoperative CTx in potentially resectable disease show that preoperative CTx is feasible and does not increase perioperative morbidity and/or mortality (Rougier et al. 1994). In most of these trials, relatively high R0 resection rates were achieved and some authors claimed that the observed survival times are better than those achieved with surgery alone (retrospective comparison with historical controls). However, similarly high resection rates and similar survival times were also reported with surgery alone. Therefore, these trials do not help to answer the question of whether preoperative CTx improves the prognosis of gastric cancer patients.

The most striking evidence that preoperative CTx improves the prognosis of patients with localized gastric cancer comes from trials in which preoperative CTx was administered to patients with "unresectable" LAGC.

The term "unresectable" comprises different clinical situations and should therefore be defined more precisely. First, gastric cancer may be judged to be unresectable for technical reasons by an experienced surgeon on the basis of an explorative laparotomy. At the moment this definition is the most reliable one, although we are well aware that a tumor considered to be unresectable by one surgeon may be regarded as resectable by another. A less precise definition of unresectability, used in a number of recently published trials, includes those tumors which are deemed "unresectable" after clinical staging procedures such as endoscopy (due to tumor size or location, e.g., carcinoma in the cardia) or computed tomography (due to infiltration of the tumor into adjacent structures or enlarged lymph nodes) (Rougier et al. 1994; Kang et al. 1992). Because of the relatively low sensitivity and specificity of these conventional diagnostic procedures, potentially resectable and unresectable gastric cancers are then grouped under the term "unresectable." This may result in misleading interpretations of the clinical value of an investigational treatment such as preoperative CTx. Therefore, if a clinical staging is the basis for future trials with preoperative CTx in LAGC, we should define these cancers as "potentially unresectable" gastric cancer. To date, this can be done at best by endoscopic ultrasound (EUS), and by surgical laparoscopy and lavage as recently reported by Fink and coworkers (1995).

Preoperative Chemotherapy in Clinically Staged Locally Advanced and Potentially Unresectable Gastric Cancer

Three abstracts and five papers have been published so far, dealing with preoperative CTx in clinically staged, potentially unresectable gastric cancer (Table 1). One publication is a more casuistic report (Bonatsos 1985). The results of CTx and subsequent surgery in patients with LAGC were reported in three CTx trials which included patients with distant metastases as well (Lerner et al. 1992; Roelofs et al. 1993; Yonemura et al. 1993). Three prospective phase II and one randomized phase III trial included only LAGC patients (Rougier et al. 1994; Kang et al. 1992; Fink et al. 1995; Schwartz et al. 1993). Two trials from Japan are not included in this analysis because detailed data on the outcome of the patients treated preoperatively with two different CTx regimens are lacking in both abstracts (Sugiyama et al. 1993; Nakajima et al. 1993).

Bonatsos et al. reported on five patients with unresectable tumors treated with 5-fluorouracil, doxorubicin, and mitomycin C (FAM) (Bonatsos et al. 1985). In three of the four patients responding to CTx (one complete and three partial remissions), secondary tumor resection was possible; one of them remained disease-free after 2 years.

In the trial of Lerner et al., 36 patients with advanced gastric cancer, including a subgroup of 13 patients with locally advanced unresectable tumors, received etoposide, doxorubicin, and cisplatin (EAP) (Lerner et al. 1992). Of these 13 patients, five underwent surgery after three cycles of EAP; their response to CTx was not recorded, but a complete (R0) tumor resection could be performed in only one of them. This patient had a pathologically confirmed complete remission lasting 12 months.

The results of a European multicenter trial with an alternating chemotherapy program consisting of methotrexate/5-FU/cisplatin/4-epidoxorubicin (FEMTX-P) were reported by Roelofs et al. (1993). The study population consisted of 36 patients with distant metastases and 14 with LAGC alone. The

Table 1. Results of preoperative chemotherapy and surgery in clinically staged potentially unresectable gastric cancer

Reference	Chemotherapy regimen	Patients (*n*)	Major responses (*n*) (%)	R0 (*n*) (%)	Survival (Years)	Recurrence after R0 (*n*)
Bonatsos et al. (1985)	2× FAM	5	4	ns	2 (2/5)	1/3
Lerner et al. (1992)	3× EAP	13	ns	1 (8)	ns	1
Roelofs et al. (1993)	4× FEMTX-P	14	7 (50)	4 (29)	ns	ns
Fink et al. (1995)	3–4× EAP	27	17 (63)	24 (89)	2 (all, 30%) (R0, 36%)	17
Rougier et al. (1993)	3× DDP/FU	28[a]	15/27 (56)	23/28 (82)	2 (42%)	13
Schwartz et al. (1993)	3× FAMTX + CDDP/ + CDDP/5-FU postoperatively	23	ns	13 (57)	NA	4 in 6 months
Kang et al. (1992)	3× PER	24	ns	(63)	ns	ns

RO, total resection; *ns*, not statch; *NA*, not available. See text for other abbreviations
[a] Twenty-eight patients who underwent operation (27 with 3 cycles of DDP/FU and one with <3 cycles of chemotherapy)

latter group received four cycles of FEMTX-P preoperatively. Seven objective responses were observed and four patients (29%) had a R0 resection. Follow-up data were not available.

At the Gustave Roussy Institute, Rougier et al. (1994) tested the combination of preoperative cisplatin/5-FU in 30 patients with LAGC. The definition of LAGC was based on the findings at explorative laparotomy (four patients), enlarged lymph nodes in the coeliac area on computed tomography (CT) scans (26 patients), tumor size exceeding 7 cm (15 patients), or by tumor location in the cardia (15 patients). Response to chemotherapy could be evaluated in 27 patients after three cycles of cisplatin/5-FU. They reported one complete and 14 partial responses (the overall response rate was 56%), and in 12 patients the disease had stabilized. Of note is the fact that in no case had the tumor progressed during CTx. A subgroup analysis of the response to CTx indicated that patients with tumors in the cardia and fewer than 50% of independent tumor cells (signet ring cell carcinoma) in the biopsy specimens were more likely to achieve a remission. In contrast, an objective response occurred in only one of six evaluable patients with linitis plastica. Twenty-eight patients underwent surgery and 82% of them (23/28) had a R0 resection – which corresponds to 77% of the total patient population. The R0 resection rate was markedly higher in patients who had an objective response to chemotherapy (86%) compared to patients without a tumor response (33%). Two out of four patients with primarily unresectable tumors (as determined by explorative laparotomy) responded to CTx and subsequently underwent R0 resection. Neither morbidity nor mortality was higher after preoperative CTx than after surgery alone. The relapse rate of patients who were disease-free after preoperative cisplatin/5-FU plus surgery was 72%. The 4-year survival rate was 20% (6/30).

An important contribution towards a more precise definition of locally advanced disease was made by Fink et al. (1995). In their trial with preoperative EAP, the only patients entered were those who had T3/T4 tumors as defined by EUS, comprising stage IIIA/IIIB/IV. Additionally, all patients underwent surgical laparoscopy with peritoneal lavage in order to exclude peritoneal carcinosis, which can be expected in approximately 20%–25% of such patients. During laparoscopy an ultrasound scan of the liver was obtained. Three cycles of EAP were planned and a fourth cycle was given to patients who had a continued response after the third EAP cycle. Surgery included a standard lymphadenectomy of lymph node compartments I and II. A major clinical response was observed in 17 (63%) of 27 patients who received at least two cycles of EAP. Nine patients (33%) had a minor response or no change. Tumor progression during CTx occurred in one patient only. Twenty-seven patients underwent surgery and a R0 resection was performed in 24 out of a total of 30 patients, which corresponds to a R0 resection rate of 80% among the entire patient population. Despite the extensive resections there was no postoperative 30-day or 90-day mortality. This high R0 resection rate markedly exceeds the R0 resection rate (41%) in patients with locally advanced tumors who underwent primary resection in the German Gastric Cancer Carcinoma study (Roder et al. 1993). A matched-pair analysis provided by the authors (patients with R0 resection after CTx versus similar patients with R0 resection but no prior CTx) indicated a clear survival benefit of preoperative CTx for their patients, partly attributed to a reduction of distant failures. The median survival times in this study were 17 months for all patients, 19 months for those with surgical resection, and 24 months after R0 resection. The 2-year actuarial survival rates were 30%, 32%, and 36% in the total patient population, in patients who had resection, and in patients who underwent a R0 resection, respectively.

Endoscopic ultrasonography was used as the clinical staging procedure in the trial by Schwartz et al. (1993). Twenty-nine eligible patients with T3/T4 NX M0 (all clinical stage III) were entered. The treatment consisted of three cycles of preoperative FAMTX (5-FU, doxorubicin, methotrexate) and, to address the peritoneal failure problem, three cycles of postoperative intraperitoneal 5-FU/cisplatin. Of the 23 patients who completed the treatment, 18 underwent surgery, and a R0 resection was possible in 13 (56%). CTx-induced downstaging was confirmed in 33% of the patients undergoing surgery. No postoperative deaths occurred, but two patients died of CTx-related complications. Long-term results are not yet available.

In a randomized trial, Kang et al. (1992) investigated the effect of two or three cycles of neoadjuvant cisplatin/etoposide/5-FU (PEF) versus surgery alone. Fifty-one patients were entered in the study. The "curative" resection rate of operated patients was 75% (15/20) after preoperative CTx and 56% (15/27) with surgery alone. Based on these results and on the markedly lower frequency of advanced stages (histopathologic workup of resected specimens) after preoperative CTx, the authors are continuing patient accrual.

Similar observations were made by Yonemura et al. (1993) who performed a randomized trial with preoperative cisplatin, mitomycin, etoposide, UFt [a combination of 1-(2-tetrahydrofuryl)-5-fluorouracil and uracil, PMUE] and postoperative PMUE versus primary surgery plus postoperative PMUE. Fifty-four patients with high-grade, advanced gastric cancer (Japanese staging) including patients with peritoneal and hepatic metastases as well as involvement of paraaortic lymph nodes were entered in the study. The authors stated that preoperative CTx was feasible, that it induced downstaging, and that it allowed a higher R0 resection rate as well as significantly better survival after resection. However, the results of this trial remain inconclusive because of the mixed patient population.

Preoperative Chemotherapy in Surgically Staged Locally Advanced and Unresectable Gastric Cancer

Three groups have reported their treatment results with preoperative chemotherapy in patients with unresectable LAGC as defined by an experienced surgeon during explorative laparotomy (Wilke et al. 1989; Plukker et al. 1991; Wilke et al. 1990; Popiela et al. 1992) (Table 2).

In a multicenter trial, the results of which were reported by Wilke et al. (1989, 1990), 35 patients with unresectable LAGC received two to four cycles of EAP and in the case of tumor response to CTx a second operation and resection of residual tumor was planned as well as two cycles of postoperative EAP for consolidation. Of the 35 patients, 28 had newly diagnosed gastric cancer, two had local recurrences after an earlier R0 resection and five had gross residual disease after palliative surgery. For this trial patients were also eligible if they had paraaortic lymph nodes (28 patients) or local peritoneal spread or both. The overall response rate after CTx was 69% (24/35) and 20 patients with an objective response underwent a second operation for control. Six patients had a pathologically complete remission as confirmed by gastrectomy and lymphadenectomy (three patients) or by laparotomy and multiple biopsies (three patients). A R0 resection was performed in ten patients with microscopic or macroscopic residual disease after EAP, a R1 resection (positive oral resection margins) in three patients and no resection in one patient. The R0 resection rate among the 28 patients with newly diagnosed LAGC was 48%. Of 21 patients who were disease free after chemotherapy alone (two patients with clinically complete remission who refused surgery), after preoperative CTx plus surgery (16 patients), or after preoperative CTx, surgery and postoperative CTx (three patients), 14 developed recurrences. Locoregional failure with or without peritoneal carcinomatosis as the first site of relapse was observed in 11, liver metastases in one, and isolated CNS metastases in two patients. The median survival time for all patients was 16 months, and for patients who were disease-free after the whole treatment program it was 24 months. Six patients are still alive after an observation time of 5–8 years. One patient was lost to follow-up 5 years

Table 2. Results of preoperative chemotherapy plus surgery in surgically staged unresectable gastric cancer

References	Chemotherapy regimen	Patients (*n*)	Major responses (*n*) (%)	R0 (*n*) (%)	Years of survival (%)	Recurrence after R0
Wilke et al. (1989; 1990)	2–5× EAP + (1–2×) postoperatively	35	24 (69)	13/28[a] (46)	5 (33)[b] (20)[c]	8[a] 14[b]
Plukker et al. (1991)	4× MTX/FU	17	ns	8 (47)	4 (12)	6
Popiela et al. (1992)	2–3× EAP	10	7 (70)	7 (70)	ns	ns

RO, total resection; *ns*, not stated. See text for other abbreviations
[a] Only patients with newly diagnosed gastric cancer (no recurrences, no prior R2 resection)
[b] Recurrences and 5-year survival rate of 21 patients disease-free after chemotherapy ± surgery ± postoperative chemotherapy
[c] The 5-year survival rate of all 35 patients

after surgery. The long-term survival at 5 years is 20% for all patients and 33% for those 21 patients who were without evidence of disease after CTx, either with or without surgery. No chemotherapy- or surgery-related mortality was observed.

Plukker et al. (1991) administered four cycles of methotrexate and 5-FU to 20 patients with stage IIIb or IV. The determination of unresectability was done by an explorative laparotomy in 17 patients. Three patients were considered to be "incurable" on the basis of a CT scan because of massive invasion of adjacent structures and involved distant, abdominal lymph nodes more than 3 cm away from the primary tumor. Seventeen patients finished four courses of preoperative CTx and 14 of them underwent a second laparotomy. A complete tumor-free (R0) resection was possible in 8/17 (47%) patients, six of whom died of recurrent disease (five locoregional) at a median of 22 months after initiation of chemotherapy. Two patients were still disease-free after 54 and 41 months, respectively.

Popiela et al. (1992) reported on 10 patients with surgically staged unresectable gastric cancer who received two to three cycles of preoperative EAP. Seven patients responded to CTx and could subsequently undergo a R0 resection. No patient died postoperatively. Follow-up and survival data are not available.

Summary and Future Perspectives

Local control and distant metastases are the two major problems associated with surgical treatment of locally advanced gastric cancer which, despite these problems, clearly remains the cornerstone of treatment for this challenging tumor. Therefore treatment modalities together with surgery are not only of high interest but are also urgently warranted if the poor prognosis of LAGC is to be improved.

During the past decades, postoperative CTx after complete tumor resection and perioperative CTx/RTx (radiotherapy) were investigated; however, the assumed benefit of these approaches, if any, was marginal (Caudrey 1992; Popiela et al. 1992). Whether it will improve with new, active CTx regimens, better timing of postoperative CTx, modern irradiation techniques, or the combination of these measures has to be investigated.

Available clinical data indicate that preoperative treatment, especially preoperative CTx, might be a therapeutic tool worth studying. Current experiences with preoperative CTx for LAGC is still limited to a few phase II and III trials with somewhat impressive results in surgically staged unresectable tumors. In patients with clinically staged "unresectable" disease, the results are frequently inconclusive.

The most striking evidence that preoperative CTx has the potential to improve the prognosis of gastric cancer patients comes from trials in which the only patients studied where those with surgically staged (explorative laparotomy) unresectable disease (Wilke et al. 1989; Plukker et al. 1991; Wilke et al. 1990; Popiela et al. 1992). Summarizing the findings of these trials, the following can be stated:

- Preoperative CTx is feasible and does not increase the postoperative morbidity or mortality compared to surgery alone.
- An active CTx regimen may induce significant tumor regression and thereby offer the possibility of a R0 resection in 40%–50% of the patients with a primarily unresectable disease. This results in an improved median survival and even in long-term survival of some patients with an otherwise fatal outcome.
- If there is a response to CTx, tumor resection should also be tried in those cases in which the intraoperative appearance of local tumor spread seems to exclude a resection with curative intention. Postchemotherapy changes in the former tumor area, such as fibrosis and inflammatory alterations, may mimic a vital tumor.
- In these trials, locoregional failure was the predominant primary site of recurrence (70%–80%) after R0 resection. Therefore extended surgery is mandatory independent of the degree of tumor regression after preoperative CTx.
- It cannot be expected that preoperative systemic CTx and subsequent surgery will solve the problem of local or intraperitoneal failure sufficiently. Therefore additional treatment options, such as intraoperative irradiation (IORT), preoperative CTx/RTx, and intraperitoneal CTx must be investigated.

Similar conclusions with respect to feasibility of preoperative CTx, its ability to induce tumor regression, and its perioperative morbiditiy and mortality can be drawn from preoperative CTx trials with clinically staged, potentially unresectable LAGC (Rougier et al. 1994; Kang et al. 1992; Fink et al. 1995; Schwartz et al. 1993). Estimating the impact of preoperative CTx on the R0 resection rate and survival is, however, difficult in this particular patient population. Patients with surgically staged unresectable tumors can serve as their own controls at the time of the second-look operation. Therefore the question of whether the patient benefited from preoperative CTx is relatively easy to answer. After clinical staging, this benefit can be demonstrated only for carefully and accurately staged tumors, and when compared with the results after surgery alone. Unfortunately, conclusive randomized trials dealing with this issue are lacking (Kang et al. 1992; Yonemura et al. 1993). However, randomization of treatment strategies might miss the true benefit of a particular treatment if there is an imbalance in prognostic factors. The most important prognostic factor related to surgery is the TNM classification; but neither CT scans, ultrasound scans, nor endoscopy enable us to define T/N with an acceptable accuracy. Therefore staging procedures in future gastric cancer trials comparing preoperative treatment versus surgery alone, or with postoperative therapy, should generally include EUS.

Laparoscopy, especially surgical laparoscopy plus intraabdominal lavage, represents another important staging method. It helps to avoid the inclusion of patients with peritoneal carcinomatosis (approximately 20% of patients with clinically locoregional confined tumors) in preoperative trials; peritoneal carcinomatosis is frequently not detectable by other means (J. Ajani, personal communication).

Nevertheless, in most reported phase II and phase III trials, the authors state that preoperative CTx for clinically staged, potentially unresectable gastric cancer seems to increase the R0 resection rate and also improve survival when compared to historical controls. This was most obvious in the study of Fink et al. (1995), who employed EUS and surgical laparoscopy as pretherapeutic diagnostic tools. To date, the available results with preoperative CTx in LAGC provide us with sufficient argument to investigate this approach versus primary surgery in well-designed randomized trials.

How should CTx be performed in the preoperative setting? The phase II trials with preoperative CTx for locally advanced disease indicate that CTx should be administered as intensively as possible (using hematopoietic growth factors if necessary) until maximum response is achieved (usually after four cycles). In addition extensive surgery is mandatory even after CTx-induced tumor reduction. Last but not least, these trials showed that after such an approach, most relapses occurred intraabdominally (locoregionally, peritoneal carcinomatosis). This finding should urge us to search for additional treatment modalities such as preoperative CTx/RTx, IORT, or intraperitoneal chemotherapy (Takahashi and Abe 1986; Hagiwara 1992) in future trials.

How should surgery be performed in perioperative trials? Although, the benefit of extended surgery seems to be more obvious at earlier stages (<IIIB) of tumor development, radical surgery of the tumor-bearing organ as well as the resection of the N2 compartment should be performed. Surgical quality control by the pathologist (number of resected lymph nodes) and quality control of the pathologist should also be included in future studies.

Are there prognostic factors related to chemotherapy which should be taken into consideration for stratification? Although not prospectively proven, there is evidence that female gender, diffuse-type histology according to the Lauren classification, proximal tumor localization, and linitis plastica may negatively influence the outcome of perioperative chemotherapy.

The coming years should reveal whether the small steps that have been taken with the current, more active chemotherapy regimens for advanced disease will indeed be relevant to the curative treatment of early and locally advanced stages of gastric cancer.

References

Bonatsos C, Aust J, Meisner D, Poiesz B, Comis R (1985) Preoperative chemotherapy for patients with locally advanced gastric carcinoma. Proc Am Soc Clin Oncol 4:83

Caudrey M (1992) Gastric cancer: radiotherapy and approaches to locally unresectable or recurrent disease. In: Ahlgren JD, MacDonald JS (eds) Gastrointestinal oncology. Lippincott, Philadelphia, pp 181–187

Fink U, Schuhmacher C, Stein HJ, Busch R, Peussner H, Dittler H-J, Helmberger H, Böttcher K, Siewert JR (1995) Preoperative chemotherapy for stage III–IV gastric carcinoma: feasibility, response and outcome after complete resection. Br J Surg 82:1248–1252

Hagiwara A, Takahashi T, Kojima O, Sawai K, Yamaguchi T, Yamane T, Taniguchi H, Kitamura K, Noguchi A, Seiki K, Sakakura C (1992) Prophylaxis with carbon-absorbed mitomycin against peritoneal recurrence of gastric cancer. Lancet 339:629–631

Kang YK, Choi DW, Kim CM, Lee JL, Hong WS, Paik NS, Moon NM, Lee JO, Kim YK, Kang TW (1992) The effect of neoadjuvant chemotherapy on the surgical outcome of locally advanced gastric adenocarcinoma: interim report of a randomized trial. Proc Am Soc Clin Oncol 11:173

Lerner A, Gonin R, Steele GD, Mayer RJ (1992) Etoposide, doxorubicin, and cisplatin chemotherapy for advanced gastric adenocarcinoma: Results of a phase II trial. J Clin Oncol 10:536–540

Meyer HJ, Jähne J, Wilke H, Pichlmayr R (1991) Surgical treatment of gastric cancer: Retrospective survey of 1704 operated cases with special reference to total gastrectomy as operation of choice. Semin Surg Oncol 7:356–364

Nakajima T, Ishihara S, Hashimoto H, Kitamura Y, Nakajima Y, Fujii M, Tokunaga A, Matai K, Anzai H, Nishi M (1993) Neoadjuvant chemotherapy for inoperable gastric cancer via local and general delivery routes (FLEP therapy). Proceedings of the 4th international conference on chemotherapy, Paris

Plukker JTh, Mulder NH, Sleijfer DTh, Grondt J, Verschueren RCJ (1991) Chemotherapy and surgery for locally advanced cancer of the cardia and fundus: phase II study with methotrexate and 5-fluorouracil. Br J Surg 78:955–958

Popiela T, Kulig J, Skucinski J, Scepanik A, Tabor J, Plaskocinski P, Nowak M (1992) Advances in treatment of seriously advanced gastric cancer using aggressive EAP chemotherapy. In: Proceedings of an international symposium on gastric cancer, 25–26 May, 1992, pp 108–116

Roder JD, Böttcher K, Siewert JR, Busch R, Hermanek P, Meyer HJ (1993) Prognostic factors in gastric carcinoma. Cancer 72:2089–2097

Roelofs EJM, Wagener DJTh, Conroy Th, Wils J, Burghouts JTH, Fickers M, De Graeff A, Lalisang F, Paillot B (1993) Phase II study of sequential high-dose methotrexate (MTX) and 5-fluorouracil (F) alternated with epirubicin (E) and cisplatin (P) (FEMTX-P) in advanced gastric cancer. Ann Oncol 4:426–428

Rougier P, Lasser P, Ducreux M, Mahjoubi M, Bellefqih S, Elias D (1994) Preoperative chemotherapy of locally advanced gastric cancer. Ann Oncol 5 [Suppl 2]:59–68

Schein PS (1992) Gastric cancer: Approaches to adjuvant therapy. In: Ahlgren JD, MacDonald JS (eds) Gastrointestinal oncology. Lippincott, Philadelphia, pp 189–193

Schwartz G, Kelsen D, Christman K, Saltz L, Toomosi F, Friedrich C, Lauwers G, Yao TJ, Karpeh M, Brennan M, Gerdes H (1993) A phase II study of neoadjuvant FAMTX (5-fluorouracil (5-FU)/Adriamycin/methotrexate) and postoperative intraperitoneal (i.p.) 5-FU and cisplatin (CDDP) in high risk patients with gastric cancer (GC). Proc Am Soc Clin Oncol 12:195

Sugiyama K, Sato H, Hoshi M, Urushiyama M, Ishisoka K, Kanamaru R (1993) Neoadjuvant chemotherapy for advanced gastric cancer: a pilot study with angiotensin II induced drug delivery system. Proceedings of the 4th international conference on Chemotherapy, Paris

Takahashi M, Abe M (1986) Intraoperaive radiotherapy for carcinoma of the stomach. Eur J Surg Oncol 12:247–250

Wilke H, Preusser P, Fink U, Gunzer U, Meyer HJ, Meyer J, Siewert JR, Achterrath W, Lenaz L, Knipp H, Schmoll H-J (1989) Preoperative chemotherapy in locally advanced and nonresectable gastric cancer: A phase II study with etoposide, doxorubicin, and cisplatin. J Clin Oncol 7:1318–1326
Wilke H, Preusser P, Fink U, Achterrath W, Meyer HJ, Stahl M, Lenaz L, Meyer J, Siewert JR, Geerlings H, Köhne-Wömpner CH, Harstrick A, Schmoll H-J (1990) New developments in the treatment of gastric carcinoma. Semin Oncol 17 [Suppl 2]:61–70
Yonemura Y, Sawa T, Kinoshita K, Matsuki N, Fushida S, Tanaka S, Ohoyama S, Takashima T, Kimura H, Kamata T, Fuijmura T, Sugiyama K, Shima K, Miyazaki I (1993) Neoadjuvant chemotherapy for high-grade advanced gastric cancer. World J Surg 17:256–262

Current Aspects of Sphincter Preservation in the Surgical Therapy of Rectal Cancer

P.M. Schlag

Robert-Rössle Hospital, Humboldt University, Lindenberger Weg 80, 13122 Berlin, Germany

Treatment of rectal cancer has changed fundamentally over the past 10 years. In the 1970s and 1980s the majority of patients with carcinoma of the rectum were still treated by operative abdominoperineal excision, as proposed by Miles in 1908. For the patients, this resulted in a definitive loss of continence and the formation of an end colostomy located in the left iliac fossa. The rationale of this radical and mutilating approach was that only by such a procedure could tumor relapse be safely avoided. Apart from these deficits in knowledge on tumor biology, the limited and hitherto insufficiently developed operative techniques further restricted the possibilities of restitution of intestinal continuity in the small pelvis or in the supraanal region. With the rediscovery of pathoanatomical and pathophysiological knowledge comprehensively presented by Westhues as early as in the 1930s, a reorientation process set in which led to new surgical concepts for the therapy of rectal cancer (Westhues 1934). The key fact supporting this is that intramural tumor dissemination beyond 2 cm towards the distal end of the rectum is extremely uncommon. The lymphatic drainage of the rectum, beginning at the levator level, primarily follows a central direction. Therefore, to avoid local recurrence, safety margins are less determinative distally than laterally (Stelzner 1995; Mac Farlanc ct al. 1993; Hermanek and Gall 1981). At the same time operative techniqucs have been developed allowing for a safe anastomosis deep in the small pelvis (Eigler 1991; Gall 1991; Schumpelick and Braun 1991). According to tumor biology the probability of lymphatic metastasis depends on the size and even more so on the depth of invasion and the degree of differentiation of the tumor (Brodsky et al. 1992; Cohen 1993), making it feasible to treat selected tumors in the distal third of the rectum exclusively by local excision. These developments have had the consequence that sphincter-saving treatment is possible in more than 70% of all rectal carcinoma patients without increased risk of recurrence. The relevant treatment strategies along with their indications and their results are presented and analyzed in the following.

Recent Results in Cancer Research, Vol. 142

Anterior Resection of the Rectum

Westhues' (1934) aforementioned observations had the effect that tumors of the upper third of the rectum were soon to be treated by anterior resection. The technical requirements for this procedure could easily be met since continuity of the large intestine can usually be restored transabdominally without problems even if a distal safety margin of 5 cm is maintained. Neither are any problems to be expected in the dissection of the lymphatic drainage areas, for which the inferior mesenteric artery and vein should be ligated just below the offshoot of the left colic artery and vein (Herfarth and Hohenberger 1989). If a tumor is located in the upper third of the rectum, the remaining portion of descending colon is usually mobile enough to achieve a sufficiently tension-free anastomosis, even if a distal safety margin of 5 cm is maintained. Consequently, for this tumor location, there was early agreement that a more radical distal dissection, including dissection of the sphincter appartus, does not yield a greater chance for cure. Anterior resection and thereby sphincter preservation soon became standard procedure in these cases. However, rectal carcinomas are only located at this high level in 20%–30% of cases. Therefore, the portion of anterior resections was low in comparison to the total number of surgically treated rectal cancer patients. Survival rates corresponded with those of sigmoid carcinomas. Continence largely unaffected in these patients since the rectal ampulla remains surgically unscathed.

Low Anterior Resection

Controversies in sphincter-saving rectal resections mainly arise from tumors located in the mid- and distal thirds of the rectum (Nicholls et al. 1979; Schlag and Slisow 1995). Numerous investigations have shown that the anterior resection of tumors located as low as the levator level is sufficiently radical. This level represents the anatomical boundary between the phylogenically discernible visceral and somatic part of the human being (Stelzner 1995). As a consequence, the lymphatic drainage cephalad to this level is directed strictly towards the viscera, i.e., intraabdominally, whereas drainage caudad to this level is directed towards the perineum and the inguen. Under these circumstances, the relevant lymphatic drainage regions of rectal tumors located above the levator level can be radically removed through the abdominal approach. There, complete removal of the entire mesorectum is of utmost importance (Mac Farlane et al. 1993). The dissection can be achieved transabdominally, i.e., anteriorly, with the same precision as through an additional perineal access. Only when the direction of lymphatic drainage is reversed due to compromise by a massive proximal lymphogenic metastasis, should perineal and inguinal metastases be considered. In such situations, however, regional operative options for cure are restricted. The safety margin in the rectum itself depends on the probability of distal intramural tumor cell propagation, which is influenced by the macroscopic growth pattern and the grade of the tumors (Slisow et al. 1993). A distal safety margin of 2 cm is usually sufficient for polypoid, highly differentiated adenocarcinomas (G1), whereas in ulcerating and especially in poorly differentiated tumors (G3) and mucinous carcinomas, margins of 3–4 cm are mandatory. Under favorable conditions, tumors located 4–5 cm and, in unfavorable morphology, from 6 cm above the anal verge are radically resectable and sphincter preserving using the abdominal approach.

For the restoration of continence, however, not only is the resectional level an important criterion but also the possibilities of a technically feasible and safe restoration of continuity. Especially the narrow and deep male pelvis can make a transabdominal anastomotic procedure difficult to perform. Mechanical suturing devices, especially double stapling, constitute a further improvement in this field. Using a linear staper, movable in two planes, the remaining rectal stump can be closed and the anastomosis performed using a circular stapling gun. After insertion of the separate head part of the apparatus into the proximal colon and fixation by a purse string suture, the gun itself is inserted transanally with the guiding pin positioned to perforate the closed rectum at the suture line. The head and plate are approximated and the anastomotic mechanism activated. Alternatively, the anastomosis can be achieved by transanal manual suturing (Schumpelick and Braun 1991). For this purpose two Parks' retractors are inserted to dilate the anal canal. The proximal colon is shifted to this region and anastomosis is achieved by interrupted seromuscular sutures which, in their distal portions, include parts of the external sphincter. To establish the anastomosis after low anterior resection, sufficient mobilization of the colon across the left flexure up to the midtransverse colon is necessary. If, after this step, the colon were shifted, a preserved main stem of the inferior mesenteric artery would be an obstruction. For this reason and more so for the sake of the required complete dissection of the mesenteric lymphatic drainage area, the separation of the main stem of the inferior mesenteric artery should be programmatic. The blood supply of the colonic segment to be anastomosed is then provided entirely by the middle colic artery via Riolan's anastomosis.

Transsphincteric Resection

It may be difficult to determine the intended safety margin transabdominally, especially in tumors positioned low in the distal third of the rectum which are resectable according to the principles mentioned above. In these cases it is advisable to determine the resection line primarily through a transanal approach and to incise the rectum in the upper sphincteric area (Hohenberger et al. 1992). The intended safety margin can be directly visualized. The remaining dissection of the mesenteric lymphatic pathways together with the complete dissection of the mesorectal tissue is achieved through an anterior access.

Reanastomosis in transsphincteric resection, however, requires a transanal manual suture with the possibility to initially evert the anastomosic line and then to reposition it after completion.

Pouch Formation to Improve Continence

A sphincter-preserving procedure should always be accompanied by thorough preoperative sphincteromanometric assessment (Braun et al. 1988). In latent sphincteric insufficiency, unsatisfactory results are likely to be expected, especially in the very low anterior resections. In impaired sphincteric function and in borderline surgical-oncological indications for sphincter preservation, abdominoperineal excision of the rectum is recommended. In each case of evident sphincter weakness pre- and postoperative sphincter training, including electrophysiological stimulation, should be carried out to improve the functional results. Apart from neurogenic and muscular mechanisms, continence is also determined by the capacity of the rectal ampulla. Under recognition of these pathophysiological facts surgical attempts to reconstruct a reservoir can be of benefit for continence (Schlag and Slisow 1995; Parc et al. 1986). The formation of a colon pouch is especially recommended in elderly patients. Due to the higher incidence of partial sphincteric insufficiency and shorter overall survival in this age group, it is less likely that this group of patients will adapt to the coloanal anastomosis as quickly as younger patients with a sufficient sphincter. With the interposition of a colon-J-pouch, faster functional adaptation can be expected. It is important to realize that the pouch volume should be kept small so as not to induce constipation by thickening of stool. Another advantage of a pouch reconstruction is the accompanying lower incidence of anastomotic dehiscence. This may be due to the technically necessary lateroterminal formation of the anastomosis. Our own comparative studies between direct coloanal and pouch–anal anastomoses have shown there to be a clear advantage of the pouch with respect to compliance, stool frequency, reservoir, and rate of continence (Kroesen et al. 1995). The technical requirements of the formation of a colon pouch do not unduly prolong the operation. Since there is evidence that pouch formation has a positive effect on the healing of anastomosis, this procedure is prefered in elderly patients with subclinical sphincter insufficiency. Another special problem in the preservation of continence is the necessity of performing a total proctocolectomy in patients with familial polyposis who have a high risk of rectal cancer. As long as there is no indication for ileorectal anastomosis, ileostomy can only be prevented by creating a pouch–anal anastomosis (Herfarth and Stern 1991). Here, a larger reservoir volume for the collection of liquid ileal stool than a colon pouch may be necessary. Especially in familial polyposis coli, ileopouch–anal anastomosis can provide favorable functional results and should be viewed differently from the same procedure in ulcerative colitis with its higher complication rate. Therefore, the colon pouch as well as the ileum pouch constitute a further step towards preservation and improvement of the sphincteric function in colorectal surgery.

Local Sphincter-Saving Procedures

Despite the above-mentioned recent developments, there is still an indication for rectal resection in tumors which are 0–5 cm above the dentate line if they are of a certain size and degree of differentiation. Besides maintaining sufficient safety margins, the removal of potentially tumorous glands is only possible in these cases by rectal excision. The likelihood of lymphogenic metastasis depends largely on grading, tumorous infiltration of the intestinal wall, and on the size of the tumors (Silsow et al. 1991). Based on these facts the question was raised as to whether in selected patients with advantageous tumor criteria, local excision would yield results which are as good as those in conventional, extensive abdominoperineal tumor excision. Technically, local tumor excision can be achieved, via posterior rectotomy or transanally. Because of the higher morbidity, posterior rectotomy has been abandoned in the local treatment of rectal cancer. Instead, the transanal access is now widely used and can be achieved by anal retractors, transanal microsurgery (Bueß et al. 1984), or through special specula which have been developed in our department (Schlag and Slisow 1995). A precondition for good results is a full-thickness, monobloc resection under the maintenance of a safety margin of at least 0.5 cm. Tumors of up to 9 cm^2 can be resected, whereby in 90% of the cases R0 can be achieved histologically. The resulting defect can be oversewn transanally. The low postoperative morbidity of this procedure as compared to abdominoperineal excision is even more pronounced knowing that mostly high risk groups of patients have previously been treated by this local procedure. The local recurrence rate after local excision is below 10%. In our own experience there has been no difference in recurrence-free and overall survival in patients with well-differentiated pT1 and pT2 tumors, comparing local with abdominoperineal excision. Tumors graded G3 or 4, however, have a local recurrence rate of more than 25% within the first 12 postoperative months if excised locally. With a view to total survival, the results for local excision in patients with pT1G1 and pT2G1 tumors are very encouraging and by no means worse than the results of abdominoperineal excision (Mac Farlane et al. 1993). Therefore, in pT1 and pT2 tumors with a high degree of differentiation and, conventionally, located such that only an abdominoperineal excision would have been feasible, today's surgical standard should be local excision. A precondition, however, is that on endosonographic rectal examination the tumors appear to be limited to the submucosa or to the luminally sided layers of the circular muscles of the rectum. Also, enlarged or suspicious lymph nodes in the peritumorous tissue or pararectal space have to be excluded endosonographically (Glaser et al. 1990). Cases in which local excision does not produce definitive R0-resection, abdominoperineal excision should follow. Whether postoperative radiation will yield similarly good results and whether preoperative radiochemotherapy will raise the rate of local resectability in rectal carcinomas of the distal third (Bannon et al. 1995) will have to be demonstrated in carefully planned randomized studies in the future.

The indication for abdominoperineal excision has been narrowed and the numbers of patients subjected to it reduced in the most recent years. Today the operation is indicated only in locally advanced carcinomas of the distal third of the rectum (uT3 and uT4), in patients in whom the tumor has infiltrated the sphincter apparatus with preexisting, severe sphincteric insufficiency. In patients in whom sphincter preservation is impossible, surgical methods designed to replace the functions of the sphincter should be considered.

Sphincteroplasty

For patients in whom the sphincter apparatus must be removed for oncological reasons, an alternative to the formation of an abdominal colostomy is to create a perineal colostomy in combination with a sphincteroplasty. The formation of a neosphincter by transposition of parts of the gluteus maximus or gracilis muscles has been unsatisfactory up to now since the striated muscles, unlike the smooth muscles, are incapable of generating a permanent tone. For this reason implantable electronic simulating devices are being worked on at present (Cavina et al. 1990; Geerdes et al. 1995).

In our hospital, a different method of neosphincter formation is being tested in cooperation with the Research Institute of Proctology in Moscow (Fedorov et al. 1989). This method consists of ample mobilization of the left hemicolon under preservation of the vascular arcades. After abdominoperineal rectal excision the mobile colon is pulled into the perineal wound. Then, the muscularis propria layer of a 10- to 12-cm-long colonic segment free of fatty tissue is separated from the mucosa. The resulting seromuscular tube is trimmed in a spiral fashion to form a band which remains connected with the intestinal wall at its base from where it is supplied by microcirculation. The distal colon is then enveloped by this seromuscular band and inserted into the perineum to form the colostomy. The seromuscular cuff acts as the internal sphincter. Supported by pelvic floor exercise and electrostimulation of the perineum, the patients learn to perceive the urge to defecate and to distinguish bowel gases from stool. After a training period of 3 months patients are able to regulate the emptying of their bowels by a conscious activation of their gluteal and thigh muscles. The perineal colostomy with the neosphincter can also be formed secondarily, after prior abdominoperineal excision.

References

Bannon JP, Marks GJ, Mohiuddin et al (1995) Radical and local excisional methods of sphincter-sparing surgery after high-dose radiation for cancer of the distal 3 cm of the rectum. Ann Surg Oncol 2:221

Braun J, Steinau G, Schumpelick V (1988) Anorektale Funktionsdiagnostik: präoperativer Aussagewert zur Kontinenzleistung nach tiefer anteriorer Rektumresektion mit kolo-analer Anastomose. Zentralbl Chir 113:1120

Brodsky JT, Richard GK, Cohen AM et al (1992) Variables correlated with the risk of lymph node metastasis in early rectal cancer. Cancer 69:332

Bueß G, Hutter F, Theiß et al (1984) Das System für die transanale endoskopische Rectumoperation. Chirurg 55:677

Cavina E, Seccia M, Evangelista G, Chiarugi M, Buccianti P, Tortora A, Chirico A (1990) Perineal colostomy and electrostimulated gracilis "neosphincter" after abdomino-perineal resection of the colon and anorectum – a surgical experience and follow-up study in 47 cases. Int J Colorec Dis 5:6

Cohen AM (1993) Colon J-Pouch rectal reconstruction after total or subtotal proctectomy. World J Surg 17:267

Eigler FW (1991) Die peranale Anastomose nach tiefer Rektumresektion. Chirurg 62:12

Fedorov VD, Odaryuk TS, Shelygin YA, Tsarkov PV, Frolov SA (1989) Method of creation of a smooth-muscle cuff at the site of the perineal colostomy after exstirpation of the rectum. Dis Col Rect 32:562

Gall FP (1991) Die tiefe Rectumresektion – transabdominaler Zugang. Chirurg 62:1

Geerdes BP, Zoetmulder FAN, Baeten CGMI (1995) Double dynamic graciloplasty and coloperineal pull-through after abdomino-perineal resection. Eur J Cancer 31A:1248

Glaser F, Friedl P, Ditfurt B, Schlag P, Herfarth C (1990) Influence of endorectal ultrasound on surgical treatment of rectal cancer. Eur J Surg 16:304

Herfarth C, Hohenberger P (1989) Lymphadenektomie bei der Primärtherapie colorectaler Carcinome. Chirurg 60:139

Herfarth C, Stern J (1991) Ileum-pouch: Indikation, Technik und Langzeitergebnisse. Dtsch Med Wochenschr 116:1485

Hermanek P, Gall FP (1981) Der aborale Sicherheitsabstand bei sphinctererhaltenden Rektumresektionen. Chirurg 52:25

Hohenberger W, Hermanek P Jr, Hermanek P, Gall FP (1992) Decision-making in Curative Rectum Carcinoma Surgery. Onkologie 15:209

Kroesen AJ, Stern J, Buhr HJ, Herfarth C (1995) Incontinence after ileo-anal pouch anastomosis – diagnostic criteria and therapeutic sequelae. Chirurg 66(4): 385

Mac Farlane JK, Ryall RDH, Heald RJ (1993) Mesorectal excision for rectal cancer. Lancet 341:457

Miles WE (1908) A method of performing abdomino perineal excision for carcinomas of the rectum and terminal portion of the pelvic colon. Lancet 2:1812

Nicholls RJ, Ritchie JK, Wadsworth J et al (1979) Total excision or restorative resection carcinoma of the middle third of the rectum. Br J Surg 66:625

Parc R, Tiret E, Frileux P et al (1986) Resection and colo-anal anastomosis with colonic reservoir for rectal carcinoma. Br J Surg 73:139

Schlag PM, Slisow W (1995) Operatives Konzept beim Rektumkarzinom. Onkologe 1:18

Schumpelick V, Braun J (1991) Rectumresektion mit coloanaler Anastomose. Chirurug 62:25

Slisow W, Seifart AW, Marx G et al (1991) Stellenwert der lokalen Exzision von kleinflächigen, tiefsitzenden Rektumkarzinomen mit kurativer Zielstellung. Zentralbl Chir 116:1245
Slisow W, Kolbow C, Fischer J (1993) Perioperative klinisch-pathomorphologische Beurteilung des pararektalen Lymphknotenstatus und ihr Beitrag zur definitiven Entscheidung für eine lokale Exstripation des Rektumkarzinomas. Zentralbl Chir 118:197
Stelzner F (1995) Ergebnisse und Erkenntnisse bei 328 Radikaloperationen des Rectumcarcinoms durch einen Operateur. Vergleichend anatomische Untersuchungen mit Brachydanio rerio und Latimeria chalumnae. Chirurg 12:1169
Westhues H (1934) Die pathologisch-anatomischen Grundlagen des Rektumkarzinoms. Thieme, Leipzig

Preoperative and Postoperative Radiotherapy in Rectal Carcinoma

V. Budach, L. Schlenger, and P. Feyer

Department of Radiotherapy, Medical School Charité Berlin, Schumannstr. 20/21, 10117 Berlin, Germany

Abstract

Surgery is the initial treatment of choice for most patients with rectal neoplasms. The objectives are to remove of tumor and drain the primary nodes. In stage I disease the surgical approach is thought to be sufficiently effective. However, at least in the case of abdominoperineal resection, this causes considerable morbidity. Therefore, at the present time, there are efforts to reduce the extent of the resection by applying other treatment modalities in stage I disease. After curative resection in stage II/III disease a considerable number of patients suffer from local recurrence or distant metastases. In these patients adjuvant therapy is currently recommended. In locally advanced disease, primary resection is not feasible. Different treatment settings which apply combinations of all treatment modalities are possible. The article reviews the literature and shows future directions.

Introduction

Adenocarcinoma of the rectum occurs in an estimated 24000 people each year in the Federal Republic of Germany (Wittekind and Tannapfel 1995). Of these patients, 35% present with stage-I disease, 25% with stage-II and stage-III, respectively, and the remaining 15% with stage-IV disease (Fig. 1). The mortality is about 30% (Boring et al. 1992).

The most useful prognostic factors are the extent of disease penetration through the bowel wall, the lymph node involvement, and the distance of the tumor from the anal verge (Rich et al. 1983; Schild et al. 1989b). The tumor grade and venous or lymphatic invasion are also important prognostic factors (Abulafi and Williams 1994). In patients with inferiorly situated rectal cancer who are considered for sphincter-saving treatment, clinical mobility, size, and morphology of the lesions are predictors of prognosis (Papillon 1982).

Recent Results in Cancer Research, Vol. 142

Modified Astler-Coller staging criteria	AJCC staging criteria	
A	Stage 1	T1, N0, M0
B1		T2, N0, M0
B2	Stage II	T3, N0, M0
B3		T4, N0, M0
C1	Stage III	T1-2, N1-3, M0
C2		T3, N1-3, M0
C3		T4, N1-3, M0
D	Stage IV	T any, N any, M1

TNM staging criteria

T1	Involves the submucosa but does not invade the muscularis propria
T2	Invades but does not penetrate the muscularis propria
T3	Penetrates through the muscularis propria; may penetrate into the serosa (if present) or pericolic fat but not into the free peritoneal cavity; nor does it invade other organs
T4	Invades other organs, or involves the free peritoneal cavity
N0	No nodal metastases
N1	One to three pericolic or perirectal nodes involved
N2	Four or more pericolic or perirectal nodes involved
N3	Involvement of any regional node along a named vascular trunk
M0	No distant metastases
M1	Distant metastases present

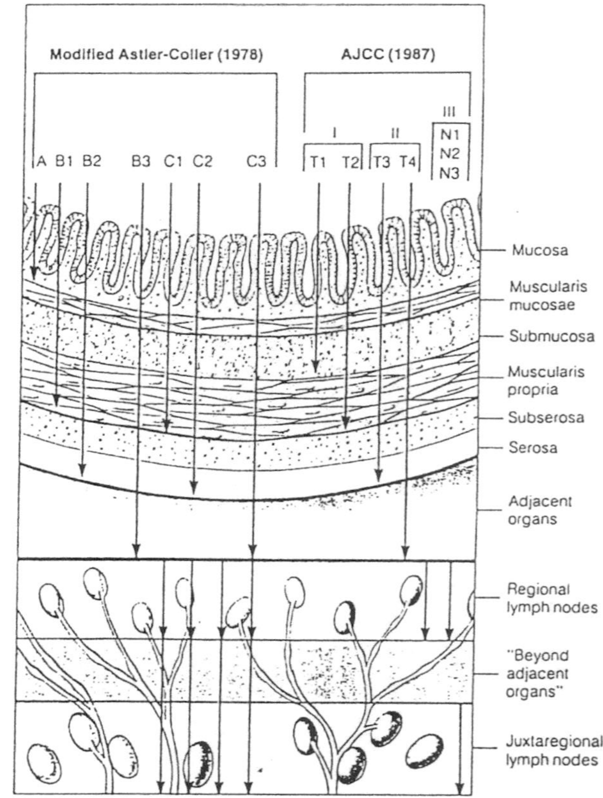

Fig. 1. Modified Astler-Coller system for staging colorectal cancer compared with the tumor-node-metastasis (TNM)-based classification of the American Joint Commission on Cancer (AJCC). (Vaughn and Haller 1993)

Intraoperative tumor perforation doubles the risk of local recurrence. If there is tumor at the resection margins, local recurrence will occur in 85% (Quirke et al. 1986). In summary, after curative resection for Duke's A, B, or C rectal tumors there will be a local recurrence in 1–25%, 5–45%, and 15–50% of cases, respectively (Table 1; Fig. 2).

Therapeutic Strategies

Stage-I Rectal Cancer (T_{1-3a} N_0 M_0 or Duke's A–B_1)

In general, for stage-I disease the surgical approach is considered to be sufficiently effective. There are alternative techniques available, however, such as low anterior resection, abdominoperineal resection, or, for selected patients, less toxic procedures such as transanal resections.

Table 1. Dependency of local recurrences and 5-year survival on tumor stage

AJCC Stage		mod. Astler Coller	Local recurrences (%)	5-Year survival (%)
(1987)		(1978)	(Cummings 1992)	(O'Connell 1994)
I	$T_{1-2}N_0M_0$	A–B_1	1–25%	85–95%
II	$T_{3-4}N_0M_0$	B_2–B_3	5–45%	60–80%
III	$T_xN_{1-3}M_0$	C*	15–50%	30–60%
IV	$T_xN_xM_1$	D	ns	<5%

AJCC, American Joint Comission on Cancer; *mod.*, modified; *C**, Astler Coller stage C1: cancer has not extended beyond muscularis propria, Astler Coller stage C2: cancer has extended completely through muscularis propria

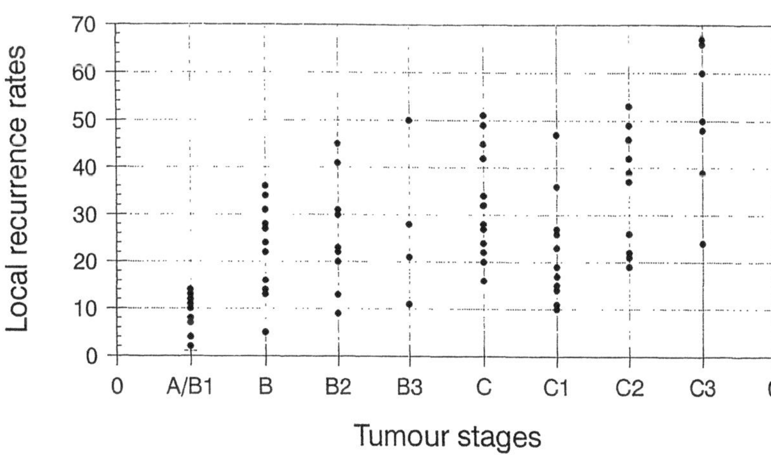

Fig. 2. Local recurrences in rectal carcinoma after radical surgery. Dependence on stage at surgery. (Cionini and Papi 1990)

If the tumor is located in the upper third of the rectum an anterior resection is indicated. Tumors of the middle or lower third of the rectum should be resected only by a low anterior resection if the distance to the anastomosis is sufficiently large; about 2 cm in exophytic well-differentiated tumors but at least 3 cm in ulcerative, undifferentiated carcinomas. Otherwise, an abdominoperineal resection should be carried out.

For small, inferiorly situated rectal neoplasms without involvement of lymph nodes, which accounts for about 5–10% of all rectal carcinomas, the abdominoperineal resection causes considerable but unnecessary morbidity. A recent study suggests that in these patients high-dose preoperative radiotherapy may allow resection of the primary tumor with a high rate of sphincter preservation (Mohiuddin and Marks 1991). According to further phase-II studies, this holds true for T1G1 tumors without venous invasion (Bailey et al. 1992; Willet et al. 1994). Other authors also suggest applying the sphincter-saving procedure to T2G1 and T1G2 tumors if they are smaller than 9 cm^2 (Slisow et al. 1991). In the case of T3G1, T2G2, and T1G3 tumors, the local excision should be combined with radiotherapy plus/minus 5-fluorouracil (5-FU) (Minsky et al. 1989). Unfortunately, there are no prospective randomized studies which compare local resection plus adjuvant therapy with wide resection.

For well-differentiated tumors less than 3 cm in size and without deep ulceration, tumor fixation, or palpable lymph nodes, endocavitary radiation can be curative. For this purpose special equipment and expertise are needed (Sischy et al. 1984; Kodner et al. 1993).

In any case, histological confirmation of total tumor removal by the margin status, frequent examinations, and the progress of the tumor markers CEA and CA 19-9 must be carried out. If there is any doubt about local recurrence then abdominoperineal resection should be performed (Schlag and Slisow 1995).

Stage-II Rectal Cancer (T_{3b} N_0 M_0–T_x $N_{1\text{-}3}$ M_0; Dukes B_2–C)

Curative resection has priority in the therapy of stage-II and -III rectal neoplasms. In recent years, the rate of curative resections has increased up to 80% (Krook et al. 1991; Gall and Hermanek 1992). However, after curative resection 5–45% of Duke's B and 15–50% of Duke's C patients will suffer local recurrences (Cummings 1992) and 30% distant metastases (Hermanek 1992). The 5-year survival is up to 62% in stage II and 48% in stage III. This is the reason for a number of attempts to improve the prognosis of stage-II and -III rectal neoplasms (Sack et al. 1990).

Postoperative Radiotherapy

The advantage of the postoperative approach to adjuvant therapy of rectal cancer is that it allows consideration of pathologic factors in the selection of patients for this treatment. In trials of preoperative radiation therapy, 22–37% of the patients randomized to surgery alone had tumors limited to the bowel wall and therefore were at low risk for recurrence. An additional 8–14% were found at surgery to have distant metastases (Rider et al. 1977; MRC 1984; Cedermark et al. 1985). Overall, an estimated 30–50% of all patients were unlikely to benefit from the preoperative treatment.

The potential disadvantages of postoperative radiation therapy are the risks associated with the irradiation of increased amounts of small bowel usually located in the pelvis after removal of the rectum. Additionally, the theoretical possibility of relative hypoxia, and, therefore, of relative radioresistance of residual cancer cells due to vascular disruption during surgery exists, and the fact that any tumor cells that spread outside the pelvis during surgery will be beyond the limits of radiation fields. Most phase-II studies (Table 2) showed a reduction of local recurrences in stage-II and -III rectal cancer by about 20% if postoperative radiation therapy was used after resection (Withers et al. 1981; Vigliotti et al. 1987; Feigen et al. 1988; Schild et al. 1989b). The best results for postoperative radiotherapy were reported by Tepper et al. (1987). When compared with a historical control group, local recurrence rates following postoperative radiotherapy with up to 45 Gy were reduced to 50%, with the exception of nodal positive T_4 tumors.

In contrast to the retrospective trials, only one of three prospective randomized studies employing postoperative radiation therapy (Table 3) showed a small significant reduction in local recurrences of nodal positive, mobile, rectal cancers ($p = 0.06$) (Fisher et al. 1988). No survival advantages were detected.

Preoperative Radiotherapy

Theoretical advantages of preoperative irradiation are the potential to damage malignant cells that may spread locally or distantly at surgery and the reduction in size of the primary tumor (down-staging) and involved regional lymph nodes, thus facilitating resection. Moreover, preoperative irradiation decreases the likelihood of late radiation enteritis due to the lesser volumes of small bowel generally present in the pelvis when the rectum and sigmoid colon have not yet been removed.

The difficulties in selecting only those patients for preoperative radiation who are at high risk of pelvic recurrence should be reduced by improved diagnostic facilities. Disadvantages could arise from the delay of definite surgical resection and from difficulty in determining pathologic factors following radiotherapy.

Randomized studies (Table 4) using single-shot preoperative radiotherapy of 5 Gy or, conventionally fractionated, low-dose (15–24 Gy) preoperative radiotherapy showed neither a decrease in local recurrence rate nor an increase in survival (Rider et al. 1977; Stearns 1980; MRC 1984). Only Roswit et al. (1975) observed advantages to overall survival by this approach. This was shown later to be due to a random error. More nodal positive patients were

Table 2. Postoperative radiotherapy – nonrandomized trials

	No. of patients	Doses (TD/Fx/Days)	Volume	5-YS (%)		Local recurrences (%)		Disease-free survival (%)		Comments
				(SRT)	(S)	(SRT)	(S)	(SRT)	(S)	
Withers et al. (1981) stage: B2C2	73	45 Gy/25/35 plus 6/3/3	Pelvis small volume boost	No difference		9%	25%	ns	ns	Historical control, actuarial analysis
Vigliotti et al. (1987) stage	105	40–50 Gy/n.s/ns ± 6–10 Gy Boost	ap/pa (92%)	55	ns	14	ns	40	ns	Historical control
B1				100	ns	ns	ns	ns	ns	
B2				62	ns	4	13	ns	ns	
B3	37			50	ns	31	26	ns	ns	
C1				65	ns	ns	ns	ns	ns	
C2				50	ns	18	30	ns	ns	
C3	62			60	ns	20	49	ns	ns	
Tepper et al. (1987) stage:	165	45 Gy/25/35 + >=5.4 Gy/3/3	4 fields to the middle of L5	53	ns	ns	ns	50	ns	Historical control
B1	3			100		0	8	100	n.s	
B2	53			71	ns	9	23	76	47	
B3	7			67	ns	0	53	69	27	
C1	10			90	ns	20	50	69	25	
C2	77			39	ns	21	47	34	27	
C3	15			17	ns	53	67	13	0	
Feigen et al. (1988) stage: B2C1C2	97	24/12/16	posterior pelvis	41	ns	49	ns	ns	ns	Actuarial analysis
Schild et al. (1989b) stage:	139	3.8–64.6//		ns	ns	ns	ns	ns	ns	Chemotherapy was added to radiation therapy in 44 patients
B2B3	36			79	ns	19	ns	ns	ns	
C1	20			89	ns	10	ns	ns	ns	
C2/C3	83			42	ns	25	ns	ns	ns	

5-YS, 5-Year survival; *TD*, total dose; *Fx*, fractions; *SRT*, surgery plus postoperative radiotherapy; *S*, surgery alone; *ap/pa*, anterior-posterior; *ns*, not stated

Table 3. Postoperative radiotherapy – randomized trials

Trials	No. of patients	Doses (TD/Fx/Days)	Volume	Interval to surgery (d)	5-YS (%)		Local recurrences (%)		Comments
					(SRT)	(S)	(SRT)	(S)	
GITSG (1985) stage: B2, C1, C2	108	40–48 Gy/ 20–27/31–38	Pelvis (ap/pa)	60–82	46	36	20	24	No significant advantage in terms of survival, treatment faults in 58% of the SRT-arm
Balslev et al. (1986)	494	50 Gy/25/35, 2 weeks rest after 30 Gy	Pelvis				8	9	– Median time to local recurrence: stage B, 12 months; stage C: 6 vs 18 months ($p = 0.01$)
stage B:	276		(3-field)	<30	ns	ns	6	6	– Short follow-up
stage C:	218						10	13	– 43% of all patients were not randomized – Few local recurrences after surgery alone for N+
Fisher et al. (1988) [NSABP R01] stage: B, C	368	47 Gy/26/36	Pelvis (ap/pa)	<75	41	43	16	25	– 5 years' follow-up – $p < 0.06$ for local recurrences

5-YS, 5-Year survival; *TD*, total dose; *Fr*, fractions; *d*, days; *SRT*, surgery plus postoperative radiotherapy; *S*, surgery alone; *ap/pa*, anterior – posterior opposed fields; *ns*, not stated

Table 4. Preoperative radiotherapy of resectable rectal cancer – randomized trials

Trials	No. of patients	Dose (TD/Fx/Days)	Volume	Interval to surgery (d)	5-YS (%) (SRT)	5-YS (%) (S)	Local recurrences (%) (SRT)	Local recurrences (%) (S)	Metastases (%) (SRT)	Metastases (%) (S)	Comments
Rider et al. (1977)	125	5 Gy/1/1	Pelvis, 15 × 13 cm	same day	36	38	ns	ns	ns	ns	
Stearns (1980)	790	20 Gy/8/10	Pelvis, 16 × 18 cm	2–42	57	58	11	17	ns	ns	
Roswit et al. (1975) [VASOG I]	700 (all)	20 Gy/10/14 plus 5 Gy/10/14 perineal	Pelvis, 20 × 20 cm	14 (average)	35	29	ns	ns	ns	ns	All patients
stage: A–C	453 (R_0)				49	39	ns	ns	ns	ns	After curative resection: $p = 0.04$
II. Report of an MRC Working Party (1984)	850	5 Gy/1/1 or 20 Gy/10/14	Pelvis, 15 × 18 cm	<7	42 40	38 ns	45 47	43 ns	48 49	50 ns	Actuarial dates of all patients after 5 years' follow-up
Higgins et al. (1986) [VASOG II] stage: LAD	361	31.5 Gy/18/24	Pelvis + para-aortic to L-2	<5	50[a] no difference		ns	ns	ns	ns	[a]After curative abdominoperineal resection
Dahl et al. (1990) [Norway]	300 (all) 259 (R_0)	31.5 Gy/18/24	Pelvis + para-aortic to L-2	14–21	58 61	57 64	17 14	26 23	26 18	26 17	Median follow-up: 54 months after curative resection
Gerard et al. (1985, 1988) [EORTC]	410 (all)	34.5 Gy/15/19	Pelvis + para-aortic to L-2	4–15	62	60	15*	35*	23	22	All patients: $p < 0.05$ for local recurrence, after curative resection: $p = 0.08$
stage: B/C	341 (R_0)				69	59 ($p < 0.08$)					
Stockholm Rectal Cancer Study Group (1990) stage: A–D	679	25.5 Gy/5/5–7	Pelvis + para-aortic to L-2	1–7	55	50	11* ($p < 0.001$)	25*	17	23	After curative resection median follow-up: 53 months, $p < 0.05$ for local recurrences
Reis Neto et al. (1989)	66	40 Gy/20/28	Pelvis	ns	71	29	15	47	15	33	After curative resection
stage: A–C											No statistics available
Kligerman et al. (1972)	31	46 Gy/23/31	Pelvis + para-aortic to L-2	28	41	25	8	0	ns	ns	All patients small number of patients

5-YS, 5-Year survival; *TD*, total dose; *Fx*, fractions; *SRT*, surgery plus preoperative radiotherapy; *S*, surgery alone; *ns*, not stated
* Fields with gray background demonstrate significance

treated by surgery alone. Accelerated radiotherapy (25.5 Gy) in the preoperative setting can reduce the rate of local recurrences without influencing the survival (Stockholm Rectal Cancer Study Group 1990). Similar results could be achieved by conventionally fractionated, moderate, preoperative doses (Higgins et al. 1986; Gerard et al. 1988; Dahl et al. 1990). Dahl et al. (1990) even showed down-staging of lymph node involvement. The data of Gerard et al. (1988) suggested an improvement in overall survival which could not be confirmed statistically. Reis Neto et al. (1989) did not use any statistical methods to test their results.

Except for the Stockholm study (Stockholm Rectal Cancer Study Group 1990), none of the randomized trials revealed an increased postoperative morbidity or mortality. The Stockholm study demonstrated that the postoperative mortality was increased up to 7% as compared with 2% from surgery alone, which is attributed to single fractions as high as 5.1 Gy and limited to patients older than 75 years.

In summary, preoperative radiotherapy causes down-staging of the tumor, reduction of local recurrences, and prolongation of the disease-free interval without increased morbidity or mortality compared with surgery alone. Unfortunately, there is a lack of studies investigating high-dose preoperative radiotherapy (45–50 Gy), which can be expected to have even better results. Phase-II studies (Table 5) employing such a dose schedule suggest a benefit for survival in addition to the advantages mentioned previously. Preoperative irradiation with 45–50 Gy should be recommended as treatment of choice for inferiorly situated and adherent lesions in an attempt to avoid permanent colostomy.

Pre- Versus Postoperative Radiotherapy

To date there has been only one prospective randomized trial comparing preoperative with postoperative radiotherapy (Frykholm et al. 1993) (Table 6). A total of 236 patients were allocated to receive high single-dose preoperative irradiation (total dosage 25.5 Gy during 5–7 days) and 235 patients were assigned to receive postoperative irradiation to a dosage level of 60 Gy in 8 weeks with conventional fractionation. In the postoperative treatment arm radiotherapy was given only to a high-risk group of patients (Astler-Coller stages B2, C1, and C2), whereas in the preoperative treatment arm all patients received radiotherapy. After a minimum follow-up of 5 years, the local recurrence rate was significantly lower after preoperative than after postoperative radiotherapy (13% versus 22%; $p = 0.02$). No difference in overall survival was noted.

The perioperative mortality was similar in both arms (preoperative, 3%; postoperative 5%). The rate of perineal wound infections was higher after preoperative radiotherapy (33% vs. 18%), however, no other significant differences were noted in the occurrence of acute side effects.

Table 5. Preoperative radiotherapy – nonrandomized trials

	No. of patients	Dose (TD/Fx/Days)	Volume	Interval to S (d)	5 YS (%)		Local recurrences (%)		Metastases (%)		Comments
					(SRT)	(S)	(SRT)	(S)	(SRT)	(S)	
Pujol et al (1978)	116	40 Gy/18/24	Pelvis 13 × 13 cm	2–5	59	44	10	11	ns	ns	Historical control, one center
Stevens et al. (1976)	57	50–60 Gy/24–30/40–56	Tumor 10 × 10 cm ap/pa	28–49	53[a]	38[a]	15	ns	16	ns	Historical control, one center
Mendenhall et al. (1985)	71	35–45 Gy//35	ns	ns	71	41	8	29	ns	ns	Historical control, one center
Reed et al. (1988)	40	40–45 Gy//	ns	ns	68 ($p < 0.05$)	52	9	31	12	27	– Historical control, one center – Disease-free survival: 84% vs 53% ($p < 0.005$)
Tobin et al. (1991) fixed tumors	134	45 Gy/25/35 +/– 4.8 to 9.6 Gy Boost	4 fields from L-5/S-1 to Tuber ischiadicus	28–42 days	92 (A/B1) 63 (B2/C)	ns	6 (A/B1) 21 (B2/C)	ns	3 (A/B1) 29 (B2/C)	ns	

5-YS, 5-Year survival; *TD*, total dose; *Fx*, fractions; *SRT*, surgery plus preoperative radiotherapy; *S*, surgery alone; *ns*, not stated; *ap/pa*, anterior-posterior.
[a] After curative surgery.

Table 6. Preoperative versus postoperative radiotherapy – randomized trial

	No. of patients	Dose (TD/Fx/Days)	Volume	Interval to S (d)	5-YS (%)	Local recurrences (%)
Trykeholm et al. (1993) [Uppsala, multicenter study]	471 (all)					
preop: all patients		25.5 Gy/5/5–7	Posterior pelvis	<7	No difference	13
postop: B2, C1, C2		40 Gy/20/28 + 10–14 days rest + 20 Gy/ 10/14 boost	Anus to L-4 (3-field)	<= 42 ($n = 62$) 43–56 ($n = 26$) 56–95 ($n = 27$)	($p = 0.05$)	22 ($p = 0.02$)

5-YS, 5-Year survival; *TD*, total dose; *Fx*, fractions; *d*, days; *postop*, postoperative; *preop*, preoperative

Table 7. Postoperative chemotherapy – randomized trials

		No. of patients	Dose (TD/Fx/Days)	5-YS (%)	Local recurrences (%)	Metastases (%)	Comments
GITSG 7175 (1985) T3, 4; N+	Surgery	58		36	21	31	– Follow-up 80 months
	5FU/ MeCCNU	48		46	18	19	– No improvement by the addition of chemotherapy
NSABP R01 Fisher et al. (1988)	Surgery	173		43	25	ns	Increase of disease-free survival with postoperative chemotherapy (p = 0.006)
	MOF	177		53 ($p = 0.05$)	21 (not significant)	No difference	
	Radiotherapy	178	47 Gy/26/36	41	16 ($p = 0.06$)	⇑	
Hafström (1990)	Surgery	56		34	ns	ns	
	MOF	43		49	ns	ns	

5-YS, 5-Year survival; *TD*, total dose; *Fx*, fractions; *S*, surgery alone; *d*, days; *MOF*, MeCCNU/vincristine/ 5-FU; ⇑, increased

The cumulative risk of developing a bowel obstruction was significantly increased after postoperative radiotherapy. Among the patients alive after preoperative radiotherapy, significant morbidity of the bowel was noted in 11%, of the urinary bladder in 2%, and of the skin in 6%. In the postoperatively treated group the corresponding figures were 15%, 6%, and 15%, respectively. In conclusion, preoperative, short-term, high-dose radiotherapy decreases the local recurrence rate relative to postoperative radiotherapy, without evidence of increased late morbidity after a follow-up of 5–10 years.

Postoperative Chemotherapy

Three randomized studies have been completed which evaluate, also the use of postoperative chemotherapy (GITSG 1985; Fisher et al. 1988; Hafström et al. 1990) (Table 7). All studies showed an increase in overall survival of 10–15% when compared with surgery alone. A significant survival advantage was, however, observed only for men younger than 65 years (Fisher et al. 1988). The risk of local recurrence was not reduced by postoperative chemotherapy.

Previously, the combination of 5-FU with semustine (MeCCNU) was used in an adjuvant setting. However, a study of the GITSG (1992) comparing MeCCNU/5-FU with 5-FU alone showed increased toxicity from the combination therapy without an increase in efficacy. Furthermore, MeCCNU has a mutagenic potential. Therefore, its use should be discontinued (Hermann 1994). There are still questions unanswered concerning the scheduling and duration of 5-FU treatment and its modulation by folinic acid and/or levamisole.

Radio/Chemotherapy

Postoperative radio/chemotherapy combines advantages of both single modalities. Likewise, the rate of local recurrence can be diminished substantially by up to 50% and the 5-year-survival increased by 10% (GITSG 1985, 1992; Krook et al. 1991; O'Connell et al. 1993; Rockette et al. 1994) (Table 8).

It has to be considered that some of these trials did not meet the demands of modern surgery and the surgical procedure was not documented sufficiently. So the rate of local recurrence after surgery alone is sometimes relatively high. In addition, no stratification for TNM criteria was carried out. An analysis of patients treated with postoperative chemotherapy and radiation therapy suggests that more patients may develop chronic bowel dysfunction in comparison to those who undergo surgical resection alone (Kollmorgen et al. 1994).

Nevertheless, according to the NIH (1990), postoperative radio/chemotherapy ranks as standard therapy in stage-II and -III rectal cancer (Fig. 3). Today, for superiorly situated and nonadherent lesions postoperative irradiation plus chemotherapy can be recommended as treatment of choice.

The only study which tested combined radio/chemotherapy in the preoperative setting was carried out by the EORTC (Boulis-Wassif et al. 1984) (Table 9). Because of increased postoperative mortality the overall survival was shortened by the preoperative radio/chemotherapy. Additionally, there was neither a reduction in local recurrences nor one in distant metastases with the adjuvant therapy. After preoperative radio/chemotherapy only the rates of liver metastases and of cancer specific deaths were lower in comparison to surgery alone. However, this advantage was not significant.

These effects are caused partially by a low total dose (34.5 Gy), high single fractions (2.3 Gy), and inappropriately large fields (anterior-posterior opposed (ap/pa) pelvis + para-aortic lymph nodes). If optimized dose schedules and techniques are used, an increase in efficacy and a reduction of side effects should be possible. At present, this approach is being applied in ongoing trials of the NSABP and the EORTC.

Table 8. Postoperative radiotherapy plus/minus chemotherapy – randomized trials

Trials		No. of patients	Dose (TD/Fx/Days)	5-YS (%)	Local recurrences (%)	Metastases (%)	Comments
GITSG 7175 (1985) T3, 4; N+	Surgery	58		36	21	31	– Follow-up 80 months – Disease-free survival significantly prolonged after combined therapy versus surgery alone
	Radiotherapy	50	40–48 Gy/20–28/31–38	46	19	28	
	5-FU/MeCCNU	48	5-FU/MeCCNU	46	18	19	
	RT + 5-FU/MeCCNU	46	40–44 Gy/20–28/31–38 + 5-FU/MeCCNU	56 ($p < 0.05$ vs surgery alone)	7 (not significant vs surgery alone)	22	
NCCTC/Mayo 794751; Krook et al. (1991) T3–4; N+	Radiotherapy	100	45/25/35 ± 5.4/3/3 Boost	38	25	46	Follow-up: >7 years
	Radiotherapy + 5-FU/MeCCNU	104		49 ($p = 0.025$)	13.5 ($p = 0.036$)	28.8 ($p = 0.011$)	
GITSG 7180 (1992)	Radio/chemotherapy + 5-FU	104	41.4 Gy/23/31	68	17	26	Disease-free survival increased in the treatment arm with 5-FU ($p = 0.2$)
	Radio/chemotherapy + 5-FU/MeCCNU	95		54 ($p = 0.58$) 3-year survival	17	40 ($p = 0.05$)	
NCCTG 864751 (intergroup) O'Connell (1994)	Radio/chemotherapy (5-FU bolus) plus 5-FU or 5-FU/MeCCNU	332	45 Gy/25/35 + 5.4/3/3 Boost ± 3.6/2/2 smaall Boost	60	No significant difference ($p = 0.11$)	40	– Median follow-up: 46 months – Increased time to relapse after continuous infusion of 5-FU ($p = 0.01$)
	Radio/chemotherapy (5-FU continosly) plus 5-FU or 5-FU/MeCCNU	328		70 ($p = 0.005$)		31 ($p = 0.03$)	
NSABP R02 Rockette (1994)	Radiotherapy + MOF or 5-FU/LV	741 (all)	ns	81	7	ns	Follow-up: 42.9 months
	MOF or 5-FU/LV			81	11 ($p < 0.05$)		

5-YS, 5-Year survival; *TD*, total dose; *Fx*, fractions; *MOF*, MeCCNU, vincristine, 5-FU; *5-FU/LV*, 5-FU, leucovorin; *ns*, not stated

Table 9. Preoperative radiotherapy plus chemotherapy – randomized trials

	No. of patients	Dose (TD/Fx/Days)	Volume	5-YS (%)	Local recurrences (%)	Metastases (%)	Comments
Boulis-Wassif et al.	121	34.5 Gy/15/18	Pelvis (ap/pa)	59	15	No difference	– More side effects
(1984) [EORTC] stage T2–4; Nx; M0	126	34.5 Gy/15/18 + 5-FU 10 mg/kg i.v. bolus injection day 1–4	plus para-aortic lymph nodes	46 ($p = 0.06$)	15		and postop. mortality – Fewer liver metastases and cancer-specific deaths ($p = 0.07$)

5-YS, 5-Year survival; *TD*, total dose; *Fx*, fractions; *RT*, radiotherapy; *Cht*, chemotherapy; *ap/pa*, anterior – posterior opposed fields

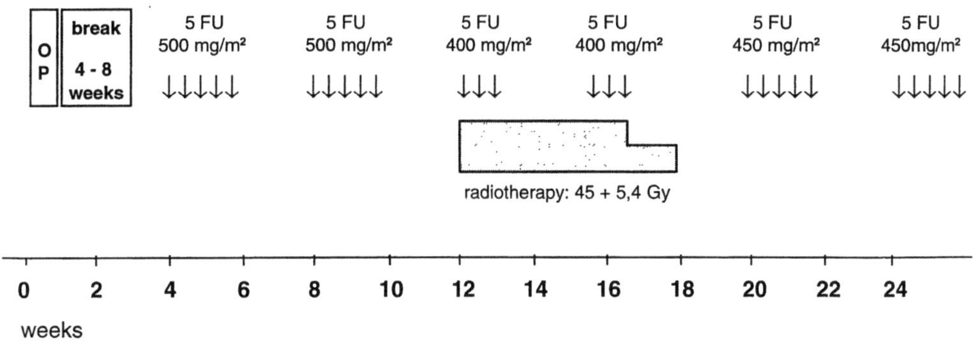

Fig. 3. Adjuvant therapy of rectal cancer stage II + III (pT3/4 or pN+), NIH recommendation, 1990

Locally Advanced Rectal Neoplasms

Since the surgeon's assessment plays the major role in deciding resectability, this group is not defined precisely. The clinical staging system by Mohiuddin et al. (1993), which differentiates between mobile, adherent or fixed tumors and frozen pelvis may help in the accurate assessment of rectal neoplasms.

External-beam radiation therapy alone or in combination with chemotherapy/hyperthermia provides effective palliation and prolongation of life but has only a minimal curative impact in patients with locally advanced unresectable rectal cancer (Martenson and Gunderson 1992). At the Mayo Clinic, 65 patients with advanced colorectal cancer were treated in a randomized trial using radiation therapy (35–40 Gy) with or without 5-FU (Moertel et al. 1969). Progression-free survival, duration of palliation, and overall survival were better in the arm with combined modality.

In the case of macroscopic residuals, postoperative radiotherapy results in an overall survival rate of 24% and local control of 24–85%. In the case of microscopic remnants, local control can be achieved in 30% (Schild et al. 1989a)–84% (Ghossein et al. 1981) with postoperative radiotherapy. This wide range of results may relate to the manner in which local failure was defined and the short duration of follow-up in some series (Martenson 1992).

After preoperative radiotherapy, 50–75% of locally advanced rectal neoplasms can be resected. The overall rate of local control is between 36% and 45% in resected patients. The overall survival is between 25% and 35% (Emami et al. 1982; Dosoretz et al. 1983; Påhlman et al. 1985).

The addition of chemotherapy increases the possibility of subsequent tumor resection by up to 90% without increasing the perioperative morbidity or mortality. The rate of complete remission after preoperative radio/chemotherapy is 20%. After 36 months' follow-up the local control rate and the overall survival were better than after preoperative radiotherapy alone (Minsky et al. 1991, 1993). Shumate (1993) noted an increased number of sphincter-saving procedures after preoperative radio/chemotherapy.

Hyperthermia, another modality used to intensify the treatment of advanced rectal neoplasms is discussed elsewhere in this book.

Intraoperative radiotherapy (IORT) has also been used to improve results in the treatment of unresectable rectal neoplasms (Tepper et al. 1986; Gundersson 1983, 1988; Willet et al. 1991). After combined external (45–55 Gy) and intraoperative (10–20 Gy) radiotherapy the overall survival is about 53–60% and the local control rate is increased to 88%.

Radiation Techniques

Doses of 45 Gy in 4.5 weeks or 50 Gy in 6 weeks are well tolerated and there are no severe complications. In patients with rectal cancer, internal iliac and presacral nodes are at risk for metastatic involvement. Since these lymph nodes are not a standard part of the dissection for rectal cancer they should be treated, as well as the primary tumor, with 45–50 Gy. After perineal resection the entire perineum should be included within the radiation therapy, since most data suggest that perineal failure after perineal resection can be decreased from approximately 20% to 2% by adjuvant radiotherapy. External iliac lymph nodes should be included in the initial radiation therapy only if pelvic organs with external iliac drainage (prostate, upper vagina, bladder, uterus) are involved by direct extension.

In general, computerized tomograpy (CT) is used to estimate the treatment volume as well as the organs at risk (Fig. 4), and CT-guided treatment planning (three dimensional) is performed. As standard, a three- or four-field wedge technique should be used to spare as much small bowel as possible. Bladder distention, prone position, and belly board are useful techniques to displace the small bowel out of the pelvis. The width of ap/pa fields should cover the pelvic inlet with a 1.0–1.5 cm margin. The superior margin of the field is usually the inferior margin of L-5. In patients who have had an anterior resection, the usual inferior margin is 5.0 cm below the former margin of the tumor. After perineal resection the inferior margin is 1.0 cm below the perineal scar.

The rectum and perirectal tissue lie just anterior to the sacrum and coccyx. Therefore, the posterior field margin should be at least 1.5–2.0 cm behind the anterior bony sacral margin. In locally advanced tumors the entire sacral canal should be included to avoid local recurrence from tumor spreading along nerve roots. The anterior margin can be shaped to reduce the dose for the

Fig. 4a–f. Treatment settings of a patient with locally advanced rectal cancer after abdominoperineal resection. **a** ap/pa Field of the standard three- or four-field wedge technique; **b** lateral field of the standard three- or four-field wedge technique; **c** dose distribution; **d** three-dimensional CT-guided treatment planning; **e** dose-volume histogram concerning bladder and target volume; **f** beam's-eye view after three-dimensional treatment planning (plotted at distance = 68 cm)

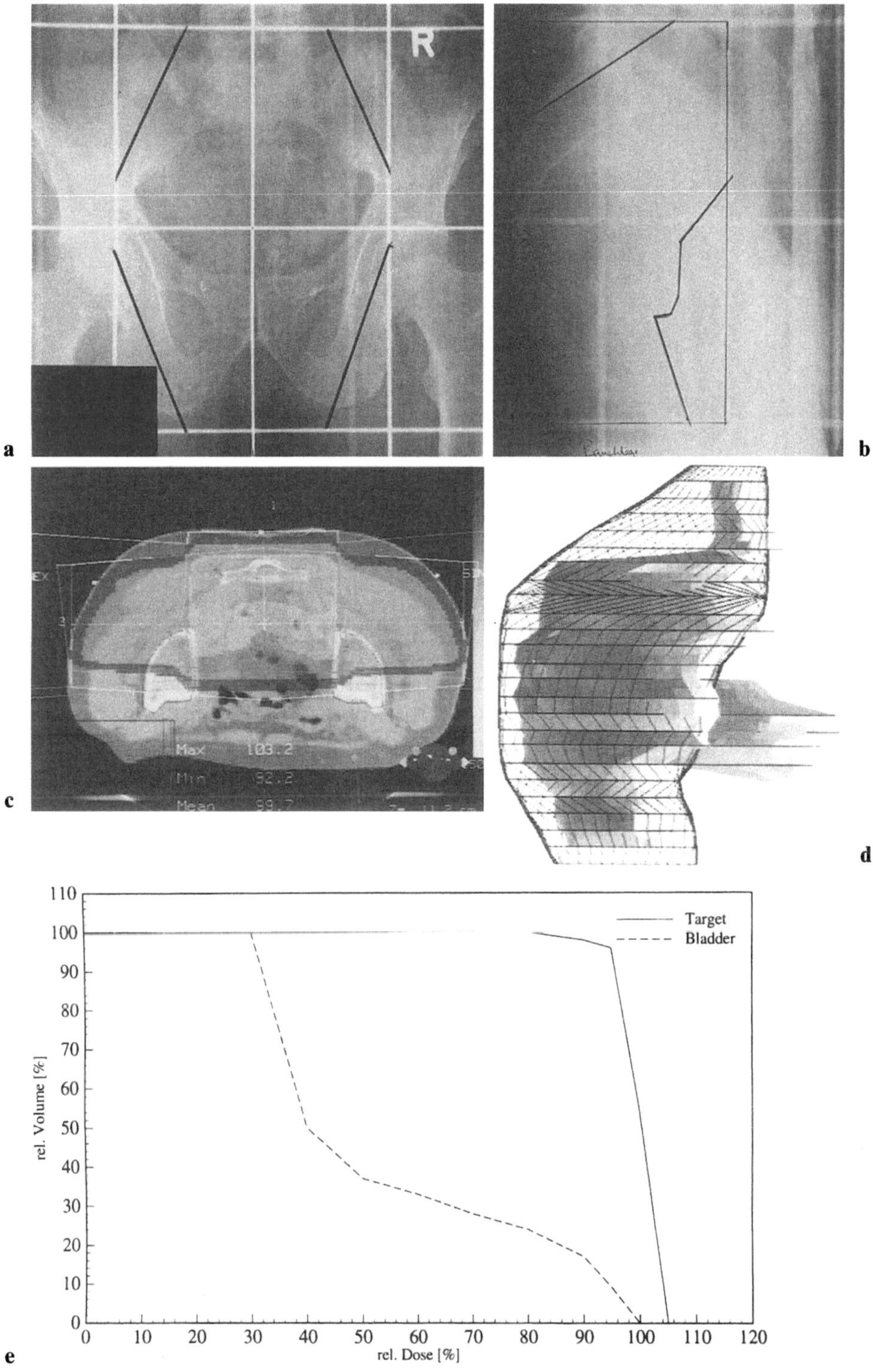
a
R
b
c
Max 103.2
Min 92.2
Mean 99.7
d
e
Target
Bladder
rel. Volume [%]
rel. Dose [%]
0
10
20
30
40
50
60
70
80
90
100
110
120

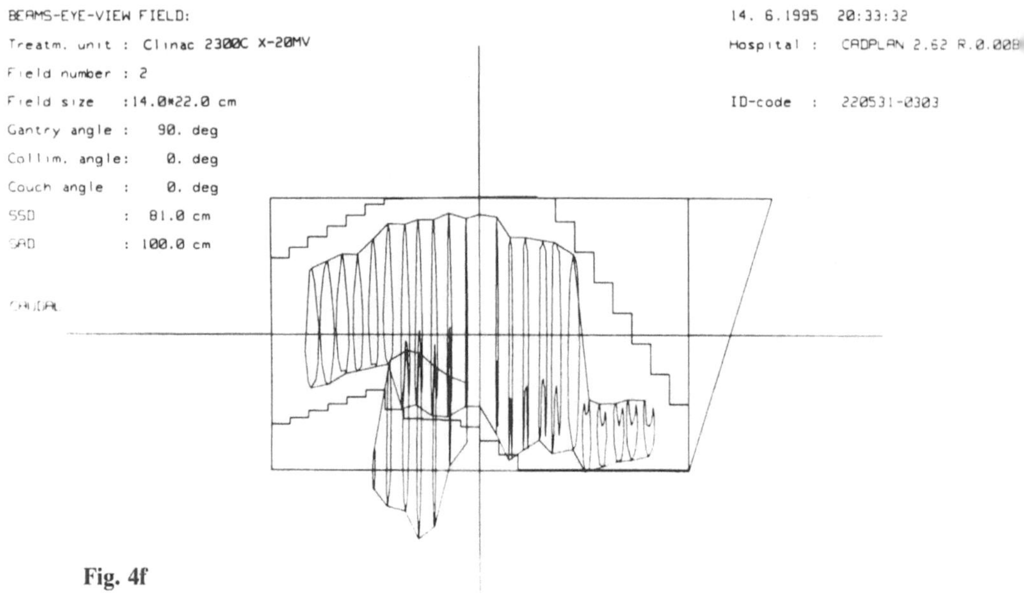

Fig. 4f

femoral heads and the bladder inferiorly and for the small bowel superiorly (Gundersson 1985).

Until now there is no proven advantage to include the para-aortic lymph nodes within the radiation therapy fields. Doing so results in a considerable increase in small bowel obstruction, requiring reoperation (Withers 1981).

Conclusion

In an adjuvant situation, radiotherapy diminishes the rate of local recurrences and increases the disease-free interval, whereas the prognosis is not altered significantly. Radiotherapy in the postoperative setting should still be considered as treatment of choice for nonadherent superiorly situated rectal neoplasms, since function-preserving resections are available. In the preoperative setting, until now, radiotherapy has been prospectively tested only in the low- and medium-dose range. This results in a down-staging and thereby allows less aggressive surgery without colostomy. Preoperative radiotherapy can be advocated for inferiorly situated and adherent lesions. The toxicity of preoperative irradiation is less pronounced than that of the postoperative approach. The value of higher preoperative radiation doses should be determined in prospectively randomized trials, as should the schedule and duration of the accompanying 5-FU therapy and its modulation by folinic Acid and/or levamisole.

In unresectable rectal carcinoma preoperative radiotherapy is effective, but it should be combined with IORT, chemotherapy, or hyperthermia. Further studies in locally advanced situations are also needed.

References

Abulafi AM, Williams NS (1994) Local recurrence of colorectal cancer: the problem, mechanisms, management and adjuvant therapy. Br J Surg 81:7–19

Bailey HR, Huval WV, Max E et al (1992) Local excision of carcinoma of the rectum for cure. Surgery 111:555–561

Balslev I, Pederson M, Teglbjaerg PS, Hanberg-Soerensen F, Bone J, Jacobsen NO, Overgaard J, Sell A, Bertelsen K, Hage E, Hansen L, Kronborg O, Hoestrup H, Noergaard-Pedersen B (1986) Postoperative radiotherapy in Duke's B and C carcinoma of the rectum and rectosigmoid. Cancer 58:22–28

Boring CC, Squires TS, Tong T (1992) Cancer statistics [published erratum appears in CA Cancer J Clin Mar–Apr 42:127–128]. CA Cancer J Clin 42:19–38

Boulis-Wassif S, Gerard A, Loygue J, Camelot D, Buyse M, Duez N (1984) Final results of a randomized trial on the treatment of rectal cancer with preoperative radiotherapy alone or in combination with 5-fluorouracil, followed by radical surgery. Cancer 53:1811–1818

Brizel HE, Tepperman BS (1984) Postoperative adjuvant irradiation for adenocarcinoma of the rectum and sigmoid. Am J Clin Oncol 7:679

Cedermark B, Theire NO, Rieger A (1985) Preoperative short-term radiotherapy in rectal carcinoma. A preliminary report of a prospective randomized study. Cancer 55:1182–1185

Cionini L, Papi MG (1990) Update on and perspectives of radiotherapy in the treatment of colonic carcinoma. Ann Ital Chir 61(5):499–507

Cummings BJ (1992) Adjuvant radiation therapy for colorectal cancer. Cancer [Suppl] 70:1372–1383

Dahl O, Horn A, Morild I et al (1990) Low-dose preoperative radiation postpones recurrences in operable rectal cancer: results of a randomized multicenter trial in western Norway. Cancer 66:2286–2294

Dosoretz DE, Gunderson LL, Hedberg S et al (1983) Preoperative irradiation for unresectable rectal and rectosigmoid carcinomas. Cancer 52:814

Emami B, Pilepich M, Willet C et al (1982) Effects of preoperative irradiation on resectability of colorectal carcinomas. Int J Radiat Oncol Biol Phys 8:1295

Feigen M, Cummings B, Hawkins N, Keane T, O'Sullivan B, Wong S (1988) Low dose postoperative adjuvant radiation therapy for rectal cancer is ineffective. Radiother Oncol 13:181–186

Fisher B, Wolmark N, Rockette H et al (1988) Postoperative adjuvant chemotherapy or radiation therapy for rectal cancer: Results from NSABP Protocal R-01. J Natl Cancer Inst 80:21–29

Frykholm GJ, Glimelius B, Påhlman L (1993) Preoperative or postoperative irradiation in adenocarcinoma of the rectum: final treatment results of a randomized trial and an evaluation of late secondary effects. Dis Colon Rectum 36:564–572

Gall FP, Hermanek P (1992) Wandel und derzeitiger Stand der chirurgischen Behandlung des colorectalen Karzinoms. Chirurg 63:227–231

Gastrointestinal Tumor Study Group (1985) Prolongation of the disease-free interval in surgically treated rectal carcinoma. N Engl J Med 312:1465–1472

Gastrointestinal Tumor Study Group (1992) Radiation therapy and fluorouracil with or without semustine for the treatment of patients with surgical adjuvant adenocarcinoma of the rectum. J Clin Oncol 10:549–557

Gerard A, Loygue J et al (1984) Final results of a randomized trial on the treatment of rectal cancer with preoperative radiotherapy alone or in combination with 5-fluorouracil, followed by radical surgery. Trial by the EORTC Gastrointestinal Tract Cancer Cooperative Group. Cancer 53:1811–1818

Gerard A, Berrod L, Pene F, Loygne J, Laugier A, Bruckner R, Camelot G, Arnaud JP, Metzger U, Buyse M (1985) Interim analysis of a phase III study on preoperative radiation therapy in resectable rectal carcinoma. Trial of the Gastrointestinal Tract Cancer Cooperative Group of the European Organization for Research on Treatment of Cancer (EORTC). Cancer 55(10):2373–2379

Gerard A, Buyse M, Nordlinger B et al (1988) Preoperative radiotherapy as adjuvant treatment in rectal cancer. Final results of a randomized study of the EORTC. Ann Surg 208:606–614

Ghossein NA, Samala EC, Alpert S, Deluca FR, Ragins H, Turner SS, Stacey P, Flax H (1981) Elective postoperative radiotherapy after incomplete resection of colorectal cancer. Dis Colon Rectum 24:252–256

Gundersson LL, Cohen AC, Dosoretz DD, Shipley WU, Hedberg SE, Wood WC, Rodkey GV, Suit HD (1983) Residual, unresectable or recurrent colorectal cancer: external beam irradiation and intraoperative electron beam boost ± resection. Int J Radiat Oncol Biol Phys 9:1597–1606

Gundersson LL, Russell HJ, Llewellyn et al (1985) Treatment planning for colorectal cancer: radiation and surgical techniques and value of small-bowel films. Int J Radiat Oncol Biol Phys 11:1379

Gundersson LL, Martin JK, Beart RW, Nagorney DM, Fieck JM, Wieand HS, Martiny A, O'Connell MJ, Martenson JA, Mcllrath DC (1988) Intraoperative and external beam irradiation for locally advanced colorectal cancer. Ann Surg 207:52–60

Hafström L, Domellöf L, Rudenstam CM, Norryd C, Bergman L, Nilsson T, Hansson K, Wählby L, Asklöf G, Kugelberg C, and the Swedish Gastrointestinal Tumour Adjuvant Therapy Group (1990) Adjuvant chemotherapy with 5-fluororacil, vincristine and CCNU for patients with Duke's C colorectal cancer. Br J Surg 77:1345

Hermanek P (1992) Prognosefaktoren nach Resektion kolorektaler Karzinome. In: Schmoll HJ, Pichlmayr R (eds) Aktuelle Therapie gastrointestinaler Tumoren. Springer, Berlin Heidelberg New York, pp 206–213

Hermann R (1994) Systemic treatment of colorectal cancer. Eur J Cancer 30A:404–409

Higgins GA, Humphrey EW, Dwight RW et al (1986) Preoperative radiation and surgery for cancer of the rectum. Veterans Administration Surgical Oncology Group Trial II. Cancer 58:352–359

Hoskins RB, Gunderson LL, Dosoretz DE et al (1985) Adjuvant postoperative radiotherapy in carcinoma of the rectum and rectosigmoid. Cancer 55:61

Kligerman MM, Urdaneta N, Knowlton A, Vidone R, Hartman PR, Vera R (1972) Preoperative irradiation of rectosigmoid carcinoma including regional lymph nodes. AJR 114:498–503

Kodner IJ, Gilley MT, Shemesh EI et al (1993) Radiation therapy as definitive treatment for selected invasive rectal cancer. Surgery 114:850–857

Kollmorgen CF, Meagher AP, Wolff BG et al (1994) The long-term effect of adjuvant postoperative chemoradiotherapy for rectal carcinoma on bowel function. Ann Surg 220:676–682

Krook J, Moertel CG, Gunderson LL, Wieand HS, Collins RT, Beart RW, Kubista TP, Poon MA, Meyers WC, Mailliard JA, Twito DI, Morton RF, Veeder MH, Witzig TE, Cha S, Vidyarthi SC (1991) Effective surgical adjuvant therapy for high-risk rectal carcinoma. N Engl J Med 324:709–715

Martenson JA Jr, Gunderson LL (1992) Colon and rectum. In: Perez CA, Brady LW (eds) Principles and practice of radiation oncology, 2nd edn. Lippincott, Philadelphia, pp 1000–1014

Mendenhall WM, Million RR, Bland KL, Pfaff WW, Copeland EM (1985) Preoperative radiation therapy for clinically resectable adenocarcinoma of the rectum. Ann Surg 202(2):215–222

Minsky BD, Rich T, Recht A (1989) Selection criteria for local excision with or without adjuvant radiation therapy for rectal cancer. Cancer 63:1421
Minsky BD, Kemeny N, Cohen AM, Enker WE, Kelsen DP, Reichman B, Saltz L, Sigurdson ER, Frankel J (1991) Preoperative high dose leucovorin/5-fluorouracil and radiation therapy for unresectable rectal cancer. Cancer 67:2859–2866
Minsky BD, Cohen AM, Kemeny N, Enker WE, Kelsen DP, Schwartz G, Saltz L, Dougherty J, Frankel J, Wiseberg J (1993) Preoperative combined 5-FU low dose leucovorin and sequential radiation therapy for unresectable rectal cancer. Int J Radiat Oncol Biol Phys 25:821–827
Moertel CG, Childs DS Jr, Reitemeier RJ et al (1969) Combined 5-fluorouracil and supervoltage radiation therapy of locally unresectable gastrointestinal cancer. Lancet 2:865
Mohiuddin M, Marks G (1991) High dose preoperative irradiation for cancer of the rectum, 1976–1988. Int J Radiat Oncol Biol Phys 20:37–43
Mohiuddin M, Ahmad N, Marks G (1993) A selective approach to adjunctive therapy for cancer of the rectum. Int J Radiat Oncol Biol Phys 27:765–772
MRC; Second Report of an MRC Working Party (1984) The evaluation of low dose pre-operative x-ray therapy in the management of operable rectal cancer: results of randomly controlled trial. Br J Surg 71:21–25
NIH Consensus Conference (1990) Adjuvant therapy for patients with colon and rectal cancer. JAMA 264:1444–1450
O'Connell MJ (1994) Surgical adjuvant therapy of colorectal cancer. In: American Society of Clinical Oncology (eds) Educational book, pp 157–161
O'Connell MJ, Maillard J, Macdouald J, Haller D, Mayer R, Wieand H (1993) An intergroup trial of intensive course 5FU and low dose leucovorin as adjuvant therapy for high risk colon cancer. Proc ASCO 12:190
O'Connell MJ, Martenson JA, Wieand HS et al (1994) Improving adjuvant therapy for rectal cancer by combining protracted-infusion fluorouracil with radiation therapy after curative resection. N Engl J Med 331:502–507
Påhlman L, Glimelius B (1990) Pre- or postoperative radiotherapy in rectal or rectosigmoid carcinoma. Ann Surg 211:187–195
Påhlman L, Glimelius B, Ginman C et al (1985) Preoperative irradiation of primarily non-resectable adenocarcinoma of the rectum and rectosigmoid. Acta Radiol Oncol 24:35
Papillon J (1982) Rectal and anal cancers: conservative treatment by irradiation – an alternative to radical surgery. Springer, Berlin Heidelberg New York
Pujol H, Solassol C, Gary-Bobo J (1978) La radiotherapie preoperatoire des cancers du rectum, actualisation des resultats. A propos de 179 cas. Chirurgie 104:606–611
Quirke P, Durdey P, Dixon MF, Williams NS (1986) Local recurrence of rectal adenocarcinoma due to inadequate surgical resection. Histopathological study of lateral tumour spread and surgical excision. Lancet 2:996–999
Reed WP, Garls L, Park WC, Stark AJ (1988) Long-term results and complications of preoperative radiation in the treatment of rectal cancer. Surgery 103(2):161–167
Reis Neto JA, Quilici FA, Res JA Jr (1989) A comparison of nonoperative versus preoperative radiotherapy in rectal carcinoma: a 10-year randomized trial. Dis Colon Rectum 32:702
Rich T, Gunderson LL, Lew R, Galdabini JJ, Cohen AM, Donaldson G (1983) Patterns of recurrence after potentially curative surgery. Cancer 52:1317–1329
Rider WD, Palmer JA, Mahoney LJ, Robertson CT (1977) Preoperative radiation in operable cancer of the rectum: report of the Toronto trial. Can J Surg 20:335–338
Rockette H, Deutsch M, Petrelli N et al (1994) Effect of postoperative radiation therapy (RTX) when used with adjuvant chemotherapy in Duke's B and C rectal cancer. Results from NSABP R-02. Proc Am Soc Clin Oncol 13:193

Roswit B, Higgins GA, Keehn J (1975) Preoperative irradiation for carcinoma of the rectum and rectosigmoid colon: report of a National Veterans Administration randomized study. Cancer 35:1597–1602

Sack H, Bamberg M, Budach V (1990) Adjuvante Strahlentherapie beim Rektumkarzinom. Langenbecks Arch Chir [Suppl II] (Kongreßbericht 1990):169–173

Schild SE, Martenson JA jr, Gunderson LL, Dozois RR (1989a) Long-term survival and patterns of failure after postoperative radiation therapy for subtotally resected rectal adenocarcinoma. Int J Radiat Oncol Biol Phys 16:459–463

Schild SE, Martenson JA jr, Gunderson LL et al (1989b) Postoperative adjuvant therapy of rectal cancer: an analysis of disease control, survival, and prognostic factors. Int J Radiat Oncol Biol Phys 17(1):55–62

Schlag PM, Slisow W (1995) Operatives Konzept beim Rektumkarzinom. Onkologe 1:18–22

Second Report of an MRC Working Party (1984) The evaluation of low dose preoperative X-ray therapy in the management of operable rectal cancer: results of a randomly controlled trial. Br J Surg 71:21–25

Shumate CR, Rich TA, Skibber JM, Ajani JA, Ota DM (1993) Preoperative chemotherapy and radiation therapy for locally advanced primary and recurrent rectal carcinoma. A report of surgical morbidity. Cancer 71:3690–3696

Sischy B, Graney MJ, Hinson EJ (1984) Endocavitary irradiation for adenocarcinoma of the rectum. Ca-A Cancer J Clin 34:333–339

Slisow W, Seifert W, Marx G (1991) Stellenwert der lokalen Exstirpation von kleinflächigen tiefsitzenden Rektumkarzinomen mit kurativer Zielsetzung. Zentralbl Chir 116:1245

Stearns MW (1980) Pre- or postoperative radiation in resectable tumors. In: Welvaart K, Blumgart LH, Kreuning J (eds) Colorectal cancer. Leiden University Press, The Hague, pp 153–159

Stevens KR, Allen CV, Fletcher WS (1976) Preoperative radiotherapy for adenocarcinoma of the rectosigmoid. Cancer 37:2866–2874

Stockholm Rectal Cancer Study Group (1990) Preoperative short-term radiation therapy in operable rectal carcinoma. A prospective randomized trial. Cancer 66:49–55

Tepper JE, Cohen AM, Wood WC et al (1986) Intraoperative electron beam radiotherapy in the treatment of unresectable rectal cancer. Arch Surg 121:421

Tepper JE, Cohen AM, Wood WC, Orlow EL, Hedberg SE (1987) Postoperative radiation therapy of rectal cancer. Int J Radiat Oncol Biol Phys 13:5–10

Tobin RL, Mohiudon M, Marks G (1991) Preoperative irradiation for cancer of the rectum with extrarectal fixation. Int J Radiat Oncol Biol Phys 21:1127–1132

Vaughn DJ, Haller DG (1993) Adjuvant therapy for colorectal cancer. Adv Oncol 9(2):22–29

Vigliotti A, Rich TA, Romsdahl MM, Withers HR, Oswald MJ (1987) Postoperative adjuvant radiotherapy for adenocarcinoma of the rectum and rectosigmoid. Int J Radiat Oncol Biol Phys 13:999–1006

Willet CG, Shellito PC, Tepper JE, Eliseo R, Convery K, Wood WC (1991) Intraoperative electron beam radiation therapy for primary locally advanced rectal and rectosigmoid carcinoma. J Clin Oncol 9:843–849

Willet CG, Compton CC, Shellito PC et al (1994) Selection factors for local excision or abdominoperineal resection of early-stage rectal cancer. Cancer 73:2716–2720

Withers HR, Cuasay L, Mason KA, Romsdahl MM, Saxton J (1981) Elective radiation therapy in the curative treatment of cancer of the rectum and rectosigmoid colon. In: Stroehlein JR, Romsdahl MM (eds) Gastrointestinal cancer. Raven, New York, pp 351–362

Wittekind C, Tannapfel A (1995) Ätiologie, Pathogenese und Pathologie des Rektumkarzinoms. Onkologe 1:4–9

Zucali R, Gadani G, Lattuada A (1987) Adjuvant irradiation after radical surgery of cancer of the rectum and rectosigmoid colon. Radiother Oncol 8:19

Hyperthermia in the Multimodal Therapy of Advanced Rectal Carcinomas

P. Wust[1], J. Gellermann[1], B. Rau[2], J. Löffel[3], A. Speidel[3], H. Stahl[1], H. Riess[3], T.J. Vogl[1], R. Felix[1], and P.M. Schlag[2]

[1] Department of Radiation Oncology, Rudolf Virchow University Clinic, Augustenburger Platz 1, 13344 Berlin, Germany
[2] Department of Surgery, Robert-Rössle Hospital, Humboldt University, Lindenberger Weg 80, 13122 Berlin, Germany
[3] Department of Medical Oncology, Rudolf Virchow University Clinic, Augustenburger Platz 1, 13344 Berlin, Germany

Abstract

The synergistic effects of hyperthermia (raising temperatures to 40°C and above) when combined with radiotherapy and cytotoxic drugs and a modulation of immunological phenomena have been demonstrated in the laboratory. Pre-clinical data relating to hyperthermia are summed up, along with their implications for clinical application. Controlled studies of local and regional hyperthermia have been performed during recent years, and these show us that the adjunction of hyperthermia provides at least an improvement of local control compared with radiotherapy alone. Current clinical results are summarized. Therapy systems based on radiowave irradiation have been commercially available for regional hyperthermia of the pelvis since the mid 1980s. This technology allows us to perform sufficiently tolerable and effective regional hyperthermia on rectal carcinomas. Used as part of curative preoperative and postoperative multimodal therapeutic strategies, hyperthermia can lead to improvement in local control (resectability, down-staging, progression-free time, recurrence rate), at least for certain risk groups. The preoperative radio-chemo-thermotherapy of advanced primary and recurring rectal carcinoma, uT3/4, was tested in a phase-I/II study of 20 patients. Therapy procedure, acute toxicity, thermal parameters, and response are described and discussed for this patient group. The regimen proved to be sufficiently tolerable, and complications did not occur. Tumor resection was performed on 14 of the 20 patients; 13 of the procedures were R0-resections and one was an R2 resection. In 64% of the resected rectal carcinomas, histopathological down-staging of the pretherapeutic endosonographical stadium was achieved; in three of the patients, despite continued non-resectability, local control has now been maintained for more than 12 months. In two patients with nonresectable rectal carcinomas, local progress was seen during the neoadjuvant combination therapy.

Recent Results in Cancer Research, Vol. 142

Introduction

Endosonography is currently recognized as the most accurate method of preoperative staging for rectal carcinomas (Glaser et al. 1990). There is no doubt that preoperative radiotherapy (+/– chemotherapy) is indicated for the advanced stages uT3/4 and N+ (and for recurrent tumors) (Molls and Fink 1994). In cases where tumors have been potentially resectable, pre- and postoperative (neo)adjuvant therapy courses have been used and studied.

Postoperative treatment courses have the advantage of enabling precise histopathological staging. In the stages Duke's B (pT3-4, i.e., penetration of muscularis mucosae) and Duke's C (N+, i.e., locoregional lymph node metastases), postoperative radiochemotherapy is the recommended standard form of therapy (Gastrointestinal Tumor Study Group 1985; Fischer et al. 1988; Krook et al. 1991). In the variance analysis by Krook et al. 1991, the level of lymph node invasion (N1-2) proved to be an independent prognostic determinant of locoregional recurrence; the histological characteristics L+ (lymphangiosis carcinomatosa) and V+ (vessel invasion) are also risk factors. For these reasons, a protocal has been developed which includes regional hyperthermia for treating this high-risk group (N+, L+, V+), in addition to the established radiochemotherapy (Fig. 1b).

In advanced nonresectable rectal carcinomas, local control is a great problem for patients. Note that the term "nonresectable" is not clearly defined and depends on the opinion of the surgeon concerned; as an orientation guide we can use the clinical stages of Mason (Mohiuddin et al. 1993; see Table 1), which range from fully mobile tumors to tumors that are completely fixed to their surroundings (stages I–IV). The relevant workgroups of the German Cancer Society recommend preoperative radiotherapy, or better still, radiochemotherapy, as a standard approach toward nonresectable tumors (Konsensus 1994).

The numerous studies to date on preoperative radiotherapy for nonresectable rectal carcinomas show a resectability rate of 40–64% and a low rate of complete remissions (<10%). In comparison with historical groups, the addition of chemotherapy appears to increase resectability to 80–90% and complete remissions to perhaps as much as 20% (Minsky et al. 1991, 1993). For certain risk groups, the local recurrence rate can still be a dominant problem; in clinical stage IV, local failure of 50% is still evident despite preoperative radiotherapy (Mohiuddin et al. 1993). At clinical stages II/III (Table 1) and for the group of distal rectal carcinomas (<6cm ab ano), Ahmad et al. (1993) found that local control was strongly dependent on radiation dose after preoperative radiotherapy and potential curative surgical intervention. We can conclude that, at least for this risk group, intensification of preoperative therapy or local therapy is required adjunctive to surgery. As well as discussing intraoperative radiotherapy (Willett et al. 1991), we have started to evaluate regional hyperthermia in a preoperative multimodal course of therapy for treating locally advanced and nonresectable rectal carcinomas (Fig. 1a).

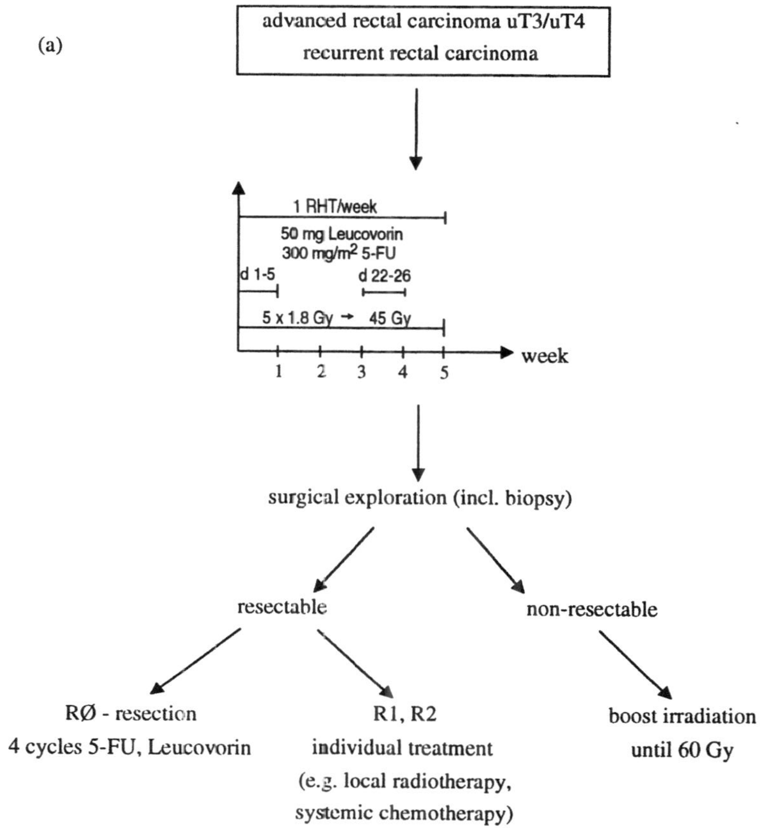

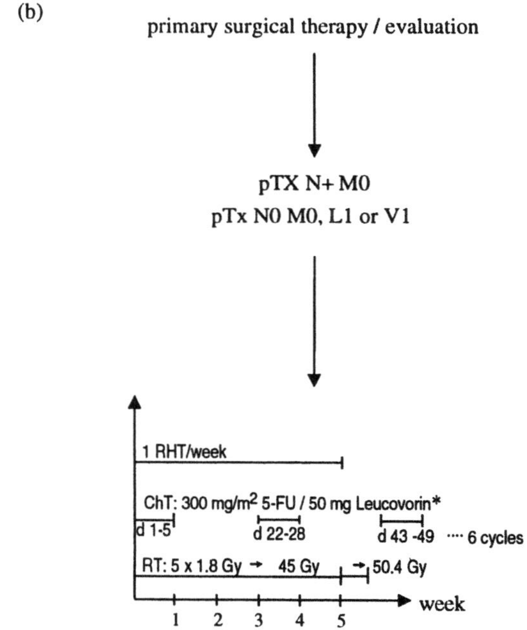

* dose escalation according to toxicity

Fig. 1a,b. Preoperative (**a**) and postoperative (**b**) radio-chemo-thermotherapy as currently performed at Rudolf Virchow Clinic (study leadership: P. Schlag and H. Riess)

Table 1. Clinical staging of rectal cancer

Stage	Condition of tumor	Resectability
CS I	Mobile	Resectable
CS II	Tethered	↓
CS III	Fixated	
CS IV	Frozen pelvis	Nonresectable

Hyperthermia in Multimodal Therapy

Preclinical Data for Hyperthermia

In vitro and in vivo investigations have given clear evidence that increasing temperature can result in a supra-additive enhancement of the effects of radiation and certain cytotoxic drugs (Table 2) (Hahn 1982; Dewey 1984; Hall 1988; Engelhardt 1987; Streffer and van Beuningen 1987; Herman et al. 1988). Additionally, hyperthermia has been found to affect effector cells in the immune system (natural killer, or NK cells) and biological response modifiers (Table 2) (Robins et al. 1993; Hanson et al. 1983, Niitsu et al. 1988, Grovemen et al. 1984).

When applications are timed closely together (ideally simultaneously), even moderate temperatures of 40.5°–41°C can enhance the effect of radiation and chemotherapeutics, as biological experiments have shown (Mills and Meyn 1981, 1983). The term used is the *sensitizing effect* of hyperthermia. The biochemical mechanisms of this amplifying effect are still being studied. Radiation sensitization is due mainly to the influence hyperthermia has on repair enzymes (recovery from sublethal or potentially lethal radiation damage) (Dewey 1989; Jung and Dikomey 1987; Spiro et al. 1982), whereas the interaction with cytotoxic drugs has other causes as well, such as the increase in cellular uptake, modification of intracellular distribution, metabolizm of the drug, and the increase in reaction rate at specific DNA sites of action (Bull 1984; Hall 1988).

Even when time intervals between radiation/cytotoxic administration and hyperthermia increase by as little as 1 h, the sensitizing effect drops significantly. At this point, hyperthermia can be seen to have a direct cytotoxic effect, which is however achieved only at temperatures of at least 42°, better 43°C (Dewey et al. 1977; Overgaard 1980; Hall and Roizin-Towle 1984). Increasing the temperature leads to several effects on cellular macromolecules (Streffer 1985; Wong and Dewey 1982; Roti-Roti and Winward 1978; Arancia et al. 1986), until finally these heat-induced lesions combine in a statistical process to kill cells (Roti-Roti and Laszlo 1988). A definite place of effect has not yet been identified (Streffer 1990).

The survival rate of mammalian cells (typically defined using the clonogenity in a colony-forming assay) is determined by the temperature and

Table 2. Sensitizing effects of hyperthermia

Supra-additive
Cytostatica
Doxorubicin, epidoxorubicin
Cisplatin, carboplatin
Cyclophosphamide, ifosfamide
BCNU, CCNU, ACNU
Melphalan
Mitoxantrone
Mitomycin C
Bleomycin
Biological response modifier
Tumor necrosis factor
Interleukins
Interferons
Radiotherapy
Additive
5-Fluorouracil
Methotrexate
Etoposide

exposure time (Henle and Dethlefsen 1978). The thermal dose (TD) is defined as follows: for a given temperature during time t, the equivalent time t_{equ} is found during which the same number of cells would be killed if the temperature were a particular reference temperature (normally 43°C). This dose is measured in min equ 43°C (minutes equivalent 43°C) (Sapareto 1988; Sapozink 1986). The thermal sensitivity fluctuates considerably from cell line to cell line (Henle and Roti-Roti 1988; Jordan et al. 1994). In order to achieve a clinically useful in vitro cell-killing effect, the cells must be incubated at 42°–43°C for at least 30–60 min. Guidelines for hyperthermia on human tumors have been derived from this (minimum tumor temperature T_{min} 43°C). For many types of cells, the thermal survival curves display a "shoulder" (analogue to the radiation dose-effect curve). These data can be described by postulation of a two-step process inside the cell, which corresponds to a second-order kinetic reaction characteristic (Jung 1986).

Analogue dose-effect curves (tumor growth time against exposure time at various temperatures) have also been demonstrated on a tumor model (e.g., on C3H/tif mammary carcinomas in mice, Overgaard 1987); the concept of thermal dose is therefore applicable to the in vivo situation.

The sensitizing and the cytotoxic effect of hyperthermia on tumor cells is not necessarily any different from the effect on normal tissue cells. We therefore cannot draw any conclusions all from the biological in vitro experiments about how a therapeutic gain is to be derived from radio/chemo-thermotherapy, or about how a synergetic effect (beyond the additive effect) is supposed to result from sequential application. However, combination therapy may have advantages that result from the interaction between the specific tumor physiology (as opposed to normal tissue) and the heat therapy and radio/chemotherapy (Vaupel 1990; Emami and Song 1984; Song 1984; Overgaard 1980, 1981). In the animal model, tumors display areas of chronic hypoxia, acidosis, and substrate deficiency (Reinhold and Endrich 1986; Vaupel et al. 1989). In this environment the cells are more sensitive to heat, at least under in vitro conditions (Gerweck 1988; Freeman et al. 1981), and also the sensitizing effect is amplified to a small extent (Holahan et al. 1984). On the other hand, the cells can be seen to adapt to the low pH value (Hahn and Shiu 1986). The formation of this tumor environment is a result of insufficient blood supply, and these badly perfused areas are therefore heated up more readily during in vivo hyperthermia. These cells, in particular, are suspected to have an environment-related radioresistance and can also demonstrate a reduced sensitivity towards chemotherapy (at least pharmacokinetically speaking).

If this environment-related cell resistance contributed significantly to the therapy failures, then the benefit of additional hyperthermia would be particularly high. However, the influence of persistent hypoxia on radioincurability is disputed (Thames and Hendry 1987; Trott 1984), because of what were, in fact, disappointing results in the clinical application of hypoxic cell sensitizers (e.g., misonidazole) and hyperbaric oxygen therapy (Henk 1986). For this reason, radiotherapeutic approaches are concentrating in particular on the development of new hyperfractionated, accelerated fractionation schemes based on the working hypothesis that the survival of a uniform, quickly proliferating cell population is a critical factor in the success of radiotherapy (Peters et al. 1988).

Meanwhile, current data on proliferation behavior (Wilson et al. 1988) and O_2 supply (Gatenby et al. 1989; Hoeckel et al. 1991) in human tumors, as well as the clinical data produced to date (Dische 1989; Dische and Saunders 1989) all suggest that both factors – persistent hypoxia and repopulation – can play a part in therapy failure. There is clinical evidence that persistent hypoxia affects advanced tumors such as N3 lymph node metastases (Valdagni et al. 1988a; Mendenhall et al. 1984) and stage-III cervical carcinomas (Watson et al. 1978; Hoeckel et al. 1991), which is understandable because of the increasing heterogeneity of tumors with increasing volume.

Under these conditions, it is imperative for oncology as a whole that we continue to develop measurement methods that allow estimation of tumor biology and identification of the most effective therapy. Methods used so far are flow cytometry (bromodesoxyuridine method, Wilson et al. 1988) and invasive methods of measuring the tumor environment (pO_2 and pH probes, Gatenby et al. 1989; Molls and Feldmann 1991; v d Zee et al. 1989; Hoeckel et al. 1991), ^{31}P spectroscopy (Ng et al. 1989), positron emission tomography (Strauss 1991), and dynamic magnetic resonance tomography.

Accordingly, the biological justification for hyperthermia is based on the interaction between thermosensitivity and resistance (as opposed to complementary therapy) with regard to tumor environment factors. This was concluded mainly from in vivo data from numerous tumor models (Vaupel 1990; Reinhold and Endrich 1986; Vaupel et al. 1989). Iso- and xenotransplanted model tumors, which generally grow quickly, display clear tissue acidosis, which increases under hyperthermia. This is related to the characteristic vulnerability of the tumor microcirculation in experimental tumors which increases the chances of a temperature rise causing vascular collapse or stasis.

There are, however, justified doubts as to whether this applies to human tumors, which are on average less acidic; in fact, MR spectroscopic measurements show that the intracellular pH values are often above neutral (Vaupel et al. 1989; Semmler et al. 1988). Vascular collapse seldom occurs in human tumors; indeed, most tumors display vessel regulation comparable to that of normal tissue, i.e., a generally small rise in perfusion with increasing temperature (Waterman et al. 1987; Wust et al. 1995a).

Finally, there are other factors that influence the cytotoxicity and sensitizing effect of hyperthermia, such as the possible development of thermotolerance (Henle and Dethlefsen 1978; Nielsen et al. 1982, 1983) and its dependence on temperature, rate of temperature increase, environmental factors (Dikomey et al. 1988; Mooibroek et al. 1988), and the special temperature-time curve (step-down heating; Jung 1989; Lindegaard and Overgaard 1987; chronically induced thermotolerance; Jung et al. 1986).

The interaction between cytotoxic substances and temperature increase has not yet been examined thoroughly (Herman et al. 1988). However, the introduction of chemo-thermotherapy would appear to have particularly good prospects; its principle advantage over radio-thermotherapy in the clinic is the fact that the two modalities can be applied simultaneously. With correct timing, the full sensitizing effect of hyperthermia can be used in this way. The temperatures required for this work are lower (e.g., 41°C).

To summarize, the variability of the thermal effect from cell line to cell line and from model tumor to model tumor leads us to the conclusion that predicting the therapeutic effect on human tumors is extremely difficult. Influential environmental factors and thermal history also complicate the picture. There are additional unclarities with regard to tumor physiology, particularly of human tumors, the biological behavior of which differs in many ways from that of animal experimental tumors. The wealth of laboratory experiments involving hyperthermia must therefore be interpreted with care when they are being applied to the clinical situation; they can supply no more than general guidelines on such things as the optimum thermal dose. It is particularly worth remembering that most of the biological investigations (generally one session) did not take into account the fractionation schemes applied to patients. Basically, new phenomena must not be excluded from consideration, such as the influence of previous hyperthermia on the next radiotherapy and/or chemotherapy session (through changes in blood perfusion or necrosis formation, which modulate the tumor environment or the pharmacokinetics).

An understanding of the molecular-biological effects within the cell during heating is vital. This includes in particular the signal events at mRNA level, and proteins which lead to expression and modulation of heat-shock proteins, cytokines, and proto-oncogenes (Laszlo et al. 1992; Lindquist and Craig 1988). Of particular interest are heat-induced molecular-biological mechanisms that are active on the membrane of the cell and therefore potentially initiate immunological reactions through association with antigen determinants, e.g., tumor-specific tumor reactions through activation of T lymphocytes (Multhoff et al. 1994). Only by explaining these mechanisms can we understand observed thermotolerance, sensitization, resistance development against certain noxae, and immune system responses on a cellular level. These effects can then be used for the refinement of therapeutic strategies.

Practical Implementation of Regional Hyperthermia

The promising results obtained in preclinical examinations have been inspiring people to develop hyperthermia systems since the beginning of the 1980s. The most significant of these systems are aimed at depositing electromagnetic energy in the tumor.

In the beginning simple high-frequency prototypes were developed that were based on the capacitive and inductive methods. They worked in the quasistatic range, i.e., below 30 MHz, usually at 13.56 or 27.12 MHz (approved ISM frequencies).

Using the capacitive method (Fig. 2a), an electrical field is generated, preferably perpendicular to the surface of the body, i.e., exactly perpendicular to the fat/muscle interface. As field maxima occur under these conditions, this is certainly not the best direction in which to polarize the E field – in fact it may even be the worst. These systems are used, nevertheless, especially in Japan and France. Used on slim patients and in certain anatomical regions, they can actually be very efficient, even advantageous.

Using the inductive method (Fig. 2b), energy is supplied primarily by an alternating magnetic field which is directed parallel to the coil axis and associated with a perpendicular circular electrical field. The power transferred in this way drops to zero at the coil axis, and this proved to be such a serious disadvantage to the prototypes that this type of system never established itself in clinical practice.

Since the beginning of the 1980s, systems have been designed based on the group-source principle, and these establish an electric field polarized parallel to the patient axis. The most advanced system of this type is the BSD 2000 system with the SIGMA phased-array applicator (shown in Fig. 2c with an elliptical phantom). The ring applicator comprises four pairs of biconical dipole antennas arranged equidistantly in a circle inside a Plexiglas ring. These antennas are fed in phase and amplitude by four broad-band power amplifiers (Wust et al. 1995b).

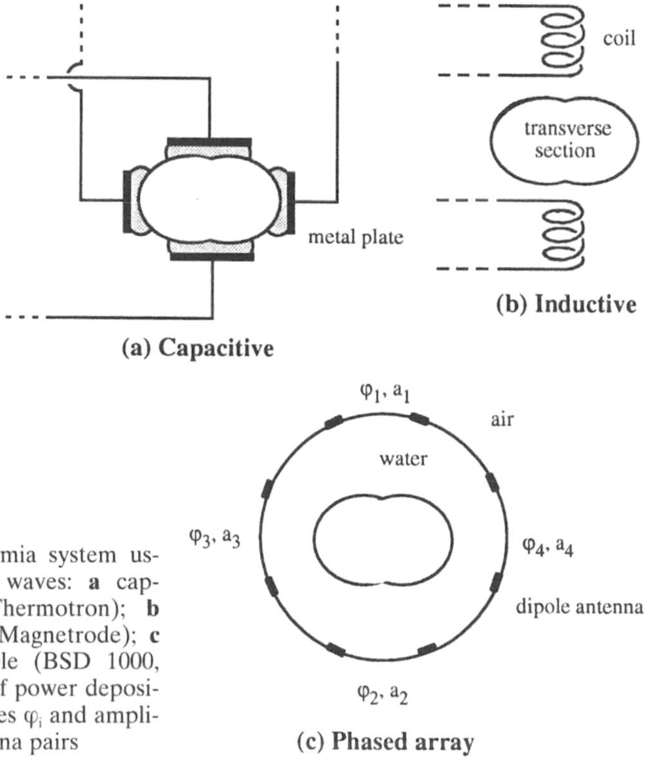

Fig. 2a–c. Hyperthermia system using electromagnetic waves: **a** capacitive principle (Thermotron); **b** inductive principle (Magnetrode); **c** group-source principle (BSD 1000, BSD 2000): control of power deposition patterns by phases φ_i and amplitudes a_i of four antenna pairs

Other systems in clinical use based on the group-source principle are the TEM applicator (DeLeeuw and Lagendijk 1987), the 4-waveguide applicator (van Dijk et al. 1989), and the BSD 1000 (predecessor of the BSD 2000) (Turner 1984). These systems differ basically in the treatment volume and in the way the patient is positioned. Larger applicators are used for larger treatment volumes (generally at lower frequency) and, clinically speaking, go hand in hand with increased systemic stress. They have the advantage (TEM applicator) of causing less local discomfort. When the TEM applicator is used, the patient is placed in water; the open arrangement has advantages for coupling and performing control measurements.

With the SIGMA applicator, the patient is completely surrounded by a water bolus, and the water pressure can sometimes give rise to position-related discomfort. Figure 3 shows the SIGMA applicator in clinical use. The most comprehensive range of clinical experience has been gathered for the BSD 2000 system's SIGMA applicator; despite some disadvantages, it has proven to be the most practical in clinical use (Wust et al. 1995a; Issels et al. 1990, Feldmann et al. 1993). Comparisons between thermal parameters such as maximum and minimum tumor temperature and index temperatures show that the BSD system is superior to the TEM applicator, the 4-wave

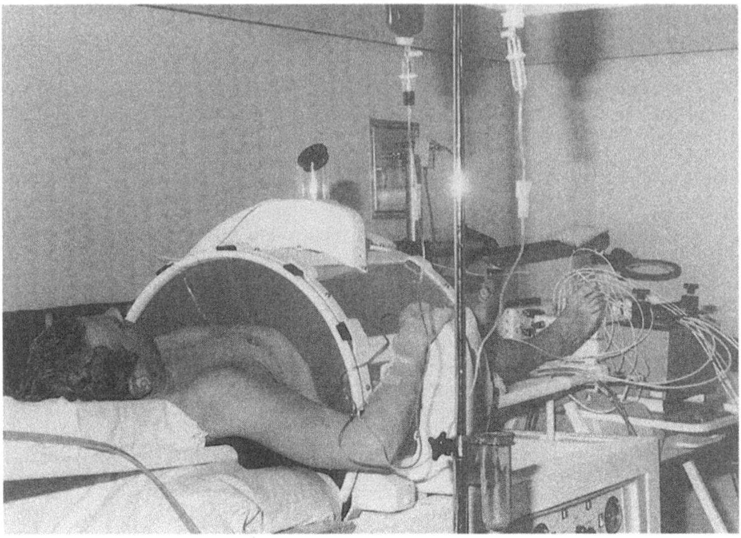

Fig. 3. Patient in SIGMA applicator

guide applicator, capacitive systems, and ultrasound systems (Wust et al. 1995b).

Current methodical research is concentrated on improving measurement techniques for quality control before therapy (Wust et al. 1994, 1995d) and control during therapy (Wust et al. 1995c). The development of planning systems in hyperthermia is also being pushed hard (Seebass et al. 1993). Wust et al. (1995b,c) provide a critical look at currently available technology and possible ways of developing it using newly evolved measurement methods and computer algorithms.

Clinical Experience with Hyperthermia

The first hyperthermia devices were developed for application to the surface of the body and were used to treat selected superficial tumors (local hyperthermia). A heterogeneous patient group was treated. Many of the patients had several similar lesions each (e.g., skin metastases of a malignant melanoma), so it was possible to compare different therapies on each patient. As far as tumor regression was concerned, the comparisons on individual patients and with members of control collectives consistently showed the superiority of combined therapy (radio-thermotherapy) over radiotherapy alone (Overgaard 1989b; Meyer 1984). Various techniques were used, such as ultrasound and microwave; the tumor manifestations treated were adapted to the techniques available. The studies confirmed the biological effectiveness of hyperthermia, and in this respect they were encouraging; they also provided a wealth of information on prognostic factors, therapy parameters, and dose-effect curves (Arcangeli et al. 1985; Oleson et al. 1984; Valdagni et al. 1988b; Overgaard 1989b; Leopold et al. 1993).

In this work, hyperthermia was being used mainly as relapse therapy or for palliation. It was used in combination therapies, bimodally with radiotherapy (of which we have the most experience, e.g., Perez et al. 1986, 1989a; van der Zee et al. 1988; Urbon et al. 1990; Scott et al. 1983, 1988; Feldmann et al. 1988, 1993; Lindholm et al. 1987; Hofman et al. 1989) and with chemotherapy (Herman et al. 1989; Pilepich et al. 1989; Issels et al. 1990, 1991). Trimodal therapies were also used (Herman et al. 1990), this being the type of which we have the least experience. Some of these studies have only limited oncological value, as the survival period of the patients treated was influenced only marginally.

As a result, people began to consider ways in which hyperthermia could be used together with radiotherapy in order to achieve improved local control while performing curative therapies (Kapp 1986; Overgaard 1989b). It is well known that about 30% of cancer patients die from the local complications of their illness, and an estimated half (i.e., 15%) of these would profit from improved local control (Suit 1982).

When it is part of a curative therapy scheme, hyperthermia can be used both preoperatively (neoadjuvantly) and as a primary therapy (in cases of nonresectability or medical inoperability). In special cases it can also be used postoperatively (e.g., if macroscopic or microscopic tumor residues are identified, or for high-risk groups in adjuvant applications). This has already been discussed for rectal carcinomas above. For other locally advanced organ tumors, treatment begins with preoperative (neoadjuvant) chemotherapy, followed by tumor resection, adding radiotherapy as a consolidating local therapy. This type of approach has been suggested for tumors such as locally advanced (primary inoperable) bladder carcinomas (Scher 1990), cervical carcinomas (Sardi et al. 1990), mammary carcinomas (Sorace and Lippmann 1988), and for soft-tissue sarcomas (Rousse et al. 1987).

Preoperative therapy can improve the conditions for surgical local therapy through down-staging (e.g., organ-preserving operations), sometimes even enabling resectability. Apart from this, local advanced tumor stages are often characterized by occult distant metastases (e.g., more than 50% in high-risk soft-tissue sarcomas). For this reason, it is logically consistent to begin with systemic therapy as early as possible in order to influence the survival time. The response of the primary tumor is also an in vivo estimate of its sensitivity. Despite the positive aspects mentioned, the occasionally unsatisfactory response of locally advanced primary tumors (with high cell burden and heterogeneity) presents a limiting factor for preoperative therapy, which gives hyperthermia an important role in this modern oncological concept.

Indications have been established for the primary treatment of superficial tumors, for which local hyperthermia is part of a potentially curative therapy approach. Several multicenter phase-III studies have been initiated by the

ESHO (European Society of Hyperthermic Oncology), the RTOG (Radiation Therapy Oncology Group), and the MRC (Medical Research Centre, Great Britain) (Overgaard 1989a); ESHO 1-85 (advanced mammary carcinomas), ESHO 2-85 (cervical lymph node metastases), ESHO 3-85 (malignant melanomas), ESHO 4-86 (interstitial tongue-base carcinomas, ESHO 5-88 (recurrent mammary carcinomas, pre-irradiated), RTOG 81-04 (various recurrent tumors), RTOG 84-11 (mammary carcinomas, head-neck tumors, soft-tissue sarcomas), RTOG 84-19 (interstitial, various locations), MRC 1 (advanced mammary carcinomas), MRC 2/3 (chest wall, cervical lymph nodes with or without pre-irradiation). Monocenter phase-III studies on smaller groups of patients were performed for cervical lymph node metastases by Valdagni et al. in 1988 and 1993, and for advanced head-neck tumors by Datta et al. in 1990.

Two phase-III studies concerning regional hyperthermia of deep-seated pelvic tumors were started in Rotterdam and Amsterdam in 1990. In these studies, hyperthermia is applied in addition to standard radiotherapy to treat inoperable bladder carcinomas (T3–4), cervical carcinomas (stages IIB distal, IIIB, IV), and rectal carcinomas (primary nonresectable or recurrent) (study leader: J. van der Zee, Dr. Daniel Hoed Cancer Center, Rotterdam).

In 1990 and 1991, Issels et al. drew up a preoperative therapy approach using combined thermo-chemotherapy for treating high-risk sarcomas (>8 cm, deep-seated, extracompartimental, G-II/III, recurrent). Following a successful phase-II study, 1994 saw the introduction of a multicenter phase-III study using a modified therapy protocol (study leader: R.D. Issels, Großhadern Clinic, Munich).

Phase I/II of preoperative radiochemotherapy for advanced rectal carcinomas as shown in Fig. 1a is now also almost completely finished; randomization was introduced in July, 1994 (study leaders: P. Schlag and H. Riess, Rudolf Virchow Clinic, Berlin; see below).

In retrospect, there have been two main difficulties with performing phase-II studies involving hyperthermia. In the first randomized study, which was completed as far back as 1988 (RTOG 81-04, 300 patients), the combination of radiotherapy and hyperthermia was shown to improve tumor response only for the group with tumor sizes of 3 cm or less (80% response after 12 months compared with 15% using radiotherapy alone). No difference was found in the remission rate for tumors larger than 3 cm (Perez et al. 1989b). The results suggest that hyperthermic treatment of large tumors was not effective due to inadequate technology, combined with ineffective thermometry, and this underlines how important sufficient technical quality control is (see for example Shrivastava et al. 1988). Starting a phase-III study too early can produce misleading results if the methods used are not evaluated in a well-conceived phase-II study.

Some of the studies suffered from difficulties in patient recruitment and from lack of acceptance in many of the institutions. This was related to developments in oncological therapy that were not taken into account in the protocols produced. For example, nonresectable mammary carcinomas (ESHO

1-85) are now rarely subjected to primary radiotherapy. As metastasis often occurs in these patients, we need a systemic therapy to increase the length of time the patients survive (see above). In such cases, the combination of initial neoadjuvant chemotherapy followed by consolidating local therapy (surgical provision and/or radiotherapy is a promising approach; Henderson et al. 1989). Combined simultaneous radiochemotherapy with accelerated fractionation schemes is now the standard therapeutic approach for treating and locally controlling inoperable advanced ENT carcinomas (ESHO 2-85) (Al-Sarraft 1988; Wendt et al. 1989; Budach et al. 1992; Wust et al. 1996). Most of the studies mentioned have now either been terminated for the reasons given or completed with sufficient numbers of patients (see Table 3).

A joint statistical evaluation of phase-III studies involving more than 300 patients with recurrent mammary carcinomas (ESHO 5-88, MRC 1, 2) showed a statistically significant improvement in response with combined radiotherapy and hyperthermia (CR rate 60%) compared with radiotherapy alone (CR rate 40%). Survival rates were not influenced to a statistically significant extent (Vernon et al. 1994).

The multicenter phase-III study concerning metastasized or recurrent malignant melanomas ESHO 3-85 and involving 134 lesions in 71 patients was completed in April 1992 (Overgaard 1994). The tumors treated using combined therapy were shown to respond more readily (CR rate 68%) than those treated with radiotherapy alone (CR rate 32%), and the chances of local control for 5 years were better, too (46% compared with 28%).

An interim analysis of the Dutch 129-patient phase-III study of advanced pelvic tumors (van der Zee et al. 1993) showed improved local control (CR after 1 year) for the group treated with combined therapy (58% against 37%). The results obtained for bladder carcinomas (79% against 41%) and cervical carcinomas (78% against 56%) were altogether more pleasing. The worst

Table 3. Phase-III studies on local and regional hyperthermia

Coordinator	Tomor	Status	Local control	Survival	Reference
Valdagni	Lymph nodes	Closed	Significant	N. sign.	Valdagni et al. 1988a
Datta	Head and neck	Closed	Significant	N. sign.	Datta et al. 1990
ESHO 1-85	Breast	Closed	N. sign.	N. sign.	González González 1994
ESHO 2-85	Lymph nodes	Closed	N. sign.	N. sign.	Overgaard 1994
ESHO 3-85	Melanoma	Closed	Significant	Significant	Overgaard 1994
ESHO 5-88 +MRC 1, 2	Recurrent breast	Closed	Significant	N. sign.	Vernon et al. 1994
Rotterdam + Amsterdam	Pelvic	Interim analysis	Significant	N. sign.	van der Zee et al. 1993
Munich	Soft-tissue sarcomas	Open	–	–	Issels et al. 1995
Berlin	Rectal cancer	Open	–	–	Schlag and Riess 1994

results were obtained for rectal carcinomas (19% against 13%, not significant). However, as we mentioned above, complete remission of advanced rectal carcinomas is extremely difficult to bring about, with regard to both CT/MRT progress (decrease in tumor size) and the histopathological findings after resection; the length of time local control can be maintained is therefore the decisive parameter. The ESHO 1-85 and 2-85 studies were terminated because not enough patients were recruited, and the results were negative (table 3).

In all, the results show that combining radiotherapy and hyperthermia helps to achieve better local control. Despite this proof of effectiveness, the areas of indication for hyperthermia within oncological therapy schemes are not yet properly defined.

In spite of its being proven to be effective, clinical application of hyperthermia is sometimes drawn into question or at least restricted if the cost in terms of money, staff requirement, and patient discomfort/risk are large and potential success small. Of central importance is the oncological concept, which must clearly be seen to be of benefit to the patient group concerned. However, acceptance also depends on the technical maturity of the therapy system and all associated logistical steps. Problems in actually performing hyperthermia will be discussed further on in this paper.

Materials and Methods (Phase-I/II Study)

In a phase-I/II study, 20 patients with advanced (uT3–4) and/or recurrent rectal carcinomas underwent multimodal preoperative therapy comprising radiotherapy (planned target volume dose 45 Gy), chemotherapy (5-FU and low doses of folinic acid), and thermotherapy (regional hyperthermia using the BSD 2000 system). The therapy protocol is shown in Fig. 1a. Apart from the regional hyperthermia, it corresponds to the recommendations made by the member workgroups of the German Cancer Society at a consensus meeting during the German Cancer Congress in Hamburg, 1994. The pretherapeutic UICC stages, which were ascertained using endosonography, other imaging modalities, and clinically, are shown in Table 4. Most of the tumors were advanced, with infiltration of the surrounding structures (T4).

Regional hyperthermia was performed at weekly intervals throughout the entire 5–6 week preoperative cycle. The BSD 2000's SIGMA ring applicator was used; Fig. 3 shows a patient in the ring applicator. Figure 2c shows the circular arrangement of the four pairs of antennas in the transverse plane around the patient. Regional hyperthermia was administered using a standard setting at 90 MHz with a 20°–40° phase delay in the bottom pair of antennas and a 5°–20° delay in the side pairs (supine position of patient). Two-dimensionally, this phase delay shifts the pattern caudally into the presacral space. This setup is shown in Fig. 4 using a lamp phantom, which provides an image of the power distribution. The central plane (antenna bases) was generally aligned with the central plane of the irradiation fields (which contains the isocenter).

Table 4. Endosonographic staging of 20 patients awaiting preoperative therapy (phase-I/II study)

Stage		Patients (%)
Primary advanced (%)		70
uT3	25	
uT4	45	
Recurrent (%)		30
uT2	5	
uT3	10	
uT4/cT4	15	
M0	80	
M1 (liver)	15	
M1 (lungs)	5	

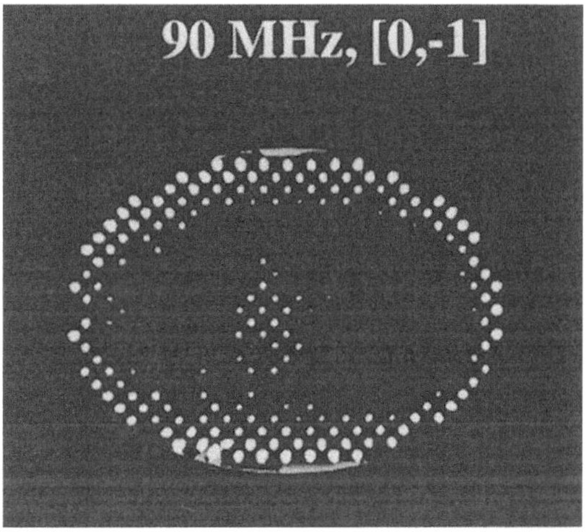

Fig. 4. Visualising the power distribution in a lamp phantom for a standard setting used on rectal carcinomas (maneuvered dorsally)

Thermometry was performed by inserting a Teflon catheter with an external diameter of 1.8mm (Angiomed) noninvasively into the rectum, into the tumor region and beyond. The patient lay on his left side during positioning procedure. In cases where the rectal carcinoma was located somewhat proximally, a rectoscope was used. The catheter's tumor contact path was reconstructed with the help of CT documentation and parameters determined endoscopically. Only for presacral recurrent tumors after abodominoperineal rectum extirpation was a catheter implanted transgluteally under CT monitoring (i.e., invasively; Fig. 5).

Temperature/position curves were regularly plotted using a scanning system driven by a stepping motor. The data collected was later analyzed to obtain the time-based index temperatures T_{20}, T_{50}, T_{90} and the minimum and maximum contact termperatures in the tumor. The data trasfer and evaluation program was developed by Basu and Bierbass in 1994. T_x is the temperature

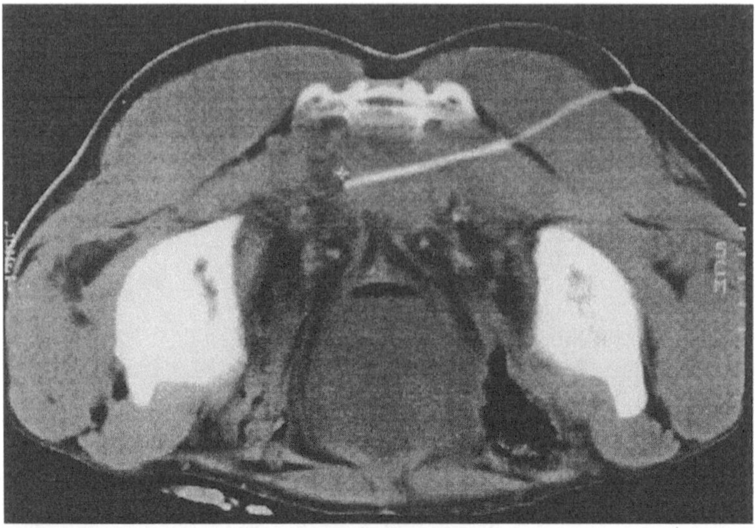

a

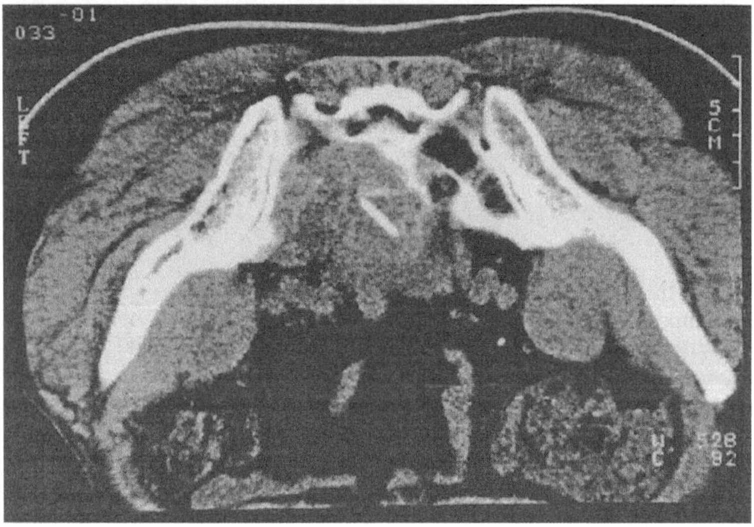

b

Fig. 5a,b. CT scans of transgluteally implanted thermometry catheters in a presacral recurrent rectal carcinoma. **a** Implantation in the transverse plane; implantation from caudal (with inclined gantry during CT guidance) above which x% of the time-averaged temperatures assigned to tumor contact measurement points climbed during the acutal therapeutic period. The therapeutic period begins when at least one measurement point has reached 41°C, or at the latest after 30 min, and ends when the therapy ends. Generally speaking, a therapeutic period of 60 min is aimed for (starting when a measurement point reaches 41°C). These guidelines are based on standard regional hyperthermia procedures (see Issels et al. 1990, 1991; Feldmann et al. 1993; Wust et al. 1995a). Data for thermal comparison are available for more than 50 patients with advanced pelvic tumors for which intratumoral (transcutaneous or intraoperatively implanted) catheters were used for measuring the temperature. Temperature is measured using a high-frequency inert temperature-dependent resistance via a high-resistance lead (known as a Bowman thermistor).

The radiotherapy was performed using an open table-top device and with the patient in prone position (Mak et al. 1994). A planning CT was done on each patient in this particular position. All were irradiated using the three-field technique and lateral wedge filters. Standard shields were used to protect lateral field corners, dorsal soft tissues (skin, rima ani), and, where necessary, cranial ventral sections of the small intestine. The upper field border was positioned at S-1 (lower edge), occasionally at L-5 (lower edge) if the rectal carcinoma was proximally located. The candal ventral border was determined by the position of the primary tumor and the infiltration into the surroundings (especially prostate). Generally speaking, the ventral field boundary passed through the central third of the head of the femur. Images of the small intestine were obtained using Gastrografin in order to document and block the sections of the small intestine situated in the field of radiation. Fractionation was 5 × 1.8 Gy in the reference point (isocenter) with a maximum of less than 2 Gy. This resulted in a target volume dose of nearly 45 Gy and a maximum dose of less than 50 Gy.

Chemotherapy using 5-FU (300 mg/m^2) and folinic acid (50 mg) was performed on days 1–5 and 22–26 in the form of a short infusion about half an hour before irradiation or during regional hyperthermia. Radiotherapy is normally carried out as soon as possible after hyperthermia.

Side effects were documented using the WHO score system, at weekly intervals and during hyperthermia treatment. Routine CT examinations were performed before and after the multimodal therapy. Some of the patients were given pre- and posttherapeutic MRT examinations, both with and without contrast agent (T1- as well as T2-weighted sequences).

Results (Phase-I/II Study)

Preoperative therapy was performed to plan in 90% of the patients. The planned number of hyperthermia sessions was reached in 80% of the patients, and only one of the patients refused to continue hyperthermia after the first session. The acute toxicity in the intestine and bladder and on the skin was not negligible) (Table 5). Diarrhea requiring therapy (grade III) caused radiotherapy to be interrupted in six patients; with one patient, therapy was interrupted because of a skin reaction III (moist epitheliolysis) in the rima ani. In 30% of patients, tenderness or aching was reported at predilection sites (suprapubic region, inguinal region, thigh, lateral gluteal region). This discomfort was interpreted as being a musculoskeletal syndrome, which arises as a result of "hot spot" formation, or excessive increases in E-field strength at electrical interfaces. These hot spots develop because of the currently limited controllability of electrical field distributions. Generally speaking, discomfort ceases after a few days without any consequences.

Hot spot phenomena are particularly troublesome, as they limit increases in total power and therefore prevent the tumor region from being heated effectively. Methods of omitting these hot spots are based on increasing the number of antennas (the phase and amplitude of each antenna can be controlled); this makes the E-field distribution easier to control (Wust et al. 1995f).

The temperatures reached along the tumor contact path are listed in Table 6. The tumor contact temperatures are lower than the temperatures measured intratumorally. The best hyperthermia treatment for all of the 20 patients is marked "best" in Table 6. Clearly, potentially effective hyperthermia is possible in most patients, with contact temperatures ≥42°C in 55% and ≥41°C in 95% of those treated. However, the endoluminal contact measurement is an indicator solely of regionally sufficient power levels; it is therefore not surprising that none of the thermal parameters listed in Table 6 could be correlated to a statistically significant extent with the response (Table 7). Then again, this may have been because the patient group was too small and heterogeneous. We shall have to wait for further results from the study.

Performing regional hyperthermia without intratumoral temperature measurement is justifiable, because extensive experience has been gathered

Table 5. Toxicity in 20 patients receiving preoperative radio-chemo-thermotherapy

Location	Grade	Percent
Intestine	0	20
	I	25
	II	20
	III	35
	IV	–
Skin	I	40
	II	40
	III	20
	IV	–
Bladder		25
Musculoskeletal syndrome		30
Hyperthermia discontinued/refused		15

Table 6. Thermal parameters at endoluminal thermometry catheters from 105 regional hyperthermia (HT) sessions for rectal cancer in 20 patients[a]

Variable	Mean (range)
T_{min} (°C)	39.5 (38.5–40.6)
$T_{min/best}$	40.2 (38.8–41.7)
T_{90} (°C)	39.8 (38.9–40.8)
$T_{90/best}$	40.4 (39.3–41.7)
T_{50} (°C)	40.7 (39.8–41.5)
$T_{50/best}$	41.2 (40.5–42.0)
T_{20} (°C)	41.1 (40.2–41.8)
$T_{20/best}$	41.6 (40.7–42.4)
T_{max} (°C)	41.4 (40.5–42.5)
$T_{max/best}$	42.1 (40.9–43.0)
Number of HT/patients	5.3 (2–10)

[a] All HT: ⩾42°C in 30%, ⩾41°C in 71%, ⩾40.5°C in 86%; best HT: ⩾42°C in 55%, ⩾41.5°C in 80%, ⩾41°C in 95%

Table 7. Response of 20 patients to combination therapy (phase-I/II study)

Modality			Patients (%)
Surgery			
Resection (14/20 patients)			70
– Rø resection (13/14 patients)		95%	
down-staging in 9/14 patients		65%	
uT4 → ypTø:	2 patients		
uT4 → ypT2:	2 patients		
uT4 → ypT3:	1 patients		
uT3 → ypT2:	2 patients		
uT2 → ypTX:	1 patients		
uT3N1 → ypT3Nø:	1 patients		
– R2 resection in 1/14 patients			5
No resection (6/20 patients)			30
– nonresectable		20%	
– surgery refused		5%	
– clinical reasons		5%	
Computerized tomography			
Regression			30
No change			70
Endosonography ($n = 18$)			
Regression			61
No change			22
Progression			17

concerning hyperthermia on pelvic tumors using invasive temperature measurement. Clinical experience and methodical parallel research (simulation studies, phantom measurements) show the standard setting described above to be the best way of using the equipment available. More advanced control methods that would require invasive temperature measurement to monitor them are currently few and far between – further technological development is first required (Wust et al. 1996b).

Table 7 provides an outline of response to preoperative therapy. The histopathological findings and the distributions seen using CT and endosonography were evaluated. Of the primary advanced and recurrent rectal carcinomas 65% (13 patients) were operated on in an R0 resection. In nine of the 13 R0-resected patients, histopathological down-staging was seen when compared with the initial endosonographic image (Table 7). In two cases, a histologically complete remission of the primary tumor was even achieved. No operation was performed on six patients (see Table 7). In cases where tumor resection was not possible, we attempted (after as short a break as possible – 1–2 weeks) to achieve a boost in the tumor region, up to a total target volume dose of around 60 Gy (in four patients). In two of these patients, hyperthermia was also performed during this second series. After a second treatment course, three of these patients have enjoyed clinical remission for periods of now more than 1 year. The periods of observation are, in all, too short for us to start drawing conclusions about the duration of local control or about how survival chances are being affected. In CT scans, 30% of the patients were shown to have an objectively verifiable decrease in tumor size or reduction in wall thickness (see Fig. 6, for example). Five patients suffered from inital pains in the presacral or anal region, and in all cases the multimodal therapy led to a significant drop in discomfort symptoms.

Discussion

For a high-risk group of rectal carcinomas, or for nonresectable cases, at least, there is evidence to support an intensification of the preoperative radiochemotherapy recommended as standard therapy. Hyperthermia is particularly practical and patient friendly when used on this type of tumor, because it is possible to measure the temperature endoluminally (in tumor contact). However, it is not yet clear whether these temperature-related parameters can be treated as indicators of the effectiveness of thermotherapy – the existing data on uniform patient groups (e.g., primary advanced stages uT4) and the observation periods are not yet sufficient.

The acute toxicity of preoperative radio-chemo-thermotherapy (Fig. 1a) is acceptable (Table 5). There are nevertheless some ways of increasing the level of tolerance. The combination of radiotherapy and 5-FU/leucovorin chemotherapy increases the toxicity in the intestine (colitis), particularly in the small intestine (diarrhea, enteritis). We must therefore strive for more careful conforming adaptation of the isodose distribution to the target volume, while

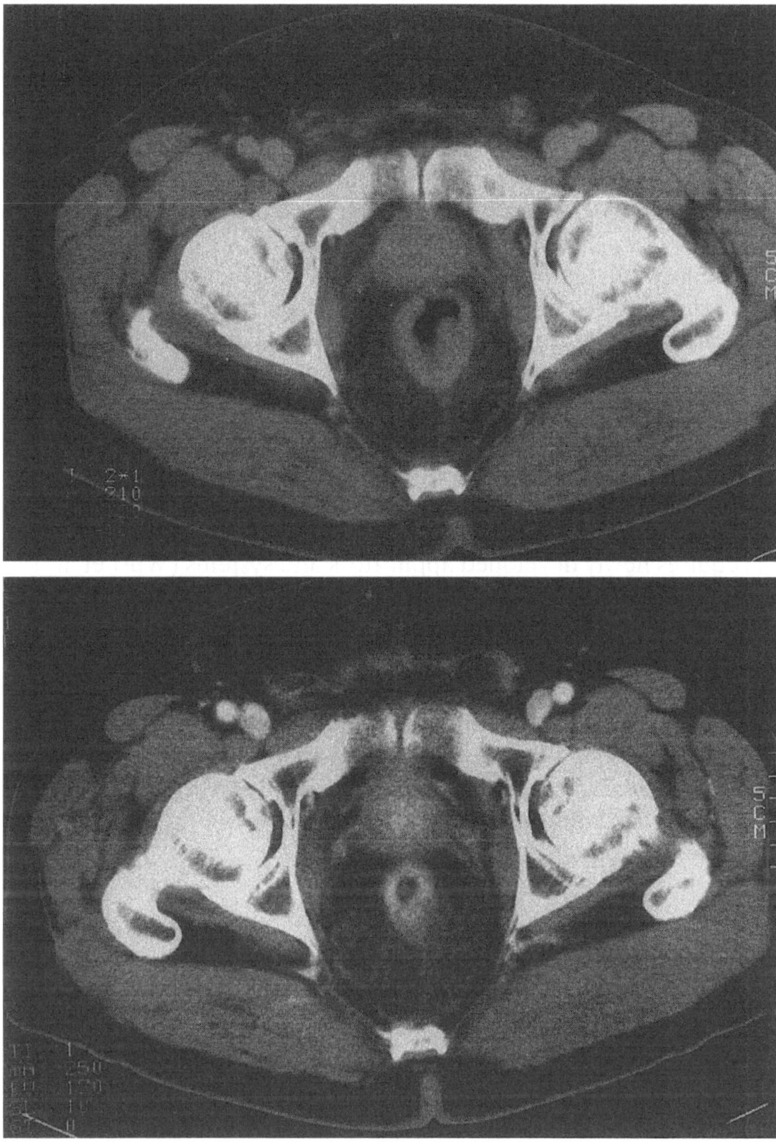

a

b

Fig. 6a,b. CT scans of a rectal carcinoma before (**a**) and after (**b**) preoperative radio-chemo-thermotherapy. Clear decrease in tumor size and wall thickness; seminal vesicles easier to demarcate from surroundings

omitting the relevant portions of the small intestine. This can be done using conformative irradiation techniques and CT-supported planning (with small-intestine contrasting). Irradiation planning involving rectal carcinomas is currently performed using the 3-D planning system HELAX, together with standard blockings.

In 20% of cases, serious skin reactions (WHO III) with moist epitheliolysis occurred around the rima ani. This is probably connected with hyperthermic sensitization increasing radiogenic skin reactions, as temperatures of 42°–43°C are often measured in the rima ani during hyperthermia. For this reason, a special cooling pipe has been developed which connects to the water circulation system (diameter 2 cm). It runs across the perineum and along the entire rima ani, and water flows through it which has been cooled to less than 10°C.

The maximum tumor contact temperatures achieved and the corresponding index temperatures (Table 6), as well as the frequency of musculoskeletal syndrome resulting from hot-spot formation (Table 5), all underline the importance of continuing to improve the technology and methods used in hyperthermia. Ways of improving these factors lie in standardization of quality assurance for existing systems using visualizing phantoms (Wust et al. 1994, 1995d), controlling the power distribution in existing and future systems by measuring the electrical field using electro-optical sensors (Wust et al. 1995c), and the development of antenna systems with a higher level of flexibility. This last requires newly developed applicators and systems (Wust et al. 1996b). All these stages in development can be realized only if we have fast algorithms for calculating E-fields and temperatures, as well as efficient, patient-specific hyperthermia planning systems.

Acknowledgement. The authors are very grateful for valuable financial support of their research by the *Berliner Sparkassenstiftung Medizin*, the *Maria Sonnenfeld-Gedächtnisstiftung* the *Deutsche Krebshilfe* (M7/94Fe9), and the *Deutsche Forschungsgemeinschaft* (SFB 273).

References

Ahmad NR, Marks G, Mohiuddin M (1993) High-dose preoperative radiation for cancer of the rectum: impact of radiation dose on patterns of failure and survival. Int J Radiat Oncol Biol Phys 27:773–778

A1-Sarraf M (1988) Head and neck cancer: chemotherapy concepts. Semin Oncol 15:70–85

Arancia G, Malorni W, Mariutti G, Trovaluski P (1986) Effect of hyperthermia on the plasma membrane structure of Chinese hamster V79 fibroblasts: a quantitative freeze-fracture study. Radiat Res 106:47–55

Arcangeli G, Arcangeli GC, Guerra A, Lovisolo G, Cividalli A, Marino C, Mauro F (1985) Tumour response to heat and radiation: prognostic variables in the treatment of neck node metastases from head and neck cancer. Int J Hyperthermia 1:207–217

Basu O, Bierbass J (1994) HTHERM – hyperthermia program for processing BSD data. Contact author for copy, Fax-No.: 0201/7235942

Budach V, Dinges S, Stüben G, Unger A, Jahnke K, Sack H (1992) Simultaneous radiochemotherapy of locally advanced ENT tumours – results of a pilot study. J Cancer Res Clin Oncol 118 [Suppl] (Abstract):2101

Bull JMC (1984) An update on the anticancer effect of a combination of chemotherapy and hyperthermia. Cancer Res 44:4853–4856

Daly PF, Cohen JS (1989) Magnetic resonance spectroscopy of tumors and potential in vivo applications: a review. Cancer Res 49:770–779

Datta NR, Bose AK, Kapoor HK, Gupta S (1990) Head and neck cancers: results of thermoradiotherapy versus radiotherapy. Int J Hyperthermia 6:479–486

DeLeeuw AAC, Lagendijk JJW (1987) Design of a clinical deep-body hyperthermia system based on the "coaxial TEM" applicator. Int J Hyperthermia 3:413–421

Dewey WC, Hopwood LE, Sapareto SA, Gerweck LE (1977) Cellular responses to combinations of hyperthermia and radiation. Radiology 123:463–474

Dewey WC (1984) Interaction of heat with radiation and chemotherapy. Cancer Res 44:4714–4720

Dewey WC (1985) Mechanism of thermal radiosenzitation. In: Urano M, Douple E (eds) Biology of thermal potentiation of radiotherapy. VSP, Utrecht, pp 1–15

Dikomey E, Eickhoff J, Jung H (1988) Effect of pH on development and decay of thermotolerance in CHO cells using fractionated heating at 43°C. Int J Hyperthermia 4:555–565

Dische S (1989) Keynote address: hypoxic cell sensitizers: clinical developments. Int J Radiat Oncol Biol Phys 16:1057-1060

Dische S, Saunders MI (1989) Continuous hyperfractionated, accelerated radiotherapy (CHART). Br J Cancer 59:325–326

Emami B, Song CW (1984) Physiological mechanisms in hyperthermia: a review. Int J Radiat Oncol Biol Phys 10:289–295

Engelhardt R (1987) Hyperthermia and drugs. In: Streffer C (ed) Hyperthermia and the therapy of malignant tumors. Springer, Berlin Heidelberg New York, pp 136–203

Feldmann HJ, Molls M, Baumhoer W, Müller R-D, Sack H (1988) Radiatio und Hyperthermie in der Behandlung oberflächlicher und halbtiefer Tumoren. Wärmeprofile, Wärmedosen, Tumorrückbildung. Strahlenther Onkol 164:602–609

Feldmann HJ, Molls M, Heinemann H-G, Romanowski R, Stuschke M, Sack H (1993) Thermoradiotherapy in locally advanced deep-seated tumors – thermal parameters and treatment results. Radiother Oncol 26:38–44

Fisher B, Wolmark N, Rockette H, Redmond C, Deutsch M, Wickerham DL, Fisher ER, Caplan R, Jones J, Lerner H, Gordon P, Feldmann M, Cruz A, Legault-Poisson S, Wexler M, Lawrence W, Robidoux A (1988) Postoperative adjuvant chemotherapy or radiation therapy for rectal cancer: results from NSABP protocol R-01. J Natl Cancer Inst 80:21–29

Freeman ML, Holahan EV, Highfield DP, Raaphorst GP, Spiro IJ, Dewey WC (1981) The effect of pH on hyperthermic and X-ray induced cell killing. Int J Radiat Oncol Biol Phys 7:211–216

Gastrointestinal Tumor Study Group (1985) Prolongation of the disease-free interval in surgically treated rectal carcinoma. N Engl J Med 312

Gatenby RA, Kessler HB, Rosenblum JS, Coia LR, Moldofsky RJ, Hartz WH, Broder GJ (1989) Oxygen distribution in squamous cell carcinoma metastases and its relationship to outcome of radiation therapy. Int J Radiat Oncol Biol Phys 14:831–838

Gerweck LE (1988) Modifiers of thermal effects: environmental factors. In: Urano M, Douple E (eds) Thermal effects on cells and tissues. VSP, Utrecht 83–98

Glaser F, Schlag P, Herfarth C (1990) Endorectal ultrasonography for the assessment of invasion of rectal tumors and lymph node involvement. Br J Surg 77:883–887

Groveman DS, Borden EC, Merritt JA, Robins HI, Steeves RA, Bryan GT (1984) Augmented antiproliferative effects of interferons at elevated temperatures. Cancer Res 44:5517–5521

González González D (1994) ESHO 1-85: Radiotherapy versus radiotherapy plus hyperthermia in locally advanced breast cancer. Joint Meeting of the European Society for Radiation Biology and Hyperthermic Oncology, June 1–4, 1994, Abstracts, p 17

Hahn GM (1982) Hyperthermia and cancer. Plenum, New York
Hahn GM, Shiu EC (1986) Adaption to low pH modifies thermal and thermo-chemical response of mammalian cells. Int J Hyperthermia 4:379–388
Hall EJ, Roizin-Towle L (1984) Biological effects of heat. Cancer Res 44:4708–4713
Hall EJ (1988) Radiobiology for the radiologist. Lippincott, Philadelphia
Hanson DF, Murphy PA, Silicano R, Shin HS (1983) The effect of temperature on the activation of thymocytes by interleukin 1 and 2. J Immunol 130 (1):216–221
Henderson IC, Harris JR, Kinne DW, Hellman S (1989) Cancer of the breast. In: DeVita VT, Hellman S, Rosenberg SA (eds) Cancer: principles and practice of oncology, 3rd edn. Lippincott, Philadelphia, pp 1242–1268
Henk JM (1986) Late results of trial of hyperbaric oxygen and radiotherapy in head and neck cancer: a rationale for hypoxic cell sensitizers? Int J Radiat Oncol Biol Phys 12:1339–1341
Henle KJ, Dethlefsen LA (1978) Heat fractionation and thermotolerance. A review. Cancer Res 38:1843–1851
Henle KJ, Roti-Roti JL (1988) Response of cultured mammalian cells to hyperthermia. VSP, Utredit, pp 57–82
Herman TS, Teicher BA, Jochelson M, Clark J, Svensson G, Coleman CN (1988) Rationale for use of local hyperthermia with radiation therapy and selected anticancer drugs in locally advanced human malignancies. Int J Hyperthermia 4:143–158
Herman TS, Jochelson MS, Teicher BA, Scott PJ, Hansen J, Clark JR, Pfeffer MR, Gelwan LE, Molnar-Griffin BJ, Fraser SM, Svennson G, Bornstein BA, Ryan L, Coleman CN (1989) A phase I-II trial of cisplatin, hyperthermia and radiation in patients with locally advanced malignancies. Int J Radiat Oncol Biol Phys 17:1273–1279
Herman TS, Teicher BA, Holden SA (1990) Trimodality therapy (drug/hyperthermia/radiation) with BCNU or mitomycin C. Int J Radiat Oncol Biol Phys 18:375–382
Hoeckel M, Schlenger K, Knoop C, Vaupel P (1991) Oxygenation of carcinomas of the uterine cervix: evaluation by computerized O_2 tension measurements. Cancer Res. 51:3316–3322
Hofman P, Knol RGF, Lagendijk JJW, Schipper J (1989) Thermoradiotherapy of primary breast carcinoma. Int J Hyperthermia 5:1–11
Holahan EV, Highfield DP, Holahan PK, Dewey WC (1984) Hyperthermic killing and hyperthermic radiosensitization in Chinese hamster ovary cells: effects of pH and thermal tolerance. Radiat Res 97:108–131
Issels RD, Prenninger SW, Nagele A, Boehm E, Sauer H, Jauch K-W, Denecke H, Berger H, Peter K, Wilmanns W (1990) Ifosfamide plus etoposide combined with regional hyperthermia in patients with locally advanced sarcomas: a phase-II study. J Clin Oncology 8:1818–1829
Issels RD, Mittermüller J, Gerl A, Simon W, Ortmaier A, Denzlinger C, Sauer H, Wilmanns W (1991) Improvement of local control by regional hyperthermia combined with systemic chemotherapy (ifosfamide plus etoposide) in advanced sarcomas: updated report on 65 patients. J Cancer Res Clin Oncol 117 [Suppl IV]:S141–S147
Issels RD (1995) Klinikum Großhadern, Department of Medical Oncology, Marchioninistr. 15, D-81337 München, Germany (Protocol)
Jordan A, Wust P, Scholz R, Vogl T, Felix R (1996) Heat sensitivity of the human colonic adenocarcinoma cell lines WiDr and SW620. Int J Hyperthermia (in review)
Jung H (1986) A generalized concept for cell killing by heat. Radiat Res 106:56–72
Jung H (1989) Step-down heating of CHO cells at 37.5–39°C. Int J Hyperthermia 5:665–673
Jung H, Dikomey E, Zywietz F (1986) Ausmaß und zeitliche Entwicklung der Thermoresistenz und deren Einfluß auf die Strahlenempfindlichkeit von soliden

Transplantationstumoren. In: Lokale Hyperthermie Streffer C, Herbst M, Schwabe H (eds) Deutscher Ärzte-Verlag, Cologner
Jung H, Dikomey E (1987) Some basic effects in cellular thermobiology. In: Issels RD, Wilmanns W (eds) Application of hyperthermia in the treatment of cancer Springer, Berlin Heidelberg New York, pp 104–112
Kapp DS (1986) Site and disease selection for hyperthermia clinical trials. Int J Hyperthermia 2:139–156
Konsensus der CAO, AIO und ARO zur adjuvanten Therapie bei Kolon- und Rektumkarzinom vom 11.3.1994. Onkologie 17:291–293
Krook JE, Moertel CG, Gunderson LL, Wieand HS, Collins RT, Beart RW, Kubista TP, Poon MA, Meyers WC, Mailliard JA, Twito DI, Morton RF, Veeder MH, Witzig TE, Cha S, Vidyarthi SC (1991) Effective surgical adjuvant therapy for high-risk rectal carcinoma. N Engl J Med 324
Laszlo A, Wright W, Roti RJ (1992) Initial characterization of heat-induced excess nuclear proteins in HeLa cells. J Cell Physiol 151:519–524
Leopold KA, Dewhirst MW, Sammulski TV, Dodge RK, George SL, Blivin JL, Prosnitz LR, Oleson JR (1993) Cumulative minutes with T_{90} greater than $Temp_{Index}$ is predictive of response of superficial malignancies to hyperthermia and radiation. Int J Radiat Oncol Biol Phys 25:841–847
Lindegaard JC, Overgaard J (1987) Factors of importance for the development of the step-down heating effect in a C3H mammary carcinoma in vivo. Int J Hyperthermia 3:79–91
Lindholm C-E, Kjellen E, Nilsson P, Hertzman S (1987) Microwave-induced hyperthermia and radiotherapy in human superficial tumours: clinical results with a comparative study of combined treatment versus radiotherapy alone. Int J Hyperthermia 3:393–411
Lindquist S, Craig EA (1988) The heat shock proteins. Annu Rev Genet 22:631–636
Mak AC, Rich TA, Schultheiss TE, Kavanagh B, Ota DM, Romsdahl MM (1994) Late complications of postoperative radiation therapy for cancer of the rectum and rectosigmoid. Int J Radiat Oncol Biol Phys 28:597–603
Meyer JL (1984) The clinical efficacy of localized hyperthermia. Cancer Res 44:4745–4751
Mendenhall WM, Million RR, Bova FJ (1984) Analysis of time-dose factors in clinically positive neck nodes treated with irradiation alone in squamous cell carcinoma of the head and neck. Int J Radiat Oncol Biol Phys 10:639–643
Mills MD, Meyn RE (1981) Effects of hyperthermia on repair of radiation-induced DNA strand breaks. Radiat Res 87:314–328
Mills MD, Meyn RE (1983) Hyperthermic potentiation of unrejoined DNA strand breaks following irradiation. Radiat Res 95:327–338
Minsky BD, Kemeny N, Cohen AM, Enker WE, Kelsen DP, Reichman B, Saltz L, Sigurdson ER, Frankel J (1991) Preoperative high-dose leucovorin/5-fluoruracil and radiation therapy for unresectable rectal cancer. Cancer 67:2859–2866
Minsky BD, Cohen AM, Kemeny N, Enker WE, Kelsen DP, Schwartz G, Saltz L, Dougherty J, Frankel J, Wiseberg J (1993) Pre-operative combined 5-FU low-dose leucovorin and sequential radiation therapy for unresectable rectal cancer. Int J Radiat Oncol Biol Phys 25:821–827
Mohiuddin M, Ahmad N, Marks G (1993) A selective approach to adjunctive therapy for cancer of the rectum. Int J Radiat Oncol Biol Phys 27:765–772
Molls M, Feldmann HJ (1991) Clinical investigations on blood flow in malignant tumors of the pelvis and the abdomen. In: Vaupel P, Jain RK (eds) Tumor blood supply and metabolic microenvironment: characterization and implications for therapy Fischer, Stuttgart, Funktionsanalyse biologischer Systeme Bd.20, pp 143–153
Molls M, Fink U (1994) Perioperative radiotherapy +/– chemotherapy in rectal cancer. Ann Oncol 5

Mooibroek J, Dikomey E, Zywietz F (1988) Thermotolerance kinetics and growth rate changes in the R1H tumour heated at 43°C. Int J Hyperthermia 4:677–686

Multhoff G, Botzler C, Wiesnet M, Issels RD (1994) Selective cell surface expression of an immunogenic determinant associated with a 72kd heat shock protein (HSP). Joint Meeting of the European Society for Radiation Biology and Hyperthermic Oncology, June 1–4, 1994, Abstracts, p 127

Ng TC, Majors AW, Vijayakumar S et al (1989) Human neoplasm pH and response to radiation therapy: P-31 MR spectroscopy studies in situ. Radiology 170:875–878

Nielsen OS, Henle KJ, Overgaard J (1982) Arrhenius analysis of survival curves from thermotolerant and step-down heated L1A2 cells in vitro. Radiat Res 91:468–482

Nielsen OS, Overgaard J, Kamura T (1983) Influence of thermotolerance on the interaction between hyperthermia and radiation in a solid tumour in vivo. Br J Radiology 56:267–273

Niitsu Y, Watanabe N, Umeno H, Sone H, Neda H, Yamauchi N, Maeda M, Urushizaki I (1988) Synergistic effects of recombinant human tumor necrosis factor and hyperthermia on in vitro cytotoxicity and artificial metastasis. Cancer Res 48:654–657

Oleson JR, Sim DA, Manning MR (1984) Analysis of prognostic variables in hyperthermia treatment of 161 patients. Int J Radiat Oncol Biol Phys 10:2231–2239

Overgaard (1980) Simultaneous and sequential hyperthermia and radiation treatment of an experimental tumor and its surrounding normal tissue in vivo. Int J Radiat Oncol Biol Phys 6:1507–1517

Overgaard J (1981) Fractionated radiation and hyperthermia: experimental and clinical studies. Cancer 48:1116–1123

Overgaard J (1987) Some problems related to the clinical use of thermal isoeffect doses. Int J Hyperthermia 3:329–336

Overgaard J (1989) The current and potential role of hyperthermia in radiotherapy. Int J Radiat Oncol Biol Phys 16:535–549

Overgaard J (1990) Clinical trials with hyperthermia and radiotherapy. In: Gautherie M (ed) Biological basis of oncologic thermotherapy. Springer, Berlin Heidelberg New York, pp 57–62

Overgaard J (1994) ESHO 3-85: assessment of the efficacy of hyperthermia as adjuvant to radiation therapy in the treatment of metastatic malignant melanomas. Joint Meeting of European Societies of Radiation Biology (ESRB) and Hyperthermic Oncology (ESHO), 1–4 June 1994, Amsterdam, Abstract Book, p 19

Perez CA, Kuske RR, Emami B, Fineberg B (1986) Irradiation alone or combined with hyperthermia in the treatment of recurrent carcinoma of the breast in the chest wall: a nonrandomized comparison. Int J Hyperthermia 2:179–188

Perez CA, Emami B, Kuske RR, Hornback N, Pajak T, Kasdorf P (1989a): Irradiation and hyperthermia in the treatment of recurrent carcinoma of the breast in the chest wall MIR and RTOG experience. In: Sugahara T, Saito M (eds) Hyperthermic oncology 1988, vol 2, Taylor and Francis, London, 422–425

Perez CA, Gillespie B, Pajak T, Hornback NB, Emami B, Rubin P (1989b) Quality assurance problems in clinical hyperthermia and their impact on therapeutic outcome: a report by the Radiation Therapy Oncology Group. Int J Radiat Oncol Biol Phys 16:551–558

Peters LJ, Ang KK, Thames HD (1988) Accelerated fractionation in the radiation treatment of head and neck cancer. Acta Oncologica 27:185–194

Pilepich MV, Jones KG, Emami BN, Perez CA, Fields JN, Myerson RJ (1989) Interaction of bleomycin and hyperthermia – results of a clinical pilot study. Int J Radiat Oncol Biol Phys 16:211–213

Reinhold HS, Endrich B (1986) Invited review: tumour microcirculation as a target for hyperthermia. Int J Hyperthermia 2:111–137

Robins HL, Cohen JD, Schmitt CL (1993) Phase I clinical trial of carboplatin and 41.8°C whole-body hyperthermia in cancer patients. J Clin Oncol 9:1787–1794
Roti-Roti JL, Winward RT (1978) The effects of hyperthermia on the protein-to-DNA ratio of isolated HeLa cell chromatin. Radiat Res 74:159–169
Roti-Roti JL, Laszlo A (1988) The effects of hyperthermia on cellular macromolecules. In: Urano M, Douple E (eds) Thermal effects on cells and tissues. VSP, Utrecht, pp 13–56
Rouesse J, Friedman S, Sevin DM et al (1987) Pre-operative induction chemotherapy in the treament of locally advanced soft tissue sarcomas. Cancer 60:296–301
Sapareto SA (1988) Practical concepts of thermal dose. In: Urano M, Douple E (eds) Thermal effects on cells and tissues. VSP, Utrecht, pp 201–212
Sapozink MD (1986) The application of thermal dose in clinical trials. Int J Hyperthermia 2:157–164
Sardi JF, DiPaola GR, Giaroli A, Sananes C, Rueda NG, Cachau A, Burlando S (1990) Results of a phase-II trial with neoadjuvant chemotherapy in carcinoma of the cervix uteri. Gynecol Oncol. 31:245–261
Scher HI (1990) Chemotherapy for invasive bladder cancer: neoadjuvant versus adjuvant. Sem Oncol 17:555–565
Schlag P, Riess H (1994) Virchow-Klinikum, Departments of Surgery and Medical Oncology, Lindenberger Weg 80, D-13122 Berlin, Germany (Protocol)
Scott RS, Johnson RJR, Kowal H, Krishnamsetty M, Story K, Clay L (1983) Hyperthermia in combination with radiotherapy: a review of five years' experience in the treatment of superficial tumors. Int J Radiat Oncol Biol Phys 9:1327–1333
Scott R, Gillespie B, Perez CA, Hornback NB, Johnson R, Emami B, Bauer M, Pakuris E (1988) Hyperthermia in combination with definitive radiation therapy: results of a phase-I/II PTOG study. Int J Radiat Oncol Biol Phys 15:711–716
Seebass M, Sullivan D, Wust P, Deuflhard P, Felix R (1993) The Berlin hyperthermia treatment planning program. Konrad-Zuse-Zentrum, Preprint SC 93-35
Semmler W, Gademann G, Bachert-Baumann P, Zabel H-J, Lorenz WJ, Kaick G van (1988) Monitoring human tumor response to therapy by means of P-31 MR spectroscopy. Radiology 166:533–539
Shrivastava PN, Saylor TK, Matloubieh AY, Paliwal BR (1988) Hyperthermia quality assurance results. Int J Hyperthermia 4:25–37
Song CW (1984) Effect of local hyperthermia on blood flow and microenvironment: a review. Cancer Research 44:4721–4730
Spiro IJ, Denman DL, Dewey WC (1982) Effects of hyperthermia on CHO DNA polymerases α and β. Radiat Res 89:134–149
Strauss LG (1991) Positron emission tomography (PET) for therapy management. In: Breit A (ed) Advanced radiation therapy: tumor response monitoring and treatment planning. Springer, Berlin Heidelberg New York, pp 25–28
Streffer C (1985) Review: metabolic changes during and after hyperthermia. Int J Hyperthermia 1:305–319
Streffer C, Beuningen D van (1987) The biological basis for tumour therapy by hyperthermia and radiation. In: Streffer C (ed) Hyperthermia and the therapy of malignant tumors. Springer, Berlin Heidelberg New York, pp 24–70
Streffer C (1990) Biological basis of thermotherapy (with special reference to oncology), In: Gautherie M (ed) Biological basis of oncologic thermotherapy. Springer, Berlin Heidelberg New York, pp 1–71
Suit HD (1982) Potential for improving survival rates for the cancer patient by increasing the efficacy of treatment of the primary lesion. Cancer 50:1227–1234
Thames HD, Hendry JH (1987) Fractionation in radiotherapy. Taylor and Francis, London
Turner PF (1984) Regional hyperthermia with an annular phased array. IEEE Trans Biomed Eng 31:106–114

Urbon J, Murthy AK, Taylor SG, Hendrickson FR, Lanzl LH (1990) Retrospective analysis of hyperthermia for use in the palliative treatment of cancer: a multimodality evaluation. Int J Radiat Oncol Biol Phys 18:155–163

Valdagni R, Amichetti M (1993) Report of long-term follow-up in a randomized trial comparing radiation therapy and radiation therapy plus hyperthermia to metastatic lymph nodes in stage-IV head and neck patients. Int J Radiat Oncol Biol Phys 28:163–169

Valdgni R, Amichetti M, Pani G (1988a) Radical radiation alone versus radical radiation plus microwave hyperthermia for N3 (TNM-UICC) neck nodes: a prospective randomized clinical trial. Int J Radiat Oncol Biol Phys 15:13–24

Valdagni R, Liu F-F, Kapp DS (1988b) Important prognostic factors influencing outcome of combined radiation and hyperthermia. Int J Radiat Oncol Biol Phys 15:959–972

van Dijk JDP, Gonzales-Gonzales D, Blank LECM (1989) Deep local hyperthermia with a four aperture array system of large waveguide radiators. Results of simulation and clinical application. In: Hyperthermic oncology 1988, vol 1: Summary papers, Sugahara T, Saito M (eds) Taylor and Francis, London, pp 573–575

van der Zee J, Treurniet-Donker AD, The SK, Helle PA, Seldenrath JJ, Meerwaldt JH, Wijaalen AJ, Berg AP, van den, Rhoon GC, van Broekmeyer-Reurink MP, Reinhold HS (1988) Low-dose reirradiation in combination with hyperthermia: a palliative treatment for patients with breast cancer in previously irradiated areas. Int J Radiat Oncol Biol Phys 15:1407–1413

van der Zee J, Broekmeyer-Reurink MP, Berg AP, van den, Geel BN van, Jansen RFM, Kroon BBR, Wijk J van, Hagenbeek A (1989) Temperature distribution and pH changes during hyperthermic regional isolation perfusion. Eur J Cancer Clin Oncol 25:1157–1163

van der Zee J, Gonzalez-Gonzalez D, van Putten WLJ, Hart AAM, Koper PCM, Treurniet-Donker AD, Wijnmaalen AJ, van Dijk JDP, van Rhoon GC (1993) Hyperthermia combined with radiotherapy in deep seated tumors-a phase III trial. In: Hyperthermia in clinical oncology, November 25–27, 1993, Book of Abstracts, p 41

Vaupel P, Kallinowski F, Okunieff P (1989) Blood flow, oxygen and nutrient supply, and metabolic microenvironment of human tumors: a review Cancer Res 49:6449–6465

Vaupel P (1990) Pathophysiological mechanisms of hyperthermia in cancer therapy. In: Gautherie M (ed) Biological bassis of oncologic thermotherapy Springer, Berlin Heidelberg New York, pp 73–134

Vaupel P, Kallinowski F, Okunieff P (1989) Blood flow, oxygen and nutrient supply and metabolic microenvironment of human tumors: a review. Cancer Res 49:6449–6465

Vernon CC, van der Zee J, Lui FF (1994) Collaborative phase-III superficial hyperthermia trial. Joint Meeting of European Societies of Radiation Biology (ESRB) and Hyperthermic Oncology (ESHO), June 1–4, 1994, Amsterdam, Abstract Book, p 16

Waterman FM, Nerlinger RE, Moylan DJ, Leeper DB (1987) Response of human tumor blood flow to local hyperthermia. Int J Radiat Oncol Biol Phys 13:75–82

Watson ER, Halnan KE, Dische S, Saunders MI, Code IS, McEwen JB, Wienik G, Perricis DJ, Sutherland I (1978) Hyperbaric oxygen and radiotherapy: a Medical Research Council trail in carcinoma of the cervix. Br J Radiol 51:879–887

Wendt TG, Hartenstein RC, Wustrow TPU, Lissner J (1989) Cisplatin, flourouracil with leucovorin calcium enhancement, and synchronous accelerated radiotherapy in the management of locally advanced head and neck cancer: a phase-II study. J Clinical Oncology 7:471–476

Willett CG, Shellito PC, Tepper JE, Eliseo R, Convery K, Wood WC (1991) Intraoperative electron beam radiation therapy for recurrent locally advanced rectal or rectosigmoid carcinoma. Cancer 67:1504–1508
Wilson GD, McNally NJ, Dische S, Saunders MI, Des Rochers C, Lewis AA, Bennett MH (1988) Measurement of cell kinetics in human tumours in vivo using bromodeoxyuridine incorporation and flow cytometry. Br J Cancer 58:423–431
Wong RSL, Dewey WC (1982) Molecular studies on the hyperthermic inhibition of DNA synthesis in Chinese hamster ovary cells. Radiat Res 92:370–395
Wust P, Fähling H, Jordan A, Nadobny J, Seebass J, Seebass M, Felix R (1994) Development and testing of SAR-visualizing phantoms for quality control in RF hyperthermia. Int J Hyperthermia 10:127–142
Wust P, Stahl H, Löffel J, Seebass M, Riess H, Felix R (1995a) Clinical, physiological and anatomical determinants for temperature elevations in radiofrequency hyperthermia. Int J Hyperthermia 11:151–167
Wust P, Seebass M, Nadobny J, Felix R (1995b) Electromagnetic deep heating technology. In: Seegenschmiedt MH, Fessenden P, Vernon CC (eds) Principles and practice of thermoradiotherapy and thermochemotherapy. Springer, Berlin Heidelberg New York: 219–251
Wust P, Meier T, Seebass M, Fähling H, Petermann K, Felix R (1995c) Noninvasive prediction of SAR distributions with an electro-optical E-field sensor. Int J Hyperthermia 11:295–310
Wust P, Fähling Felix RH, Rahman S, Issels RD, Feldmann H, van Rhoon G, van der Zee J (1995d) Quality control of the SIGMA applicator using a lamp phantom: a four-center comparison. Int J Hyperthermia 11:755–767
Wust P, Stahl H, Dieckmann K, Scheller S, Löffel J, Riess H, Jahnke V, Bier J, Felix R (1996a) Local hyperthermia of N2/N3 cervical lymph node metastases: correlation of technical and thermal parameters with response. Int J Radiat Oncol Biol Phys 34:635–646
Wust P, Nadobny J, Seebass M, Deuflhard P, Mönich G, Felix R (1996b) Simulation studies promote technological development of phased-array radiofrequency hyperthermia. Int J Hyperthermia (in press)

Adjuvant Treatment of Colon and Rectal Cancer: Impact of Chemotherapy, Radiotherapy, and Immunotherapy on Routine Postsurgical Patient Management

K.H. Link[1], L. Staib[1], E.-D. Kreuser[2], and H.G. Beger[1] for the Forschungsgruppe Onkologie Gastrointestinaler Tumoren (FOGT)

[1] Department of General Surgery, University Hospital of Ulm, Steinhövelstraße 9, 89075 Ulm, Germany
[2] Department of Hematology and Oncology, Benjamin Franklin University, Hindenburgdamm 30, 12200 Berlin, Germany

Abstract

Colon cancer patients with UICC stage III or T4 N0 M0 stage II should receive postoperative adjuvant therapy, since relapse rates are high and surgical outcome has been improved by adjuvant treatment. The standard treatment is 5-fluourouracil plus levamisole; an alternative option is the combination of 5-fluourouracil and folinic acid. Stage II (T3 N0 M0) colon cancer patients should not receive adjuvant treatment outside of studies. Rectal cancer patients of stage II or III should receive postoperative radiochemotherapy with 45–54.4 Gy and 5-fluourouracil as standard treatment. Patients not eligible for radiotherapy may receive adjuvant chemotherapy only. Studies need to be conducted to improve adjuvant therapy in colorectal cancer. All qualified patients should be treated within these studies requiring sufficient patient numbers, as well as comparable surgical procedures, proper patient selection and stratification criteria, drug and dose intensities.

Intraportal infusion may be as effective as systemic adjuvant treatment; the tumor type and stage for which benefit from this kind of treatment is consistently significant needs to be defined, since intraportal infusion of all resectable colorectal cancers is overtreatment.

Both surgery and histopathological staging may be improved in some centers, and these require standardization and quality control.

Introduction

The adjuvant treatment of colon and rectum cancers, the second most common malignancy among human cancers, was not established as a standard procedure until 1987. Many studies using 5-fluorourocil (5-FU) and other drugs had been conducted, but with negative results. The only study indicating a benefit from adjuvant postoperative therapy was published by the Gastrointestinal Tumor Study Group for Rectal Cancer (GITSG 1985, 1986; Douglass 1987; Douglass et al. 1988; Buyse et al. 1988). This study clearly indicated that the combination of local irradiation and systemic chemotherapy reduces relapse rates and increases survival in patients with rectal cancer undergoing surgery with curative intend. After a history of disappointments, Windle and coworkers (1987) were the first to demonstrate an adjuvant treatment effect in colon and rectal cancer patients with postoperative systemic treatment using 5-FU+levamisole (Ergamisol). Since then the treatment concepts with radiochemotherapy for rectal cancer patients (Krook et al. 1991) and 5-FU+levamisole for colon cancer (Moertel et al. 1990) have been proven in independent studies, and adjuvant therapy has become established in colon and rectal cancer. The treatment modalities that have proven to be active are recommended for the disease stages whose spontaneous postoperative courses are significantly improved by adjuvant therapy (NIH 1990; Beger et al. 1994). Efforts have since been started to amend the adjuvant treatment outcome. Many studies have been inaugurated with the aim either to reproduce the previous results by the same treatment or to test new drug combinations. Most of these studies have respected the different biology of colon and rectal cancers. The two tumor entities received systemic treatment, and rectal cancers, in addition, were treated by pelvic irradiation. As a result of these scientific efforts the outcome in surgical treatment of colorectal cancer has been improved, and multimodal treatment has been substantially increased, at least in the United States (Steele 1994).

We describe the indications and therapeutic options for adjuvant treatment, report the established results as a base for routine treatment, and analyze the newest tendencies regarding their impact on standard treatment strategies of the future.

Epidemiology and Tumor Biology

Incidence, Survival Rates

Large bowel cancer is the second most common malignancy in the Western World (Silverberg and Lubera 1989). In 1989, 151 000 new colorectal carcinoma patients were diagnosed in the United States, and 61 000 patients died of their disease (Silverberg and Lubera 1989). The incidence of colon cancers in the United States (107 000 per year) is 2.4 times higher than that of rectal cancers (44 000 per year). The average patient age at diagnosis is 69.9 years for colon and 67.1 for rectal cancer (Steele 1994). The overall 5-year survival rates in the United States are 50%–55% for all stages of colon cancers and 44%–54% for rectal cancers (Steele 1994). There is no doubt that complete surgical resection is the standard therapy with the only option of cure in 10%–95% of patients (MacDonald 1987). The 5-year survival rates after curative resection clearly depend on the tumor stage and are reported to be overall 63%–80% in colon cancer (Minsky et al. 1988) and 67% in rectal cancer (Bethune 1987).

Survival rates after R0 resection decrease with increasing primary tumor penetration through the bowel wall and with lymph node metastasis. The UICC stage dependent survival rates after complete tumor resection are listed in Table 1. Up to 100% of resectable patients with the earliest stage (I) have an option for cure. The 5-year survival rates of colon cancer stage II (63%–90%) are higher than those in stage II rectal cancer (51%–69%). The prognosis in stage III is comparable for colon and rectal cancer (33%–76% vs. 30%–62%). The stage-dependent crude 5-year survival rates of rectal cancer patients ($n = 927$, 1978–1994) treated in the Department of General Surgery at Ulm University are 91% (I), 69% (II), 35% (III), and 1% (IV). Obviously there is great variation in reported survival rates within each stage, providing evidence that surgical standards may differ although staging is identical. Unfortunately, fewer than 70% of patients presenting with large bowel cancer have an option for resection with curative intend. Among colorectal cancer patients 30% have synchronous metastatic disease, and only 0%–22% of these are curable (Russell et al. 1984; MacDonald 1987; Hermanek 1989). While the overall survival rates in North America have risen minimally for colorectal cancer over recent decades (Minsky et al. 1988; Silverberg and Lubera 1989), survival after resection has improved significantly in German centers, with an increase in 5-year actuarial survival rates for resected colon cancer patients from 48% to 68% and from 42% to 66% for rectal cancer patients (Gall and Hermanek 1992). Similar trends have been observed in the United Kingdom for colon but not for rectal cancer (Slaney et al. 1991).

Table 1. Stage-dependent actuarial 5-year survival rates after curative resection of colon and rectal cancers

Tumor	Stage	5-year survival rates		
Colon	I	92%–93%[a]	100%[d]	70%[e]
	II	64%–90%[a]	72%–89%[d]	63%[e]
	III	33%–76%[a]	37%–65%[d]	46%[e]
	IV	<5%[b]	0%–19%[d]	12%[e]
Rectum	I	91%[c]	80%–100%[d]	70%[e]
	II	69%[c]	51%–67%[d]	55%[e]
	III	35%–62%[c]	30%–55%[d]	41%[e]
	IV	<5%[b]	0%–19%[d]	12%[e]

[a] Minsky et al. (1988)
[b] Soybel et al. (1987)
[c] Bethune (1987)
[d] Hermanek (1989)
[e] Steele (1994)

Prognostic Factors and Patterns of Relapse

The prognosis of nonmetastasized colorectal cancers clearly depends on whether the tumor can be resected. In colon cancers of stages I–III, the resectability rate may be 96.5% (Hermanek et al. 1994). In the case of resectability, the R classification is a significant surgical therapy related prognostic factor. R0 resections may be obtained in 61%–81% of primarily resectable patients and differ within surgical centers (Hermanek et al. 1994, 1995).

Primary tumor stage, lymph node metastasis, and distant metastasis are the most established pathological (tumor-related) prognostic factors, and these are reflected in the UICC classification system. As seen in Tables 2 and 3, the events of serosal invasion and lymph node metastasis have a significant effect on the incidence of relapses that determine the further patient course. In keeping with these literature results, the prognosis of our colorectal cancer patients also clearly depends on UICC stages. Between January 1978 and

Table 2. Stage-dependent relapse rates after curative resection of colon cancer

Duke stage[a]	T	N	M	UICC stage[b]	Relapse (%)	
					a[b]	b[c]
A	1	0	0	I	1	8
B_1	2	0	0	I	9	7
B_2	3	0	0	II	32	14
B_3	4	0	0	II	61	42
C_1	1–2	1–3	0	III	45	22
C_2	3	1–3	0	III	60	51
C_3	4	1–3	0	III	88	67

[a] Modified according to Gunderson (1976)
[b] $n = 550$, Russell et al. (1984)
[c] $n = 188$, Minsky et al. (1988)

Table 3. Stage-dependent relapse rates after curative resection of rectal cancer

Duke stage[a]	T	N	M	UICC	Relapse[b] (%)
A	1	0	0	I	12
B_1	2	0	0	I	19
B_2	3	0	0	II	32
C_1	1–2	1–3	0	III	36
C_2	3	1–3	0	III	64

[a] Modified according to Astler-Coller (1954)
[b] $n = 430$, Bethune (1987)

September 1995, 1981 patients were treated at the Department of General Surgery, University of Ulm, for colon and rectal cancer. Colon cancer patients (n = 1019) had the following stages: stage I 15%, II 38%, III 23%, IV 21%, unknown 2%; in rectal cancer patients (n = 962) the stage distributions were I 24%, II 25%, III 20%, IV 17%, and unknown 13%. The median age was 64 years in both colon (range 18–94 years) and rectal cancer (range 23–91 years). The resection rate was 95% (colon) and 90.4% (rectum). Of the 1162 colorectal cancer patients primarily resected for cure at our Department 33% developed progressive disease during their postoperative follow-up. The relapse rates in stage I were 13%, II 34%, and III 61%. Only 6% of patients with relapse remained free of recurrence after surgical removal of the recurrent tumor. Thus the cure rate is clearly limited when either local relapse or distant metastasis occurs (Safi et al. 1993; Kelly and Daly 1992). The only option to improve the fate of advanced stage colorectal cancer patients is an effective adjuvant treatment in addition to optimal primary tumor surgery. When adjuvant therapy is chosen as part of a multimodal treatment, it is essential to select only patients with a high risk for disease progression to prevent overtreatment. Currently the UICC classification is the only basis for patient selection. In addition to the UICC system, the impact of a variety of prognostic factors determined by the biology of the tumor and characteristics of the host still need to be confirmed (Siewert and Fink 1992; O'Connell et al. 1992b). Stage-dependent relapse rates differ significantly between institutes. These results underline the recent caveat that the surgeon himself may also be a significant prognostic factor (McArdle and Hole 1991; Hermanek et al. 1994, 1995).

Colon and rectal cancers have a different biology. This fact should be respected whenever new adjuvant therapy strategies are being developed. When comparing all resectable cancers of the colon and rectum, relapse rates seem to be higher in rectal than in colon cancer (Metzger et al. 1987; Kelly and Daly 1992). Colon and rectal cancer have a different pattern of progression, influenced by the pathways of metastases, on the one hand, and surgical limits, on the other. In colon cancer, metastases are spread via the portal venous system and the lymphatic drainage or by intraperitoneal tumor dissemination. In rectal cancer, depending on the location of the primary tumor, tumor cells metastasize either hematogenously via the portal system or via the inferior vena cava, or along the centripedal and lateral lymphatic network (Weiss and Ward 1991).

The tumor cell deposits in lymphatic vessels of the mesenterium ("lateral and distal spread"), in addition to direct continuity of tumor tissue in and through the bowel wall may well be responsible for local relapses (Heald and Karanjia 1992). Transperitoneal spread may cause peritoneal carcinosis as in colon cancer (Heald and Karanjia 1992). Implantation of tumor cell deposits during surgery, especially if the tumor is disrupted, may be a major reason for local relapse (Heald and Karanjia 1992; Hermanek et al. 1994, 1995).

Large prospective randomized adjuvant trials register the first sites of relapse in untreated control groups. In these reports the liver was the first site of relápse in colon cancer patients (16.2%), followed by the peritoneum (8.9%), extrahepatic metastasis (7.6%), and local relapse (3.9%). The high rate of local relapse as first site of progression in rectal cancer patients (24.5%) is due to the fact that extensive surgical resection of the primary tumor with its lymphatic network in the pelvis is surgically more limited than in surgery of colon cancers. In rectal cancer patients the liver (11.4%) and lungs (12.0%) as first sites of relapse are second to local relapses (Wolmark et al. 1988; Fisher et al. 1988). The bone, brain, and extra-abdominal lymph nodes are extremely rare first sites of metastatic disease manifestation in colon cancer, while 1%–1.6% of rectal cancer patients have metastases in the bone, soft tissue, and other locations as first sites of relapse (Fisher et al. 1988; Wolmark et al. 1988).

Isolated Local and Distant Relapse/Metastases

Tumor relapses may be biologically confined to the relapse site. This biological behavior justifies extensive surgical procedures for removing recurrence or metastases, especially in cases of anastomotic relapses and isolated liver metastases. However, since the surgical cure rate in these relapsed cases is too low, a prospective regional intensive adjuvant treatment started after primary tumor removal and directed to the most relevant first sites of relapse may influence the progression rate and pattern for the benefit of the patient. Radiation or intraportal/intra-arterial chemotherapy to the liver could be effective treatment options in this sense. These treatments might be applied either alone or in combination with systemic treatment. To decide on the modality of regional therapy and the target site, the biological relevance of isolated local or distant relapses of colon and of rectal cancers must be well respected.

Progressive colon cancer patients rarely present with isolated locoregional disease, such as anastomotic recurrence, regional tumor growth in the tumor bed, or regional lymph nodes. As indicated in Table 4, these recurrence sites

Table 4. Local and combined local/distant relapses after curative resection of colon and rectal cancers

Tumor	UICC stage	Local only	Combined local/distant
Colon	I	7%–8%[a]	7%–8%[a]
	II	0%–4%[a]	14%–43%[a]
	III	0%–7%[a]	22%–67%[a]
Rectum	I	6%–17%[b]	12%–18%[b]
	II	13%–24%[b]	32%[b]
	III	3%–50%[b]	37%–64%[b]

[a] Minsky et al. (1988)
[b] Bethune (1987)

are often combined with distant metastasis (Minsky et al. 1988; Russell et al. 1984). Isolated liver metastasis is a more frequent event in colon cancer. The liver is the only site of metastasis in 32% of the patients presenting with (synchronous) metastatic disease and in 22% of patients developing (metachronous) disease progression after previous radical primary tumor resection (Russell et al. 1984). Liver failure is the cause of death in 25% of patients with metastatic disease (Taylor 1962).

In rectal cancer there is the risk of both isolated regional recurrence and the evolving of distant metastasis. Local relapses are reported in 6%–64% after radical rectal cancer surgery (Bethune 1987) and can be confined to the pelvis in up to 50% (Table 4).

Even among experienced surgeons the figures of local relapse rates in rectal cancer vary considerably, and in most published controlled adjuvant trails the local recurrence rates of the surgical control arm exceed 20% (range 17%–42%; Pahlman and Glimelius 1992).

Local relapses are a mostly painful cause of death in 20%–25% of relapsed rectal cancer patients (Welch and Donaldson 1979).

Adjuvant Chemotherapy and/or Radiotherapy

Much emphasis has been put on clinical research trying to improve the prognosis of colorectal cancer after initial radical tumor resection (R0). The postoperative course in R0 resected patients can be influenced by chemo-, radio-, and immunotherapy either alone or in combination. When conducting adjuvant treatment, the following biological principles should be respected according to the NIH Consensus Conference (1990):

- Even in case of radical (R0) primary tumor resection occult vital tumor cells can be present either in the circulation (intravascular, intralymphatic), or microscopic tumor cell nests can be manifested as micrometastasis locoregionally or at distant sites.
- Chemotherapy is most effective if the tumor burden is minimal, and cell kinetics are optimal (Goldie and Coldman 1986).
- Adjuvant therapy should be conducted with agents whose effectiveness against the tumor is proven.
- Cytotoxic therapy shows a dose-response relationship and therefore must be administered in maximally tolerated doses, and the duration of therapy must be sufficient to eradicate all tumor cells.
- The risk-benefit ratio for therapy must be favorable for individuals who may remain asymptomatic for their natural life expectancy after tumor resection.

The primary aim of adjuvant therapy should be prolongation of disease-free survival, and the secondary aim is to prevent recurrences and thereby improve quality of life as long as possible. Below, the various strategies of adjuvant therapy in colon and rectal cancer are analyzed and their impact on survival after radical tumor surgery is discussed.

Local Regional Treatments

Local regional adjuvant treatments in colon and rectum cancer, such as radiation therapy, intraportal hepatic infusion, and intraperitoneal therapy, have been advocated to reduce the risk for local spread, avoiding systemic side effects.

In colon cancer, *intraperitoneal* chemotherapy or intraperitoneal treatment with isotopes and total abdominal radiation have been studied by various groups. Since isolated recurrence or metastasis is a rare event, and biologically relevant in colon cancer only in case of liver metastasis, the locoregional (intraperitoneal) treatment concepts have had no major success unless a systemic treatment component was added (Russell et al. 1984; Douglass 1987; Sugarbaker et al. 1985).

Postoperative adjuvant intraperitoneal chemotherapy may be effective after cytoreductive surgery, for example, in malignant pseudomyxoma or in colon cancers with high risk of peritoneal carcinomatosis (Sugarbaker 1991). In rectal cancer, irradiation alone, although of proven benefit in the palliative situation concerning pain and tumor volume reduction (Romsdahl and Withers 1978; Stevens et al. 1976; Fisher et al. 1988; Douglass 1987; Mayer et al. 1989) has no significant adjuvant advantage on survival or formation of distant metastasis (Gunderson 1976; Cummings 1992). Adjuvant *radiation alone*, delivered either before or after surgical resection, may reduce the risk for local recurrence (Fisher et al. 1988; Douglass 1987; Gerard et al. 1988; Bleiberg 1990; Cummings 1992) and, although reduction of mortality could be about 10%, significant prolongation of life by this single treatment is very unlikely (Gray et al. 1991). If, despite these data, the patient or physician rejects chemotherapy and prefers adjuvant radiation treatment only, postoperative radiation is recommended, since only patients at risk with exact tumor staging should receive this single-modality regional treatment (Bleiberg 1990). Although preoperative radiotherapy may reduce relapse rates more effectively, the postoperative surgical morbidity and mortality may be increased (Cedermark et al. 1995), and overtreatment of nonadvanced stages is very likely. To avoid overtreatment a sufficient endosonographic primary tumor staging is mandatory for the indication of preoperative radiotherapy or radiochemotherapy. If patients younger than 80 years receive this treatment, as performed in the Stockholm II trial, preoperative radiotherapy seems to reduce local recurrence rates and extends disease-free suvival significantly (Cedermark et al. 1995).

The only locoregional adjuvant treatment approach that has improved survival significantly in several studies, early postoperative *intraportal infusion* therapy, should be discussed in detail. As mentioned above, the liver is a frequent first site of metastasis in colon and rectal cancers and is the only target organ in 22%–34% (Russell et al. 1984). If liver metastasis is detected early and can be resected, the 5-year survival rate, as reported in a large retrospective collective review, may be 30% (Hughes et al. 1988), and 87% of resected patients who were disease-free at 5 years remained disease-free, with a median follow-up of 12.5 years (Leslie et al. 1995). This experience clearly shows that prevention of liver metastasis can improve the cure rate of resected colon and rectal cancer patients. Since (a) systemic adjuvant therapy with 5-FU alone is ineffective (Buyse et al. 1988), (b) fluoropyrimidines show a clear concentration-response behavior in cytotoxicity at all infusion times (Link et al. 1988), and (c) perioperatively generated intraportal micrometastases receive their supply by the portal vein (Archer and Gray 1990; Ackerman 1994), various groups have tested immediate postoperative intraportal infusion chemotherapy as adjuvant treatment. Most trials have infused 5-FU alone or in combination with mitomycin C (MMC). The results of this adjuvant modality are summarized in Table 5.

In four of eight studies a significant improvement of survival rates was obtained. Since the frequency of liver metastases was significantly reduced in only two of the eight intraportal studies, the adjuvant treatment benefit of intraportal infusion more likely contributes to the systemic treatment compo-

Table 5. Results of intraportal infusion for adjuvant chemotherapy of colon (C) and rectal (R) cancer in control (Cont) and treated (Ther) patients

Reference	*n*	Duke stage	Liver metastases		Relapse		Survival	
			Cont	Ther	Cont	Ther	Cont	Ther
Taylor et al. (1985)	244 CR	A–C	17%	4%*	–	–	–	–*
Gray et al. (1987)	232 C	B, C	–	–	–	–	61%	81*
Metzger et al. (1994)	505 CR	A–C	21%	18%**	45%	39%*	55%	66%*
Ryan et al. (1988)	232 CR	A–C	–	–	–	–	–**	
Wereldsma et al. (1990)	304 CR	A–C	23%	7%*	37%	19%*	66%	73%**
Wolmark et al. (1990)	901 C	A–C	6%	7%**	18%	15%**	73%	81**
Beart et al. (1990)	219 C	B, C	13%	15%**	–	–	68%	68%**
Fielding et al. (1992)	398 CR	A–C	n.s.**		–	–	73%–79%	82%**

* $p \leq 0.05$; ** $p > 0.05$

nent and not to the locoregional approach only (Metzger et al. 1994). Taylor et al. (1985) were the first to show a significant survival benefit, and they also demonstrated a significant reduction in liver metastasis in colon and rectal cancer patients. Metzger et al. (1994) reported that in the SAKK trial, this significant reduction in liver metastasis rate was not achieved; survival, however, was extended to a significant level after 8 years of follow-up. The risk reduction in both the SAKK study and an Australian trial was most pronounced in patients with positive lymph nodes (stage III) and in those with colon cancer (Metzger et al. 1994; Gray et al. 1987). While Fielding et al. (1992) confirmed the survival advantage in the subset of lymph node positive patients, without seeing a significant reduction of liver metastases or increase in overall survival of the whole treated group, Taylor et al. (1985) found a survival advantage in the Duke B colon cancer subcategory but not in rectal cancer or colon cancer Duke C. An improvement in disease-free but not overall survival by intraportal infusion – without significant reduction in liver metastases – was reported by Wolmark for the NSABP in 1990 (Wolmark et al. 1990). This extension of disease-free suvival had finally translated into a significant prolongation of overall-survival (Wolmark et al. 1993a). However, the incidence of liver metastases was not reduced in the NSABP trial, and the liver was the first site of treatment failure in 33% of control group relapses and in 46% of relapses in the group receiving portal vein 5-FU and heparin (Wolmark et al. 1993a). Surprisingly, a Dutch trial reported by Wereldsma et al. (1990) observed a significant reduction in liver metastasis in colorectal cancer patients without impact on survival improvement. Beart et al. (1990) reported neither a reduction in liver metastases nor an improvement in survival rates. The total relapse rate was significantly reduced in two studies (Metzger et al. 1994; Wereldsma et al. 1990). During intraportal infusion anticoagulants were administered to prevent catheter and portal vein thrombosis. The portal infusion of heparin alone or urokinase resulted in no survival or relapse rate differences compared to surgical controls (Fielding et al. 1992; Wereldsma et al. 1990).

The hypothesis that systemic drug levels contribute significantly to the positive adjuvant treatment effect of intraportal infusion of 5-FU with or without MMC is supported indirectly by the observation that intraportal 5-fluodeoxyuridine (5-FUDR) has no impact on intra- or extrahepatic relapse rates or on survival (Schlag et al. 1990). The different results obtained with 5-FU and 5-FUDR intraportal infusion may be due the fact that with 5-FU the hepatic extraction rate is low enough to allow systemic drug levels, while 5-FUDR is nearly completely extracted by the liver (Wagner et al. 1986). The combination of intraportal high and systemic lower 5-FU levels might lead to a significant adjuvant treatment effect, so that intraportal 5-FUDR may be regarded as an exclusively regional treatment, such as radiation in rectal cancer. Most interestingly, in contrast to the intraportal infusion arm, perioperative systemic treatment with 5-FU in the three-arm study of Gray et al. (1987) did not extent survival, indicating that systemic drug levels alone are not sufficient to exert a significant adjuvant effect. Furthermore, experimental studies show that intra-arterial perioperative drug delivery (in addition to intraportal infusion) can reduce liver metastases and extend survival (Sutanto-Ward et al. 1992).

Although portal vein infusion of 5-FU appears to be at least as effective as systemic 5-FU and levamisole (Gray et al. 1991), and a significant risk reduction for death has been demonstrated in a meta-analysis (Piedbois et al. 1995), the contradictary results on the reduction of colorectal liver metastases by intraportal infusion prevented the NIH Consensus Conference to recommend this treatment approach for standard therapy in colon and rectal cancer. In addition, while the long-term overall survival curves after 5-FU plus levamisole in colon cancer remain different (Moertel et al. 1995), those of the SAKK intraportal study converged after 7 years (Laffer 1995). Intraportal infusion with 5-FU MMC is part of prospective randomized trials conducted either by SAKK or the EORTC. Further trials will clarify whether the intraportal route is necessary for perioperative drug delivery (Wolmark et al. 1993a).

Systemic Treatment (Alone or in Combination with Radiotherapy)

Obviously, regional treatments to the major sites of disease recurrence or progression are not sufficient to prolong life after complete resection of colon and rectal cancers, although the biology of disease progression in the postoperative course may be changed. Considering the fact that the major proportion of progressive patients have multilocal metastases, an effective systemic treatment principle, either chemo- or immunotherapy, is a prerequisite for effective adjuvant treatment of both colon and rectal cancers. In each tumor entity the addition of a regional treatment component may enhance the effect of systemic therapy.

Systemic Adjuvant Treatment in Colon Cancer

The history of systemic adjuvant treatment in colon and rectal cancer dates back to 1956, when nitrogen mustard was administered perioperatively in rectal cancer surgery (Mrazek et al. 1959). It remained frustrating until several trials in the late 1980s provided positive results. Up to 1988 many controlled trials testing *adjuvant systemic chemotherapy* in colon and rectal cancer produced no consistant success although noncontrolled studies gave evidence that survival may be improved by adjuvant treatment (Douglass 1987; Buyse et al. 1988). A meta-analysis of systemic 5-FU adjuvant treatment in colorectal cancer resulted in a marginal 5-year survival benefit of 3.4% vs. untreated controls ($p = 0.04$; Buyse et al. 1988), and an update of this review suggested that adjuvant chemotherapy may reduce mortality by about 10%–15% (Gray et al. 1991), which was at a statistically marginally significant level. A major criticism of these studies is the suboptimal dosing and timing of adjuvant treatment. The 5-FU doses/dose intensities in many trials may have been too low. Sufficient dose intensity, however, is the prerequisite for effective systemic chemotherapy (Hryniuk et al. 1987; Arbuck 1989). Timing of the treatment start may also be important. If systemic 5-FU treatment is started in the immediate postoperative phase, an adjuvant treatment effect seems to be possible even with a single 5-FU intravenous treatment (Li and Ross 1976). The impact of 5-FU dose and timing is still hypothetical and needs to be confirmed in appropriate studies.

Since 1987 significant achievements in adjuvant treatment for *colon cancer* have been reported (Table 6). Windle et al. (1987) were the first to obtain a significant survival benefit with immediate perioperative treatment using 5-FU+levamisole compared to untreated controls or to the patients receiving 5-FU only. These authors also showed that levamisole improves antitumor cell immune reactions. Since then two studies have confirmed or supported the adjuvant benefit of 5-FU+levamisole treatment. In addition, sufficient evidence has been provided by several studies that 5-FU modulations with either folinic acid or interferon-alpha prolong disease free and overall survival. Laurie and coworkers tested 5-FU+levamisole vs. levamisole alone or no adjuvant treatment in colorectal carcinoma patients of Duke stage B and C. They came to the conclusion that 5-FU+levamisole reduces cancer recurrence rates significantly. The improvement in overall survival reached significance only for stage C patients treated with levamisole+5-FU in subset analysis (Laurie et al. 1989; Moertel 1992). Subsequently Moertel reported for the Intergroup that treating only colon cancer patients of stage C improves relapse rates and overall survival times to a highly significant level (Moertel et al. 1990). The final analysis of this study with 929 eligible patients followed up for 5 years or more showed that 5-FU+levamisole reduced the recurrence rate by 40% ($p < 0.0001$) and the death rate by 33% ($p = 0.0007$). Levamisole alone had no adjuvant treatment effect and reduced recurrence and death rates by only 2% and 6%, respectively. The adjuvant treatment with 5-FU+levamisole, with few exceptions, had a mild toxicitiy; patient compliance was excellent, and there was no evidence of late side effects (Moertel et al. 1995). Relapses were reduced in all sites but not locoregionally. Since the curves are not convergent after long-term observation, the statement that recurrences are prevented and not delayed, and that death rates are reduced, is highly objective and relevant. Up to now there has been no proven adjuvant treatment benefit of 5-FU+levamisole in colon cancers of Duke stage B (UICC II).

The impact of levamisole in this adjuvant treatment concept remains somewhat unclear and may be due to immuno- or biochemical modulation (Moertel 1992, 1994; Moertel et al. 1995; AbdAlla et al. 1995). Except for the Windle et al. (1987) study no randomized trial has compared 5-FU+levamisole vs. 5-FU alone to test whether the addition of levamisole to 5-FU is important. Levamisole may influence the immune response. As mentioned above, Windle et al. (1987) demonstrated that the anti-colon cancer cellular immune response

Table 6. Results of systemic adjuvant treatment in colon and rectal cancer and of radiochemotherapy in rectal cancer in control (Cont) and treated (Ther) patients

Reference	*n*	Therapy	Relapse		Survival	
			Cont	Ther	Cont	Ther
Colon cancer stage III						
Wolmark et al. (1988)[a,b]	773	5-FU+MeCCNU+VCR	49%	42%*	59%	67%*
Hafström et al. (1990)[c]	205	5-FU+CCNU+VCR	55%	59%	52%	48%
Moertel et al. (1990)[b]	619	5-FU+levamisole	53%	37%*	55%	71%*
Moertel et al. (1995)[b]	619	5-FU+levamisole	56%	39%*	47%	60%*
O'Connell et al. (1993a)[a,b]	309	5-FU+FA	36%	23%*	71%	75%
Wolmark et al. (1993b)[a,b,d]	1041	5-FU+FA	33%	25%*	77%	84%*
Francini et al. (1994)[a,d]	118	5-FU+FA	59%	33%*	43%	69%*
IMPACT (Marsoni 1995)[a,b]	1493	5-FU+FA	30%	22%*	78%	83%*
Rectal cancer stages II und III						
Fisher et al. (1988)[a]	371	5-FU+MeCCNU+VCR	70%	58%*	43%	53%*
Hafström et al. (1990)[c]	77	5-FU+CCNU+VCR	71%	56%	34%	49%
GITSG (1986)[a]	104	5-FU+MeCCNU+RT	53%	29%*	43%	59%*
Krook et al. (1991)[a,d]	204	5-FU+MeCCNU+RT	63%	42%*	47%	58%*
O'Connell et al. (1993b)[a,d]	664	5-FU Cont+RT	44%	33%*	68%	76%*
Colon and rectal cancer stages I–III						
Windle et al. (1987)[a]	96	5-FU+levamisole	–	–	48%	68%*
Laurie et al. (1989)[a,b]	271	5-FU+levamisole	55%	40%*	57%	63%
Ito et al. (1990)[a,d]	149	MMC+carmofur	–	–	66%	79%*
Frasci et al. (1994)[d,e]	108	5-FU+interferon-alpha	53%	35%*	46%	64%*
Metzger et al. (1994)[b]	533	5-FU+MMC i.p.	52%	43%*	55%	66%*
Riethmüller et al. (1994)[b]	189	Mab 17-1A	67%	49%*	49%	64%*

* $p < 0.05$
[a] Prospective randomized controlled study
[b] Stage II and III patients
[c] Subgroup analysis from a prospective randomized controlled study
[d] Comparison to chemotherapy or radiotherapy
[e] Stage III patients

of operated patients is reconstituted postoperatively at a higher rate than in operated or 5-FU treated patients. Since then ample evidence has been collected that levamisole has a dose-dependent immune-stimulating effect, and that tumor burden effects (inversely) the immune response to levamisole, supporting its use in the adjuvant – not in the palliative – situation (Hamilton et al. 1990; Janik et al. 1993; Taylor et al. 1993; AbdAlla et al. 1995). The optimal timing and dose of levamisole has not yet been determined, and current doses are below the optimal immune stimulatory dose (Janik et al. 1993).

Although "chemoimmunotherapy" with 5-FU+levamisole seemed to be superior to 5-FU monotherapy, recent studies have shown that combination chemotherapy or 5-FU modulations may be as effective as 5-FU+levamisole (Table 6). In 1988 the NSABP (Wolmark et al. 1988) significantly reduced relapse and improved survival rates in resected colon cancer patients by systemic combination therapy with 5-FU+methyl-lomustine (MeCCNU) + vincristine (VCR). This positive adjuvant effect was not reproduced by Hafström et al. (1990), who used a similar protocol with 5-FU+CCNU+VCR, or other groups combining 5-FU with MeCCNU (for review see Hartung et al. 1993). The benefit of the NSABP protocol was no longer apparent after 8 years (Wolmark et al. 1993b). In an Italian cooperative study the overall survival after adjuvant treatment with 5-FU and CCNU was significantly *lower* than in untreated controls (Marangolo et al. 1989). In the subsequent NSABP study (Wolmark et al. 1993b) relapse and survival rates were improved significantly by the 5-FU+FA modulation compared to the previously successful combination chemotherapy control arm (Wolmark et al. 1993a). A significant reduction in relapses (O'Connell et al. 1993a; Erlichman et al. 1994; Marsoni 1995) and improvement in survival (Erlichman et al. 1994) with the combination of 5-FU+FA compared to untreated controls in randomized studies was reported independently by a North American–European Group which pooled data from three study centers (Erlichman et al. 1994; Marsoni 1995) and the Mayo Clinic (O'Connell et al. 1993a), confirming the findings of Wolmark et al. (1993b). Marsoni and others (Marsoni 1995; O'Connell et al. 1993a; Wolmark et al. 1993b) have included UICC stage II and III colon cancers. The compliance of the adjuvant 5-FU+FA treatment was well and 80% of the European, Canadian and NSABP trial patients completed the planned treatment (Marsoni 1995; Wolmark et al. 1993b).

Francini et al. (1994) induced a significant reduction of recurrence and death rates by adjuvant 5-FU and FA treatment in UICC II and III colon cancer, which had been started less than 3 weeks after surgery and lasted for 12 cycles (1 year). Toxicity was acceptable. In subset analyses treatment with 5-FU+FA was effective in stage III but not in stage II patients. On the other hand, in the NSABP protocol there was no significant treatment interaction between Duke stage and the benefits of chemotherapy (Wolmark et al. 1993b).

In a nonrandomized case-control study Frasci et al. (1994) compared the adjuvant treatment with 5-FU+interferon-alpha vs. their previous 5-FU monotherapy protocol for adjuvant treatment of patients from the same institution. The combination of 5-FU+interferon-alpha reduced relapse rates and increased survival rates vs. 5-FU alone at a significant level and with no major difference in toxicity. The significant improvement of the adjuvant treatment with 5-FU+FA or 5-FU+interferon-alpha can most probably be attributed to the higher activity (response rates) of the 5-FU modulation protocols vs. 5-FU alone, as demonstrated in the palliative treatment of advanced colorectal cancer (Einhorn 1989; Arbuck 1989; Köhne-Wömpner et al. 1992). This advantage of 5-FU+FA vs. 5-FU alone in the palliative situation was pronounced at minimal tumor loads (Poon et al. 1989). In a Japanese randomized study comparing postoperative MMC vs. MMC plus carmofur in colorectal cancers of UICC stages I–III, the patients treated with MMC plus carmofur had a significantly longer 5-year survival rate (79.3%) than the patient group treated with MMC only (65.7%). Again, the highest benefit was obtained in stage III patients (Ito et al. 1990, 1995).

Systemic Chemotherapy With and Without Irradiation in Rectal Cancer

Rectal cancer patients may receive radiation, chemotherapy, or their combination, radiochemotherapy, for adjuvant treatment. While radiation alone does not prolong life significantly in resected rectal cancer patients, the adjuvant effect of *chemotherapy* as a single treatment modality up to now remains an unsettled question. Windle et al. (1987), Laurie et al. (1989), Metzger et al. (1994) and Frasci et al. (1994) included rectal cancer patients in their studies (Table 6). In subgroup analyses Laurie et al (1989) and Metzger et al. (1994) obtained evidence that colon cancer patients of UICC stage III profit more from systemic adjuvant treatment than rectal cancer patients, indicating that their chemotherapy protocols were less or not effective in rectal cancer. In the Frasci et al. (1994) study rectal cancer patients treated with 5-FU+interferon-alpha had a 5-year survival rate of 53% vs. 40% in the patients receiving 5-FU. However, this positive tendency was statistically not significant since the patient number was low. However, the 5-year survival rates in 5-FU+interferon-alpha treated rectal cancer patients were similar to those of trials with combined chemoradiation treatment. This study indicates that 5-FU+interferon-alpha is very likely to be active as systemic adjuvant treatment in colon and rectal cancer patients. This hypothesis must be tested in a properly designed randomized study (Frasci et al. 1994). Another trial indicating that systemic chemotherapy has an adjuvant therapeutic effect was conducted by the NSABP (Fisher et al. 1988). This three-arm randomized trial of the NSABP compared controls vs. postoperative adjuvant chemotherapy with 5-FU, MeCCNU, and VCR vs. postoperative radiation alone and demonstrated a significant activity of adjuvant chemotherapy in rectal cancer (Tables 6, 7). The survival advantage in this study obtained by adjuvant chemotherapy alone was not overwhelming, and the local relapse rate was not reduced by

Table 7. Adjuvant chemotherapy (Chemo), radiotherapy (Rad), and chemoradiotherapy of rectal cancer in prospective studies with control (Cont) and treated (Ther) patients

Reference	*n*	Duke stage	Therapy		Local relapse		Survival	
			Rad	Chemo	Cont	Ther	Cont	Ther
GITSG (1985, 1986)	104	B2+C	+	+	24%	11%*	43%	59%*
Krook et al. (1991)	204	B2+C	+	+	25%[a]	14%*	47%[a]	58%*
Fisher et al. (1988)	371	B+C	+	–	25%	16%*	43%	41%
Fisher et al. (1988)	371	B+C	–	+	25%	21%	43%	53%*

* $p < 0.05$
[a] Radiotherapy alone as control

systemic adjuvant treatment. However, unlike in the adjuvant NSABP colon study, the survival benefit was retained at 8 years of follow-up (Wolmark et al. 1993b). A Swedish group using 5-FU+CCNU+VCR did not reproduce this significant adjuvant treatment effect, but it must be noted that this study showed a positive tendency with low patient numbers at relatively high relapse rates (Hafström et al. 1990). Further studies with 5-FU+MeCCNU for adjuvant chemotherapy of rectal cancer have also been negative (Hartung et al. 1993).

In the radiation therapy group of the NSABP study (Fisher et al. 1988) the local relapse rate was reduced significantly, however, without impact on survival (Table 7). The results of this single treatment modality study suggest that the *combination of radiation and chemotherapy* should be more effective than either radio- or chemotherapy alone. This was first confirmed by the GITSG in 1985 and 1986 (Tables 6, 7). This four-arm randomized trial with 202 prospectively randomized patients compared chemotherapy with 5-FU+MeCCNU to radiotherapy, radiochemotherapy, and surgery only. Disease-free and overall survival was significantly increased by *radiochemotherapy* (Gastrointestinal Tumor Study Group 1985, 1986; Douglass et al. 1988). The cooperative study of the Mayo Clinic, of Duke university, and of NCCTG (Krook et al. 1991) confirmed that the combination of radiochemotherapy reduces recurrence rates and increases survival significantly compared to radiotherapy alone in rectal cancer (Tables 6, 7). In this study radiochemotherapy also led to a significant reduction in local and overall recurrences and distant metastases compared to radiotherapy alone. The 5- and 7-year overall survival rates were 58% and 53% in the radiochemotherapy group vs. 47% and 38% in the group receiving radiation alone. Severe side effects were enteritis requiring treatment in 4.4%, rectal perforation in 1/202 patients, and severe pelvic fibrosis in 2/202 patients (Moertel 1992). To prevent the small bowel problems which occur in 6%–7% of patients under pelvic irradiation the pelvic inlet should be closed surgically (Steele 1991; Thom et al. 1992).

The NCCTG, as the GITSG, used 5-FU+MeCCNU in addition to radiotherapy. Since MeCCNU is toxic and may induce hematological malignancies, the impact of this drug in adjuvant combination therapy with 5-FU was studied critically. The GITSG and the NCCTG found independently that 5-FU+radiation is as effective as 5-FU+MeCCNU+radiation (O'Connell et al. 1991; Gastrointestinal Tumor Study Group 1992) so that MeCCNU can clearly be omitted. The enhancement of adjuvant (systemic) effectivity can be improved by a better timing of the 5-FU administration together with radiotherapy. The NCCTG demonstrated that continuous 5-FU infusion during radiotherapy is significantly superior to bolus 5-FU, resulting in an increase of disease free- and overall survival at similar local control rates in both arms (Table 6; O'Connell et al. 1993b). Deducting from mono- and multimodality trials for adjuvant therapy in rectal cancer, one can conclude that chemotherapy contributes to a reduction in distant metastases and increase in survival. Radiotherapy decreases local relapses with a prospective palliative effect (Schmoll 1994a). Thus, both the improvement in chemotherapeutic protocols and the optimization of radiation dose and strategy is mandatory in adjuvant multimodal therapy of rectal cancer.

Recent studies have examined the feasibility and impact of the combination with 5-FU+FA and radiotherapy delivered either before or after rectal cancer surgery. Minsky et al. (1993) demonstrated that preoperative chemoradiation with 5-FU+FA plus radiotherapy is feasible, seems to downstage rectal cancer, and increases local control and probably survival rates. These authors also reported that 5-FU+FA plus radiotherapy delivered after rectal cancer surgery is relatively well tolerated (Minsky et al. 1991). Thus, this 5-FU modulation therapy is suitable not only for postoperative but also for preoperative radiochemotherapy. In combined modality programs radiotherapy should be delivered at full doses of 45 Gy or more and chemotherapy at dose levels that have proven effective in metastatic disease (Minsky et al. 1993).

Radiotherapy with or without chemotherapy seems to improve the results of *local excision* in early stage rectal cancer. This observation must be verified with appropriate studies defining also the role of additional chemotherapy (Cummings 1992; Minsky 1993). The local control rate seems to be inversely correlated to the primary tumor stage (T category) and is influenced by radiation dose.

Systemic (adjuvant) chemotherapy in colon cancer and chemoradiation in rectal cancer are far from perfect since the absolute improvements in relapse and survival rates range between 7%–26% and 4%–26% (Table 6). These results may be improved by strengthening the host's immune defense.

Adjuvant Immunotherapy

General Remarks

Immunotherapy or biological response modifier (BRM) therapy is gaining increasing acceptance as a fourth column of colorectal cancer therapy, along with surgery, chemotherapy, and radiation therapy. Easy (outpatient) administration, inexpensive therapy courses, and few side effects make biological therapies attractive for patients and physicians, but in this young and rapidly developing field much more valid clinical experience is needed (Hoover et al. 1993). To avoid enthusiastic anticipation of immunotherapeutic modalities, the hopes and realities of adjuvant immunotherapy are discussed below.

The general concept of immunotherapy includes the recognition and subsequent eradication of the patient's tumor or, in the adjuvant situation, of micrometastatic spread by the patient's immune system. This can be achieved by a direct antiproliferative effect of the BRM (e.g., interferon-alpha), or more often by an indirect biological effect on the tumor cell through boosting of the immune response against antigens, cytokine cascade activation, or activation of lymphocytes, macrophages, monocytes, or granulocytes. Since many different approaches to immunotherapy have been studied in animal and human tumor models, a clearcut classification of immunotherapy into five main categories is advisable (Table 8, Mitchell 1992). Examples of these therapy forms are discussed in detail in a later section.

Table 8. Categories of immunotherapy (adapted from Mitchell 1992)

Category of Immunotherapy	Effect	Examples
Active-specific	Activation of specific effector cells (CTL, Ab-bound macrophages) by tumor antigens	Tumor cell lysates Tumor cell extracts Synthetic tumor antigens
Active-unspecific	Activation of unspecific effector cells (macrophages, NK cells) by microbial or chemical adjuvants	Bacille Calmette-Guérin, methylene diphosphate Pertussis toxin Endotoxin Interferon-alpha Interferon-beta
Passive	Administration of antibodies or "carriers" for antitumor "factors"	Monoclonal antibodies Immunoconjugates
Adoptive	Transfer of immune-active cells (or informational molecules)	Lymphokine-activated killer cells Interleukin-2 Granulocyte-macrophage colony-stimulating factors
Restorative	Restoration of defective immune functions Inhibition of suppressor factors	Levamisole Cyclophosphamide H_2 receptor antagonists Prostaglandin synthetase inhibitors
Cell-modulatory	Upregulation of tumor-associated antigens or MHC antigens on tumor cells	Interferon-gamma Levamisole (+5-FU)

Up to now most adjuvant studies involving immunotherapeutic strategies have been disappointing. Obviously, although experimental results have been positive, clinical immunotherapy is still in the learning phase. Only recently it has been understood that in spite of parallels substantial differences also exist between chemotherapy and immunotherapy regarding administration form and schedule, dose escalation, and handling of toxicities (Creekmore et al. 1991). Several reasons have been recognized for the discouraging results after uncritical or experimental immunotherapy:

- Testing was carried out in nonrandomized clinical trials.
- Immunotherapy was applied in immuno*in*competent patients with high tumor burden.
- Treatment schedules were too short.
- Preparations for immune therapy were little purified, not well characterized, and tested in insufficient amounts.
- Clinical trials were based on wrong conclusions from insufficient animal models.
- No immunological therapy monitoring was included.

Taking these points into account, it is not surprising that in colorectal cancer up to now there has been only one study confirming substantial evidence that adjuvant passive immunotherapy with a monoclonal antibody (Mab 17-1A) significantly prolongs life (Riethmüller et al. 1994; Tables 6, 9). The different categories of immunotherapy and their clinical significance (Table 8) are discussed below.

Active Unspecific Immunotherapy

Despite initially enthusiastic reports (Rosenberg et al. 1989) single unspecific immune stimulators such as interferons, interleukins, and bacterial preparations (Grundmann et al. 1988) have failed to prove their beneficial effect in clinical trials of colorectal cancer immunotherapy (John et al. 1993). Single BRM treatment, as with interleukin-2, may play a supportive role in perioperative colonic surgery if impaired natural killer cell function needs to be restored (Deehan et al. 1994; Nichols et al. 1993). In experimental models metastasis was prevented by chemoimmunotherapy with, for example, 5-FU or MMC combined with OK-432 (Klein et al. 1986). Results with clinical significance can be expected in protocols in which active unspecific immunotherapy, such as interferon-alpha (Frasci et al. 1994) but not BCG (Table 9), is combined with chemotherapy or other forms of immunotherapy.

Active Specific Immunotherapy

Active-specific immunotherapy (ASI) is understood as the administration of a tumor vaccine. This contains autologous or allogeneic tumor-associated anti-

Table 9. Results of adjuvant trials in colon (C) and rectal (R) cancers involving specific and nonspecific immunotherapies

Chemotherapy	Immunotherapy	Reference	Tumor type	Relapse reduction	Survival extension
5-FU	LEV	Moertel et al. (1990)	C	+	+
5-FU	LEV	Windle et al. (1987)	CR	+	+
5-FU	LEV	Laurie et al. (1989)	CR	+	+
5-FU+RT	MER	Robinson et al. (1982)	C	(+)	(+)
–	BCG	Wolmark et al. (1988)	C	–	(+)
–	LEV	Arnaud et al. (1989)	C	–	–
–	MER	GITSG (1984)	C	–	–
MMC+5-FU	PSK	Mitomi and Noto (1990)	CR	+	+
–	Vacc	Wunderlich et al. (1985)	CR	(+)	(+)
–	ASI	Hoover et al. (1985)	CR	+	+
	ASI	Hoover et al. (1993)	C	+	+
	ASI	Hoover et al. (1993)	R	–	–
5-FU+MeCCNU	BCG	Pannetiere et al. (1988)	CR	–	–
5-FU+MeCCNU	MER	GITSG (1984)	CR	–	–
5-FU+MeCCNU	BCG	McPherson et al. (1984)	CR	–	–
–	Mab 17-1A	Riethmüller et al. (1994)	CR	+	+
5-FU	IFN-α	Frasci et al. (1994)	CR	+	+

ASI, Active-specific immunotherapy; BCG, bacille Calmette-Guérin; LEV, levamisole; MER, methanol-extracted residue; PSK, protein-bound plant polysaccharide from coriolus versicolor; Vacc, vaccine with inactivated allogeneic tumor cells. Adjuvant treatment effect: +, significant; –, not significant; (+), questionable

gens (e.g., as cell lysates) or, more recently, synthetically produced tumor-associated antigens. These antigens are mixed with an unspecific adjuvant (ALUM, bacille Calmette-Guérin, or detoxified endotoxins) which is very important for the amplification of a specific immune response (Staib et al. 1994b). Clinically active tumor vaccines have been demonstrated mainly in melanoma treatment (Mitchell et al. 1990; Barth et al. 1994). Great public attention was drawn to a study published by Hoover et al. (1985, 1993) (Table 9) who used a mixture of autologous tumor cells and BCG administered subcutaneously as an adjuvant immunotherapy in resected colorectal cancer patients. Initially it seemed that recurrence rates were reduced, and that life was prolonged. The outcome of this promising trial was disappointing. In a final report no statistically significant improvement of survival or disease-free survival was achieved by ASI. In a subset analysis colon cancer patients seemed to profit with a significant improvement of disease-free and overall survival, whereas rectal cancer patients did not profit from ASI (Hoover et al. 1993; Hanna et al. 1991). Although this subset analysis indicated a positive effect of immunotherapy in colon cancer patients, the study was heavily criticized and the method of subset analysis rejected (Moertel 1993). Meanwhile, a randomized phase III study has been designed by the ECOG to confirm the suggested adjuvant therapeutic benefit of ASI in combination with chemotherapy (5-FU and levamisole) in colon cancer patients (Hoover et al. 1993).

In a nonrandomized trial a German group observed life prolongation and a delayed-type hypersensitivity skin reaction with an Epstein-Barr virus transformed autologous tumor vaccine (without an immunological adjuvant) in curatively resected colorectal cancer patients compared to historical controls (Lehner et al. 1990). Follow-up observations of this study are still awaited. Immunization with inactivated allogeneic tumor cells in an earlier protocol from Austria (Wunderlich et al. 1985) had no adjuvant treatment effect (Table 9) although in a subgroup analysis lymph node positive patients had a significant survival benefit.

So far, in spite of this experimentally cogent concept, no active tumor vaccine has been described which can be recommended for adjuvant use in colorectal cancer.

Passive Immunotherapy

A German group successfully tested passive immunotherapy with the monoclonal antibody Mab 17-1A for postoperative adjuvant treatment in colorectal cancer patients. In this multicenter trial with 189 patients, Riethmüller et al. (1994) reduced the overall death rate by 30% ($p = 0.04$) and recurrence by 27% ($p = 0.03$; Table 9). The effect of the adjuvant antibody therapy was most pronounced in preventing distant metastases, but not of local relapses. The antibody treatment was tolerated well and no severe life-threatening, noncontrollable toxic reactions were described. Colon and rectal cancer patients with positive lymph nodes were included (UICC stage III), and rectal cancer patients did not have routine radiotherapy. Although the results reached statistical significance, patient numbers were surprisingly low. The study had a high rate of ineligible patients and awaits confirmation by a second trial with the same design. Due to these weaknesses monoclonal antibody treatment with Mab 17-1A must be regarded as an experimental approach (Schlag 1994).

Adoptive Immunotherapy

The transfer of immune active cells or information molecules such as interleukin-2 and growth factors have provided experimentally impressive results in solid tumors. Although adoptive immunotherapy with lymphokine-activated killer cells and interleukin-2 induced remission rates of 17% in metastasized colorectal cancer patients (Rosenberg et al. 1988, 1989), this combination has not been tried in the adjuvant situation because of its high toxicity. The experimental set-up of lymphokine-activated killer cell transfer is rather expensive and complicated.

Restorative Immunotherapy

Recent studies have shown that an activated intact immune system, measured by cytotoxicity of patients' mononuclear cells against autologous tumor cells or tumor cell lines of identical histology (Vanky et al. 1986; Staib et al. 1994a) is correlated with a better prognosis. Niimoto et al. (1990) found in a patient group receiving postoperative chemoimmunotherapy that an active immune system is a significant positive prognostic factor. After major surgery in gastrointestinal tract cancer natural killer cell function is impaired for at least 10 days postoperatively (Houvenaeghel et al. 1994; Schäfer et al. 1994). On the other hand, the observation that intraoperative blood transfusions facilitate relapses in colorectal cancer patients (Foster et al. 1985; Harder et al. 1988) provides indirect evidence that a suppressed immune system is a negative prognostic factor. Therefore restoration of an impaired immune system postoperatively might contribute to reducing recurrence rates and improving survival. Levamisole has been shown (only in combination with 5-FU; Tables 6, 9) to be active in adjuvant colorectal cancer treatment (Laurie et al. 1989; Windle et al. 1987). Although this combination has been recommended widely, the effect of levamisole remains to be confirmed in a second randomized trial comparing 5-FU+levamisole vs. 5-FU alone (Janik et al. 1993; AbdAlla et al. 1995), as mentioned above. Suppressor cell function can be selectively decreased by a single injection of cyclophosphamide. Although clinically used in melanoma immunotherapy protocols (Mitchell 1988), this has not been described so far in colorectal cancer.

Cell Modulatory Immunotherapy

HLA class I levels have been found to be decreased in colon cancer cells (AbdAlla et al. 1995). Upregulation of MHC antigens that are usually presented in context with tumor-associated antigens to competent immune cells can facilitate tumor cell recognition and killing experimentally (Staib et al. 1993). There may be a cell modulatory effect of levamisole when combined with 5-FU as levamisole reverses the 5-FU induced generalized inhibition of RNA synthesis of HLA antigens. Another potentially cell-modulatory BRM with proven upregulatory effect on tumor cells (Staib et al. 1993), interferon-gamma, has been tested so far in adjuvant colorectal cancer treatment with immunological but not clinical effect (O'Connell et al. 1992a). Again, single BRM administration may lack clinical efficiency, and combination immunotherapy is more likely to restore defeciencies in the immune cascade of tumor cell rejection.

Combination Immunotherapy

The use of defined BRM such as interferon-alpha or interleukin-2 together with other cytokines or monoclonal antibodies has been propagated for adjuvant therapy (Hersh 1987). Combining BRMs or different functional characteristics seems to be favorable. There is experimental evidence that the combination of interleukin-2 and interferon-alpha exerts a synergistic effect at a minimal tumor load (Igo et al. 1988; Rosenberg et al. 1988; Talmadge et al. 1984; Bubenik 1990). Although the combination of interleukin-2 (high-dose) and interferon-alpha (low-dose) is not effective in advanced metastasized colorectal cancer (Hirsh et al. 1990), there may be an adjuvant treatment benefit since a high proportion of effector vs. target cells is essential for effective anticancer immunotherapy (Talmadge et al. 1984; Bubenik 1990). A combination of these two substances with chemotherapy may be even more beneficial (Hirsh et al. 1990; Shau 1988). Another approach is the combination of Mab 17-1A with granulocyte-macrophage colony-stimulating factor as enhancer, which has been reported to induce long-lasting complete remissions in a few cases of advanced colorectal cancer (Ragnhammer et al. 1993).

Combination of Chemotherapy with Immunotherapy

Any combination of chemotherapy with immunotherapy in its various forms requires exact knowledge of pharmacokinetics, effect profiles, and interactions of both substance groups with the immune system to achieve a synergistic effect (Mitchell 1988). Experimentally it has been reported that the effects of BRM are potentiated by prior chemotherapy (Weisenthal et al. 1991). Historically, various studies using unspecific immunomodulators together with chemotherapy or with chemotherapy plus radiation have been conducted in colorectal cancer patients, and most groups claim that their treatment concept was active. However, with few exceptions these studies have had insufficient designs to confirm the beneficial effect of adjuvant active unspecific immunotherapy on a significant basis (Moertel et al. 1990; Frasci et al. 1994); these are listed in Table 9 (Masucci et al. 1995). Most of these studies were not randomized, and therefore reductions in relapse rates and increases in survival times described were not conclusive.

Interferon-alpha in combination with 5-FU may contribute to an improvement in the current standard. The high toxicity of the combination of 5-FU (750 mg/m^2) with an interferon-alpha dose of 9×10^6 IU initially described by

Wadler et al. (1989), has probably prevented testing of interferon-alpha in adjuvant treatment protocols as well. However, the toxicity can be reduced by lowering the interferon-alpha dose without compromising the antitumor effect (Wadler et al. 1990, 1991). Frasci et al. (1994) used an interferon-alpha dose of 6×10^6 IU $3\times$ per week (3×10^6 IU/m^2/week) and a 5-FU dose of 450 mg/m^2 (days 1–5 every 4 weeks for six cycles). As mentioned above, the adjuvant treatment effect of the Frasci et al. protocol seemed superior to 5-FU treatment only (Tables 6, 9).

In summary, immunotherapy in the adjuvant treatment of colorectal cancer is a very attractive therapy option, but still experimental. Proven so far in (controlled) clinical trials is the benefit to levamisole and that of interferon-alpha in combination with 5-FU and passive immunotherapy with the monoclonal antibody Mab 17-1A.

Adjuvant Therapy After Resection of Colorectal Cancer Metastasis

While several protocols have confirmed that adjuvant therapy improves survival in colorectal cancer after curative primary tumor resection, there is no proven effective adjuvant treatment after resection of colorectal metastases. The indications for resection of liver and lung metastases at defined stages are clear (Rosenberg 1987). Patients with colorectal liver metastasis benefit from resection, especially if no more than three metastases must be resected, and if the tumor-free margin exceeds 1 cm (Hughes et al. 1988). The actuarial 5-year survival rate in a multi-institutional study was 33%, and the actuarial 5-year disease-free survival rate was 21%, indicating, that 79% of patients eventually developed recurrences (Hughes et al. 1988). The analysis of the recurrence pattern revealed that 40% of the patients with relapse after resection of isolated hepatic colorectal cancer metastasis had experienced a recurrence in the liver and 31% in the lungs (either alone or in combination with other organs). The liver was the only metastatic site in 16%, while this was the case for the lung in 7%. The liver and lungs, however, are the *initial* sole sites of recurrence in 28% and 14%, respectively (Hughes and Sugarbaker 1987).

Systemic adjuvant chemotherapy has not been successful after resection of liver metastases (O'Connell et al. 1985). Since relapses occur at a high rate in the liver, regional liver chemotherapy has been used for adjuvant treatment. Patt et al. (1991) reported that patients with positive resection margins and postoperative intra-arterial 5-FUDR infusion lived as long as those who had negative resection margins. The authors suggested adjuvant activity in this treatment concept without having confirmed this conclusion. Wagman et al. (1990) conducted a randomized controlled study and found that patients with 5-FUDR intra-arterial infusion had a significantly longer relapse-free survival. However, toxicity in this study was high, and two patients died of sclerosing cholangitis. A German group provided evidence that the intrahepatic relapse rate after resection of colorectal liver metastases is significantly reduced when patients with intra-arterial chemotherapy are compared to historical controls. There was a tendency toward increased disease-free and overall survival, without confirmed significant difference. Hepatobiliary toxicity in this study was high (Lorenz et al. 1993).

Although the impact of an adjuvant treatment effect with 5-FUDR hepatic arterial infusion may be verified by currently running randomized studies (Lorenz et al. 1993; Safi et al. 1995), this treatment modality will have no future due to its high hepatobiliary toxicity in form of sclerosing cholangitis and gastroduodenal ulcer formation (Hohn et al. 1988). Most probably the intra-arterial postoperative infusion of 5-FU+FA will evolve as an acceptable alternative to 5-FUDR, since in the palliative situation this combination compared to 5-FUDR is at least as effective in isolated liver metastasis with nearly no hepatic or gastrointestinal tract toxicity; in addition, potentially effective systemic 5-FU drug levels were measured during hepatic artery infusion of 5-FU+FA, while 5-FUDR is totally extracted by the liver, excluding systemic 5-FUDR levels (Link et al. 1993). While the adjuvant benefit of chemotherapy after resection of isolated colorectal liver metastases still needs to be confirmed, a combination of regional chemo- and immunotherapy probably improves the prognosis in these patients. Lykidakis et al. (1995) recently reported, that patients receiving locoregional chemoimmunotherapy to the liver lived significantly longer than those who had resection of their colorectal liver metastases only. Some evidence has been generated that active specific immunostimulation after resection of liver metastases improves the results of surgery alone (Schlag et al. 1991). The long-term follow-up in this randomized study (not available yet) will show whether the lower incidence of recurrence in the treated group translates to longer survival times.

Standard Recommendations for Adjuvant Therapy

The significant improvements achieved by adjuvant chemo-(immuno-)therapy with 5-FU+levamisole in colon cancer and radiochemotherapy in rectal cancer strongly support the inclusion of these treatments in a multimodality approach toward advanced resectable stages in colorectal cancer. The results also serve as a solid base for research on improving adjuvant therapy with more effectivity, less toxicity, and lower costs. In 1990 the NIH published its consensus on the recommendable standard adjuvant treatment for colon and rectal cancers (NIH 1990). According to this statement, colon cancer patients of UICC stage III should be offered adjuvant therapy with 5-FU and levamisole as administered in the Intergroup trial (Moertel et al. 1990) unless medical or psychosocial contraindications exist. Patients with stage II should not receive adjuvant treatment outsite clinical trials. Rectal cancer patients stage II or III should receive combined postoperative chemotherapy and radiation with 5-FU+MeCCNU and high-dose pelvic irradiation according to the NCCTG protocol (Krook et al. 1991). In 1991 the NCl corrected the recommendation for rectal cancer patients by suggesting that radiation therapy should be combined with 5-FU only. In 1994 O'Connell (1994) recommended that high-risk colon cancer patients in stage II with T4 N0 M0 lesions or stage II tumors with abnormal DNA flow cytometry should receive adjuvant treatment with 5-FU+levamisole as well since this subgroup benefitted from adjuvant 5-FU plus levamisole in the stage II arm of the Intergroup study (Moertel 1992). Based on the results of recent studies with 5-FU+FA O'Connell (1994) suggested this combination as an alternative adjuvant therapy regimen for patients with colon cancer, particularly for the individual patient who does not tolerate levamisole. A council of German oncology surgeons, medical oncologists, radiotherapists, and pathologists came to a basically identical consensus in 1994 (Beger et al. 1994): colon cancer patients of stage III should receive 5-FU and levamisole. Rectal cancer patients with T4 tumors may receive pre-operative radiochemotherapy if R0 resection seems possible on the basis of the staging before initiating radiochemotherapy. Rectal cancer patients of stages II or III should receive postoperative adjuvant radiotherapy combined with 5-FU, according to the NIH recommendations.

Current Studies and Future Developments

Both recommended standard procedures for adjuvant therapy in colon and rectal cancer are based on the combination of 5-FU with either a highly hypothetic immunotherapeutic principle (levamisole) or 5-FU with radiotherapy. The statements of the NIH Consensus Conference and the German Consensus Conference include the urgent suggestion to treat qualified patients in studies trying to improve those adjuvant treatment protocols. The activity of 5-FU and levamisole in metastatic disease has no advantage over 5-FU alone, and levamisole alone has no activity at all at this stage of disease (Hamilton et al. 1990; Moertel et al. 1995). The role of levamisole in adjuvant chemoimmunotherapy must be elucidated. Over the past decade 5-FU modulation therapies have been compared to 5-FU alone for treatment of metastatic disease, and in several randomized studies response rates and survival times were superior to those with 5-FU alone (Köhne-Wömpner et al. 1992; Arbuck 1989), suggesting that these regimens should be tested in adjuvant chemotherapy or chemoradiotherapy. In analogy to the development of adjuvant treatment in breast cancer, it can be assumed that combination chemotherapy protocols which produce significantly higher response rates than 5-FU in metastatic disease should have a better adjuvant treatment effect. Many studies are therefore underway to test the 5-FU modulations of 5-FU+FA and 5-FU+interferon-alpha with and without levamisole. In an interim analysis comparing 5-FU+levamisole vs. 5-FU+FA an Israeli group found no significant difference in relapse-free survival, but 5-FU and FA was tolerated better (Perez et al. 1995). Continuous 48-h 5-FU+FA seems to be effective in adjuvant therapy of colon cancer stage III (Koike et al. 1995).

Rectal cancers up to now have been treated with radiochemotherapy only, but not with levamisole, due mainly to the tradition in the United States that rectal cancers are treated by other groups than colon cancers. There is no reason for rectal cancers to receive a systemic treatment that differs from that for colon cancer (Wils 1992). With this aim our study group (Forschungsgruppe Onkologie Gastrointestinale Tumoren, FOGT) has initiated a trial comparing 5-FU+levamisole vs. 5-FU+FA+levamisole vs. 5-FU+interferon-alpha+levamisole as the systemic treatment principles for adjuvant therapy of colon cancer of stage III, including stage II subcategory T4 N0 M0, and rectal cancers of stages II and III. Rectal cancer patients also receive radiotherapy according to the NCCTG protocol. This trial began in 1993 and now has more than 850 patients being randomized.

Clinical research on adjuvant therapy in colorectal cancer has expanded since 1990, and a variety of other protocols (Table 10) are examining the optimal route of drug delivery (SAKK, Axis, EORTC, Kelsen et al. 1994), the optimal combination therapy (NSABP, NCCTG + Intergroup, EORTC, ACO, Mannheim) or the optimal timing of chemotherapy (Mannheim, Erlangen, SMAC, NCCTG + Intergroup, NSABP) and the combination of chemotherapy with immunotherapy (ECOG). These studies, including the intraportal infusion trials, will contribute to improving adjuvant therapy of colorectal cancer. Other studies concentrate on levamisole dosing (Moertel et al. 1994) or try to substitute levamisole by more potent immune stimulators (Taylor et al. 1993). These studies usually need great patient numbers and good discipline in patient guidance.

An important question in adjuvant treatment of rectal cancer is the timing of radio- and chemotherapy. Preoperative radiation may be more effective than postoperative radiotherapy (Molls 1994; Molls and Fink 1994; Cummings 1992; Pahlman and Glimelius 1992; Papillon 1994); however, the risk of overtreatment should not be underestimated. The extension of overall survival has not been confirmed for radiotherapy unless chemotherapy is added (Pahlman and Glimelius 1992). The Erlangen study group is comparing preoperative radiochemotherapy vs. postoperative radiochemotherapy and a Heidelberg group is trying to reduce recurrences by intraoperative radiotherapy combined with pre- or postoperative irradiation and 5-FU and FA treatment (Kallinowski et al. 1995). A Japanese group has found evidence that preoperative hyperthermia plus irradiation plus chemotherapy reduces local recurrence and lung metastases rates in rectal cancer (Korenaga et al. 1992). An additional variable in radiotherapy is the drug infusion timing concomitant with radiotherapy. Future studies in radiochemotherapy must consider that continous 5-FU infusion significantly increases disease-free survival and overall survival compared to bolus 5-FU during radiotherapy (O'Connell et al. 1993b). Other studies are under way testing continuous adjuvant 5-FU infusion during the whole adjuvant treatment vs. conventional weekly cyclus/bolus infusion protocols (e.g., SWOG 9304). One reason for the benefit of portal infusion may be the early perioperative start of treatment, while reduction in

Table 10. List of activated studies for adjuvant therapy in colon and rectal cancers in North America and Europe kh031195

North America

NSABP, USA
- NSABP R-02 males, rectal cancer
  - 5-FU+MeCCNU+VCR + RT
  - 5-FU+MeCCNU+VCR
  - 5-FU+FA + RT
  - 5-FU+FA
- NSABP R-02 females, rectal cancer
  - 5-FU+FA + RT
  - 5-FU+FA
- NSABP R-03 rectum UICC I, II, III
  - Surg, RT+5-FU+FA
  - RT+5-FU+FA, Surg, 5-FU+FA
- NSABP C-03, colon cancer
  - 5-FU+MeCCNU+VCR
  - 5-FU+FA
- NSABP C-04, colon cancer
  - 5-FU+FA
  - 5-FU+FA+LEV
  - 5-FU+LEV
- NSABP R, rectal cancer
  - 5-FU+FA preoperative
  - 5-FU+FA postoperative
- NSABP C-05, colon cancer
  - 5-FU+FA+IFNa
  - 5-FU+FA

NCCTG+INT, USA
- NCCTG-INT-0089 Part 3, colon cancer stage B, C
  - 5-FU+LEV (12m)
  - 5-FU+FA (low dose) (6m)
  - 5-FU+FA (high dose) (6m)
  - 5-FU+FA (low dose)+LEV (6m)
- NCCTG-894651, stage B2, C
  - 5-FU+LEV (6m)
  - 5-FU+LEV (12m)
  - 5-FU+LEV (6m)+FA (low dose)
  - 5-FU+LEV (12m)+FA (low dose)
- INT-0114, rectal cancer, stage B2, C
  - 5-FU, RT+5-FU
  - 5-FU+FA, RT+5-FU
  - 5-FU+LEV, RT+5-FU
  - 5-FU+FA+LEV, RT+15-FU
- INT-0144. rectal cancer UICC II, III
  - 5-FU, RT+5-FU c.i., 5-FU
  - 5-FU c.i., RT+5-FU c.i., 5-FU c.i.
  - 5-FU+FA+LEV, RT+5-FU+FA+LEV, 5-FU+FA+LEV44

EST (ECOG), USA
- EST 1290

Table 10. *Continued*

Autologous tumor vaccine
5-FU+LEV
Autologous tumor vaccine + 5-FU+LEV
EST 2288
5-FU+FA (low dose)
5-FU+FA (high dose)
5-FU+FA (low dose) + LEV
5-FU+LEV
Europe
AG Chir. Onkologie (ACO), Österr.Ges.Hämatologie/ Onkologie, Österr.Krebsge Sellschaft
Studie 90, colon Dukes C
5-FU
5-FU+LEV
5-FU+IFNα
5-FU+LEV+IFNα
Austria
Rectum
NOV into sacral cavity + CT (5-FU+FA)
RT + CT (5-FU+FA) postop
Colon
5-FU+FA i.v. + intraperitoneal
5-FU+LEV
GRECR-B, Belgium
Colon and rectum
Intraportal CT
– + 5-FU+LEV
– + 5-FU+FA+LEV
Surgery only
– + 5-FU+LEV
– + 5-FU+FA+LEV
EORTC colon and rectum UICC II+III, Brussels, Europe
EORTC-40911 (postop)
5-FU (intraportal)/5-FU (intraperitoneal)
Control
EORTC-40911 (long term)
5-FU+LEV (6m)
5-FU+FA (6m)
EORTC-40871
Control
5-FU (intraportal)
EORTC-22921 rectum (T4/T4)
RT, Surg
RT, Surg, 5-FU+FA
RT+5-FU+FA, Surg
RT+5-FU+FA, Surg, 5-FU+FA
Fondation Française de Cancerologie Digestive, France
5-FU+FA
Control

Table 10. *Continued*

FFCD, France
Rectum
RT preop
RT preop + CT preop/postop (5-FU+FA)
FNCLCC, France
Rectum
RT preop + early surgery
RT preop + late surgery
FASR, France and Italy
Colon
Intraportal CT (5-FU)
Continuous 5-FU+FA+LEV
FOGT, Germany
Colon UICC III and T4N0M0
5-FU+LEV
5-FU+FA+LEV
5-FU+IFN α+LEV
Rectum UICC II and III
5-FU+LEV + RT
5-FU+FA+LEV + RT
5-FU+IFN α+LEV + RT
Düsseldorf, Germany
Colon UICC III
5-FU+FA
5-FU+LEV
Erlangen, Germany
Chemotherapy
Chemotherapy+immunotherapy
Control
Erlangen, Germany
Rectum UICC II, III
Control
5-FU + RT
5-FU + RT, Surgery, ±5-FU (response-adapted)
Mannheim, Germany
Colon UICC III
5-FU+LEV (48 w)
5-FU+FA (48 w)
5-FU+LEV (24 w)
5-FU+FA (24 w)
Rectum UICC II, III
5-FU+FA (48 w) + RT
5-FU+FA (24 w) + RT
5-FU+FA (6 cycles) + RT
5-FU+FA (4 cycles) + RT
AXIS (UKCCCR), UK
Rectum
Control
5-FU intraportal
Radiotherapy
Radiotherapy + 5-FU intraportal
Colon

Table 10. *Continued*

		Control
		5-FU intraportal
QUASAR, UK		
	Colon	
		Control
		5-FU+FA$_{LD}$
		5-FU+FA$_{HD}$
		5-FU+FA$_{LD}$+LEV
		5-FU+FA$_{HD}$+LEV
Istituto Mario Negri, Milan, Italy		
		5-FU+FA (6m)
		5-FU intraportal (7d)
		5-FU intraportal (7d) + 5-FU+FA (6m)
GIVIO and ACOI, Italy		
	Colon	
		Intraportal CT (5-FU)
		5-FU+FA
		Intraportal CT (5-FU) + 5-FU+FA
NACCP, Netherlands		
	Colon and rectum UICC II and III	
		Control
		5-FU+LEV
NCCSG, Scandinavian countries		
	Rectum nonresectable	
		RT preop
		RT + CT (5-FU+FA) preop
Four Scandinavian trials (evaluable in an interim analysis)		
SRCSG, Stockholm, Sweden		
	Colon	
		Control
		5-FU+FA
		5-FU+FA+LEV
SCCS, Sweden		
	Colon	
		Control
		5-FU+FA
		5-FU+FA+LEV
		5-FU+LEV
NCRSG, Norway		
	Colon and rectum UICC II+III	
		5-FU+LEV
		Control
DAKREKA, Denmark		
	Colon and rectum UICC II+III	
		5-FU+LEV
		Control
SAKK 40/93, Switzerland		
	Colon and rectum	
		5-FU+MMC intraportal, 5-FU+LEV
		5-FU+MMC intraportal, 5-FU (high dose)
		5-FU+MMC intraportal, 5-FU (low dose)

colorectal liver metastases has been noted in only part of the intraportal studies. Colorectal liver metastases might be effectively inhibited by perioperative treatment with angiogenesis inhibitors (Konno et al. 1995) or lectins.

In addition to finding the most active treatment protocol, the major important issue of future research is to select patients properly according to prognostic factors relevant for adjuvant therapy other then the conventional UICC staging criteria. These prognostic factors could be genetic or molecular biological parameters determining the tumor cells' biological behavior in the patient, host factors suppressing relapses and metastasis, or molecular biological tests on sensitivity of tumor cells against fluoropyrimidines, such as the determination of the thymidilate synthase gene expression (NIH 1990; O'Connell 1994; O'Connell et al. 1992b; Lenz et al. 1993; Link et al. 1994; Schmoll 1994b; Peters et al. 1994; Witzig et al. 1991). Facing the solid data and the many questions which are still open, adjuvant therapy in colon and rectal cancer has become a well-established standard therapy, on the one hand, and research field of modern multimodal oncological treatment concepts, on the other (Moertel 1994; Moertel et al. 1995; Wils 1992; Cummings 1992). In spite of all the emphasis on adjuvant therapy in this disease it must be borne in mind that up to now only a minority of the treated patients have really profited from adjuvant therapy, and that the most significant prognostic factor is the correct surgical removal of the primary tumor and the draining lymphatic network (McArdle and Hole 1991; Hermanek et al. 1994, 1995; Myerson et al. 1995).

If it is consistently confirmed that local relapses after curative rectal cancer surgery occur in less than 5% without any adjuvant treatment (Heald and Karanjia 1992), postoperative irradiation of the pelvis may be omitted.

The benefit from adjuvant therapy must be related to the toxicity and costs of adjuvant treatment. Finally, it is important to note that colorectal cancer patients have an increased risk of developing a second large bowel cancer. Close follow-up and dietary or chemoprevention may evolve as effective "adjuvant" measure to decrease the risk for secondary polyps or cancer (Greenwald 1992). Those who perform standard adjuvant therapy or conduct research trials should be well aware of the potential toxic side effects of this treatment.

Although levamisole in the initial reports (Laurie et al. 1989; Moertel et al. 1990, 1995) is described as tolerable, it should be noted that severe neurological side effects such as multifocal leukencephalopathy (Leichman et al. 1993; Neu and Ober 1992) have been reported. Although this toxicity has been associated with levamisole, leading to arguments against 5-FU+levamisole adjuvant treatment, it should be kept in mind, that this toxic side effect has also been observed with the combination therapy with 5-FU and ranitidin (deClari 1993), and that this rare toxicity may thus be due to 5-FU. When levamisole was administered alone in the Intergroup study, side effects were low (Moertel 1992). No long-term toxicity and no increase in secondary cancers due to therapy were noted. A second side reaction of 5-FU and levamisole involves the liver function in up to 39% of the patients and may be indicated by elevated serum levels of alkaline phosphatase, aminotransferase, and bilirubin, yet without clinical consequence (Moertel 1994; Moertel et al. 1995). The toxicity of levamisole, including CNS side effects, is dose dependent (Janik et al. 1993). Studies have been initiated in which levamisole doses have been raised fivefold (Moertel 1994). This increase in levamisole, however, may lead to increased toxicity, and this is not the aim of adjuvant protocols. On the contrary, the treatment must be more compatible. The 1-year treatment of 5-FU and levamisole is too long, and 30% of the patients in the Intergroup study did not complete treatment (Moertel 1992). On the other hand, there were 20% treatment interruptions in the 5-FU+FA studies (Marsoni 1995; Wolmark et al. 1993b). As many as 19%–30% of intraportal infusion patients failed to complete treatment (Fielding et al. 1992; Laffer 1995). Currently running protocols will determine not only the most effective but also the most patient-compatible treatment principles.

Adjuvant treatment should be cost effective. In 22% of our patients and 23.5% of the United States patients the colon cancer was of stage III (Steele 1994), and 45% of our patients and 47.1% of those in the United States (Steele 1994) with rectal cancer stage II or III qualify for adjuvant therapy. Multimodal adjuvant therapy is being used increasingly in the United States, where 9% of colon cancer patients in 1985 vs. 20% in 1990 received surgery and some other adjuvant therapy (Steele 1994). In 1990, 38.9% of stage III colon cancers, 41.5% of stage II rectal cancers, and 61.3% of stage III rectal cancers received either chemotherapy, radiotherapy, or combinations in addition to surgery (Steele 1994). The costs of this additional treatment are high and should be justified – in view of health economists but not necessarily of physicians.

Regarding the socioeconomic benefit, adjuvant treatment with 5-FU+levamisole in stage III colon cancer is judged to be a very cost-effective procedure (Brown et al. 1994; Moertel 1994; Smith et al. 1993).

References

AbdAlla EE, Blair GE et al (1995) Mechanism of synergy of levamisole and flourouracil: induction of human leukocyte antigen class I in a colorectal cancer cell line. J Natl Cancer Inst 87:489–496

Ackerman NB (1994) Portal vein versus hepatic artery chemotherapy. Am J Surg 167:455–455

Arbuck SG (1989) Overview of clinical trials using 5-fluorouracil and leucovorin for the treatment of colorectal cancer. Cancer 63:1036–1044

Archer S, Gray B (1990) Intraperitoneal 5-fluorouracil infusion for treatment of both peritoneal and liver micrometastases. Surgery 108:502–507

Arnaud JP, Buyse M et al (1989) Adjuvant therapy of poor prognosis colon cancer with levamisole: results of an EORTC double-blind randomized clinical trial. Br J Surg 76:284–289

Astler VB, Coller FA (1954) The prognostic significance of direct extension of carcinoma of the colon and rectum. Ann Surg 139:846–852

Barth A, Hoon DSB et al (1994) Polyvalent melanoma cell vaccine induces delayed-type hypersensitivity and in vitro cellular immune response. Cancer Res 54:3342–3345

Beart RWJ, Moertel CG et al (1990) Adjuvant therapy for resectable colorectal carcinoma with fluorouracil administered by portal vein infusion. Arch Surg 125: 897

Beger HG, Eigler FW et al (1994) Konsensus der CAO, AIO und ARO zur adjuvanten Therapie bei Kolon- und Rektumkarzinom vom 11.3.1994. Onkologie 17:291–293

Bethune WA (1987) Carcinoma of the rectum: 508 patients with failure analysis and implication for adjuvant therapy. J Can Assoc Radiol 38:209–216

Bleiberg H (1990) The future of adjuvant treatment in gastrointestinal cancer. Eur J Surg Oncol 16:189–194

Brown ML, Nayfield SG et al (1994) Adjuvant therapy for stage III colon cancer: economics returns to research and cost-effectiveness of treatment. J Natl Cancer Inst 86:424–430

Bubenik J (1990) Local and regional immunotherapy of cancer with interleukin 2. J Cancer Res Clin Oncol 116:1–7

Buyse M, Zeleniuch JA et al (1988) Adjuvant therapy of colorectal cancer: why we still don't know. JAMA 259:3571–3578

Cedermark B, Johansson H et al (1995) The Stockholm I trial of preoperative short term radiotherapy in operable rectal carcinoma. Cancer 75:2269–2275

Creekmore SP, Urba WJ et al (1991) Principles of the clinical evaluation of biological agents. In: DeVita VTJ, Hellman S, Rosenberg SA (eds) Biologic therapy of cancer. Lippincott, Philadelphia, pp 67–86

Cummings BJ (1992) Adjuvant radiation therapy for colorectal cancer. Cancer 70:1372–1383

deClari F (1993) Beschleunigtes Auftreten einer multifokalen Leukenzephalopathie unter Fluorouracil und Ranitidin. DMW 118:1176

Deehan DJ, Heys SD et al (1994) Enhanced peri-operative natural cytotoxicity with recombinant interleukin-2 in patients undergoing colonic surgery. Eur J Surg Oncol 20:268–268

Douglass HO (1987) Adjuvant treatment in colorectal cancer: an update. World J Surg 11:478–492

Douglass HO, Stablein DM et al (1988) An organized multi-institutional interdisciplinary evaluation of role of radiation therapy alone or combined with chemotherapy in treatment of adenocarcinoma of the gastrointestinal tract. NCI Monogr 6:253–257

Einhorn LH (1989) Improvements in fluorouracil chemotherapy? J Clin Oncol 7:1377–1379

Erlichman C et al (1994). Event free and overall survival is increased by FU/FA in resected B and C colon cancer: a prospective pooled analysis of 3 randomized trials (RCTS). Proc ASCO 13:562

Fielding LP, Hittinger R et al (1992) Randomized controlled trial of adjuvant chemotherapy by portal-vein perfusion after curative resection for colorectal adenocarcinoma. Lancet 340:502–506

Fisher B, Wolmark N et al (1988) Postoperative adjuvant chemotherapy or radiation therapy for rectal cancer. Results from NSABP R-01. J Natl Cancer Inst 80:21–29

Foster RS, Costanzy MC et al (1985) Adverse relationship between blood transfusions and survival after colectomy for colon cancer. Cancer 55:1195–1201

Francini G, Petrioli R et al (1994) Folinic acid and 5-flourouracil as adjuvant chemotherapy in colorectal cancer. Gastroenterology 106:899–906

Frasci G, Leone F et al (1994) 5-flourouracil-interferon-a2b adjuvant treatment of Dukes[1] C colorectal cancer. Dis Colon Rectum 37:643–650
Gall FP, Hermanek P (1992) Wandel und derzeitiger Stand der chirurgischen Behandlung des colorectalen Carcinoms. Chirurg 63:227–234
Gastrointestinal Tumor Study Group (1984) Adjuvant therapy of colon cancer – results of a prospectively randomized trial. N Engl J Med 310:737–743
Gastrointestinal Tumor Study Group (1985). Prolongation of disease-free interval in surgically treated rectal carcinoma. N Engl J Med 312:1465–1472
Gastrointestinal Tumor Study Group (1986) Survival after postoperative combination treatment of rectal cancer (letter to the editor). N Engl J Med 315:1294–1295
Gastrointestinal Tumor Study Group (1992) Radiation therapy and fluorouracil with or without semustine for the treatment of patients with surgical adjuvant adenocarcinoma of the rectum. J Clin Oncol 10:549–557
Gerard A, Buyse M et al (1988) Preoperative radiotherapy as adjuvant treatment in rectal cancer. Ann Surg 208:606–614
Goldie JH, Coldman AJ (1986) Application of theoretical models to chemotherapy protocol design. Cancer Treat Rep 70:127–131
Gray BN, deZwart J et al (1987) The Australia and New Zealand trial of adjuvant chemotherapy in colon cancer. In: Harcourt Jovanovich B (ed) Adjuvant therapy of cancer V. Grune and Stratton, Orlando, pp 537–546
Gray R, James R et al (1991) AXIS – a suitable case for treatment. Br J Cancer 63:841–845
Greenwald P (1992) Colon cancer overview. Cancer 70:1206–1215
Grundmann R, Weber F et al (1988) Präoperative unspezifische Immunstimulation mit Proprionibacterium granulosum KP-45 bei Patienten mit colorectalem Carcinom. Chirurg 59:272–278
Gunderson LL (1976) Combined irradiation and surgery for rectal and sigmoid cancer. Curr Probl Cancer 1:40–53
Hafström L, Domellöf L et al (1990) Adjuvant chemotherapy with 5-flourouracil, vincristine and CCNU for patients with Dukes' C colorectal cancer. Br J Surg 77:1345–1348
Hamilton JM, Sznol M et al (1990) 5-Fluorouracil plus levamisole: effective adjuvant treatment for colon cancer. In: DeVita VTJ, Hellman S, Rosenberg SA (eds) Important advances in oncology. Lippincott, Philadelphia, pp 115–130
Hanna MG, Peters LC et al (1991) Immunotherapy by active specific immunization: basic principles and preclinical studies. In: DeVita VTJ, Hellman S, Rosenberg SA (eds) Biologic therapy of cancer. Lippincott, Philadelphia, pp 651–669
Harder F, Laffer U et al (1988) Nach kurativer Resektion colorectaler Carcinome wirkt die portale Chemotherapie vor allem beim nicht-bluttransfundierten Patienten. Chirurg 61:280–285
Hartung G, Diezler P et al (1993) New approaches to adjuvant therapy of colorectal carcinoma including current German activities. Onkologie 16:416–424
Heald RJ, Karanjia ND (1992) Results of radical surgery for rectal cancer. World J Surg 16:848–857
Hermanek P (1989) Aktuelle Aspekte der neuen Stadieneinteilung des colorectalen Carcinoms und ihre klinischen Konsequenzen. Chirurg 60:1–7
Hermanek P, Wiebelt H et al (1994) Langzeitergebnisse der chirurgischen Therapie des Kolonkarzinoms (Ergebnisse der Studiengruppe Kolorektales Karzinom). Chirurg 65:287–297
Hermanek P, Wiebelt H et al (1995) Prognostic factors of rectum carcinoma – experience of the German Multicentre Study SGCRC. Tumori 81[Suppl]:60–64
Hersh EM (1987) Adjuvant therapy of cancer V. The potential role of immunotherapy and biological therapy in the adjuvant therapy of cancer. In: Salmon SE (ed) Adjuvant therapy of cancer V. Grune and Stratton, Orlando, pp 47–56

Hirsh M, Lipton A et al (1990) Phase I study of interleukin-2 and interferon alpha-2a as outpatient therapy for patients with advanced malignancy. J Clin Oncol 8:1657–1663

Hohn DC, Shea WJ et al (1988) Complications and toxicities of hepatic arterial chemotherapy. Contr Oncol 29:169–180

Hoover HC, Surdyke MG et al (1985) Prospectively randomized trial of adjuvant active-specific immunotherapy for human colorectal cancer. Cancer 55:1236–1243

Hoover HC, Brandhorst JS et al (1993) Adjuvant active specific immunotherapy for human colorectal cancer: 6.5-year median follow-up of a phase III prospectively randomized trial. J Clin Oncol 11:390–399

Houvenaeghel G, Blache DO et al (1994) Immunological status, cancer and surgery. Eur J Surg Oncol 20:268–268

Hryniuk WM, Figueredo A et al (1987) Applications of dose intensity to problems in chemotherapy of breast and colorectal cancer. Semin Oncol 14:3–11

Hughes KS, Sugarbaker PH (1987) Resection of the liver for metastatic solid tumors. In: Rosenberg SA (ed) Surgical therapy of metastatic cancer. Lippincott, Philadelphia, pp 125–164

Hughes KS, Simon R et al (1988) Resection of the liver for colorectal carcinoma metastases: a multi-institutional study of indications for resection. Surgery 103:278–288

Igo M, Sakurai M et al (1988) In vivo activity of multiple injections of recombinant interleukin-2, alone, and in combination with three different types of recominant interferons in various syngeneic murine tumors. Cancer 48:260–264

Ito K, Watanabe T et al (1990). Are there any effective adjuvant chemotherapies after surgical therapy for colorectal cancer? Proc ASCO 9:124

Ito K, Koike A et al (1995) Prospective adjuvant chemotherapy of MMC and HCFU after curative resection of colorectal cancer: ten-years follow-up. Proc ASCO 14:219

Janik J, Kopp WC et al (1993) Dose-related immunologic effects of levamisole in patients with cancer. J Clin Oncol 11:125–135

John WJ, Neefe JR et al (1993) 5-Flourouracil and interferon-alpha-2a in advanced colorectal cancer. Results of two treatment schedules. Cancer 72:3191–3195

Kallinowski F, Eble MJ et al (1995) Intraoperative radiotherapy for primary and recurrent rectal cancer. Eur J Surg Oncol 21:191–194

Kelly CJ, Daly JM (1992) Colorectal cancer (principles of postoperative follow-up). Cancer 70:1397–1408

Kelsen D, Saltz L et al (1994) A phase I trial of immediate postoperative intraperitoneal floxuridine and leucovorin plus systemic 5-flourouracil and levamisole after resection of high risk colon cancer. Cancer 74:2224–2233

Klein E, Vanky F et al (1986) The effect of OK-432 on lymphocyte-mediated lysis of autologous tumor cells in patients with solid tumors. In: Micksche M, Klein E (eds) OK-432 – a biological response modifier. Professional Postgraduate Services International, pp 15–22

Köhne-Wömpner C, Schmoll HJ et al (1992) Chemotherapeutic strategies in metastatic colorectal cancer: an overview of current clinical trials. Semin Oncol 19:105–125

Koike A, Kanemitsu K et al (1995) Significant efficacy of a 48-hour infusion of 5-fluorouracil (5-FU) with leucovorin (LV) after curative resection in Dukes' C colon cancer. Proc ASCO 14:223

Konno H, Tanaka T et al (1995) Comparison of the inhibitory effect of the angiogenesis inhibitor, TNP-470, and mitomycin C on the growth and liver metastasis of human colon cancer. Int J Cancer 61:268–271

Korenaga D, Matsushima T et al (1992) Preoperative hyperthermia combined with chemotherapy and radiotherapy for patients with rectal carcinoma may prevent early local pelvic recurrence. Int J Colorectal Dis 7:206–209

Krook JE, Moertel CG et al (1991) Effective surgical adjuvant therapy for high-risk rectal carcinoma. N Engl J Med 324:709–715

Laffer UT (1995) Long-term results of single course of adjuvant intraportal chemotherapy for colorectal cancer. Swiss Group for Clinical Cancer Research (SAKK). Lancet 345:349–353

Laurie JA, Moertel CG et al (1989) Surgical adjuvant therapy of large-bowel carcinoma: an evaluation of levamisole and the combination of levamisole and fluorouracil. J Clin Oncol 7:1447–1456

Lehner B, Schlag P et al (1990) Postoperative active specific immunization in curatively resected colorectal cancer patients with a virus-modified autologous tumor cell vaccine. Cancer Immunol Immunother 32:173–178

Leichman L, Brown T et al (1993) Symptomatic, radiologic and pathologic changes in the central nervous system associated with 5-fluorouracil and levamisole. Proc ASCO 12:198

Lenz HJ, Leichman C et al (1993) Thymidylate synthase (TS) gene expression predicts response of primary gastric cancer to 5-fluorouracil. Proc ASCO 12: 199

Leslie KA, Rossi R et al (1995) Survival expectancy of patients alive 5 years after hepatic resection for metastatic colon carcinoma. Proc ASCO 14:200

Li MC, Ross ST (1976) Chemoprophylaxis for patients with colorectal cancer. Prospective study with five-year follow-up. JAMA 235:2825

Link KH, Aigner KR et al (1988) Concentration and time dependence of the toxicity of fluorinated pyrimidines to HT 29 colorectal carcinoma cells. Cancer Chemother Pharmacol 22:58–62

Link KH, Kreuser ED et al (1993) Die intraarterielle Chemotherapie mit 5-FU und Folinsäure (FA, Rescuvolin) im Therapiekonzept bei nicht resektablen kolorektalen Lebermetastasen. Tumordiagn Ther 14:224–231

Link KH, Kornmann M et al (1994) Response prediction in hepatic artery infusion with fluoropyrimidines using cell culture and polymerase chain reaction techniques. Eur J Surg Oncol 20:317–318

Lorenz M, Hottenrott C et al (1993) Adjuvante, regionale Chemotherapie nach Resektion von Lebermetastasen kolorektaler Primärtumoren. Zentralbl Chir 118:279–289

Lygidakis NJ, Ziras N et al (1995) Resection versus resection combined with adjuvant pre- and post-operative chemotherapy-immunotherapy for metastatic colorectal liver cancer. Hepatogastroenterology 42:155–161

MacDonald JS (1987) New approaches to management of colorectal carcinoma. Hosp Pract 22:185–204

Marangolo M, Pezzuoli G et al (1989) Adjuvant chemotherapy with flourouracil and CCNU in colon cancer. Results of a multicentric randomized study. Tumori 75:269–276

Marsoni S (1995) Efficacy of adjuvant fluorouracil and folinic acid in colon cancer – International Multicentre Pooled Analysis of Colon Cancer Trials (IMPACT) investigators. Lancet 345:939–944

Masucci G, Ragnhammer P et al (1995) Chemotherapy and immunotherapy of colorectal cancer. Med Oncol Tumor Pharmacother 8:207–220

Mayer RJ, O'Connell MJ et al (1989) Status of adjuvant therapy for colorectal cancer. Commentary. J Natl Cancer Inst 81:1359–1364

McArdle CS, Hole D (1991) Impact of variability among surgeons on postoperative morbidity and mortality and ultimate survival. BMJ 302:1501–1505

McPherson TA, Brzezinski WS et al (1984) Adjuvant chemoimmuno- and immunotherapy in B2 and C colorectal cancer: a single center, population-based study. In: Jones SE, Salmon SE (eds) Adjuvant therapy of cancer IV. Grune and Stratton, Orlando, pp 487–496

Metzger U, Mermillod B et al (1987) Intraportal chemotherapy in colorectal carcinoma as an adjuvant modality. World J Surg 11:452–458
Metzger U, Laffer U et al (1994) Stellenwert der portalen Perfusion beim colorectalen Carcinom. Chirurg 65:509–513
Minsky BD (1993) Clinical experience with local excision and postoperative radiation therapy for rectal cancer. Dis Colon Rectum 36:405–409
Minsky BD, Mies C et al (1988) Potentially curative surgery of colon cancer: patterns of failure and survival. J Clin Oncol 6:106–118
Minsky BD, Cohen AM et al (1991) Phase I trial of postoperative 5-FU, radiation therapy, and high dose leucovorin for resectable rectal cancer. Int J Radiat Oncol Biol Phys 22:139–145
Minsky BD, Cohen AM et al (1993) The efficacy of preoperative 5-flourouracil, high-dose leucovorin and sequential radiation therapy for unresectable cancer. Cancer 71:3486–3492
Mitchell MS (1988) Combining chemotherapy with biological response modifiers in treatment of cancer. J Natl Cancer Inst 80:1445–1450
Mitchell MS (1992) Biomodulators in cancer treatment. J Clin Pharmacol 32:2–9
Mitchell MS, Harel W et al (1990) Active-specific immunotherapy for melanoma. J Clin Oncol 8:856–869
Mitomi T, Noto T (1990) A randomized controlled study on adjuvant immuno-chemotherapy with an immunmodulator in curatively resected colorectal cancer. J Cancer Res Clin Oncol 116:872–879
Moertel CG (1992) Accomplishments in surgical adjuvant therapy for large bowel cancer. Cancer 70:1364–1371
Moertel CG (1993) Vaccine adjuvant therapy for colorectal cancer: "very dramatic" or ho-hum? J Clin Oncol 11:385–386
Moertel CG (1994) Chemotherapy for colorectal cancer. N Engl J Med 30:1136–1142
Moertel CG, Fleming TR et al (1990) Levamisole and fluorouracil for adjuvant therapy of resected colon carcinoma. N Engl J Med 322:352–538
Moertel CG, Gunderson LL et al (1994) Early evaluation of combined fluorouracil and leucovorin as a radiation enhancer for locally unresectable, residual, or recurrent gastrointestinal carcinoma. J Clin Oncol 12:21–27
Moertel CG, Fleming TR et al (1995) Fluorouracil plus levamisole as effective adjuvant therapy after resection of stage III colon carcinoma: a final report. Ann Intern Med 122:321–326
Molls M (1994) Multimodale Therapieprinzipien beim Rectumcarcinom. Prä- und postoperative Radiotherapie mit und ohne Chemotherapie beim Rectumcarcinom. Chirurg 65:569–575
Molls M, Fink U (1994) Perioperative radiotherapy +/– chemotherapy in rectal cancer. Ann Oncol 5:105–113
Mrazek R, Economou S et al (1959) Prophylactic and adjuvant use of nitrogen mustard in the surgical treatment of cancer. Ann Surg 150:745–755
Myerson RJ, Michalski JM et al (1995) Adjuvant radiation therapy for rectal carcinoma: predictors of outcome. Int J Radiat Oncol Biol Phys 32:41–50
Neu IS, Ober H (1992) Multifokale Leukenzephalopathie nach adjuvanter Therapie mit Fluorouracil und Levamisol. DMW 117:1379
Nichols PH, Ramsden CW et al (1993) Peri-operative modulation of cellular immunity in patients with colorectal cancer. Clin Exp Immunol 94:4–10
NIH Consesus Conference (1990) Adjuvant therapy for patients with colon und rectal cancer. JAMA 264:1444–1450
Niimoto M, Yanagawa E et al (1990) Prospective randomized controlled study on Bestatin in resectable gastric cancer. J Cancer Res Clin Oncol 116:1013
O'Connell MJ (1994) Surgical adjuvant therapy of colorectal cancer. In: American Society of Clinical Oncology (ed) Educational book. American Society of Clinical Oncology, Dallas, pp 158–161

O'Connell MJ, Adson MA et al (1985) Clinical trial adjuvant therapy after surgical resection of colorectal cancer metastatic to the liver. Mayo Clin Proc 60:517–520

O'Connell M, Wieand H et al (1991) Lack of value for methyl-CCNU (MeCCNU) as a component of effective rectal cancer surgical adjuvant therapy. Interim analysis of Intergroup protocol 86-47-51. Proc ASCO 10:134

O'Connell M, Wiesenfeld M et al (1992a) Interferon-gamma as postoperative surgical adjuvant therapy for colon cancer: significant immune stimulation without evidence of therapeutic effect. Proc ASCO 11:167

O'Connell MJ, Schaid DJ et al (1992b) Current status of adjuvant chemotherapy for colorectal cancer. Cancer 70:1732–1739

O'Connell M, Mailliard J et al (1993a) An Intergroup trial of intensive course 5-FU and low dose leucovorin as surgical adjuvant therapy for high risk colon cancer. Proc ASCO 12:190

O'Connell M, Martenson J et al (1993b) Protracted venous infusion (PVI) 5-fluorouracil (5FU) as a component of effective combined modality postoperative surgical adjuvant therapy for high-risk rectal cancer. Proc ASCO 12:193

Pahlman L, Glimelius B (1992) Pre-operative and post-operative radiotherapy and rectal cancer. World J Surg 16:858–865

Panettiere FJ, Goodman PJ et al (1988) Adjuvant therapy in large bowel adenocarçinoma: long-term results of a Southwest Oncology Group study. J Clin Oncol 6:947–954

Papillon J (1994) Surgical adjuvant therapy for rectal cancer: present options. Dis Colon Rectum 37:144–148

Patt YZ, Mavligit GM (1991) Arterial chemotherapy in the management of colorectal cancer. An overview. Semin Oncol 18:478–490

Perez T, Shani A et al (1995) A randomized study of 5-FU and levamisole (LM) vs 5-FU and leucovorin (LV) as adjuvant therapy of colon cancer (CC). Proc ASCO 14:214

Peters GJ, vanderWilt CL et al (1994) Thymidylate synthase inhibition after administration of fluorouracil with or without leucovorin in colon cancer patients: implications for treatment with fluorouracil. J Clin Oncol 12:2035–2042

Piedbois P, Buyse M et al (1995) Portal vein infusion is an effective adjuvant treatment for patients with colorectal cancer. Proc ASCO 14:192

Poon MA, O'Connell MJ et al (1989) Biochemical modulation of fluorouracil: evidence of significant improvement of survival and quality of life in patients with advanced colorectal carcinoma. J Clin Oncol 7:1407–1418

Ragnhammer P, Fagerberg J et al (1993) Effect of monoclonal antibody 17-1A and GM-CSF in patients with advanced colorectal carcinoma – long-lasting, complete remissions can be induced. Int J Cancer 53:751–758

Riethmüller G, Schneider-Gädicke E et al (1994) Randomised trial of monoclonal antibody 17-1A for adjuvant therapy of resected Dukes' C colorectal carcinoma. Lancet 34:1177–1183

Robinson E, Bartal A et al (1982) Combined adjuvant therapy of radically operated colorectal cancer patients (chemotherapy, radiotherapy and MER-BCG). Cancer Chemother Pharmacol 8:35–40

Romsdahl M, Withers HR (1978) Radiotherapy combined with curative surgery. Arch Surg 113:466–453

Rosenberg SA (1987) Surgical treatment of metastatic cancer. Lippincott, Philadelphia

Rosenberg SA, Schwarz SL et al (1988) Combination immunotherapy for cancer: synergistic antitumor interactions of interleukin-2, alpha interferon, and tumor-infiltrating lymphocytes. J Natl Cancer Inst 80:1393–1397

Rosenberg SA, Lotze MT et al (1989) Experience with the use of high-dose interleukin-2 in the treatment of 652 cancer patients. Am J Surg 210:474–485

Russell AH, Tong D et al (1984) Adenocarcinoma of the proximal colon. Sites of initial dissemination and patterns of recurrence following surgery alone. Cancer 53:360–367

Ryan H, Weiden P et al (1988) Adjuvant portal vein infusion for colorectal cancer: a 3-arm randomized trial. Proc ASCO 7:95

Safi F, Link KH et al (1993) Is follow-up of colorectal cancer patients worthwhile? Dis Colon Rectum 36:636–644

Safi F, Hepp G et al (1995) Simultaneous adjuvant regional and systemic chemotherapy after resection of liver metastases of colorectal cancer. Proc ASCO 14:217–217

Schäfer H, Bruns CH et al (1994) The influence of surgical trauma on natural killer cell function in patients with esophageal and gastric cancer. Eur J Surg Oncol 20:265–266

Schlag PM (1994) Adjuvante systemische Chemo- oder Immuntherapie beim Coloncarcinom. Chirurg 65:503–508

Schlag P, Saeger HD et al (1990) Adjuvant intraportal FUDR-chemotherapy in colon cancer patients. In: Salmon SE (ed) Proceedings of the 6th international conference on the adjuvant therapy of Cancer. Saunders, Philadelphia, pp 439–445

Schlag P, Hohenberger P et al (1991) Operative Möglichkeiten und therapeutische Chancen bei Lebermetastasen. Chirurg 62:715–719

Schmoll HJ (1994a) Adjuvante Chemotherapie beim Rektumcarcinom. Chirurg 65:576–584

Schmoll HJ (1994b) Colorectal carcinoma: current problems and future perspectives. Ann Oncol 515:115–121

Shau H, Kim A (1988) Suppression of lymphokine-activated killer induction by neutrophils. J Immunol 141:4395–4402

Siewert JR, Fink U (1992) Multimodale Therapieprinzipien bei Tumoren des Gastrointestinaltraktes. Chirurg 63:242–250

Silverberg E, Lubera JA (1989) Cancer statistics 1989. Cancer 39:3–39

Slaney G, Powell J et al (1991) Cancer of the large bowell: overall treatment. In: Clinical cancer monographs. MacMillan, London, pp 116–140

Smith RD, Hall J et al (1993) A cost-utility approach to the use of 5-flourouracil and levamisole as adjuvant chemotherapy for Dukes' C colonic carcinoma. Med J Aust 158:319–322

Soybel DI, Bliss DP et al (1987) Colon and rectal carcinoma. Curr Probl Cancer 11:257–356

Staib L, Harel W et al (1993) Prevention against experimental cerebral murine melanoma B16 by active immunization. Cancer Res 53:1113–1121

Staib L, Butzer U et al (1994a) Immune reactivity is reduced in patients with advanced colorectal cancer. Proc AACR 35:249

Staib L, Harel W et al (1994b) Active-specific immunotherapy for cerebral murine melanoma: which components are necessary? Proc AACR 35:514

Steele G (1991) Combined-modality therapy for rectal carcinoma – the time has come. N Engl J Med 324:764–766

Steele GD (1994) The national cancer data base report on colorectal cancer. Cancer 74:1979–1989

Stevens KR, Allen CV et al (1976) Preoperative radiotherapy for adenocarcinoma of the rectosigmoid. Cancer 37:2866–2874

Sugarbaker PH (1991) Mechanism of relapse for colorectal cancer: implications for intraperitoneal chemotherapy. J Surg Oncol [Suppl] 2:36–41

Sugarbaker PH, Gianola FJ et al (1985) Prospective, randomized trial of intravenous versus intraperitoneal 5-fluorouracil in patients with advanced primary colon or rectal cancer. Surgery 98:414–422

Sutanto-Ward E, Sigurdson ER et al (1992) Adjuvant chemotherapy for colorectal hepatic metastases: role of route of administration and timing. Surg Oncol 1:87–95

Talmadge JE, Fidler J et al (1984) The NCI preclinical screen of biological response modifiers. Behring Inst Mitt 74:189–194
Taylor DD, Gercel-Taylor C et al (1993) Enhancement of antitumor effects of combined chemoimmunotherapy. J Immunother 13:91–97
Taylor FW (1962) Cancer of the colon and rectum: a study of routes of metastases and death. Surgery 52:305–308
Taylor I, Machin D et al (1985) A randomized controlled trial of adjuvant portal vein cytotoxic perfusion in colorectal cancer. Br J Surg 72:359–363
Thom A, Baumann J et al (1992) Experience with high dose radiation therapy and the intestinal sling procedure in patients with rectal carcinoma. Cancer 70:581–584
Vanky F, Klein E et al (1986) Lysis of autologous tumor cells by blood lymphocytes tested at the time of surgery. Correlation with the postsurgical clinical course. Cancer Immunol Immunother 21:69–76
Wadler S, Schwartz EL et al (1989) Fluorouracil and recombinant alpha-2a-interferon: an active regimen against advanced colorectal carcinoma. J Clin Oncol 7:1769–1775
Wadler S, Goldmann M et al (1990) Phase I trial of 5-fluorouracil and recombinant a2a-interferon in patients with advanced colorectal carcinoma. Cancer Res 50:2056–2059
Wadler S, Lembersky B et al (1991) Phase II trial of flourouracil and recombinant interferon alfa-2a in patients with advanced colorectal carcinoma: an Eastern Cooperative Oncology Group study. J Clin Oncol 9:1806–1810
Wagman LD, Kemeny MM et al (1990) A prospective, randomized evaluation of the treatment of colorectal cancer metastatic to the liver. J Clin Oncol 8:1885–1893
Wagner JG, Gyves JW et al (1986) Steady-state nonlinear pharmacokinetics of 5-fluorouracil during hepatic arterial and intravenous infusion in cancer patients. Cancer Res 46:1499–1506
Weisenthal LM, Dill PL et al (1991) Effect of prior cancer chemotherapy on human tumor-specific cytotoxicity in vitro in response to immunopotentiating biologic response modifiers. J Natl Cancer Inst 83:37–42
Weiss L, Ward PM (1991) Metachronous and synchronous seeding of target organs in the mouse, after paracecal injection of colon-26 cancer cells: is it relevant to human metastatic colorectal carcinoma? Regional Cancer Treat 4:55–59
Welch JP, Donaldson GA (1979) The clinical correlation of autopsy study of recurrent colorectal cancer. Ann Surg 189:496–502
Wereldsma JCJ, Bruggink E et al (1990) Adjuvant portal liver infusion in colorectal cancer with 5-fluorouracil/heparin versus Urokinase versus control. Cancer 65:425–432
Wils JA (1992) Chemotherapy for gastrointestinal cancer: new hopes or new disappointments? Scand J Gastroenterol 27:87–94
Windle R, Bell P et al (1987) Five year results of a randomized trial of adjuvant 5-Fluorouracil and Levamisole in colorectal cancer. Br J Surg 74:569–572
Witzig TE, Loprinzi CL et al (1991) DNA ploidy and cell kinetic measurements as predictors of recurrence and survival in stages B2 and C colorectal carcinoma. Gastroenterology 102:1612–1619
Wolmark N, Fisher B et al (1988) Postoperative adjuvant chemotherapy or BCG for colon cancer: results from NSABP protocol C-01. J Natl Cancer Inst 80:30–36
Wolmark N, Rockette H et al (1990) Adjuvant therapy of Dukes' A, B and C adenocarcinoma of the colon with portal-vein fluorouracil hepatic infusion: preliminary results of NSABP C-02. J Clin Oncol 8:1466–1475
Wolmark N, Rockette H et al (1993a) Adjuvant therapy for carcinoma of the colon: review of NSABP clinical trials. In: Salmon SE (ed) Adjuvant therapy of cancer VII. Lippincott, Philadelphia, pp 300–306

Wolmark N, Rockette H et al (1993b) The benefit of leucovorin-modulated fluorouracil as postoperative adjuvant therapy for primary colon cancer and bowel project protocol C-03. J Clin Oncol 11:1879–1887
Wunderlich M, Schiessel R et al (1985) Effect of adjuvant chemo- or immunotherapy on the prognosis of colorectal cancer operated for cure. Br J Surg 72:107–110

Current Treatment Modalities in Advanced Colorectal Carcinoma

R.U. Hilgenfeld[1], M. Streit[2], E. Thiel[2], and E.-D. Kreuser[2]

[1] Medical Department I, St. Joseph Hospital, Bäumerplan 24, 12101 Berlin, Germany
[2] Department of Hematology/Oncology, University Medical Center Benjamin Franklin, Free University of Berlin, Hindenburgdamm 30, 12200 Berlin, Germany

Abstract

Several biochemical and immunological substances are currently being tested for their efficacy in the treatment of advanced colorectal cancer, the second-most malignant disease in the western world. Presently, a combination of 5-fluorouracil (FU) and the biochemical modulator folinic acid is considered to be the standard treatment for this malignancy, with a median response rate of 30%. A recent multi-analysis of phase III trials with methotrexate and FU versus FU alone has demonstrated a statistically significant doubling of the response rate as well as a significant survival advantage for the combination. So far, other biochemical or immunological modulators of FU have not shown a significant advantage regarding response or survival. Several new drugs such as tegafur, thymidilate synthase inhibitors, trimetrexate, or topoisomerase-I-inhibitors have been tested with promising results in preclinical and early clinical settings. While local treatment such as hepatic artery infusion has become safer, it is still more toxic than systemic treatment and showed a significant improvement of response but no survival advantage. Since all treatment strategies in advanced colorectal cancer are still palliative, quality of life is a more important endpoint in clinical trials.

Incidence, Epidemiology, and Clinical Relevance of Colorectal Carcinoma

Colorectal carcinoma (CRC) is among the most common cancer types in the western world. The incidence is high in the developed countries, with the exception of Japan, and still rising (Vogel and McPherson 1989). In the United States of America, there are approximately 150000 new cases and about 50000 fatalities per year (Boring et al. 1993). Despite several new treatment modalities, the prognosis depends largely on the extent of disease at the time of diagnosis. While surgery may be curative in earlier stages, about 50% of

Recent Results in Cancer Research, Vol. 142

patients will suffer a relapse and die within 5 years (Fleischer et al. 1989). However, it has been demonstrated that adjuvant strategies can significantly improve survival in certain stages of CRC (Moertel et al. 1990, 1992).

Prognostic Factors in Advanced Disease

Over the years, several reports have correlated prognostic factors to response or survival. So far, the only reliable prognostic factor found by several authors to be statistically significant in CRC is the performance status (for review see Graf et al. 1991). Kemeny and Braun (1983) detected no prognostic factor for response in 220 patients with advanced CRC. However, statistically significant for a poor prognosis were an elevated LDH, an abnormal CEA, a WBC >10000, a Karnofsky performance status <60%, and liver metastases. Graf et al. (1991) examined 340 patients with advanced colorectal cancer and found the hemoglobin level, the disease-free interval, the number of symptoms, and the performance status to be statistically significant prognostic factors for survival, while the main independent determinant of response was the hemoglobin level. In another retrospective analysis of 324 patients included in four chemotherapy trials, the same group found only a response to chemotherapy of 4 months duration to be associated with a statistically significant survival advantage (Graf et al. 1994a). When these prognostic factors were tested in an independent population for their relationship to survival by univariate and multivariate analyses to determine their predictive value, the group confirmed the importance of the hemoglobin level, the disease-free interval, and the Karnofsky performance status in both analyses. However, they found statistical significance for the number of symptoms only in the univariate analysis (Graf et al. 1994b). Steinberg et al. (1992) reported baseline albumin and GOT to be significant determinants of survival, while the performance status was prognostic for the response. In a recent prospective randomized trial in 142 patients with advanced colorectal cancer a Karnofsky performance status <80%, an elevated alkaline phosphatase and/or GOT, as well as no response to chemotherapy all were found to have a statistically significant negative impact on survival, using a multivariate analysis. In this study patients with a Karnofsky performance status <80% who had liver metastases and showed no response to chemotherapy had only a 10% survival rate after 7 months, while patients with a Karnofsky performance status ≥80%, response to therapy within the first 4 months of treatment, and metastases to the lung only showed a survival rate of 75% after 7 months ($p = 0.0001$; Hilgenfeld and Kreuser 1996).

Biochemical Modulation

In recent years, biochemical modulators have been introduced in the treatment of cancer patients. These are non-cytotoxic drugs which are supposed to enhance the efficacy of the main cytotoxic agent in various pathways by altering intracellular metabolism (Table 1).

5-Fluorouracil

Since it was first introduced in the treatment of cancer patients in the 1950s, 5-fluorouracil (FU) has remained the most active drug in CRC (Heidelberger et al. 1957; for overview see: Haskell et al. 1990). While phase-I/II trials disclosed a median response rate of 20% with a range of 8–54% for treatment with FU alone in patients with CRC, this response rate was reduced to 12% in randomized trials (Haskell et al. 1990; Table 2) and to 11% in a recent meta-analysis (Advanced Colorectal Cancer Meta-Analysis Project 1992).

5-Fluorouracil and Folinic Acid

The hitherto most efficient modulator in CRC is folinic acid (FA). Its use in combination with FU is based on the ability of the FU metabolite fluorodeoxyuridine monophosphate (FdUMP) to inhibit the enyzyme thymidilate synthase (TS). This results in the inhibition of thymidilate (dTMP) production and subsequently interferes with DNA synthesis. The ability of FdUMP to inhibit TS is affected by the intracellular level of 5,10-methylenetetrahydrofolate, a reduced folate. The co-administration of folinic acid as an exogenous reduced folate has been shown to enhance the cytotoxicity of FU in several preclinical models (for review see Sotos et al. 1994).

Phase-II trials in previously untreated patients showed the average median response rate for the combination of FU/FA to be between 20 and 30% (for

Table 1. Biochcmical modulators of 5-fluorouracil and mechanisms involved (modified from Sotos et al. 1994)

Modulator	Known or presumed mechanism of action
Folinic acid	Increased TS inhibition
Interferon α	Increased FU metabolism?
Methotrexate	Purine synthesis inhibition
	Increased PRPP levels
	Increased FU incorporation into RNA
Trimetrexate	Purine synthesis inhibition
	Increased PRPP levels
	Increased FU incorporation into RNA
PALA	Pyrimidine synthesis inhibition
	Increased FU incorporation into RNA
Uridine	Selective decreased FU incorporation into RNA?

Table 2. Randomized trials: 5-fluorouracil vs. 5-fluorouracil/folinic acid in colorectal carcinoma

Reference	Year	Patients enrolled[a] (*n*)	Response rate (%)		Time to disease progression (months)		Median survival (months)	
			FU	FU+FA	FU	FU+FA	FU	FU+FA
Petrelli et al.	1987	52	11 *	48	*			
Erlichman et al.	1988	125	7 *	33	2.9 *	5.1	9.6 *	12.6
Poon et al.	1989	429	10 *	43[b]	*		7.7 *	12.0
Petrelli et al.	1989	343	12 *	30[c]	6.0	8.0	11.5	13.7
Valone et al.	1989	245	17	19	4.6	5.5	11.5	11.8
Clendeninn et al.	1990	218	23	33	4.4	5.5	12.7	10.6
Doroshow et al.	1990	79	13 *	44	4.0 *	5.5	12.8(*)	14.4[d]
Labianca et al.	1991	182	10 *	22	6.0	6.0	11.0	11.0
Di Costanzo et al.	1992	119	18	16	5.0	5.3	15.5	13.3
Nobile et al.	1992	142	8 *	23	3.0	5.0	11.0	11.0
Steinke et al.	1992	122	20	30	3.0 *	8.5	7.0	10.5
Median			12.5	33	4.4	5.5	11.5	11.9

[a] For all arms
[b] Low dose of FA
[c] High dose of FA
[d] Cross-over study
* Statistically significant difference

review see Grem et al. 1987). In 7/11 randomized trials conducted from 1987 to 1992, significantly higher response rates were seen for the combination of FU and FA than for FU alone (Table 2). An analysis of the time to disease progression yielded a statistical significance for five of the trials, but only 2/11 studies showed a significantly improved survival in patients treated with the combination (Table 2). A meta-analysis of numerous randomized clinical trials comparing FU with a combination of FU/FA also revealed the latter to be associated with better response rates (23% vs. 11%; Advanced Colorectal Cancer Meta-Analysis Project, 1992). However, there was no clear evidence that the modulation of FU by FA also improved time to disease progression or survival.

While these results did not confirm the superiority of FU/FA, Poon et al. (1989) reported a considerable weight gain as well as an improvement of the performance status and the symptoms of disease in patients treated with FU/FA compared with those treated with FU only.

A randomized trial comparing two FU/FA protocols in advanced CRC was published in 1994. A 5-day FU regimen plus low-dose FA was not superior to weekly FU plus high-dose FA with regard to response rates and survival; however, the financial costs and side effects were lower (Buroker et al. 1994). Several groups investigated the efficacy and toxicity of high-dose FA and high-dose FU as a continuous infusion in patients with advanced CRC. Using a 24-h infusion of 2600 mg/m^2 FU with 500 mg/m^2 FA, Ardalan et al. (1991) reported a response rate of 30% in ten patients. To confirm these results, Weh et al. (1994) conducted a multicenter trial. Patients received 2600 mg/m² FU over 24 h weekly, preceeded by 500 mg/m² FA as a 1-h infusion. All patients had been pretreated, mostly with FU/FA and/or FU/IFN. In patients who had a partial remission or stable disease with an improved clinical condition, therapy was continued until progression occurred. Five of 57 patients (9%) achieved a PR, while 56% of patients (32/57) remained stable; 81% (30/37) of those showing an overall response (PR/SD) under this regimen had had a response before. The median duration of response was 3 months, and the median survival for all patients was 8 months (3–17+). There was one toxic death; other side effects included mucositis, nausea, diarrhea, and hand-foot syndrome (Weh et al. 1994).

Methotrexate

Methotrexate (MTX), an antimetabolite, causes an increased intracellular concentration of phosphoribosylpyrophosphate due to MTX inhibition of purine metabolism, which results in an increased formation of fluorouridyl triphosphate (FUTP) (Cadman et al. 1980). FUTP is then integrated into RNA instead of the physiologic UTP.

The proper timing of sequential MTX and FU is an important issue. Phase-II trials showed response rates of approximately 40% when MTX was administered 4–7 h before FU (Table 3). In randomized trials with FU and MTX versus FU alone, the combination was distinctly advantageous for the response and, in some reports, also for survival, when the interval between MTX and FU application was longer (Table 4). For comparison, a MTX-FU interval of only 1 h resulted in response rates of 3–28%, while a 24-h interval yielded responses in 20–32% of the patients. This trend toward better results with a longer interval was confirmed by a phase-III trial comparing a 1-h with a 24-h interval. The arm with the 24-h interval was significantly better with respect to the overall response rate (29% vs. 14.5%), the time to disease progression (9.9 months vs. 5.9 months), and the median survival (15.3 months vs. 11.4 months; Marsh et al. 1991). A recent meta-analysis of phase-III trials of sequential MTX and FU vs. FU alone found a statistically significant doubling of the response rate as well as a significant survival advantage for the combination (Advanced Colorectal Cancer Meta-Analysis Project 1994).

Phosphonacetyl-L-aspartate

In 1979, *N*-(phosphonacetyl)-L-aspartate (PALA) was introduced into clinical trials as a potent inhibitor of de novo pyrimidine biosynthesis. It inhibits the enzyme aspartate carbamyl transferase (ACTase), thus depleting cells of uridine nucleotide pools and subsequently causing an increased uptake of FU by

Table 3. 5-Fluorouracil/methotrexate in colorectal carcinoma (phase-II trials)

Reference	Year	Regimen	Interval MTX/FU (h)	No. of patients	Response rate (%)
Cantrell et al.	1982	FU/MTX/FA	1	16	6
Ajani et al.	1985	FU/MTX	1	30	3
Panasci et al.	1985	FU/MTX/FA	1	25	28
Hansen et al.	1986	FU/MTX/FA	1	26	19
Pyrhönen and Kouri	1992	FU/MTX/FA/EPI	1	85	29
Weinerman et al.	1982	FU/MTX/FA	4	29	42
Herrmann et al.	1984	FU/MTX/FA	7	20	40
Leone et al.	1986	FU/MTX	20	24	46
Leone et al.	1992	FU/MTX/FA	20	33	33
Glimelius et al.	1986	FU/MTX/FA	3/23	50	50
Kemeny et al.	1984	FU/MTX	24	43	32
Sinnige et al.	1990	FU/MTX/FA	24	20	20
Abad et al.	1991	FU/MTX/FA	24	30	40

FU, 5-Fluorouracil; *MTX*, methotrexate; *FA*, folinic acid; *EPI*, epirubicin

Table 4. 5-Fluorouracil/methotrexate versus 5-fluorouracil in advanced colorectal carcinoma (randomized trials)

Reference	Year	Regimen	Interval MTX/FU (h)	No. of Patients	RR (%)	Survival (months)
Petrelli et al.	1987	FU/MTX	4	21	5	10
		FU		19	*11	11
		FU/FA		25	*48	12
O'Connell et al.	1990	FU/MTX	7	45	7	7
		FU/FA[a]		49	*33	*14
		FU/FA[b]		42	*33	*13
Herrmann et al.	1992	FU/MTX	7	83	25	13
		FU		76	18	15
Abad et al.	1992	FU/MTX/FA	10	60	25	13
		FU/FA		56	18	13
Delfino et al.	1992	FU/MTX/FA	18	28	*18	8
		FU		33	0	11
Macchiavelli et al.	1990	FU/MTX/FA	20	60	*28	N/A
		FU		58	12	8
NGTATG[c]	1989	FU/MTX/FA	3#21	82	*24	*10
		FU		91	3	6
Kemeny et al.	1988	FU/MTX	24	17	6	10
		MOF/Strep		17	35	12
Poon et al.	1989	FU/MTX	24	39	*26	8
		FU/MTX/FA	7	39	21	8
		FU		39	10	8
Valone et al.	1989	FU/MTX	24	96	20	12
		FU		52	17	12
Marsh et al.	1991	FU/MTX/FA	24	76	*29	*15
		FU/MTX/FA	1	83	14.5	12

[a] Low-dose FA
[b] High-dose FA
[c] Nordic Gastrointestinal Tumor Adjuvant Therapy Group
RR, Response rate; *FU*, 5-fluorouracil; *MTX*, methotrexate; *FA* folinic acid; *, statistically significant; *N/A*, not applicable

RNA (Martin and Kemeny 1992). Martin et al. (1983) showed in preclinical models that PALA is more effective when given at a lower rather than at a higher dose. Clinical trials with different dosages of PALA in combination with FU have shown response rates of 10–43% (median 26%; Table 5). However, randomized trials comparing FU/PALA with FU alone are still lacking.

Immunotherapy for Advanced Colorectal Cancer

Recent years have witnessed the exploration of many new immunotherapeutic strategies in CRC. Immunotherapy can be divided into an active and a passive category. Active immunotherapy should ideally stimulate host antitumor immunity, either cellular or humoral. Numerous specific tumor vaccines have been developed and tested for this purpose (for review see Foon 1989). Active specific immunotherapy (ASI) against tumor-associated antigens is supposed to result in a host immune response with subsequent selective cytotoxicity for tumor cells (Kennett et al. 1980). Passive immunotherapy relies on the administration of biologically active agents with innate antitumor properties such as reactivity to monoclonal antibodies and conjugates (Foon 1989).

Interleukin

Interleukin 2 (rIL-2) is a 15-kDa glycoprotein secreted by T-helper lymphocytes following activation by antigens or mitogens (Morgan et al. 1976). It enhances natural cytotoxicity, mediated by natural killer (NK) and lymphokine-activated killer (LAK) cells (Grimm et al. 1983; Ortaldo et al. 1984).

Earlier clinical studies showed response rates of up to 17% in CRC after treatment with rIL-2 alone or in combination with LAK cells (Rosenberg et al.

Table 5. 5-Fluorouracil + PALA in advanced colorectal cancer

Reference	Year	PALA dose	Response rate	
			n	(%)
Ardalan et al.	1981	HD	2/18	(11)
Weiss et al.	1982	HD	2/21	(10)
Erlichman et al.	1982	HD	1/28	(4)
Presant et al.	1983	HD	2/10	(20)
Buroker et al.[a]	1985	HD	4/34	(12)
Muggia et al.	1987	HD	9/37	(24)
Ardalan et al.	1988	LD	7/19	(37)
Ahlgren et al.	1990	LD	3/10	(30)
O'Dwyer et al.	1990	LD	16/37	(43)
Kemeny et al.	1992a	LD	15/43	(35)

[a]Randomized study
HD, High dose; *LD*, low dose

1987, 1989). Hamblin et al. (1989) reported an enhanced response rate of 29% after combining rIL-2 and FU. Yang et al. (1993) reported a 44% response rate in patients treated with high doses of FU, FA, and rIL-2, but all of the patients had responded well to FU/FA before receiving IL-2. A recent randomized trial in which FU/FA was compared with a combination of FU, FA, and rIL-2 did not disclose significant differences between the two schedules. Response rates were 16% and 17%, respectively (Heys et al. 1995).

Interferon

Interferons (IFN) are a group of glycoproteins with common antiviral, immunomodulatory, and antiproliferative functions. The three main types, alpha, beta and gamma interferon, are characterized by their acid stability, cell surface receptors, and primary sequences. While the exact mechanism of action is still unknown, antiproliferative effects against various tumor cell lines and immunostimulatory effects in vivo have been reported (for review see Itri 1992). In the late 1980s, first clinical trials with FU/IFN showed promising results, especially in patients with advanced CRC who had received no prior chemotherapy (Wadler et al. 1989). The excellent results reported in this initial study were not confirmed in later trials. In 19 phase-I/II trials conducted between 1987 and 1993 with a total of 453 patients, the median response rate of FU/IFN combined was 31% (range 5–63%; Table 6). Two randomized trials

Table 6. Phase-I/II trials with 5-fluorouracil and interferon in colorectal carcinoma

Reference	Year	Response rate	
		n	(%)
Rios et al.	1987	3/16	(19)
Clark et al.	1987	1/20	(5)
Ajani et al.	1989	2/29	(7)
De Vecchis et al.	1989	3/12	(25)
Wadler et al.	1989	20/32	(63)
Kemeny et al.	1990	9/34	(26)
Pazdur et al.	1990	16/45	(35)
Douillard et al.	1991	5/16	(31)
Huberman et al.	1991	13/33	(39)
Jaiyesimi et al.	1991	4/23	(16)
Wadler et al.	1991	15/36	(42)
Bang et al.	1992	6/17	(35)
Botto et al.	1992	19/47	(40)
John et al.	1992	16/48	(33)
Pavlick et al.	1992	4/11	(36)
Weh et al.	1992	17/55	(31)
Aiba et al.	1993	6/20	(24)
Meehan et al.	1993	4/17	(24)
Pazdur et al.	1993	12/39	(31)
Median (%)			31

of FU/FA vs. FU/IFN did not show a statistically significant difference of FU/IFN regarding response, time to disease progression, or survival (Corfu-A Study Group 1995, Kreuser et al. 1995; Table 8). Recently, a prospective randomized trial was performed to determine the efficacy, toxicity, and quality of life with FU and FA compared with FU and IFN α-2b (Kreuser et al. 1995). This study, in which a total of 142 patients were treated, revealed a significantly improved quality of life in the FU/FA treatment arm compared with the patients treated with FU/IFN. Quality of life in this study was assessed with the European Organisation for Research and Treatment of Cancer (EORTC) QLQ C 30 questionnaire before and during the first 6 months of chemotherapy.

Clinical trials using "double modulation" of FU by FA and IFN did not show a clear benefit, with a median response rate of 28% (Table 7). Several randomized trials comparing the triple combination (FU/FA/IFN) with FU/FA yielded contradictory results, the double modulation showing no clear advantage in the form of higher response rates or longer survival (Table 8).

Table 7. 5-Fluorouracil, folinic acid, and interferon in colorectal carcinoma[a]

Reference	Year	Response rate	
		n	(%)
Labianca et al.	1990	4/15	(27)
Grem et al.	1991	10/22	(45)
Inoshita et al.	1991	14/46	(30)
Köhne-Wömpner et al.	1991	3/32	(9)
Piedbois et al.	1991	7/10[b]	(70)
		1/6[c]	(17)
Punt et al.	1992	5/19	(26)
Seymour et al.	1991	17/47	(26)
Taylor et al.	1991	3/14	(21)
Brunetti et al.	1992	3/17	(18)
Cascinu et al.	1992	23/45	(51)
van Hadzel et al.	1992	7/25	(28)
Kreuser et al.	1992c	18/62	(29)
Labianca et al.	1992	8/36	(22)
Lembersky et al.	1992	9/11	(82)
Moore et al.	1992	7/25	(28)
Sobrero et al.	1992	6/44	(14)
Grem et al.	1993	24/44	(54)
Sinnige et al.	1993	17/30	(57)
Auber et al.	1994	3/10	(33)
Buter et al.	1994	26/49	(53)
Pazdur et al.	1994	14/47	(30)
Median (%)			28

[a] At least ten patients included
[b] Previously untreated
[c] Pretreated

Table 8. Randomized trials including 5-fluorouracil, folinic acid, and interferon in colorectal carcinoma

Reference	No. of patients	Regimen	Response rate (%)	Time to disease progression (months)	Median survival (months)
Dufour et al. 1992	43	FU	18	5.0	N/A
		FU/IFN	24	6.9	N/A
York et al. 1993	146	FU	19	3.9+	13.6
		FU/IFN	31	4.6	12.4
Cellerino et al. 1994	131	FU	14	4.0	12.0
		FU/IFN	6	4.0	12.0
Recchia et al. 1992	72	FU/FA	45	7.0	8.2
		FU/FA/IFN	22	6.6	8.2
Kosmidis et al. 1993	95	FU/FA	19	5.8	10.0
		FU/FA/IFN	6	4.0	7.0
Pensel 1993	48	FU/FA	33	8.3	11.1
		FU/FA/IFN	42	9.9	13.2
Seymour et al. 1994	165	FU/FA	30	N/A	10.8
		FU/FA/IFN	31	N/A	10.0
Corfu-A Study Group 1995	449	FU/FA	18	6.2	11.3
		FU/IFN	21	7.3	11.0
Kreuser et al. 1996	142	FU/FA	8	3.7	7.4
		FU/IFN	8	2.2	9.3

N/A, Not applicable

Locoregional Therapy

Approximately 40% of patients with CRC will develop metastases to the liver as the primary organ during the course of their disease (Weiss et al. 1986). Therefore, several treatment approaches directed at liver metastases have been developed.

Hepatic Artery Infusion

Since the 1960s, the delivery of chemotherapy directly to the liver via hepatic artery infusion (HAI) has gained considerable interest, and is nowadays almost exclusively performed with percutaneous intra-arterial catheters and external pumps (Shepard et al. 1985). As in systemic therapy, fluoropyrimidines such as FU and fluorodeoxyuridine (FUdR) so far are the most potent cytotoxic drugs regarding response rates (Patt and Mavligit 1991). In numerous phase-II trials with FU/FUdR in patients with metastatic CRC, response rates of 5–83% were reported; the median response rate was 47% (Table 9). The survival in these studies varied between 9 and 31 months; median survival was 14.5 months. Response rates and survival in pretreated

Table 9. Locoregional chemotherapy in advanced colorectal cancer[a]

Author	Year	Drug	No. of patients enrolled	Pretreated (%)	RR (%)	Med. Surv. (months)
Balch et al.	1983	FUdR	50	40	83[c]	26
Cohen et al.	1983	FUdR[b]	50	36	51	N/A
Weiss et al.	1983	FUdR	17	85	29	31
Kemeny et al.	1984	FUdR	41	43	42	12
Niederhuber et al.	1984	FUdR	70	45	83	25
Johnson and Rivkin	1985	FUdR[b]	40	0	47	12
Schwartz et al.	1985	FUdR	25	N/A	15	18
Shepard et al.	1985	FUdR[b]	53	42	32	17
Cohen et al.	1986	FUdR[b]	36	42	70	12
Quagliuolo et al.	1987	FUdR	60	N/A	26	17
Rougier et al.	1987	FUdR	16	N/A	53	15
Scheele et al.	1991	FUdR[b]	72	0	54	13
Lorenz et al.	1992	FUdR	112		45	16
Kemeny et al.[d]	1993	FUdR	49	100	33	15
		FUdR[b]	45	100	47	19
Stagg et al.	1991	FUdR/FU	64	47	50	22
Grage et al.	1979	FU	31	0	34	10
Denck et al.	1984	FU	24	0	44	14
Thirlwell et al.	1986	FU	68	30	60	13
Wils et al.	1986	FU[b]	30	0	30	19
Cortesi et al.	1987	FU[b]	12	0	33	11
Arai et al.	1988	FU[b]	33	N/A	64	12
Schlag et al.	1988	FU	36	0	72	14
Goldberg et al.	1990	FU	20	0	5	9
Rougier et al.	1991	FU[b]	48	0	60	14

[a] Non randomized triasl
[b] Combination chemotherapy
[c] Evaluation of response by CEA value
[d] Randomized trial. *RR*, response rate; *Med. Surv.*, median survival; *N/A*, not applicable

patients were comparable. Toxicities of HAI included direct hepatic toxicity, biliary sclerosis, and gastric/duodenal irritation and ulceration. In a recent randomized trial, patients treated with dexamethasone in addition to HAI were able to receive greater dose intensity and had improved response rates while showing similar toxicity (Kemeny et al. 1992b). To enhance the efficacy of HAI, several trials combined modulators such as FA and IFN with the fluoropyrimidine. While response rates in phase-II trials were encouraging, the combination of FUdR and FA increased hepatic toxicity considerably (Kemeny et al. 1994; Patt et al. 1994). Five randomized trials conducted between 1987 and 1992 compared locoregional with systemic chemotherapy in patients with metastic CRC (Table 10). While four of them showed a significantly higher response rate for the intra-arterial treatment, only one found a

Table 10. Locoregional vs. systemic chemotherapy in advanced colorectal cancer[a]

Reference	Year	No. of patients enrolled	Response (%)			Time to disease progression (months)		Med. survival (months)		
			IA		IV	IA	IV	IA		IV
Change et al.	1987	64	62	*	17	7	9	18		12
Kemeny et al.	1987	99	50	*	20	9	5	17		12
Hohn et al.[b]	1989	143	42	*	10	13	7	17		16
Martin et al.	1990	74	48		21	5	6	12.5		10.5
Rougier et al.	1992	166	43	*	9	14.5	5.5	15	*	11

[a] Randomized trials
[b] Cross-over study
IA, Intra-arterial (HAI); *IV*, intravenous; *, statistically significant

significant improvement of survival for this treatment, and none showed a difference in time to disease progression.

Chemoembolization

Chemoembolization is a new technique performed by placing a catheter into the hepatic artery, followed by concomitant local delivery of chemotherapy and a vascular occlusion agent. In comparison to HAI, this should result in a more confined and prolonged delivery of chemotherapy. Experience with chemoembolization in metastatic CRC so far is limited. Several phase-II trials with different combinations of cytotoxic agents such as doxorubicin, mitomycin C, FU, and cisplatin have resulted in response rates from 17 to 50%; median survival was between 11 and 18 months (Daniels et al. 1992; Lang and Brown 1993; Martinelli et al. 1994).

New Drugs in the Treatment of Colorectal Cancer

Due to the unsatisfactory results obtained by treating advanced CRC with the agents described above, several new drugs are currently undergoing preclinical and clinical investigation. While some substances show promising results in preclinical and early clinical testing, many cytotoxic drugs which are effective in the treatment of other malignancies are not effective in advanced CRC (Table 11).

Tegafur

Tegafur, a prodrug to FU, is hydroxylated and converted to FU by hepatic microsomal enzymes, which may lead to a steadier level of FU in the tumor

Table 11. Substances with little or no efficacy in advanced colorectal carcinoma

Reference	Substance	Efficacy
Wadler et al. 1994	Echinomycin	1/10
Abbruzzese et al. 1991	Gemcitabine	1/26
Herrmann et al. 1995	Iododoxorubicin	0/18

(Au et al. 1979; Anttila et al. 1983) Clinical development of tegafur was discontinued in the USA because it had massive gastrointestinal and CNS side effects but no apparent therapeutic advantage over FU itself given intravenously (Friedman and Ignoffo 1980).

In a recent phase II trial at the M.D. Anderson Cancer Center, a response rate of 42% was achieved with UFT, a mixture of uracil and tegafur at a molar ratio of 4:1, combined with FA given orally (Pazdur et al. 1994). Serious side effects were not seen with this regimen. There has not yet been any report of survival data.

Thymidilate Synthase Inhibitors

ZD 1694 (Tomudex) is the most prominent new specific thymidilate synthase inhibitor; it entered clinical trials in 1992. Preliminary results suggested high activity and therefore a clinical phase II trial in advanced CRC was started in the UK in 1993. Patients were treated at a dose of 3 mg/m^2 every third week. In 176 patients the investigators found a response rate of 26% with five complete responses. Grade 3 and 4 toxicities included asthenia, nausea and vomiting, diarrhea, and leukopenia. Two toxic deaths occurred due to severe diarrhea and leukopenia (Zalcberg et al. 1995). Currently more clinical trials are underway to evaluate the combination of ZD 1694 with other cytotoxic drugs in CRC.

Trimetrexate

Trimetrexate (TMTX), like MTX, is an antifolate inhibitor of the enzyme dihydrofolate reductase (DHFR). In contrast to MTX, it does not compete with FA for cellular uptake and metabolism (Romanini et al. 1992) because of several different attributes (for review see O'Dwyer et al. 1987). In vitro studies showed a cytotoxic effect of TMTX in combination with FU/FA (Romanini et al. 1992). The combination of FU, FA, and TMTX was also found to be more cytotoxic than MTX alone. A phase-I trial in pretreated patients with colon carcinoma yielded a response rate of 20% (Conti et al. 1994). Several phase-II trials with a combination of TMTX and other modulators are presently underway.

Topoisomerase-I Inhibitors

Camptothecin (CPT) is a plant alkaloid obtained from *Camptotheca acuminata* that shows significant antitumor activity against several experimental tumors (Gallo et al. 1971). Reports of severe side effects like leukopenia, gastrointestinal toxicity, and hemorrhagic cystitis in earlier trials led to the abandonment of the drug for further clinical investigation. Camptothecin-11 (CPT-11), a CPT derivative, was first synthesized in 1983 and found to be less toxic than CPT (Kunimoto et al. 1987). Both preclinical and phase II trials have demonstrated CPT-11 activity in several malignancies (for review see Shimada et al. 1993; Matsuoka et al. 1994). A recent phase II study demonstrated some activity in CRC with a response rate of 27% (17/63 patients); however, no complete response was seen (Shimada et al. 1993).

Quality of Life

Since treatment of advanced CRC is still palliative, attention has recently shifted to the quality of life as a valid end point for clinical trials. Several investigators have attempted to assess the quality of life in patients with CRC. Scheithauer et al. (1993) reported that chemotherapy with FU, FA, and cisplatin improved both the quality of life and survival in a small number of patients compared with supportive care alone. The quality of life was measured by using a 22-item self-assessment scale. A Swedish group conducted interviews with patients treated for CRC using a questionnaire (Glimelius et al. 1994). Comparison of two treatment modalities revealed a significant difference in the quality of life, but not in the response or survival.

A more widespread instrument for assessing quality of life over time is the EORTC QLQ C 30 questionnaire, which consists of functional scales (physical state, ability to work, and cognitive, emotional, social, and global quality of life) as well as symptom scales (pain, nausea, vomiting, fatigue, dyspnea, loss of appetite, sleep disturbances, diarrhea, and constipation) (Aaronson et al. 1993). Besides this validated "core questionnaire", there are several modular supplements specifically designed for certain types of cancer (Bergman et al. 1994). In a recent randomized clinical trial comparing FU/FA and FU/IFN in advanced CRC, quality of life for the first time was a major end point of the study. In a total of 142 patients serial self-assessment revealed a significantly reduced quality of life in the FU/IFN treatment arm. This result was not expected from the physicians' rating conducted at the same time using the NCI Common Toxicity Criteria. The compliance with the quality of life self-assessment by the patients was 92%. Evaluability of the EORTC questionnaire was also high, at 88%, thereby qualifying it as a valuable instrument for assessing patients' quality of life in future randomized trials in CRC (Kreuser et al. 1995).

Conclusion

In recent years, some progress has been made in the treatment of advanced colorectal cancer. The biochemical modulation of FU with FA significantly improves the response rate compared with FU alone (30% vs. 12%). Therefore, this combination is currently considered the standard treatment despite the fact that, according to a recent meta-analysis, it has not as yet been possible to translate this advantage into improved survival. However, FU/FA offers a significant benefit regarding the quality of life compared with FU/IFN. A recent multi-analysis of phase-III trials of sequential MTX and FU vs. FU alone has demonstrated a statistically significant doubling of the response rate, as well as a small but significant survival advantage for the combination. Other biochemical modulators such as PALA cannot significantly improve the efficacy of FU. A high-dose chemotherapy with FU over 24 h in combination with FA can induce stable disease in approximately half the patients with a median survival of 8 months. The interferons and interleukin are ineffective in advanced CRC. Moreover, at this time, no immunotherapy can be recommended for treatment of advanced CRC. Several new drugs have been tested in CRC with promising results, including CPT-11. The efficacy of TMTX, FU, and FA is currently under evaluation. Locoregional treatment of liver metastases has become safer over the past few years due to new application modes and systems, but local toxicity is still higher than with systemic therapy. Moreover, the superior response rates in randomized trials of patients with locoregional treatment of liver metastases compared with systemic treatment were not translated into improved survival. It has been demonstrated that treatment in CRC should be started as early as possible when advanced or metastatic disease has been diagnosed, since a good performance status, normal alkaline phosphatase, and GOT are good prognostic factors. Due to the palliative treatment goals that are always preeminent in advanced CRC, quality of life is becoming the most important issue in clinical trials. The EORTC QLQ C 30 is a reliable and valuable instrument to demonstrate over time differences in quality fo life between treatment arms in randomized trials.

References

Aaronson NK, Ahmedzai S, Bullinger M (1993) The European Organisation for Research and Treatment of Cancer QLQ-C-30: a quality-of-life instrument for use in international clinical trials in oncology. J Natl Cancer Inst 85:333–338

Abad A, Rosell R, Pastor MC, Barnadas A, Carles J, Ribelles N, Oller B, Armengol M, Salva A, Ribas M (1991) Sequential combination of methotrexate (MTX), 5-fluorouracil (FU), and high-dose folinic acid (FA) in advanced colorectal cancer: double biochemical modulation? Am J Clin Oncol 14:393–396

Abad A, Garcia P, Grávalos C, Tusquets I, Rosell R, Perez-Manga G, Cortés-Funes H, Fabregat X, Barnadas A (1992) Phase-III trial with methotrexate, 5-FU and high-dose leucovorin (MFL) vs 5-FU, leucovorin (FL) vs 5-FU (F) in advanced and metastatic colorectal cancer. Proc Am Soc Clin Oncol 11:161 (abstract)

Abbruzzese JL, Grunewald R, Weeks EA, Gravel D, Adams T, Nowak B, Mineishi S, Tarassoff P, Satterlee W, Raber MN, Plunkett W (1991) A phase-I clinical, plasma, and cellular pharmacology study of gemcitabine. J Clin Oncol 9:491–498

Advanced Colorectal Cancer Meta-Analysis Project (1992) Modulation of fluorouracil by leucovorin in patients with advanced colorectal cancer: evidence in terms of response rates. J Clin Oncol 10:896–903

Advanced Colorectal Cancer Meta-Analysis Project (1994) Meta-analysis of randomized trials testing the biochemical modulation of fluorouracil by methotrexate in metastatic colorectal cancer. J Clin Oncol 12:960–969

Ahlgren JD, Lokich J, Schulz J, McCulloch W, Lynn J, Schein PS (1990) Protracted infusion of 5-fluorouracil (5-FU) with weekly PALA: pilot study in metastatic colorectal carcinoma. Proc Am Soc Clin Oncol 9:119 (abstract)

Aiba K, Ogawa M, Kuraishi Y, Akazawa S, Sasaki T, Sakata Y, Esaki K (1993) A combination phase-II study of 5-fluorouracil and natural-type alpha interferon in patients with advanced colorectal adenocarcinoma. Proc Am Soc Clin Oncol 12:208 (abstract)

Ajani JA, Kanojia MD, Bedikian AY, Korinek JK, Stein SH, Espinoza EG, Bodey GP (1985) Sequential methotrexate and 5-fluorouracil in the primary treatment of metastatic colorectal carcinoma. Am J Clin Oncol 8:69–71

Ajani JA, Abbruzzese JL, Faintuch JS, Blackburn R, Levin B, Boman BM (1988) Phase-II study of fludarabine phosphate in patients with advanced colorectal carcinoma. Invest New Drugs 6:47–50

Ajani JA, Rios AA, Ende K, Abbruzzese JL, Edwards C, Faintuch JS, Saks S, Gutterman JU, Levin B (1989) Phase-I and -II studies of the combination of recombinant human interferon-γ and 5-fluorouracil in patients with advanced colorectal carcinoma. J Biol Response Mod 8:140–146

Anderson H, Lund B, Bach F, Thatcher N, Walling J, Hansen HH (1994) Single-agent activity of weekly gemcitabine in advanced non-small-cell lung cancer: a phase-II study. J Clin Oncol 12:1821–1826

Anttila MI, Slotaniemi EA, Kairaluoma MI, Mokka RE, Sundquist AT (1983) Pharmacokinetics of ftorafur after intravenous and oral administration. Cancer Chemother Pharmacol 10:150–153

Arai Y, Kido C, Endo T, Miyake Y, Ariyoshi Y, Fukushima M (1988) Hepatic arterial infusion (HAI) chemotherapy for liver metastasis from colon, gastric and breast cancer (ca). Proc Am Soc Clin Oncol 7:102 (abstr)

Ardalan B, Glazer RI, Kensler TW, Jayaram HN, Pham TV, Macdonald JS, Cooney DA (1981) Synergistic effect of 5-fluorouracil and N-(phosphonacetyl)-L-aspartate on cell growth and ribonucleic acid synthesis in a human mammary carcinoma. Biochem Pharmacol 30:2045–2049

Ardalan B, Singh G, Silberman H (1988) A randomized phase-I and -II study of short-term infusion of high-dose fluorouracil with or without *N*-(phosphonacetyl)-L-aspartic acid in patients with advanced pancreatic and colorectal cancers. J Clin Oncol 6:1053–1058

Ardalan B, Chua L, Tian E, Reddy R, Sridhar K, Benedetto P, Richman S, Legaspi A, Waldman S, Morrell L, Feun L, Savaraj N, Livingstone A (1991) A phase-II study of weekly 24-hour infusion with high-dose fluorouracil with leucovorin in colorectal carcinoma. J Clin Oncol 9:625–630

Au JL, Freidman MA, Sadeed W (1979) Pharmacokinetics and metabolism of ftorafur in man. Cancer Treat Rep 63:343–350

Auber M, Lynch J, Higa G, Romero P, DeVore R, Crowell E, Rogers J, Raich P (1994) Phase-I study of 5-FU, folinic acid (FA), and recombinant interferon alpha-2 (IFN) in patients (pts) with metastatic colorectal carcinoma. Proc Am Soc Clin Oncol 13:209 (abstract)

Balch CM, Urist MM, McGregor ML (1983) Continuous regional chemotherapy for metastatic colorectal cancer using a totally implantable infusion pump. Am J Surg 145:285–290

Bang YJ, Kim HT, Suh CI, Kim SY, Heo DS, Kim NK (1992) Phase II study of 5-fluorouracil and recombinant interferon-gamma in patients with metastatic colorectal cancer. Proc Am Soc Clin Oncol 11:179 (abstract)

Bergman B, Aaronson NK, Ahmedzai S, Kaasa S, Sullivan M (1994) The EORTC-QLQ-LC 13: a modular supplement to the EORTC core quality-of-life questionnaire (QLQ-C30) for use in lung cancer clinical trials. Eur J Cancer 30:635–642

Boring CC, Squires TS, Tong T (1993) Cancer statistics, 1993. CA Cancer J Clin 43:7–26

Botto HG, Galvez C, Palao Marco F, Bonamassa M, Fabeiro MA, Marin F, Botto IS (1992) 5-Fluorouracil (5-FU) and interferon alpha 2b (INF) in advanced colo-rectal cancer: results in 47 patients. Proc Am Soc Clin Oncol 11:176 (abstract)

Brunetti I, Falcone A, Bertuccelli M, Giannessi PG, Conte PF (1992) Double 5-fluorouracil (5-FU) modulation with folinic acid (FA) and recombinant alfa 2-B interferon (IFN) in patients (PTS) with metastatic colorectal carcinoma (MCRC). Proc Am Soc Clin Oncol 11:175 (abstract)

Buroker TR, Moertel CG, Fleming TR, Everson LK, Cullinan SA, Krook JE, Mailliard JA, Marschke RF, Klaassen DL, Laurie JA, Moon MD (1985) A controlled evaluation of recent approaches to biochemical modulation or enhancement of 5-fluorouracil therapy in colorectal carcinoma. J Clin Oncol 3:1624–1631

Buroker TR, O'Connell MJ, Wieand HS, Krook JE, Gerstner JB, Mailliard JA, Schaefer PL, Levitt R, Kardinal CG, Gesme DH Jr (1994) Randomized comparison of two schedules of fluorouracil and leucovorin in the treatment of advanced colorectal cancer. J Clin Oncol 12:14–20

Buter J, Sinnige HAM, Cats A, Sleijfer DTh, Verschueren RCJ, Mulder NH (1994) Maintenance of remission on 5-fluorouracil (5-FU), leucovorin (LV) and α-2a interferon (IFNα) in advanced colorectal cancer. Proc Am Soc Clin Oncol 13:193 (abstract)

Cadman E, Heimer R, Benz C (1980) The influence of methotrexate pretreatment on 5-fluorouracil metabolism in L1210 cells. J Biol Chem 256:1695–1704

Cantrell JE Jr, Brunet R, Lagarde C, Schein PS, Smith FP (1982) Phase-II study of sequential methotrexate-5-FU therapy in advanced measurable colorectal cancer. Cancer Treat Rep 66:1563–1565

Cascinu S, Fedeli A, Luzi Fedeli L, Catalano G (1992) Double biochemical modulation of 5-fluorouracil by leucovorin and cyclic low-dose interferon alpha 2b in advanced colorectal cancer patients. Ann Oncol 3:489–491

Cellerino R, Antognoli S, Giustini L, Acito L, Marcellini M, Bavosi M, Trivisonne R, Francini G, Del Papa M, Rossi G, Testa E, Latini L, Piga A (1994) A randomised study of fluorouracil (5FU) with or without α-interferon (IFN) in advanced colorectal cancer. Proc Am Soc Clin Oncol 13:217 (abstract)

Chang AE, Schneider PD, Sugarbaker PH, Simpson C, Culnane M, Steinberg SM (1987) A prospective randomized trial of regional versus systemic continuous 5-fluorodeoxyuridine chemotherapy in the treatment of colorectal liver metastases. Ann Surg 206:685–693

Clark PI, Slevin MK, Reznek RH, Niederle N, Kurschel E, Lundell G, Cedermark B, Fallenius A, Blomgren H, Ohman U, Silfersward C, Theve NO, Wrigley PFM (1987) Two randomized phase-II trials of intermittent intravenous versus subcutaneour α-2 interferon alone (trial 1) and in combination with 5-fluorouracil (trial 2) in advanced colorectal cancer. Int J Colorect Dis 2:26–29

Clavel M, Vermorken JB, Judson I, Wagener T, Hatty S, Wanders J (1992) Gemcitabine is an active drug in patients with squamous cell carcinoma of the head and neck. Proc Am Soc Clin Oncol 11:249 (abstract)

Clendeninn NJ, Guaspari A, Laufman LR, Brenckman WD Jr, and the BW Colorectal Cancer Cooperative Group (1990) A randomized, double-blind trial of fluorouracil (FU) plus placebo (P) vs FU plus high dose oral leucovorin (LV) in colorectal cancer. J Cancer Res Clin Oncol 116 [Suppl part I]:661 (abstract)
Cohen AM, Kaufman SD, Wood WC, Greenfield AJ (1983) Regional hepatic chemotherapy using an implantable drug infusion pump. Am J Surg 145:529–533
Cohen AM, Schaeffer N, Higgins J (1986) Treatment of metastatic colorectal cancer with hepatic artery combination chemotherapy. Cancer 57:1115–1117
Collins KD, Stark GR (1971) Aspartate transcarbamylase. Interaction with the transition-state analogue N-(phosphonacetyl)-L-aspartate. J Biol Chem 246:6599–6605
Conti JA, Kemeny N, Seiter K, Goker E, Tong W, McKenzie A, Ragusa K, Bertino JR (1994) Trial of sequential trimetrexate, fluorouracil and high-dose leucovorin in previously treated patients with gastrointestinal carcinoma. J Clin Oncol 12:695–700
Corfu-A Study Group (1995) Phase-III randomized study of two fluorouracil combinations with either interferon alfa-2a or leucovorin in advanced colorectal caner. J Clin Oncol 13:921–928
Cortesi E, Aschelter AM, Marchetti P, Padovani A, Pellegrini A (1987) Three drugs treatment for regional intra-arterial therapy liver metastases from colorectal cancer. Proc Am Soc Clin Oncol 6:95 (abstr)
Daniels J, Pentecost M, Teitelbaum G, Daniels A, Paylunian C, Sternlicht M (1992) Hepatic artery chemoembolization (HAE) for carcinoma of colon using angiostat collagen and cisplatin, mitomycin, and doxorubicin: response, survival, and serum levels. Proc Am Soc Clin Oncol 11:171 (abstract)
Delfino C, Gaccia G, Maniago O (1992) 5-Fluorouracil (FU) alone versus methotrexate (M) + leucovorin (L) + FU in patients (pts) with metastatic colorectal cancer (MCC). Proc Am Soc Clin Oncol 11:177 (abstract)
Denck H (1984) Ergebnisse einer intraarteriellen intermittierenden Chemotherapie mit 5-FU bei Metastasenleber sowie inoperablen Tumoren des Gastrointestinal- und Urogenitaltrakts. Onkologie 7:167–176
De Vecchis L, Nunziata C, Ricci F, Cucchiara G, Picconi A, Bonmassar G, Lagomarsino Caprino M, Bonmassar E (1989) Immunotherapy of advanced colorectal cancer with alpha-interferon and 5-fluorouracil. J Chemother 1:128–135
Di Costanzo F, Bartolucci R, Calabresi F, Sofra M, Marzola M, Belsanti V, Boni C, Bacchi M (1992) Fluorouracil-alone versus high-dose folinic acid and fluorouracil in advanced colorectal cancer: a randomized trial of the Italian Oncology Group for Clinical Research (GOIRC). Ann Oncol 3:371–376
Doroshow JH, Mullhauf P, Leong L, Margolin K, Litchfield T, Akman S, Carr B, Bertrand M, Goldberg D, Blayney D, Odujinrin O, Delap R, Shuster J, Newman E (1990) Prospective randomized comparison of fluorouracil versus fluorouracil and high-dose continuous- infusion leucovorin calcium for the treatment of advanced measurable colorectal cancer in patients previously unexposed to dremotherapy. J Clin Oncol 8:491–501
Douillard JY, Leborgne J, Danielou JY, Lehur PA, Pottron L, Le Neel JC, Bolze JL, Jutel P (1991) Phase-II trial of 5-fluorouracil (5 FU) and recombinant alpha interferon (R IFN) (Intron A[R]) in metastatic, previously untreated colorectal cancer (CRC). Proc Am Soc Clin Oncol 10:139 (abstract)
Dufour P, Husseini F, Cure P, Olivier JP, Dumas F, Dreyfuss F, Prevot G, Cholet Ph, Audhuy B, Oberling F (1992) Randomized study of 5-fluorouracil (5-FU) versus 5-FU + alpha 2A interferon (IFN) for metastatic colorectal carcinoma. Proc Am Soc Clin Oncol 11:192 (abstract)
Erlichman C, Donehower RC, Speyer JL, Klecker R, Chabner BA (1982) Phase I-phase II trial of N-phosphonacetyl-L-aspartic acid given by intravenous infusion and 5-fluorouracil given by bolus injection. J Natl Cancer Inst 68:227–231

Erlichman C, Fine S, Wang A, Elkahim T (1988) A randomized trial of fluorouracil and folinic acid in patients with metastatic colorectal carcinoma. J Clin Oncol 6:469–475
Fleischer DE, Goldberg SB, Browning TH, Cooper JN, Friedman E, Goldner FH, Keeffe EB, Smith LE (1989) Detection and surveillance of colorectal cancer. JAMA 261:580–585
Foon KA (1989) Biological response modifiers: the new immunotherapy. Cancer Res 49:1621–1639
Friedman MA, Ignoffo RJ (1980) A review of the United States clinical experience of the fluoropyrimidine, ftorafur (NSC-148958). Cancer Treat Rev 7:205–213
Gallo RC, Whang-Peng J, Adamson RH (1971) Studies on the antitumor activity, mechanism of action, and cell cycle effects of camptothecin. J Natl Cancer Inst 46:789–795
Glimelius B, Ginman C, Graffman S, Påhlman L, Ståhle E (1986) Sequential methotrexate-5-FU-leucovorin (MFL) in advanced colorectal cancer. Eur J Cancer Clin Oncol 22:295–306
Glimelius B, Hoffmann K, Graf W, Pahlman L, Sjöden PO (1994) Quality of life during chemotherapy in patients with symptomatic advanced colorectal cancer. Cancer 73:556–562
Goldberg JA, Kerr DJ, Wilmott N, McKillop JH, McArdle CS (1990) Regional chemotherapy for colorectal liver metastases: a phase II evaluation of targeted hepatic arterial 5-fluorouracil for colorectal liver metastases. Br J Surg 77:1238–1240
Graf W, Glimelius B, Påhlman L, Bergström R (1991) Determinants of prognosis in advanced colorectal cancer. Eur J Cancer 27:1119–1123
Graf W, Påhlman L, Bergström R, Glimelius B (1994a) The relationship between an objective response to chemotherapy and survival in advanced colorectal cancer. Br J Cancer 70:559–563
Graf W, Bergström R, Påhlman L, Glimelius B (1994b) Appraisal of a model for prediction of prognosis in advanced colorectal cancer. Eur J Cancer 30A:453–457
Grage TB, Vassilopoulos PP, Shingleton WW, Jubert AV, Elias EG, Aust JB, Moss SE (1979) Results of a prospective randomized study of hepatic arterial infusion with 5-fluorouracil versus intravenous 5-fluorouracil in patients with hepatic metastases from colorectal cancer: a Central Oncology Group study. Surgery 86:550–555
Grem JL, Hoth DF, Hamilton JM, King SA, Leyland-Jones B (1987) Overview of current status and future direction of clinical trials with 5-fluorouracil in combination with folinic acid. Cancer Treat Rep 71:1249–1264
Grem JL, King SA, O'Dwyer PJ, Leyland-Jones B (1988) Biochemistry and clinical activity of *N*-(phosphonacetyl-L-aspartate: a review. Cancer Res 48:4441–4454
Grem JL, McAtee N, Murphy RF, Balis FM, Steinberg SM, Hamilton JM, Sorensen JM, Sartor O, Kramer BS, Goldstein LJ, Gay LM, Caubo KM, Goldspiel B, Allegra CJ (1991) A pilot study of interferon alfa-2a in combination with fluorouracil plus high-dose leucovorin in metastatic gastrointestinal carcinoma. J Clin Oncol 9:1811–1820
Grem JL, Jordan E, Robson ME, Binder RA, Hamilton JM, Steinberg SM, Arbuck SG, Beveridge RA, Kales AN, Miller JA, Weiss RB, McAtee N, Chen A, Goldspiel B, Saver E, Allegra CJ (1993) Phase-II study of fluorouracil, leucovorin, and interferon alfa-2a in metastatic colorectal carcinoma. J Clin Oncol 11:1737–1745
Grimm EA, Robb RJ, Roth JA, Neckers LM, Lachman LB, Wilson DJ, Rosenberg SA (1983) Lymphokine-activated killer cell phenomenon III. Evidence that IL2 is sufficient for direct activation of peripheral blood lymphocytes into lymphokine-activated killer cells. J Exp Med 158:1356–1361
Hamblin TJ, Inzani V, Sadullah S, Stevenson FK, Williamson P, Van der Plas J, Palmer P, Franks CR (1989) A phase-II trial of recombinant interleukin-2 and 5-FU chemotherapy in patients with metastatic colorectal carcinoma. Cancer Treat Rev 16 [Suppl A]:163–167

Hansen R, Ritch P, Anderson T (1986) Sequential methotrexate, 5-fluorouracil, and calcium leucovorin in colorectal carcinoma. Am J Clin Oncol 9:352–354

Haskell CM, Selch MT, Ramming KP (1990) Colon and rectum. In: Haskell DM (ed) Cancer treatment. Saunders, Philadelphia, pp 232–254

Heidelberger C, Chaudhari NK, Danenberg P, Mooren D, Griesbach L, Duschinsky R, Schnitzer RJ, Pleven E, Scheiner J (1957) Fluorinated pyrimidines, a new class of tumor-inhibitory compounds. Nature 179:663–666

Herrmann R, Spehn J, Beyer JH, von Franqué U, Schmieder A, Holzmann K, Abel U (1984) Sequential methotrexate and 5-fluorouracil: improved response rate in metastatic colorectal cancer. J Clin Oncol 2:591–594

Herrmann R, Knuth A, Kleeberg U, Middeke H, Korsten FW, Trux FA, Schmieder A, Evers C (1992) Sequential methotrexate and 5-fluorouracil (5-FU) vs 5-FU alone in metastatic colorectal cancer. Ann Oncol 3:539–543

Herrmann R, Mross K, Kleeberg U, Kreuser ED, Becher R, Edler L, Queißer W, Liati P, Kerpel-Fronius S for the Phase-II Study Group of the Association of Medical Oncology of the German Cancer Society (1995) 4′-Iodo-4′-deoxydoxorubicin (IDX) in colorectal cancer – a multicenter phase-II study. Onkologie 18:28–30

Hertel LW, Boder GB, Kroin JS, Rinzel SM, Poore GA, Todd GC, Grindey JB (1990) Evaluation of the antitumor activity of gemcitabine (2′,2′-difluoro-2′-deoxycytidine). Cancer Res 50:4417–4422

Heys SD, Eremin O, Ruggeri EM, Pein F, Rainer H, Oskam R, de Peuter RA, Palmer PA, Franks CR (1995) A phase-III study of recombinant interleukin-2,5-fluorouracil and leucovorin versus 5-fluorouracil and leucovorin in patients with unresectable or metastatic colorectal carcinoma. Eur J Cancer 31A:19–25

Hilgenfeld RU, Kreuser ED (1996) Immunological and biochemical modulation in the treatment of advanced colorectal cancer: update and future directions. In: Güntbert U, Birchmeier W (eds) Attempts to understand metastasis formation. Springer, Berlin Heidelberg New York (Current Topics in Microbiology and immunology, vol 213/III)

Hohn DC, Stagg RJ, Friedman MA, Hannigan JF Jr, Rayner A, Ignoffo RJ, Acord P, Lewis BJ (1989) A randomized trial of continuous intravenous versus hepatic intraarterial floxuridine in patients with colorectal cancer metastatic to the liver: the Northern California Oncology Group trial. J Clin Oncol 7:1646–1654

Huberman M, McClay E, Atkins M, Goldsweig H, Bonanno D, Layton M, Tessitore J (1991) Phase-II trial of 5 fluorouracil (5FU) and recombinant interferon-α-2a (IFN) in advanced colorectal cancer. Proc Am Soc Clin Oncol 10:153 (abstract)

Inoshita G, Yalavarthi P, Murthy S, Budd GT, Andresen S, Netaji B, Gibson V, Sergi J, Bukowski RM (1991) Phase-I trial of 5-FU, leucovorin (LV) and rHuIFN-alpha2a in metastatic colorectal cancer (CR Ca). Proc Am Soc Clin Oncol 10:152 (abstract)

Itri LM (1992) The interferons. Cancer 70:950–945

Jaiyesimi I, Pazdur R, Patt YZ, Ajani J, Abbruzzese JL, Daugherty K, Levin B (1991) Phase-II study of recombinant interferon alpha 2a (rIFN) and continuous infusion 5-fluorouracil (5FU) in metastatic colorectal carcinoma. Proc Am Soc Clin Oncol 10:147 (abstract)

John W, Neefe J, Smith M, Massie M, Cantrell J (1992) 5-Fluorouracil (5-FU) and interferon-α (IFN) in advanced colon cancer: The University of Kentucky experience. Proc Am Soc Clin Oncol 11:189 (abstract)

Johnson LP, Rivkin SE (1985) The implanted pump in metastatic colorectal cancer of the liver. Risk versus benefit. Am J Surg 149:595–598

Kemeny NE (1992) Is hepatic infusion of chemotherapy effective treatment for liver metastases? Yes. In: DeVita VT Jr, Hellman S, Rosenberg SA (eds) Important advances in oncology. Lippincott, Philadelphia, pp 207–227

Kemeny N, Braun DW (1983) Prognostic factors in advanced colorectal carcinoma. Am J Med 74:786–794

Kemeny NE, Ahmed T, Michaelson RA, Harper HD, Yip LC (1984a) Activity of sequential low-dose methotrexate and fluorouracil in advanced colorectal carcinoma: attempt at correlation with tissue and blood levels of phophoribosylpyrophosphate. J Clin Oncol 2:311–315

Kemeny N, Daly J, Oderman P, Shike M, Chun H, Petroni G, Geller N (1984b) Hepatic artery pump infusion: toxicity and results in patients with metastatic colorectal carcinoma. J Clin Oncol 2:595–600

Kemeny N, Daly J, Reichman B, Geller N, Botet J, Oderman P (1987) Intrahepatic or systemic infusion of fluorodeoxyuridine in patients with liver metastases from colorectal carcinoma. A randomized trial. Ann Int Med 107:459–465

Kemeny NE, Reichman B, Geller N, Hollander P (1988) Implementation of the group sequential methodology in a randomized trial in metastatic colorectal carcinoma. Am J Clin Oncol 6:84 (abstract)

Kemeny N, Younes A, Seiter K, Kelsen D, Sammarco P, Adams L, Derby S, Nurray P, Houston C (1990) Interferon alpha-2a and 5-fluorouracil for advanced colorectal carcinoma. Assessment of activity and toxicity. Cancer 66:2470–2475

Kemeny N, Costa JA, Seiter K, Niedzwiecki D, Botet J, Martin D, Costa P, Wiseberg J, McCulloch W (1992a) Biochemical modulation of bolus fluorouracil by PALA in patients with advanced colorectal cancer. J Clin Oncol 10:747–752

Kemeny N, Seiter K, Niedzwiecki D, Chapman D, Sigurdson E, Cohen A, Botet J, Oderman P (1992b) A randomized trial of intrahepatic infusion of fluorodeoxyuridine with dexamethasone versus fluorodeoxyuridine alone in the treatment of metastatic colorectal cancer. Cancer 69:327–334

Kemeny N, Cohen A, Seiter K, Conti JA, Sigurdson ER, Tao Y, Niedzwiecki D, Botet J, Budd A (1993) Randomized trial of hepatic arterial floxuridine, mitomycin, and carmustine versus floxuridine alone in previously treated patients with liver metastases from colorectal cancer. J Clin Oncol 11:330–335

Kemeny N, Conti JA, Cohen A, Campana P, Huang Y, Shi WJ, Botet J, Pulliam S, Bertino JR (1994) Phase II study of hepatic artery floxuridine, leucovorin, and dexamethasone for unresectable liver metastases from colorectal carcinoma. J Clin Oncol 12:2288–2295

Kennett RH, Jonak ZL, Bechtol KB (1980) Monoclonal antibodies against human tumor-associated antigens. In: Kennett RH, McKearn TJ, Bechtol KB (eds) Monoclonal antibodies: hybridomas: a new dimension in biological analyses. Plenum, New York, pp 55–168

Köhne-Wömpner CH, Schmoll HJ, Hiddemann W, Knipp H, Wilke H, Bodenstein H, Lohrmann HP, Preiss J, Käufer C, Fischer JT, Balleisen L, Urbanitz D, Schwark J, Schöffski P, Kreuser ED, Graubner M (1991) 5-Fluorouracil (5-FU), leucovorin (LV), alpha-2b interferon (IFN) in advanced colorectal cancer (CC): a phase-I/II study. Proc Am Soc Clin Oncol 10:159 (abstract)

Kosmidis P, Tsavaris N, Skarlos D, Pavlidis N, Beer M, Theocharis D, Samanta D, Briasoulis E, Fountzilas G (1993) Fluorouracil (5-FU) and folinic acid (FA) with or without a2b-interferon (IFN) in advanced colorectal cancer (ACC). A prospective randomized trial. Proc Am Soc Clin Oncol 12:211 (abstract)

Kreuser ED, Hilgenfeld RU, Matthias M, Hoksch B, Boewer C, Oldenkott B, Knauf WU, Boese-Landgraf J, Schalhorn A, Zeitz M, Thiel E (1992a) A phase-I trial of interferon α-2b with folinic acid and 5-fluorouracil administered by 4-hour infusion in metastatic colorectal carcinoma. Semin Oncol 19 [Suppl 3]:197–203

Kreuser ED, Wadler S, Thiel E (1992b) Interactions between cytokines and cytotoxic drugs: Putative molecular mechanisms in experimental hematology and oncology. Semin Oncol 19 [Suppl 4]:1–7

Kreuser ED, Hilgenfeld RU, Matthias M, Hoksch B, Boewer C, Oldenkott B, Lenk H, Wiener N, Boese-Landgraf J, Schalhorn A, Thiel E (1992c) A phase-II trial of interferon α-2b with folinic acid and 5-fluorouracil administered by 4-hour infusion in metastatic colorectal carcinoma. Semin Oncol 19 [Suppl 4]:57–62

Kreuser ED, Streit M, Küchler T, Matthias M, Thiel E (1995) A multicenter randomized trial with the assessment of the quality of life in patients with metastatic colorectal carcinoma given either folinic acid or interferon a-2b as a modulator of 5-fluorouracil. Proc Am Soc Clin Oncol 14:202 (abstract)

Kunimoto T, Nitta K, Tanaka T, Uehara N, Baba H, Takeuchi M, Yokokura T, Sawada S, Miyasaka T, Mutai M (1987) Antitumor activity of 7-ethyl-10-[4-(1-piperidino)-1-piperidino] carbonyloxy-camptothecin, a novel water-soluble derivative of camptothecin, against murine tumors. Cancer Res 47:5944–5947

Labianca R, Pancera G, Luporini A, Dallavalle G, Locatelli MC, Fraschini P, Luporini G (1990) Double modulation of 5-fluorouracil (5-FU) with α2b interferon (IFN) and folinic acid (FA) in advanced colorectal cancer. Ann Oncol 1 (Suppl):92 (abstract)

Labianca R, Pancera G, Aitini E, Barni S, Beretta A, Beretta GD, Cesana B, Comella G, Cozzaglio L, Cristoni M, Spagnolli P, Frontini L, Gottardi O, Martignoni G, Scapaticci R, Smerieri F, Vinci M, Zadro A, Zaniboni A, Luporini G (1991) Folinic acid + 5-fluorouracil (5-FU) versus equidose 5-FU in advanced colorectal cancer. Phase-III study of "GISCAD" (Italian Group for the Study of Digestive Tract Cancer). Ann Oncol 2:673–679

Labianca R, Giaccon G, Pancera G, Ambrosini G, Amichetti G, Barni S, Cascinu S, Martignoni G, Pavananto G, Scapaticci R, Zaniboni A, Luporini G (1992) Low-dose α2b interferon (IFN) + folinic acid (FA) + 5-fluorouracil (5FU) in advanced colorectal cancer (ACC): a phase-II study of GISCAD (Italian Group for the Study of Gastrointestinal Cancer). Proc Am Soc Clin Oncol 11:177 (abstract)

Lang EK, Brown CL (1993) Colorectal metastases to the liver: selective chemoembolization. Radiology 189:417–422

Lembersky B, Koff H, Miketic L, Posner M, Jacobs S, Carr B (1992) Phase-II trial of 5-fluorouracil (FU), leucovorin (LV) and interferon alfa-2b (IFN) in the treatment of metastatic colorectal cancer (CRC). Proc Am Soc Clin Oncol 11:186 (abstract)

Leone BA, Romero A, Rabinovich MG, Perez JE, Macchiavelli M, Strauss E (1986) Sequential therapy with methotrexate and 5-fluorouracil in the treatment of advanced colorectal carcinoma. J Clin Oncol 4:23–27

Leone B, Romero A, Rabinovich M, Vallejo C, Bianco A, Perez J, Rodriguez R, Cuevas A, Macchiavelli M, Paris A, Lacava J (1992) Double modulation of 5-fluorouracil (5-FU) by methotrexate (MTX) and leucovorin (LV) in metastatic colorectal carcinoma. Proc Am Soc Clin Oncol 11:174 (abstract)

Lorenz M, Maier P, Reimann M, Inglis R, Hottenrott C (1992) Regionale Chemotherapie von 160 Patienten mit Lebermetastasen kolorektaler Karzinome. In: Schmoll HJ, Meyer HJ, Wilke H, Pichlmayer R (eds) Aktuelle Therapie gastrointestinaler Tumoren, 1st edn. Springer, Berlin Heidelberg New York, pp 372–381

Macchiavelli M, Leone B, Romero A, Rabinovich M, Vallejo C, Bianco A, Pérez J, Rodriguez R, Cuevas M, Alvarez L, Chacon R, Hannois A (1990) Advanced colorectal carcinoma (CRC): a prospective randomized trial of sequential methotrexate (MTX) – 5-fluorouracil (5FU) vs. 5FU alone. Proc Am Soc Clin Oncol 9:102 (abstract)

Marsh JC, Bertino JR, Katz KH, Davis CA, Durivage HJ, Rome LS, Richards F 2nd, Capizzi RL, Farber LR, Pasquale DN, Stuart R, Koletsky AJ, Makuch R, O'Hollaren K (1991) The influence of drug interval on the effect of methotrexate and fluorouracil in the treatment of advanced colorectal cancer. J Clin Oncol 9:371–380, 1991

Martin DS, Kemeny NE (1992) Modulation of fluorouracil by *N*-(phosphonacetyl)-L-aspartate: a review. Semin Oncol 19:49–55

Martin DS, Stolfi RL, Sawyer RC, Spiegelman S, Casper ES, Young CW (1983) Therapeutic utility of utilizing low-dose N-(phosphonacetyl)-L aspartic acid in combination with 5-fluorouracil: a murine study with clinical relevance. Cancer Res 43:2317–2321

Martin JK Jr, O'Connell MJ, Wieand HS, Fitzgibbons RJ Jr, Mailliard JA, Rubin J, Nagorney DM, Tschetter LK, Krook JE (1990) Intra-arterial floxuridine vs systemic fluorouracil for hepatic metastases from colorectal cancer. A randomized trial. Arch Surg 125:1022–1027

Martinelli DJ, Wadler S, Bakal CW, Cynamon J, Rozenblit A, Haynes H, Kaleya R, Wiernik PH (1994) Utility of embolization or chemoembolization as second-line treatment in patients with advanced or recurrent colorectal carcinoma. Cancer 74:1706–1712

Matsuoka H, Furasawa M, Tomoda H, Seo Y, Kono A, Takeda S, Sato K (1994) Cytotoxicity of CPT-11 and SN-38 for gastrointestinal and recurrent carcinomas cultured on contract-sensitive plates. Anticancer Res 14:405–409

Meehan K, Seidler C, Gehr G, Maurer LM (1993) An outpatient regimen of 5-fluorouracil (5-FU) and recombinant interferon alpha-2b (rIFNa-2B) in metastatic adenocarcinoma of the colon (MAC). Proc Am Soc Clin Oncol 12:222 (abstract)

Moertel CG, Fleming TR, Macdonald JS, Haller DG, Laurie JA, Goodman PJ, Ungerleider JS, Emerson WA, Tormey DC, Glick JH, Veeder MH, Mailliard JA (1990) Levamisole and fluorouracil for adjuvant therapy of resected colon carcinoma. N Engl J Med 322:352–358

Moertel C, Fleming T, Macdonald J, Haller D, Laurie J (1992) The intergroup study of fluorouracil (5-FU) plus levamisole (LEV) and levamisole alone as adjuvant therapy for stage C colon cancer. Proc Am Soc Clin Oncol 11:161 (abstract)

Moore MJ, Kaizer L, Erlichman C, Bunting P, Feld R, Fine S, Myers R, Thiessen JJ, Yuan S (1992) A phase-II clinical and pharmacologic study of 5-fluorouracil (5FU) + leucovorin + interferon in advanced colorectal cancer. Proc Am Soc Clin Oncol 11:183 (abstract)

Morgan DA, Ruscetti FW, Gallo R (1976) Selective in vitro growth of T lymphocytes from normal human bone marrows. Science 193:1007–1010

Mross K, Mayer U, Hamm K, Burk K, Hossfeld DK (1990) Pharmacokinetics and metabolism of iodo-doxorubicin and doxorubicin in humans. Eur J Clin Pharmacol 39:507–513

Muggia FM, Camacho FJ, Kaplan BH, Green MD, Greenwald ES, Wernz JC, Engstrom PF (1987) Weekly 5-fluorouracil combined with PALA: toxic and therapeutic effects in colorectal cancer. Cancer Treat Rep 71:253–256

Negoro S, Fukuoka M, Kurita Y, Niitani H (1994) Results of phase-II studies of gemcitabine in non-small cell lung cancer (NSCLC) Proc Am Soc Clin Oncol 13:367 (abstract)

Niederhuber JE, Ensminger W, Gyves J, Thrall J, Walker S, Cozzi E (1984) Regional chemotherapy of colorectal cancer metastatic to the liver. Cancer 53:1336–1343

Nobile MT, Rosso R, Sertoli MR, Rubagotti A, Vidili MG, Guglielmi A, Venturini M, Canobbio L, Fassio T, Gallo L, Galligioni E, Galotti P, Bruzzi P, Sobrero A (1992) Randomised comparison of weekly bolus 5-fluorouracil with or without leucovorin in metastatic colorectal carcinoma. Eur J Cancer 28A:1823–1827

Nordic Gastrointestinal Tumor Adjuvant Therapy Group (1989) Superiority of sequential methotrexate, fluorouracil, and leucovorin to fluorouracil alone in advanced symptomatic colorectal carcinoma: a randomized trial. J Clin Oncol 7:1437–1446

O'Connell M, Poon MA, Wieand H, Moertel C, Krook J, Gerstner J (1990) Biochemical modulation of 5-fluorouracil (5FU) with leucovorin (LV): confirmatory evidence

of improved therapeutic efficacy in the treatment of advanced colorectal cancer. Proc Am Soc Clin Oncol 9:106 (abstract)
O'Dwyer PJ, DeLap RJ, King SA et al, (1987) Trimetrexate: clinical development of a nonclassical antifolate. NCI Monogr 5:105–109
O'Dwyer PJ, Paul AR, Walczak J, Weiner LM, Litwin S, Comis RL (1990) Phase-II study of biochemical modulation of fluorouracil by low-dose PALA in patients with colorectal cancer. J Clin Oncol 8:1497–1503
Ortaldo JR, Mason AT, Gerard JP, Henderson LE, Farrar W, Hopkings RF 3d, Herberman RB, Rabin H (1984) Effects of natural and recombinant IL2 on regulation of IFN gamma production and natural killer cell activity: lack of involvement of the TAC antigen for these immunoregulatory effects. J Immunol 133:779–783
Panasci L, Ford J, Margolese R (1985) A phase-II study of sequential methotrexate and fluorouracil in advanced colorectal cancer. Cancer Chemother Pharmacol 15:164–166
Patt YZ, Mavligit GM (1991) Arterial chemotherapy in the management of colorecal cancer: an overview. Semin Oncol 18:478–490
Patt YZ, Jones D, Chase J, Charnsangavej C, Chuang V, Carrasco H, Lawrence D, Roh M (1994) Hepatic arterial infusion (HAI) of recombinant intefereon-alpha (rIFNα) & 5-fluorouracil (5FU) for colorectal cancer (CRC) liver metastases refractory to intravenous (IV) 5FU & leucovorin (LCV). Proc Am Soc Clin Oncol 13:201 (abstract)
Pavlick AC, DelGaudio D, Harper H, Rosenbluth R, Pecora AL (1992) Salvage therapy with continuous infusion 5-fluorouracil and alpha interferon in patients with colorectal cancer. Proc Am Soc Clin Oncol 11:188 (abstract)
Pazdur R, Ajani JA, Patt YZ, Winn R, Jackson D, Shepard B, DuBrow R, Campos L, Quaraishi M, Faintuch J, Abbruzzese JL, Gutterman J, Levin B (1990) Phase-II study of fluorouracil and recombinant interferon alfa-2a in previously untreated advanced colorectal carcinoma. J Clin Oncol 8:2027–2031
Pazdur R, Ajani JA, Patt YZ, Gomez J, Bready B, Levin B (1993) Phase-II evaluation of recombinant alpha-2a-interferon and continuous infusion fluorouracil in previously untreated metastatic colorectal adenocarcinoma. Cancer 71:1214–1218
Pazdur R, Lassere Y, Rhodes V, Ajani JA, Sugarman SM, Patt YZ, Jones DV, Markowitz AB, Abbruzzese JL, Bready B, Levin B (1994) Phase -II trial of uracil and tegafur plus oral leucovorin: an effective oral regimen in the treatment of metastatic colorectal carcinoma. J Clin Oncol 12:2296–2300
Pazdur R, Roach R, Braud E, Osmon C, Verschraegen C, Kolbye S, Bready B, Winn R (1994) Phase-II study of folinic acid, 5-fluorouracil,and interferon alfa-2a for patients with advanced colorectal carcinoma. Proc Am Soc Clin Oncol 13:224 (abstract)
Pensel R (1993) Advanced colon cancer (ACC): a randomized trial of fluorouracil (5-FU) + folinic acid (FA) and 5-FU + FA + interferon alpha 2b (IFN). Proc Am Soc Clin Oncol 12:203 (abstract)
Petrelli N, Herrera L, Rustum Y, Burke P, Creaven P, Stulc J, Emrich LJ, Mittelman A (1987) A prospective randomized trial of 5-fluorouracil versus 5-fluorouracil and high-dose leucovorin versus 5-fluorouracil and methotrexate in previously untreated patients with advanced colorectal carcinoma. J Clin Oncol 5:1559–1565
Petrelli N, Douglass HO Jr, Herrera L, Russell D, Stablein DM, Bruckner HW, Mayer RJ, Schinella R, Green MD, Muggia FM, Megibow A, Greenwald ES, Bukowski RM, Harris J, Levin B, Gaynor E, Loutfi A, Kalser MH, Barkin JS, Benedetto P, Woolley PV, Nauta R, Weaver DW, Leichman LP (1989) The modulation of fluorouracil with leucovorin in metastatic colorectal carcinoma: a prospective randomized phase-III trial. J Clin Oncol 7:1419–1426
Piedbois P, Gimonet JF, Feuilhade F, Le Péchoux C, Lévy C, Brun B, Rotman N, Delchier JC, Blasquez M, Thill L, Fagniez PL, Bader JP, Julien M, Le Bourgeois JP

(1991) 5FU, folinic acid and alpha-2a-interferon combination in advanced gastrointestinal cancer. Proc Am Soc Clin Oncol 10:141 (abstract)

Poon MA, O'Connell MJ, Moertel CG, Wieand HS, Cullinan SA, Everson LK, Krook JE, Mailliard JA, Laurie JA, Tschetter LK, Wiesenfeld M (1989) Biochemical modulation of fluorouracil: evidence of significant improvement of survival and quality of life in patients with advanced colorectal carcinoma. J Clin Oncol 7:1407–1418

Presant CA, Ardalan B, Multhauf P, Chan C, Staples R, Green L, Browning S, Carr BI, Chang FF, Thayer W (1983) Continuous five-day infusion of PALA and 5FU: a pilot phase-II trial. Med Pediatr Oncol 11:162–163

Punt CJA, de Mulder PHM, Burghouts JTM, Wagener DJT (1992) Fluorouracil continuous infusion plus alfa interferon plus oral folinic acid in advanced colorectal cancer. Semin Oncol 19 [Suppl 3]:208–210

Pyrhönen SO, Kouri MO (1992) Phase-II study of epirubicin sequential methotrexate and 5-fluorouracil for advanced colorectal cancer. Eur J Cancer 28A:1828–1832

Quagliuolo V, Bignami P, Doci R, Civalleri D, Cosimelli M (1987) Continuous artery infusion of floxuridine for metastatic colorectal cancer. Proc ECCO 4:179 (abstr)

Recchia F, Nuzzo A, Lombardo M, Lalli A, Fabiani F, Fanini R, Di Lullo L, Venturoni L, Peretti G for the IORAM (Istituto Oncologico Regione Abruzzo e Molise) (1992) 5-Fluorouracil (5FU) and high-dose folinic acid (HDFA) chemotherapy (CT) with or without alfa 2b interferon (IFN) in advanced colorectal cancer (ACC). Preliminary report of a randomized trial. Proc Am Soc Clin Oncol 11:162 (abstract)

Rios A, Levi B, Ajani J, Abbruzzese J, Faintuch J, Ende K, Gutterman J (1987) Combination of recombinant human interferon gamma (rIFN-α) and 5-fluorouracil (5-FU) in the treatment of patients with advanced colorectal carcinoma (CRC). Proc Am Soc Clin Oncol 6:84 (abstract)

Romanini A, Li WW, Colofiore JR, Bertino JR (1992) Leucovorin enhances cytotoxicity of trimetrexate/fluorouracil, but not methotrexate/fluorouracil in CCRF-CEM cells. J Natl Cancer Inst 84:1033–1038

Rosenberg SA, Lotze MT, Muul LM, Chang AE, Avis FP, Leitman S, Linehan WM, Robertson GN, Lee RE, Rubin JT, Seipp CA, Simpson CG, White DE (1987) A progress report on the treatment of 157 patients with advanced cancer using lymphokine-activated killer cells and interleukin-2 or high-dose interleukin-2 alone. N Engl J Med 316:889–897

Rosenberg SA, Lotze MT, Yang JC, Aebersold PM, Linehan WM, Seipp CA, White DE (1989) Experience with the use of high-dose interleukin-2 in the treatment of 652 cancer patients. Ann Surg 210:474–485

Rougier P, Lasser P, Elias D, Ghosn M, Droz JP, Sidibe S, Theodore C, Lumbroso J (1987) Intra-arterial hepatic chemotherapy (IAHC) for liver metastases (LM) from colo-rectal (CR) origin. Proc Am Soc Clin Oncol 6:94 (abstr)

Rougier P, Ducreux M, Pignon JP, Elias D, Tigaud JM, Lumbroso J, Ruffie P, Lasser PH (1991) Prognostic factors in patients with liver metastases from colorectal carcinoma treated with discontinuous intra-arterial hepatic chemotherapy. Eur J Cancer 27:1226–1230

Rougier P, Laplanche A, Huguier M, Hay JM, Ollivier JM, Escat J, Salmon R, Julien M, Roullet Audy JC, Gallot D, Gouzi JL, Pailler JL, Elisa D, Lacaine F, Roos S, Rotman N, Luboinski M, Lasser P (1992) Hepatic arterial infusion of floxuridine in patients with liver metastases from colorectal carcinoma: long-term results of a prospective randomized trial. J Clin Oncol 10:1112–1118

Scheele J, Stangl R, Altendorf-Hofmann A, Gall FP (1991) Regionale Chemotherapie bei diffusen Lebermetastasen des kolorektalen Karzinoms. Zenntralbl Chir 116:1215–1235

Scheithauer W, Rosen H, Kornek GV, Sebesta C, Depisch D (1993) Randomised comparison of combination chemotherapy plus supportive care with supportive care alone in patients with metastatic colorectal cancer. Br Med J 306:752–755

Schlag P, Hohenberger P, Schwarz V, Herfarth CH (1988) Intraarterielle 5-Fluorouracil-Chemotherapie bei Lebermetastasen kolorektaler Karzinome. Med Klin 83:705–709

Schwartz SI, Jones LS, McCune CS (1985) Assessment of treatment of intrahepatic malignancies using chemotherapy via an implantable pump. Ann Surg 201:560–567

Seymour MT, Johnson PWM, Wrigley PFM, Slevin ML (1991) 5-Fluorouracil (5FU), leucovorin (LV) and α-interferon (IFNα): a new regimen suitable for randomised trial. Proc Am Soc Clin Oncol 10:160 (abstract)

Seymour MT, Slevin M, Cunningham D, Kerr D, James R, Lederman J, Perren T, McAdam W, Duffy A, Stenning S, Taylor I (1994) A randomized assessment of interferon-α2a (IFNα) as a modulator of 5-fluorouracil (5FU) and leucovorin (LV) in advanced colorectal cancer. Proc Am Soc Clin Oncol 13:209 (abstract)

Shepard KV, Levin B, Karl RC, Faintuch J, DuBrow RA, Hagle M, Cooper RM, Beschorner J, Stablein D (1985) Therapy for metastatic colorectal cancer with hepatic artery infusion chemotherapy using a subcutaneous implanted pump. J Clin Oncol 3:161–169

Shimada Y, Yoshino M, Wakui A, Nakao I, Futatsuki K, Sakata Y, Kambe M, Taguchi T, Ogawa N, and the CPT-11 Gastrointestinal Cancer Study Group (1993) Phase-II study of CPT-11, a new camptothecin derivative, in metastatic colorectal cancer. J Clin Oncol 11:909–913

Sinnige HAM, Sleijfer DT, de Vries EGE, Willemse PHB, Mulder NH (1990) Modification of 5-fluorouracil activity by high-dose methotrexate or leucovorin in advanced colorectal carcinoma. Eur J Cancer 26:625–628

Sinnige HAM, Buter J, Sleijfer DTh, Verschueren RCJ, Mulder NH (1993) Update of a phase-II study of 5-fluorouracil (5-FU), leucovorin (LV) and α-2a interferon (IF) in advanced colorectal cancer. Proc Am Soc Clin Oncol 12:206 (abstract)

Sobrero A, Nobile MT, Guglielmi A, Mori A, Aschele C, Bolli E, Tixi L, Gallo L, Parodi GC, Bruzzi P, Brema F, Rosso R (1992) Phase-II study of 5-fluorouracil plus leucovorin and interferon alpha 2b in advanced colorectal cancer. Eur J Cancer 28A:850–852

Sotos GA, Grogan L, Allegra CJ (1994) Preclinical and clinical aspects of biomodulation of 5-fluorouracil. Cancer Treat Rev 20:11–49

Stagg RJ, Venook AP, Chase JL, Lewis BJ, Warren RS, Roh M, Mulvihill SJ, Grobman BJ, Rayner AA, Hohn DC (1991) Alternating hepatic intra-arterial floxuridine and fluorouracil: a less toxic regimen for treatment of liver metastases from colorectal cancer. J Natl Cancer Inst 83:423–428

Steinberg J, Erlichman C, Gadalla T, Fine S, Wong A (1992) Prognostic factors in patients with metastatic colorectal cancer receiving 5-fluorouracil and folinic acid. Eur J Cancer 28A:1817–1820

Steinke B, Günther E, Hirschmann WD, Sondern W, Koniczek KH, Wander HE, Natt F, Wagner T, Hinrichs HF, Werdier D (1992) Fluorouracil versus folinic acid/ fluorouracil in advanced colorectal cancer – preliminary results of a randomized trial. Semin Oncol 19 [Suppl 3]:141–147

Taylor C, Modiano M, Alberts D, Marcus S, Hersh E (1991) Combination chemotherapy with 5-fluorouracil (5-FU), leucovorin (LCV) and interferon-alpha (IFN-α) in patients with adenocarcinoma. Proc Am Soc Clin Oncol 10:141 (abstract)

Thirlwell MP, Hollingsworth LM, Herba MJ, Boileau G, Boos G, MacFarlane JK (1986) Ambulatory hepatic artery infusion chemotherapy for cancer of the liver. Am J Surg 151:585–589

Valone FH, Friedman MA, Wittlinger PS, Drakes T, Eisenberg PD, Malec M, Hannigan JF, Brown BW Jr (1989) Treatment of patients wtih advanced colorectal

carcinomas with fluorouracil alone, high-dose leucovorin plus fluorouracil, or sequential methotrexate, fluorouracil, and leucovorin: a randomized trial of the Northern California Oncology Group. J Clin Oncol 7:1427–1436
Van Hazel GA, Buck M, Byrne MJ (1992) Phase-II study of the combination of 5-fluorouracil (5FU), folinic acid (FA) and alpha interferon (IFN) in metastatic colorectal adenocarcinoma (CC). Proc Am Soc Clin Oncol 11:195 (abstract)
Villa R, Zaffaroni N, Giulani FC, Colella G, Sanfilippo O, Sivestrini R (1990) Absolute and relative activities of 4′-iodo-4′-deoxydoxorubicin against human colo-rectal tumors, as evaluated by a short-term in vitro assay. Anticancer Res 10:105–108
Vogel VG, McPherson RS (1989) Dietary epidemiology of colon cancer. Hematol Oncol Clin North Am 3:35–63
Wadler S, Schwartz EL, Goldman M, Lyver A, Rader M, Zimmerman M, Itri L, Weinberg V, Wiernik PH (1989) Fluorouracil and recombinant alpha-2a-interferon: an active regimen against advanced colorectal carcinoma. J Clin Oncol 7:1769–1775
Wadler S, Lemebrsky B, Atkins M, Kirkwood J, Petrelli N (1991) Phase II trial of fluorouracil and recombinant interferon alfa-2a in patients with advanced colorectal carcinoma: an Eastern Cooperative Oncology Group Study. J Clin Oncol 9:1806–1810
Wadler S, Tenteromano L, Cazenave L, Sparano JA, Greenwald ES, Rozenblit A, Kaleya R; Wiernik PH (1994) Phase-II trial of echinomycin in patients with advanced or recurrent colorectal cancer. Cancer Chemother Pharmacol 34:266–269
Weh HJ, Platz D, Braumann D, Buggisch P, Eckardt N, Schmiegel WH, Drescher S, Kleeberg UR, Müllerleile U, Crone-Munzebrock W, Hoffmann R, Müller P, Klapdor R, Pompecki R, Erdmann H, Reichel L, Jungbluth M, Hoffmann L, Mainzer K, Hossfeld DK (1992) Phase-II trial of 5-fluorouracil and recombinant interferon alfa-2b in metastatic colorectal carcinoma. Eur J Cancer 28A:1820–1823
Weh HJ, Wilke HJ, Dierlamm J, Klaassen U, Siegmund R, Illiger HJ, Schalhorn A, Kreuser ED, Hilgenfeld RU, Steinke B, Weber W, Burkhard O, Zoller A, Pfitzner J, Subert R, Kriebel R, Hossfeld DK (1994) Weekly therapy with folinic acid (FA) and high-dose 5-fluorouracil (5-FU) 24-hour infusion in pretreated patients with metastatic colorectal carcinoma. Ann Oncol 5:233–237
Weinerman B, Schacter B, Schipper H, Bowman D, Levitt M (1982) Sequential methotrexate and 5-FU in the treatment of colorectal cancer. Cancer Treat Rep 66:1553–1555
Weiss GR, Ervin TJ, Meshad MW, Kufe DW (1982) Phase II trial of combination therapy with continuous-infusion PALA and bolus-injection 5-FU. Cancer Treat Rep 66:299–303
Weiss GR, Garnick MB, Osteen RT, Steele GD Jr, Wilson RE, Schode D, Kaplan WD, Boxt LM, Kandarpa K, Mayer RJ, Frei ET III (1983) Long-term hepatic arterial infusion of 5-fluorodeoxyuridine for liver metastases using an implantable infusion pump. J Clin Oncol 1:337–344
Weiss L, Grundmann E, Torhorst J, Hartveit F, Moberg I, Eder M, Fenoglio-Preiser CM, Napier J, Horne CH, Lopez MJ (1986) Haematogenous metastatic patterns in colonic carcinoma: an analysis of 1541 necropsies. J Pathol 150:195–203
Wils J, Schlangen J, Naus A (1986) Phase II study of hepatic artery infusion with 5-fluorouracil, adriamycin, and mitomycin C (FAM) in liver metastases from colorectal carcinoma. Recent Results Cancer Res 100:157–162
Yang JC, Shlasko E, Ritchey JL, Landry JG, White DE, Rosenberg SA (1993) Combination chemotherapy for metastatic colorectal cancer using 5-fluorouracil, leucovorin and interleukin-2. Eur J Cancer 29A:355–359
York M, Greco FA, Figlin RA, Einhorn L, Man T, Cockey L, Mott D, Light SE (1993) A randomized phase III trial comparing 5-FU with or without interferon alfa 2a for advanced colorectal cancer. Proc Am Soc Clin Oncol 12:200 (abstract)

Young JC, Shlasko E, Ritchey JL, Landry JG, White DE, Rosenberg SA (1993) Combination chemotherapy for metastatic colorectal cancer using 5-fluorouracil, leucovorin and interleukin-2. Eur J Cancer 29A:355–359

Zalcberg J, Cunningham D, Green M, Francois E, van Cutsem E, Schornagel J, Adenis A, Seymour L, Azab M (1995) The final results of a large phase II study of the potent thymidilate synthase (TS) inhibitor Tomudex (ZD1694) in advanced colorectal cancer. Proc Am Soc Clin Oncol 14:204 (abstr)

Antibody-Based Immunotherapeutic Strategies in Colorectal Cancer

E. Holz[1], R. Raab[2], and G. Riethmüller[3]

[1] Tumorzentrum München an den Medizinischen Fakultäten der Ludwig-Maximilians-Universität und der Technischen Universität, Maistr. 11, 80337 Munich, Germany
[2] Medizinische Hochschule Hannover, Klinik für Abdominal- und Transplantationschirurgie, Konstanty-Gutschow-Str. 8, 30625 Hannover, Germany
[3] Institut für Immunologie der Universität München, Goethestr. 31, 80336 Munich, Germany

Abstract

Monoclonal antibodies may well be on their way to becoming an integral part of therapy after the most recent success in prolonging overall and recurrence-free survival in patients with stage III colorectal cancer after potentially curative surgery. After a median follow-up of 5 years, antibody treatment reduced the overall death rate by 30% and decreased the recurrence rate by 27%. These results are similar with regard to efficacy but there is less toxicity with those obtained in contemporary and more recent chemotherapy trials. The key to success with high-molecular-weight substances such as immunoglobulines lies in the careful selection of the appropriate target population, i.e., patients with minimal residual disease, where only isolated tumor cells which are readily accessible to therapy are present. An argument for combining immunotherapy with chemotherapy can be made on the basis of the phenotype of individual disseminated tumor cells, which by immunocytochemistry were found to only rarely express proliferation-associated antigens and therefore are independent of the cell cycle. Further efforts to improve immunotherapy have also led to the combined clinical use of antibodies with biologic response modifiers which are known to enhance effector cell-mediated antibody-dependent cytotoxicity. Additional rationally designed clinical trials are ongoing in which specific immunotherapy is directed towards known, readily accessible, and abundant cell target structures, either alone or combined with treatment modalities which employ different action mechanisms.

Recent Results in Cancer Research, Vol. 142

Introduction and Historical Perspective

In the past 15 years, the clinical development of cancer therapy with monoclonal antibodies (mAbs) has followed essentially the same path as therapy with other small molecules, i.e., initiation with phase-I trials on terminally ill patients who present with large tumor burden, at the same time nuturing the expectation that shrinkage of large measurable tumor nodes would occur. Thus far, however, only very few and anecdotal objective clinical responses have been reported in such patients treated with antibodies (Riethmüller and Johnson 1992; Riethmüller et al. 1993). This is not surprising, since immunoglobulins, with their molecular weight of 150-kD, can hardly penetrate the solid parenchyma of bulky tumor nodes (Jain 1990). In fact, clinical trials (Pimm and Baldwin 1985) have shown that less than 1% of an infused radiolabeled mAb reaches the tumor. The restricted accessibility of tumor cells seems to be one of the major reasons why antibodies have thus far so blatantly failed in cancer. Speculations that not inaccessibility of large tumor mass, but insufficient lytic capacity of unmodified or naked antibody accounts for this negative record have led to a controversial discussion (Colnaghi et al. 1993). More encouraging results were reported with particular mAbs selected for the treatment of leukemias and lymphomas, i.e., tumors that do not form an epithelium-like parenchyma (Grossbard et al. 1992; Levy et al. 1979; Kwak et al. 1992). Yet even in these malignancies with improved accessibility of the target cells, the delicate balance of tumor mass to administered antibody appears to be critical. It is now increasingly recognized that patients presenting with minimal cancer burden or micrometastatic disease will experience the greatest benefit from treatment with mAbs. In an exemplary study by Chatal et al. (Chatal et al. 1989), patients with ovarian cancer were injected i.p. with an ^{111}In-labeled antibody (OC-125) several days before they underwent surgery. The study clearly demonstrated that uptake by large tumors was low; however, for malignant cells or cell clusters isolated from peritoneal fluid or for smaller tumor nodules, uptake of the antibody conjugate was distinctly higher.

Another indication that micrometastatic cells might be suitable targets for passive antibody therapy was provided by Schlimok et al. (1987), who demonstrated that tumor cells in the bone marrow compartment of patients with colorectal cancer can be labeled with mouse immunoglobulin in vivo. In a later report (Pantel et al. 1991), the therapeutic effects of antibody infusions over a period of several months up to 2 years were monitored by immunocytochemical analysis of bone marrow. In 12 of the 23 Dukes' C patients with clinically manifest metastases, micrometastatic cells were repeatedly identified, and clinical relapse occurred in nine of these patients.

Specificity and Safety of Antibodies

Ideally, a monoclonal antibody should specifically target the tumor cell and have minimal cross-reactivity with normal tissues. However, if the antibody cross-reacts with normal tissues it should not impair vital functions of the body. Antibodies used for radioimmunoscintigraphy or even immunotherapy often react to a similar degree with carcinoma and benign epithelial tissue in immunohistochemical studies. However, since tumor cells have penetrated the epithelial basement membrane and invaded the submucosal interstitial compartment, they should be distinctly more accessible for intravenously injected IgG antibodies than normal epithelial cells, which are shielded by the basement membrane (Mach et al. 1983; Meredith et al. 1991; Granowska et al. 1993; Welt et al. 1994). The therapeutic efficacy of antibodies is also prevented when the target antigen is shed into the blood and into the tumor environment in a form that leads to neutralization of the mAb via complex formation (Granowska et al. 1989; Beatty et al. 1986). With regard to safety, the common clinical experience is that antibodies in general are less toxic to the patient than current small-molecule chemotherapeutic agents, probably due to the protective shield of the basal membrane, which is not permeable for large molecules such as immunoglobulins.

Thus, though the 17-1A antigen is widely expressed on cells of normal simple epithelium, an "operational" in vivo tumor specificity of the 17-1A antibody can be derived from its rather benign profile of adverse events. The overall clinical safety profile of patients has been studied in numerous trials with 17-1A administered in single doses of up to 1000 mg and cumulative doses of up to 12000 mg (Khazaeli et al. 1988; Frödin et al. 1990). Adverse experiences related to treatment with 17-1A are predominantly gastrointestinal or allergic in nature and have been easily controlled or reversed without lasting tissue damage. Generally, about half of all adverse experiences reported are gastrointestinal, with frequently experienced nausea with and without vomiting, diarrhea, abdominal pain and cramping, and less frequently noted occurrences of constipation, indigestion, and bleeding. Less than 5% of adverse experiences were anaphylactic and led to cessation of treatment and/or medical intervention but did not require hospitalization of the patient. Otherwise, all adverse experiences were mild to moderate in nature and resolved with routine outpatient measures.

Mechanism of Action of Antibodies

When antibody reaches the tumor cell, its ability to exert a cytotoxic effect on its own depends on the nature of the antigen as well as on the biological activities of the antibody itself, such as its ability to activate endogenous cytotoxic mechanisms like antibody-dependent complement-mediated cytotoxicity (ADCMC) or antibody-dependent cell-mediated cytotoxicity (ADCC). The latter mechanisms can be demonstrated in vitro under experimental conditions and depends on Fc receptor-bearing cells such as lymphocytes, macrophages, and granulocytes recognizing the Fc region of cell-bound antibody which binds to the tumor antigen via its Fab domain. The mechanism by which antibody inhibits tumor growth has been the focus of numerous published reports. Human monocyte/macrophages and peripheral blood lymphocytes (PBLs) incubated with murine monoclonal antibody were capable of lysing human colorectal carcinoma target cells in the ADCC assay (Steplewski et al. 1983), although optimizing the experimental conditions of such assays remains crucial for results. Human macrophages isolated from cancer patients, as well as cultured human monocytes that express FcR receptors, bind murine IgG_{2a} antibodies much better than murine antibodies of the IgG_1, IgG_{2b}, or IgG_3 subclasses. For example, recent studies by Liesveld et al. (1991) indicate that human monocytes can mediate ADCC using 17-1A, an IgG_{2a} murine monoclonal antibody, after allowing sufficient time for in vitro maturation and activation into macrophages. The antibody-independent cell killing averaged 7.4% ± 1.7%, while the antibody-dependent cell killing steadily increased with the effector-to-target (E:T) ratio, to 63% ± 6% at an E:T ratio of 50:1. It was found that culturing of monocytes as effectors for 5–7 days produced maximum ADCC (expressed as percent cytotoxicity), since by then the E:T ratio has increased to 50:1. These data suggest that the 17-1A antibody can mediate ADCC of human colorectal cancer cells by activated macrophages. The mechanisms by which such activated macrophages recognize and can kill a variety of different tumor types is still unclear. One possibility is that direct macrophage-target cell contact involving lysosomal enzyme transfer results in tumor cell destruction, while another explanation has implicated the release of certain macrophage-secretory products, like tumor necrosis factor (TNFα) or nitrous oxide (NO) that can mediate target cell lysis. Also the induction of apoptosis in the target cell has been described in certain ADCC systems. Thus it was recently shown by Wang et al. (1994) that a CD4-antibody-mediated depletion of CD4 T cells was not induced in Fas-deficient 1pr mice, pointing to Fas-Fas ligand interaction induced or facilitated by Fc receptor-bearing cells.

ADCMC is another possible mechanism by which antibody-mediated immunotherapy can induce specific tumor cell killing. In ADCMC, the cascade of complement factors is activated by the Fc region of immunoglobulins of the IgG or IgM class. Usually, at least two molecules of IgG must bind to adjacent antigen epitopes before the complement cascade can be initiated by the intercalating C1q component (Hugli 1982; Muller-Eberhard 1975) that leads to activation of the classical complement pathway, with deposition of further complement components resulting in pore formation of the cellular membrane and death of the cellular target. These effector functions of immunoglobulins are dependent upon the isotype of the Fc portion of the antibody molecule, which differ in their capability to mediate either ADCC or ADCMC.

An example of the above has been demonstrated with 17-1A, which, in early studies, was shown to have little or no ADCMC activity (Herlyn et al. 1985; Steplewski et al. 1986). However, Fogler et al. (1988) demonstrated that 17-1A could mediate ADCMC in the prescence of other monoclonal antibodies, M77 or M79, which, by binding to different epitopes on the 17-1A antigen, allow Fc-Fc interaction as a necessary prerequisite to ADCMC.

These results have been obtained in experimental systems. However, it must be borne in mind that complement activity induced by IgG mAbs in vivo can be controlled by membrane-bound proteins such as CD59 or decay-accelerating factor (DAF), also called homologous restriction factors, dampening the cytolytic effect of autologous complement (Riethmüller and Johnson 1992).

Immune Response to Murine Monoclonal Antibodies

A human-anti-mouse antibody (HAMA) response has been observed in patients after injection of mAbs ranging from 1-mg to 1-g doses and was found to increase with repeated injections (Khazaeli et al. 1994). Patients with solid neoplasms generally have a 50–100% incidence of HAMA response when exposed to mAbs (Granowska et al. 1993; Carrasquillo et al. 1988; Scheinberg et al. 1991). Concurrent administration of interleukin (IL)-2, granulocyte-macrophage colony-stimulating factor (GM-CSF), or interferon does not appear to alter the IgG-HAMA response (Bajorin et al. 1990; Saleh et al. 1990; Chachova et al. 1994). The HAMA response is not detected prior to day 8 and usually reaches a peak at 4–6 weeks after single doses of mAb (Blottiere et al. 1991) and somewhat later after multiple injections (Riethmüller et al. 1994). Some authors have argued that the development of HAMA may preclude the efficacy of mAbs because of enhanced clearance of the antibody from the circulation, and/or neutralization via formation of antigen-antibody complexes, which subsequently could lead to a form of immune complex disease with damage of organs like kidney or lung. No such side effects, however, have so far been seen in association with HAMA formation of the IgG type, perhaps because the absolute amont of HAMA and immune complexes formed is very low. This also explains why the putative presence of HAMA does not alter the immunoreactivity of circulating antibody or the pharmacokinetics of subsequent administrations of antibody when given at high doses such as 100 mg or more (Khazaeli et al. 1988; Blottiere et al. 1991). The formation of IgE-type HAMA, however, is likely to be involved in anaphylactic reactions observed in a minority of patients.

Others have postulated that such a HAMA response favorably influences the prognosis of a patient. This is based upon clinical evidence demonstrating that various populations of anti-idiotypic (Ab2) antibodies, which are directed against antitumor antibodies bearing the internal image of the tumor antigen, will selectively stimulate specific B and/or T cells of the recipient, resulting in specific immune reactions against the original antigen (Herlyn et al. 1986).

Overall, the HAMA response appears to have all the classic features of an immune response to protein antigens. Lanzavecchia et al. (1988) demonstrated that the immune response to several murine monoclonal reagents induced MHC-restricted T-helper cell binding and proliferation, dependent upon antigen-presenting cells. They also showed that this Ig-directed T-cell response led to T-cell-mediated cytolytic activity against murine Ig-epitopes processed and presented by tumor cells. More recently, these observations were extended by Kosmas et al. (1991), who demonstrated in vitro T-cell stimulation by the $HMFG_1$ monoclonal antibody in 11 of 13 patients with ovarian cancer, thus providing evidence for circulating memory T cells present as long as 1 year after therapy. The lymphocyte response included increased expression of IL-2 receptor on responding lymphocytes.

According to the original hypothesis of Jerne, the generation of anti-id (Ab2) antibody reponse against the primary antitumor antibody (Ab1) leads to the formation of anti-anti-idiotypic (Ab3) antibodies, which are expected to react with the tumor antigen itself (Jerne 1974). The destruction of the tumor by endogenously generated Ab3 is thought to occur via ADCC or ADCMC. Ab2 antibody is directed against the variable regions of the Ab1 molecule and as such is part of the overall HAMA response. The fraction of Ab2 that could be important in immunizing the patient against tumor antigen is supposed to function as the "internal image" of the Ab1-binding site. Anti-idiotypic antibodies (Ab2) have been observed in patients treated with 17-1A (Herlyn et al. 1985, 1986a, 1986b, 1987, 1991; Frödin et al. 1991). In studies reported by Herlyn et al. (1986b), anti-id antibodies constituted 21–80% of the total human-anti-mouse antibodies in various patients, with up to 42 μg/ml of Ab2 measured. Further studies by Frödin et al. (1991) have revealed the production of Ab3 in patients treated with multiple infusions of 17-1A. Forty-three patients with metastatic colorectal carcinoma received a variable regimen, according to which different dosages and different numbers of infusions of 17-1A were administered. The doses per infusion were either 200, 400, or 500 mg, and repeat treatments varied from four to 24 per patient. In this study 95% (41/43) of the patients developed Ab2, of both the IgM and IgG classes. Of the 43 patients, 25 (47%) had detectable Ab3. The Ab3 showed in vitro binding to colorectal carcinoma cells, which was inhibited by Ab1 (17-1A). In addition, the Ab3 was able to bind directly to both human monoclonal anti-idiotypic antibodies (Ab2), as well as to polyclonal goat-anti-idiotypic antibody (Ab2). In the latter trial, patients who had detectable levels of Ab3 had a survival time greater than 80 weeks, compared with patients who did not develop Ab3 and survived for a much shorter interval, i.e., 38 weeks. This difference was statistically significant ($p < 0.001$). These data suggest that the anti-idiotypic network based upon the immunogenicity of 17-1A and leading to the production of Ab2 and Ab3 may be another mechanism of producing an anti-tumor reponse.

This is in contrast, however, to data obtained in an adjuvant trial of patients with stage-III colorectal cancer after surgical removal of their tumor (Riethmüller et al. 1994). In this adjuvant therapy trial no difference was found regarding HAMA or anti-idiotypic antibody formation between patients responding to therapy with 17-1A and nonresponders, i.e., those who relapsed or died despite therapy.

At this writing, there are observations of antigen specificity differences between the Ab1 and the Ab2-induced Ab3. For example, the reactivity of a CEA-specific Ab1 differs from a monoclonal Ab3 induced by Ab2 in staining of tumor tissue sections (Bhattacharya-Chatterjee et al. 1990). Similar epitope shifts from the original Ab1 to the Ab3 were seen in other systems (Viale et al. 1989). These findings cannot be easily explained by Ab2 mimicking the antigen. Taking these observations into consideration, the biological responses to immunization with Ab2 are not always totally compatible with an internal antigen mimicry by anti-id. In a review by Bhattacharya Chatterjee et al. (1994), structural data and considerations that are difficult to reconcile with simple antigen mimicry are covered. For example, in an attempt to understand the underlying molecular contacts involved in an imperfect mimicry by Ab2, X-ray studies of an id-anti-id complex were obtained in a lysozyme-binding system (Bentley et al. 1990). The particular Ab2 made contact to Ab1 involving 13 amino acids in its variable regions. Only seven of these 13 Ab1/Ab2 contact residues were also involved in binding of the Ab1 to its antigen lysozyme. The imperfect overlap between the lysozyme-contacting residues and the anti-id contacts may be unique to this particular Ab2, and other Ab2 may be making contacts more resembling the contacts to antigen; however, the structure of the anti-lysozyme Ab1/Ab2 complex alone hints at the limitations of a potential molecular mimicry of antigen by Ab2.

Numerous experiments have failed to produce anti-idiotype (Ab2) antibodies against CD4 antibodies (Ab1) that mimic the CD4 receptor for the gp 120 envelope protein of the HIV virus. Though a broad spectrum of anti CD4 idiotype hybridomas were raised and tested, none of them was found to react with the gp 120 (Chen 1992). Sequencing the CDR region of the idiotype and mutating the idiotypically essential epitopes revealed that CDR2 and CDR3 loops, each on their own could already constitute a idiotypic determinant (Weissenhorn et al. 1992). Furthermore, none of the ten anti-CD4 antibodies that were selected from 225 as specific reactants of the gp 120 binding loop of the CD4 receptor could be proposed on the basis of direct measurement of mab specificity and affinity as a gp 120 mimic (Davis et al. 1992).

Successful Cellular Targets of Antibodies

The elimination of isolated tumor cells from bone marrow has been demonstrated in a pilot study where the intravenous application of mAb ABL 364 resulted in specific clearance of dispersed metastatic cells in the bone marrow (Schlimok et al. 1995). ABL 364 is a murine monoclonal IgG_3 antibody directed against a Lewis Y blood group-related antigen on the cell membrane of carcinoma cells from gastrointestinal, breast, and lung tumors (Scholz et al. 1991), which displays high complement-dependent cytotoxicity. The IgG_3 subclass of murine immunoglobulins is unique among mammalian immunoglobulins because of peculiar Fc-Fc-cooperativity and is particularly effective in the activation of human complement and ADCC. Although the administration of 6 × 50 mg mAb over 2 weeks (3 doses/week, total 300 mg) to patients with advanced breast cancer resulted in no regression of solid metastases, it did induce significant eradication or reduction of dispersed cytokeratin-positive tumor cells detected in the bone marrow. A similar decrease of disseminated cells was not observed in the placebo-treated group, or in patients who received mAb but presented with cells lacking the Lewis Y-related target antigen. The antibody exerted a marked cytotoxicity on tumor cell lines when tested ex vivo with serum taken from these patients after antibody infusion. As heat treatment at 56°C for 30 min abolished the cytotoxicity of the serum completely, the observed reduction of individual tumor cells may be due to a complement-mediated cytotoxic effect of the infused antibody.

The most rigid test of efficacy of a mAb in minimal residual disease has recently been reported with mAb 17-1A in patients with colorectal cancer stage III (Dukes' C) after complete resection of the primary tumor (Riethmüller et al. 1994). It recognizes a 40-kD antigen expressed on the cell surface of a wide variety of tumors derived from different simple epithelia that is also present on epithelial cells of various normal tissues (Koprowski et al. 1979; Göttlinger et al. 1986; Goodwin et al. 1987; Shen et al. 1984; Shetye et al. 1988; Hall 1993). This was surprising at the time, since earlier in vitro studies on tumor cell lines had led to the conclusion that this mAb was highly specific (Herlyn et al. 1979). The function of the 17-1A antigen has recently been claimed to be related to cell-cell adhesion of epithelial cells (Litvinov et al. 1994). Its highly conserved structure during evolution supports the importance of its function (Velders et al. 1994).

In the adjuvant immunotherapy trial, patients received a total of 900 mg mAb 17-1A in five infusions over 20 weeks, starting at 2–3 weeks after surgery. Surgery of patients and patient selection were prospectively standardized and the stringent criteria applied led to elimination of 23 of 189 patients for the final analysis of all eligible patients. In all instances intent-to-treat analyses confirmed the results. To be included in the study, patients were required to have histologically confirmed adenocarcinoma of the colon or rectum with spread to regional lymph nodes and to have undergone curative resection with documented R_0 status (= microscopically and macroscopically tumor free) post surgery. A dynamic randomization procedure was performed by an independent biometric institution and all patients were stratified according to the most common prognostic variables for colorectal cancer, thus leading to well-balanced study groups. The target sample size for the study was a minimum of 150 patients to ensure detection of a potential benefit of 20% for treated patients regarding overall and disease-free survival.

Data of a historic control group of 67 patients, selected post hoc from 107 screened patients of one participating center who matched the entry criteria of the study, were analyzed and compared with data of the prospective immunotherapy trial. Patients had curative (R_0) surgery for stage-III colorectal cancer performed at the *Medizinische Hochschule Hannover* during the period from

December 1980 until January 1985, had no further therapy after surgery, and were followed up until December 1991. The patient characteristics of this historic control group are listed, together with those of the study population, in Table 1.

After a median follow-up of 5 years, antibody therapy reduced overall death rate by 30% and decreased the recurrence rate by 27% (Fig. 1a,b); these results are confirmed after a median follow-up of 7 years. Analysis of the historic control group and comparison with the obtained trial results provides further credence to the finding that the treatment effect observed with mAb 17-1A is real and not due to a prognostically worse control group, as might be derived from the early initial separation of the Kaplan-Meier overall survival curves. Retrospective, descriptive subgroup analyses of all 96 colon cancer patients and all 70 rectal cancer patients are underpowered because of the small patient numbers per treatment group. Yet the data of these subgroup analyses demonstrate a clear trend toward a treatment benefit with 17-1A as compared with no further therapy.

When analyzing the *pattern of recurrence*, it is interesting to note that the antibody did not prevent locoregional recurrence of disease, largely believed to be due to occult tumor left behind after surgery. On the other hand, the antibody was effective in eliminating isolated dispersed cells in the periphery, thus preventing outgrowth of distant metastases.

The importance of selecting patients with no detectable tumor burden after primary surgery cannot be sufficiently emphasized. In another randomized controlled trial (Büchler et al. 1991) of adjuvant immunotherapy in patients

Table 1. Clinical and pathological characteristics of eligible patients in prospective immunotherapy trial and historic controls

Factor	No. of patients		
	17-1A	Observation	Historic controls
Age			
<61 years	50	47	37
≥61 years	40	29	30
Sex			
Male	45	37	41
Female	45	39	26
Location of primary tumor			
Colon	53	43	35
Rectum	37	33	32
Depth of invasion			
T1	1	1	1
T2	15	8	3
T3	72	63	58
T4	2	4	5
Nodal involvement			
N1	61	52	63
N2	29	24	4

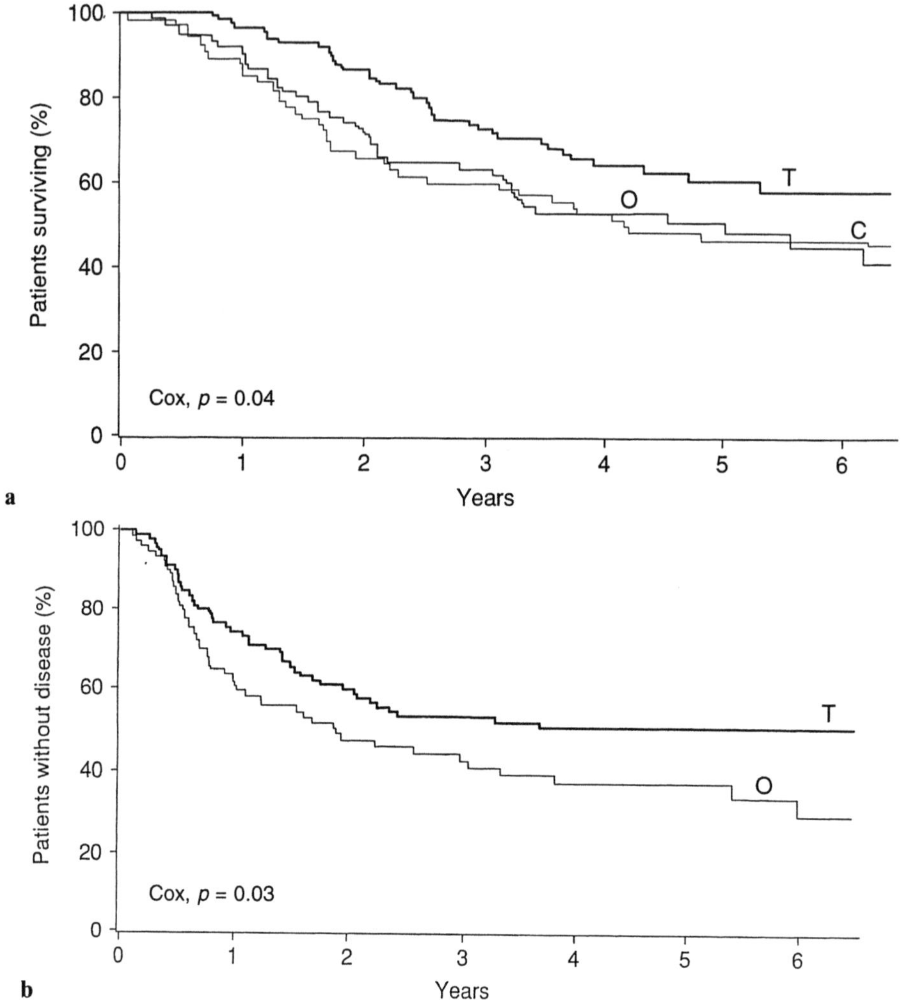

Fig. 1. a Overall survival at 5-year median follow-up for eligible patients treated with 17-1A (*T, thick line*), observed patients (*O, medium line*), and historic control (*C, thin line*) from Hanover. Log rank: T-C, $p = 0.04$; O-C, $p = 0.97$; T-O, $p = 0.05$; Cox: T-O, $p = 0.04$. **b** Disease-free survival for treated group (*thick line*) and observed patients (*thin line*). Log rank: T-O, $p = 0.05$; Cox: T-O, $p = 0.03$

with resected pancreatic cancer using mAb 493/32, a murine IgG_1 isotype which recognizes a carbohydrate epitope on pancreatic cancer cells and mediates ADCC in vitro, no statistically significant difference was detected regarding overall survival for treated and observed groups. This may be explained primarily by the fact that resection in pancreatic cancer is often only a palliative procedure, leaving tumor remnants at least at a microscopic level (R_1 resection according to UICC 1987). In the quoted study, this is underlined by the fact that only 28% of patients showed normalization of serum CA 19-9 after Whipple resection. When elevated, this has proved to be a highly sensitive marker for tumor cells remaining after resection (Safi et al. 1988). Another problem of this clinical study is the low patient number (61 eligible patients), which would require an absolute improved median survival of the treated group of more than 26% in order to become statistically significant, a somewhat overly aggressive goal.

The results obtained with 17-1A antibody therapy in colorectal cancer are similar to the benefit obtained in contemporary and more recent (radio-) chemotherapy trials at better toxicity and therefore may be considered a valuable new treatment alternative (see Table 2; Windle et al. 1987; Laurie et al. 1989; GITSG 1985; Krook et al. 1991; O'Connell et al. 1993, 1994; Moertel et al. 1990, 1995; Erlichmann et al. 1994; Wolmark et al. 1993; SAKK 1995). The trial was initiated in May 1985, and since then adjuvant radio(-chemo)therapy for colorectal cancer has become common practice. Therefore, the data obtained so far will need confirmation in clinical trials with radio(-chemo)therapy as a control arm.

Combination Therapy with Antibodies

Several facts speak for combining immunotherapeutic with conventional treatment modalities. For example, an argument for combining radiation with antibody therapy is that radiation is largely regarded as effective local tumor control, but as having no effect on overall survival when applied alone, while antibody therapy appears to be particularly effective against distant metastases. Thus, adjuvant systemic therapy when combined with post surgical immuno- or chemotherapy may confer additional benefit by reducing the rate of distant metastases. In the trial cited above, the reduction of distant metastases in patients with Dukes' C colorectal cancer has been particularly impressive (Riethmüller et al. 1994). Since murine 17-1A has been proven comparatively safe relative to systemic cancer chemotherapies, a carefully timed combination with radio- or chemotherapy may become a promising treatment alternative.

A further argument for combining immunotherapy with chemotherapy can be derived from studying the biology of individual microdisseminated tumor cells by an immunocytochemical method (Lindemann et al. 1992; Schlimok et al. 1990). For example isolated tumor cells in bone marrow of patients with breast, non-small-cell lung (NSCLC), or gastrointestinal cancer rarely expressed proliferation-associated markers such as Ki-67 or p 120 (Pantel et al. 1993a,b) and thus are believed to be in the Go phase of cell cycle. Though the authors are cautious with conclusions, since the number of detectable carcinoma cells per patient is rather small, these observations may provide another argument for combining immunotherapy, active also on resting cells, with chemotherapy, directed against proliferating cells. Currently, two large trials in colon cancer, stage III, have been initiated in Europe and the US (Table 3), and a rectal cancer trial involving 17-1A in combination with radiation therapy

Table 2. Overview of published studies of adjuvant therapy of colorectal cancer

Study group Publication year	Tumor location	Treatment groups	Tumor stage	Patient number per group	Follow-up time median (years)	Recurrence rate per group (%)	Mortality per group (%)	Significant reduction (+) in	
								Recurrence rate	Mortality
Windle et al. 1987	Colon plus rectum	• No treatment	I + II + III	45	≥5.0	44	NA	NA	–
		• FU		42		52			–
		• FU/levamisole		44		32			+
Laurie et al. 1989	Colon plus rectum	• No treatment	II	49	7.75	NA	NA	–	–
		• Levamisole		45				–	–
		• FU/levamisole		45				–	–
			III	86	7.75	NA	NA	–	–
				85				–	–
				91				+	+
Riethmüller et al. 1994	Colon plus rectum	• No treatment	III	76	5.0	67	51	–	–
		• 17-1A antibody		90		49	36	+	+
GITSG 7175 1985	Rectum	• No treatment	II	21	6.5 (survivors)	33	64	–	–
		• XRT		19		32	54	–	–
		• FU/MeCCNU		16		19	54	–	–
		• XRT + FU/MeCCNU		16		25	44	+	–
			III	37	6.5 (survivors)	68			
				31		58			
				32		59			

				30		37			
Krook et al. NCCTG 794751 1991	Rectum	• XRT	II + III	100	≥7.0	62	62	–	–
		• XRT + FU/MeCCNU		104		42	47	+	+
O'Connell et al. 1994	Rectum	• XRT + FU/MeCCNU (bolus)	II + III	112	≥2.0	NA	NA	–	–
		• XRT + FU/MeCCNU (PVI)		114				+	+
		• XRT + FU (bolus)		198				–	–
		• XRT + FU (PVI)		111				+	+
Moertel et al. 1990	Colon	• No treatment	II	318 (total)	3.0	NA	NA	NA	NA
		• Levamisole	III	315	3.0	49	36	–	–
		• FU/levamisole		310		47	35	–	–
				304		34	26	+	+
Moertel et al. 1995					6.5	56	53	–	–
						56	51	–	–
						39	40	+	+
Erlichman et al. 1994	Colon	• No treatment	(II) III	798	3.1	37	22	–	–
		• FU/FA		695		28	17	+	+
Wolmark et al. NSABP C-03	Colon	• MOF	II + III	524	3	36	23	–	–
		• FU/leucovorin		521		27	16	+	+
O'Connell et al. 1993	Colon	• No treatment	II + III	151	3.5	36	29	–	–
		• FU/leucovorin		158		23	25	+	–
SAKK 1995	Colon plus rectum	• No treatment	I + II + III	253	8	52	45	–	–
		• Fu/mitomycin (intraportal)		252		43	34	+	+

and chemotherapy is being planned, with results of these trials anticipated toward the end of 1999.

Efforts to improve immunotherapy have led to the introduction of novel cytokines into preclinical and clinical studies of combinations of cytokines and monoclonal antibodies (Eisenthal et al. 1990; Massuci et al. 1990; Ragnhammar et al. 1993). There is ample preclinical evidence that cytokines can enhance effector cell-mediated ADCC (Liesveld et al. 1991). Also the efficacy of mAbs can be augmented when the full cytotoxic capacity of effector cells is exploited by stimulation with cytokines (Ragnhammar et al. 1994; Masucci and Mellstedt 1991).

In a clinical study of patients with advanced solid tumors (Ragnhammar et al. 1993), the combination of mAb 17-1A and GM-CSF was evaluated in 20 patients, leading in two to a complete response and in one patient to a partial response. Together with the "stable disease" responses, an overall clinical response rate of 30% was reported. These results were obtained at minor toxicity to the patients. Bajorin et al. (1990) reported the use of low-dose IL-2 together with R24 and observed one partial response among 20 treated patients with metastatic melanoma. When a higher-dose IL-2 regimen was used together with R24 and monthly low-dose cyclophosphamide in patients with melanoma (Creekmore et al. 1992), ten of 23 evaluable patients had partial responses. However, toxicities related to IL-2 and reported in this trial were substantial and included hypotension, fever, and renal and pulmonary toxicities.

Though this selection of phase-I clinical studies shows that there may be a merit to combining mAbs with cytokines for the treatment of cancer, further comparative studies are needed to define the optimal agents, their dose, and the schedule of administration.

Conclusions and Perspectives

While it is clear that accessibility of the tumor cells should be a major consideration for the successful application of antibody therapy in solid tumors,

Table 3. Current studies with 17-1A in resected stage-III colon cancer

Study	Treatment groups	Estimated patient number per group	Estimated median follow-up (years)	Estimated mortality (%)
US phase III	• FU/levamisole	900	2.1	30
	• 17-1A + FU/levamisole	900		23
European phase III	• 17-1A	900	2.1	30
	• FU/leucovorin	900		30
	• 17-1A + FU/leucovorin	900		23

other biological aspects also need to be taken in account. *Heterogeneity of tumor cells* is one of the major obstacles to any antigen-targeting therapy: To cope with antigen heterogeneity, which increases with tumor progression, a carefully selected combination of antibodies directed to genetically independently controlled membrane antigens should be applied as early as possible, i.e., immediately after removal of the primary tumor. Published data demonstrate that selected pairs of antibodies directed against different epitopes of a particular antigen exhibit up to a 100-fold synergistic increase in cell killing in vitro (Fogler et al. 1988) or in vivo (Quin et al. 1987), or result in augmented binding (Saito et al. 1991; Mujoo et al. 1991; Casalini 1991). Another obstacle to overcome is the insufficient presence of activated effector cells at the site of the tumor cells. Preclinical studies have demonstrated (Ragnhammar et al. 1994; Masucci et al. 1991; Creekmore et al. 1992) that biological response modifiers (BRMs) such as GM-CSF and IL-2 can enhance effector cell activity. GM-CSF will enhance the total number of monocytes and granulocytes and will activate these cells for ADCC; IL-2 will expand and activate the natural killer cell population, which can also mediate ADCC. Both cytokines can trigger synthesis of other potentially helpful BRMs.

Finally, combinations of mAbs and BRMs may become the mainstay of future immunotherapy, since both the target structures on tumor cells and the effector cell arm become optimized. Other options are the use of *bispecific antibodies* which recruit cytotoxic T cells for potent tumor cell elimination or antibodies would consist of human or "humanized" versions of the parental murine antibodies. Since normal epithelial cells of the gastrointestinal tract appear to be less accessible to cytotoxic antibodies due to the dense basal membrane, which is quasi-impermeable to nonsecretory immunoglobulin, an absolute specificity for therapeutic antibodies appears less critical. Indeed, toxicity to normal epithelia has been negligible in all trials reported thus far. Although the inactivation of complement by membrane-bound homologous restriction factors also present on tumor cells may contribute to the resistance of the tumor cells to lysis, it may be possible to eventually inhibit these factors (Lachman 1991). As demonstrated by several studies (Lindemann et al. 1992; Schlimok et al. 1987), micrometastatic cells can be reproducibly identified in individual patients over time, thus offering a new way to monitor micrometastasis. Such monitoring will be mandatory for a more expeditious development of an effective passive antibody therapy. Furthermore, new diagnostic techniques such as PCR may replace the more laborious immunocytological methods (Gerhard et al. 1994).

In conclusion, monoclonal antibodies, which are exquisitely specific and versatile tools and capable of harnessing powerful natural effector mechanisms, have been shown to present a new immunological strategy if applied to a suitable target such as minimal residual disease. The task ahead is to consolidate their role and define their place together with and amidst other treatment modalities.

References

Bajorin DF, Chapman PB, Wong G et al (1990) Phase-I evaluation of a combination of monoclonal antibody R24 and interleukin 2 in patients with metastatic melanoma. Cancer Res 50:7490–7495

Beatty JD, Duda RB, Williams L et al (1986) Preoperative imaging of colorectal carcinoma with 111-In-labelled anticarcinoembryonic antigen monoclonal antibody. Cancer Res 46:6494–6502

Bentley GA, Boulot G, Riottot MM et al (1990) Three-dimensional structure of an idiotope-anti-idiotope complex. Nature 348:254

Bhattacharya-Chatterjee M, Mukerjee S, Biddle W et al (1990) Murine monoclonal anti-idiotype antibody as a potential network antigen for human carcino-embryonic antigen. J Immunol 145:2758

Bhattacharya-Chatterjee M, Foon KA, Köhler H (1994) Review. Idiotypic antibody immunotherapy of cancer. Cancer Immunol Immunother 38:75–82

Blottière HM, Steplewski Z, Herlyn D et al (1991) Human anti-murine immunoglobulin responses and immune functions in cancer patients receiving murine monoclonal antibody therapy. Hum Antibod Hybridomas 2:16–25

Büchler M, Friess H, Schultheiss K-H et al (1991) A randomized controlled trial of adjuvant immunotherapy (murine monoclonal antibody 494/32) in resectable pancreatic cancer. Cancer 68:1507–1512

Carrasquillo JA, Sugarbaker P, Colcher D et al (1988) Radioimmunoscintigraphy of colon cancer with iodine-131-labeled B72.3 monoclonal antibody. J Nucl Med 29:1022–1030

Casalini P, Mezzanzanica D, Canevari S et al (1991) Use of combination of monclonal antibodies directed against three distinct epitopes of a tumor-associated antigen – analysis of cell binding and internalization. Int J Cancer 48:284–290

Chachoua A, Oratz R, Liebes L et al (1994) Phase-Ib trial of granulocyte-macrophage colony-stimulating factor combined with murine monoclonal antibody R24 in patients with metastatic melanoma. J Immunother 16:132–141

Chatal JF, Saccavini J-C, Gestin J-F et al (1989) Biodistribution of indium-111-labeled OC 125 monoclonal antibody intraperitoneally injected into patients operated on for ovarian carcinomas. Cancer Res 49:3087–3094

Chen Y-H (1992) Herstellung und Charakterisierung anti-idiotypischer Antikörper gegen monoklonale CD4-Antikörper als Grundlage einer HIV-Vakzineentwicklung. Doctoral thesis University of Munich

Colnaghi MI, Ménard S, Canevari S (1993) Evoluation of the therapeutic use of new monoclonal antibodies. Curr Op Oncol 5:1035–1042

Creekmore S, Urba W, Kopp W et al (1992) Phase-Ib/II trial of R24 antibody and interleukin-2 in melanoma. Proc Am Soc Clin Oncol 11:1186

Davis SJ, Schockmel GA, Somoza C et al (1992) Antibody and HIV-1 gp 120 recognition of CD4 undermines the concept of mimicry between antibodies and receptors. Nature 358

Eisenthal A, Cameron RB, Rosenberg SA (1990) Induction of antibody-dependent cellular cytotoxicity in vivo by IFN-α and its antitumor efficacy against established B16 melanoma liver metastases when combined with specific anti-B16 monoclonal antibody. J Immunol 144(11):4463–4471

Erlichmann C, Marsoni S, Seitz JF et al (1994) Event-free and overall survival is increased by FUFA in resected B and C colon cancer: a prospective pooled analysis of 3 randomized trials. Proc Am Soc Clin Oncol 13:194

Fogler WE, Klinger MR, Abraham KG et al (1988) Enhanced cytotoxicity against colon carcinoma by combinations of noncompeting monoclonal antibodies to the 17-1A antigen. Cancer Res 48:6303–6308

Frödin JE, Lefvert AK, Mellstedt H (1990) Pharmacokinetics of the mouse monoclonal antibody 17-1A in cancer patients receiving various treatment schedules. Cancer Res 50:4866–4871

Frödin JE, Faxas ME, Hagström B et al (1991) Induction of anti-idiotypic (ab2) and anti-anti-idiotypic (ab3) antibodies in patients treated with the mouse monoclonal antibody 17-1A (ab1). Relation to the clinical outcome – an important antitumoral effector function? Hybridoma 10:421–431

Gerhard M, Juhl H, Kalthoff H et al (1994) Specific detection of carcinoembryonic antigen-expressing tumor cells in bone marrow aspirates by polymerase chain reaction. J Clin Oncol 12(4):725–729

GITSG (1985) Prolongation of the disease-free interval in surgically treated rectal carcinoma. N Engl J Med 312(23):1465–1472

Göttlinger HG, Funke I, Johnson JP et al (1986) The epithelial cell surface antigen 17-1A, a target for antibody-mediated tumor therapy: its biochemical nature, tissue distribution and recognition by different monoclonal antibodies. Int J Cancer 38:47–53

Goodwin RA, Tuttle SE, Bucci DM et al (1987) Tumor-associated antigen expression of primary and metastatic colon carcinomas detected by monoclonal antibody 17-1A. Am J Clin Pathol 88:462–467

Granowska M, Jass JR, Britton KE et al (1989) A prospective study of the use of ^{111}In-labeled monoclonal antibody against carcino-embryonic antigen in colorectal cancer and of some biological factors affecting its uptake. Int J Colorectal Dis 4:97–108

Granowska M, Britton KE, Mather SJ et al (1993) Radioimmunoscintigraphy with technetium-99m-labelled monoclonal antibody, 1A3, in colorectal cancer. Eur J Nuc Med 20(8):690–698

Grossbard ML, Press OW, Appelbaum FR et al (1992) Monoclonal antibody-based therapies of leukemia and lymphoma. Blood 80(4):863–878

Hall WC (1993) Cross-reactivity of mouse monoclonal antibody 17-1A with human tissues. Immunopathology report to Centocor (No. IMo83)

Herlyn M, Steplewski Z, Herlyn D et al (1976) Colorectal carcinoma-specific antigen: detection by means of monoclonal antibodies. Proc Natl Acad Sci USA 76(3): 1438–1442

Herlyn D, Lubeck M, Sears H et al (1985) Specific detection of anti-idiotypic immune responses in cancer patients treated with murine monoclonal antibody. J Immunol Methods 85:27–38

Herlyn D, Ross AH, Koprowski H (1986a) Anti-idiotypic antibodies bear the internal image of a human tumor antigen. Science 232:100–102

Herlyn D, Sears H, Iliopoulous D et al (1986b) Anti-idiotypic antibodies to monoclonal antibody CO17-1A. Hybridoma 5[Suppl 1]:S51–S58

Herlyn D, Ross AH, Iliopoulos D et al (1987) Induction of specific immunity to human colon carcinoma by anti-idiotypic antibodies to monoclonal antibody CO17-1A. Eur J Immunol 17:1649–1652

Herlyn D, Benden A, Kane M et al (1991) Anti-idiotype cancer vaccines: pre-clinical and clinical studies. In Vivo 5:615–624

Hugli TE (1982) Complement. In: Baron S (ed) Medical microbiology. Addison-Wesley, Menlo Park, pp 31–44

Jain RK (1990) Physiological barriers to delivery of monoclonal antibodies and other macromolecules in tumors. Cancer Res 50:814s–819s

Jerne NK (1974) Towards a network theory of the immune system. Ann Inst Pasteur Immunol 125C:373–389

Khazaeli MB, Saleh MN, Wheeler RH et al (1988) Phase-I trial of multiple large doses of murine monoclonal antibody CO17-1A. II. Pharmacokinetics and immune response. J Natl Cancer Inst 80(12):937–942

Khazaeli MB, Conry RM, LoBuglio AF (1994) Human immune response to monoclonal antibodies. J Immunother 15:42–52
Koprowski H, Steplewski Z, Mitchell K et al (1979) Colorectal carcinoma antigens detected by hybridoma antibodies. Somat Cell Genet 5(6):957–972
Kosmas C, Epenetos AA, Courtenay-Luck NS (1991) T-cell proliferation following monoclonal antibody treatment. In: Epenetos A (ed) Monoclonal antibodies, applications in clinical oncology. Chapman and Hall Medical, London, pp 273–281
Krook JE, Moertel CG, Gunderson LL et al (1991) Effective surgical adjuvant therapy for high-risk rectal carcinoma. N Engl J Med 324(11):709–715
Kwak LW, Campbell MJ, Czerwinski DK et al (1992) Induction of immune responses in patients with B-cell lymphoma against the surface-immunoglobulin idiotype expressed by their tumors. N Engl J Med 327(17):1209–1215
Lachman PJ (1991) The control of homologous lysis. Immunol Today 12:312–315
Lanzavecchia A, Abrignani S, Scheidegger D et al (1988) Antibodies as antigens. The use of mouse monoclonal antibodies of focus human T cells against selected targets J Exp Med 167:345–352
Laurie JA, Moertel CG, Fleming TR et al (1987) Surgical adjuvant therapy of large-bowel carcinoma: an evaluation of levamisole and the combination of levamisole and fluorouracil. J Clin Oncol 7:1447–1456
Levy PC, Shaw GM, LoBuglio AF (1979) Human monocyte, lymphocyte, and granulocyte antibody-dependent cell-mediated cytotoxicity toward tumor cells. I. General characteristics of cytolysis. J Immunol 123:594–599
Liesveld JL, Frediani KE, Winslow JM et al (1991) Cytokine effects and role of adhesive proteins and Fc receptors in human macrophage-mediated antibody-dependent cellular cytotoxicity. J Cell Biochem 45:381–390
Lindemann F, Schlimok G, Dirschedl P et al (1992) Prognostic significance of micrometastatic tumour cells in bone marrow of colorectal cancer patients. Lancet 340:685–689
Litvinov SV, Velders MP, Bakker HA (1994) Ep-CAM: a human epithelial antigen is a homophilic cell-cell adhesion molecule. J Cell Biol 125(2):437–446
Mach JP, Chatal JF, Lumbroso JD et al (1983) Tumor localization in patients by radiolabeled monoclonal antibodies against colon carcinoma. Cancer Res 43:5593–5600
Masucci G, Ragnhammar P, Wersäll P et al (1990) Granulocyte-monocyte colony-stimulating factor augments the interleukin-2-induced cytotoxic activity of human lymphocytes in the absence and presence of mouse or chimeric monoclonal antibodies (mAb 17-1A). Cancer Immunol Immunother 31:231–235
Masucci G, Mellstedt H (1991) Combinations of IL-2, GM-CSF, IL-4, IFN-α and TFN-α increase the antibody-dependent cellular cytotoxicity (ADCC) of blood mononuclear cells in presence of either mouse or chimeric MAb 17-1A – a preclinical evaluation. Cancer J 4(3):168–173
Meredith RF, LoBuglio AF, Plott WE (1991) Pharmacokinetics, immune response, and biodstribution of iodine-131-labeled chimeric mouse/human IgG1,k 17-1A monoclonal antibody. J Nucl Med 32:1162–1168
Moertel CG, Fleming TR, MacDonald JS et al (1990) Levamisole and fluorouracil for adjuvant therapy of resected colon carcinoma. N Engl J Med 322(6):352–358
Moertel CG, Fleming TR, Macdonald JS et al (1995) Fluorouracil plus levamisole as effective adjuvant therapy after resection of stage-III colon carcinoma: a final report. Ann Intern Med 122:321–326
Mujoo K, Rosenblum MG, Murray JL et al (1991) Augmented binding of radiolabeled monoclonal antibodies to melanoma cells using specific antibody combinations. Cancer Res 51:2768–2772

Muller-Ėberhard HJ (1975) Complement. Ann Rev Biochem 44:697–724
O'Connell M, Mailliard J, Macdonald J et al (1993) An intergroup trial of intensive course 5FU and low dose leucovorin as surgical adjuvant therapy for high risk colon cancer. Proc ASCO 12:197
O'Connell MJ, Martenson JA, Wieand HS et al (1994) Improving adjuvant therapy for rectal cancer by combining protracted-infusion fluorouracil with radiation therapy after curative surgery. N Engl J Med 331:502–507
Pantel K, Schlimok G, Kutter D et al (1991) Frequent down-regulation of major histocompatibility class-I antigen expression on individual micrometastatic carcinoma cells. Cancer Res 51:4712–4715
Pantel K, Izbicki JR, Angstwurm M et al (1993a) Immunocytological detection of bone marrow micrometastasis in operable non-small cell lung cancer. Cancer Res 53:1027–1031
Pantel K, Schlimok G, Braun S et al (1993b) Differential expression of proliferation-associated molecules in individual micrometastatic carcinoma cells. J Natl Cancer Inst 85(17):1419–1424
Pimm MW, Baldwin RW (1985) Localization of an antitumor monoclonal antibody in human tumor xenographs: kinetic and quantitative studies with the 791T/36 antibody. In: Baldwin RW, Byers VS (eds) Monoclonal antibodies for cancer detection and therapy. Academic Press, New York, pp 97–128
Quin S, Cobbald S, Tighe H et al (1987) CD4 Monoclonal antibody pairs for immunosuppression and tolerance induction. Eur J Immunol 17:1159–1165
Ragnhammar P, Fagerberg J, Frödin JE et al (1993) Effect of monoclonal antibody 17-1A and GM-CSF in patients with advanced colorectal carcinoma – long-lasting, complete remissions can be induced. Int J Cancer 53:751–758
Ragnhammar P, Frödin JE, Trotta PP et al (1994) Cytotoxicity of white blood cells activated by granulocyte-colony-stimulating factor, granulocyte/macrophage-colony-stimulating factor and macrophage-colony-stimulating factor against tumor cells in the presence of various monoclonal antibodies. Cancer Immunol Immunother 391:254–262
Riethmüller G, Johnson JP (1992) Monoclonal antibodies in the detection and therapy of micrometastatic epithelial cancers. Curr Op Immun 4:647–655
Riethmüller G, Schneider-Gädicke E, Johnson JP (1993) Monoclonal antibodies in cancer therapy. Curr Op Immun 5:732–739
Riethmüller G, Schneider-Gädicke E, Schlimok G et al (1994) Randomised trial of monoclonal antibody for adjuvant therapy of resected Dukes' C colorectal carcinoma. Lancet 343:1177–1183
Safi F, Roscher R, Beger HG (1988) Prognostic value CA-19-9 determination in resected pancreatic carcinoma. Cancer 3:279–286
Saito S, Inque T, Kawase I et al (1991) Two monoclonal antibodies against small-cell lung cancer show existence of synergism in binding. Cancer Immunol Immunother 33:165–170
SAKK (1995) Long-term results of single course of adjuvant intraportal chemotherapy for colorectal cancer. Lancet 345:349–353
Saleh MN, LoBuglio AF, Wheeler RH et al (1990) A phase-II trial of murine monoclonal antibody 17-1A and γ-IFN-clinical and immunological data. Cancer Immunol Immunother 32:185–190
Scheinberg DA, Lovett D, Divgi CR et al (1991) A phase-I trial of monoclonal antibody M195 in acute myelogenous leukemia: specific bone marrow targeting and internalization of radionuclide. J Clin Oncol 9:478–490
Schlimok G, Funke I, Holzmann B et al (1987) Micrometastatic cancer cells in bone marrow: in vitro detection with anti-cytokeratin and in vivo labelling with 17-1A monoclonal antibodies. Proc Natl Acad Sci USA 84:8672–8676

Schlimok G, Funke I, Bock B et al (1990) Epithelial tumor cells in bone marrow of patients with colorectal cancer: immunocytochemical detection, phenotypic characterization, and prognostic significance. J Clin Oncol 8:831–837
Schlimok G, Pantel K, Loibner H et al (1995) Reduction of metastatic carcinoma cells in bone marrow by intravenously administered monoclonal antibody: towards a novel surrogate test to monitor adjuvant therapies of solid tumors. Eur J Cancer 31A(11):1799–1803
Scholz D, Lubeck M, Loibner H et al (1991) Biological activity in the human system of isotype variants of oligosaccharide-Y-specific murine monoclonal antibodies. Cancer Immunol Immunother 33:153–157
Shen JW, Atkinson B, Koprowski H et al (1984) Binding of murine immunoglobulin to human tissues after immunotherapy with anticolorectal carcinoma monoclonal antibody. Int J Cancer 33:465–468
Shetye J, Frödin JE, Christensson B et al (1988) Immunohistochemical monitoring of metastatic colorectal carcinoma in patients treated with monoclonal antibodies (MAb 17-1A). Cancer Immunol Immunother 27:154–162
Steplewski Z, Lubeck MD, Koprowski H (1983) Human macrophages armed with murine immunoglobulin G2a antibodies to tumors destroy human cancer cells. Science 221:865–867
Steplewski Z, Herlyn D, Lubeck M et al (1986) Mechanisms of tumor growth inhibition. Hybridoma 5:S59–S64
Velders MP, Litvinov SV, Warnaar SO et al (1994) New chimeric antipancarcinoma monoclonal antibody with superior cytotoxicity-mediating potency. Cancer Res 54:1753–1759
Viale G, Flamini G, Grassi F et al (1989) Idiotypic replica of an anti-human tumor-associated antigen monoclonal antibody. J Immunol 143:4338
Wang Z, Dudhane A, Orlikowsky T et al (1994) CD4 engagement induces Fas antigen-dependent apoptosis of T cells in vivo. Eur J Immunol 24:1549–1552
Weissenhorn W, Chen YH, Riethmüller G et al (1992) VH-related idiotypes detected by site-directed mutagenesis. A study induced by the failure to find CD4 anti-idiotypic antibodies mimicking the cellular receptor of HIV. J Immunol 149(4): 1237–1241
Welt S, Divgi C, Kemeny N et al (1994) Phase-I/II study of iodine 131-labeled monoclonal antibody A33 in patients with advanced colon cancer. J Clin Oncol 12(8): 1561–1571
Windle R, Bell PR and Shaw D (1987) Five-year results of a randomized trial of adjuvant 5-fluorouracil and levamisole in colorectal cancer. Br J Surg 74:569–572
Wolmark N, Rockette H et al (1993) The benefit of leucovorin-modulated flourouracil as postoperative adjuvant therapy for primary colon cancer: results from national surgical adjuvant breast and bowel project protocol C-03. J Clin Oncol 11:1879–1887

Surgical Concepts for Therapy of Pancreatic Neoplasms

H. Keck, J.M. Langrehr, V. Henneken, M. Knoop, and P. Neuhaus

Department of Surgery, Virchow Clinic, Free University Berlin, Augustenburger Platz 1, 13353 Berlin, Germany

Abstract

Surgical treatment of pancreatic malignomas has improved dramatically over the past decades, which is illustrated by the decrease in perioperative mortality to 1%–2%. This has made it possible to widen the indication for pancreatic resection and the extent of the surgical intervention. Experience with pancreatic resection for neoplasms at our center using standard surgical techniques during the last decade is reviewed, with special focus on the cases with partial resection of the portal vein. Perioperative morbidity has decreased below 5% and 5-year survival rates reach 60% for stage I tumors and 15%–25% for stage II and III tumors. The authors conclude that surgical therapy for pancreatic neoplasms is safe and yields a considerably higher quality of life for the patient and therefore should be considered in all patients with this disease entity.

Introduction

Pancreatic carcinomas have become one of the most frequent neoplasms over the past few decades. This is reflected by the annual statistic report of the National Institute of Cancer of the United States of America, listing carcinomas of the pancreas in fourth place in western civilized countries (National Cancer Institute). However, the steep rise in the occurrence of pancreatic carcinomas may also reflect the advanced diagnostic tools and more invasive evaluation of the patient.

While epidemiologic studies have revealed that exposure to several factors, including toxic agents such as alcohol, may foster the development of pancreatic cancer, the etiology of this entity is still unclear (Farrow and Davis 1990; Fisher et al. 1990; Hirayama 1989; Lowenfels et al. 1993; Offerhaus et al. 1988). Furthermore, the biology of this specific cancer, its growth patterns, and

Recent Results in Cancer Research, Vol. 142

metastatic behavior are not well understood, and because of the localization of the tumor, clinical symptoms are often detected late in the course of the disease (Grace et al. 1986). These factors are the leading reasons why the overall prognosis for patients with pancreatic neoplasm is still poor.

Standard conservative therapeutic concepts, such as chemotherapy using various drugs and regimens, have shown disappointing results (Arbuck 1990; Cullinan et al. 1989; Hurdis et al. 1986; Wils 1989), and sole external radiation has also not been able to ameliorate the prognosis (Glaser et al. 1993; Moertel et al. 1981). Furthermore, with the recently employed method of intraoperative radiation therapy (IORT), improved results were observed initially. However, the number of cases has been small so far, and after 2 years of follow-up the results were similar to those with surgical therapy alone (Tuckson et al. 1988), and survivial rates have not significantly increased (Gunderson et al. 1987; Roldan et al. 1988). Therefore, especially in the cases of biliary stenosis due to the tumor growth, surgical concepts still constitute the fundamental principle in treatment of pancreatic neoplasms (Beger and Bittner 1986; Connolly et al. 1987; Trede 1987; Warshaw and Fernandez Del Castillo 1992).

Despite many described modifications, the partial duodenopancreatectomy, or Kausch-Whipple procedure, still represents the standard surgical procedure used in most centers around the world, accounting for as much as 90% of the cases in some. Therefore, this contribution describes our experience with of this procedure for patients with carcinoma of the pancreatic head and considers the results in patients undergoing an extended Kausch-Whipple procedure including resection of major venous vessels.

Patients, Materials, and Methods

Between August 1985 and April 1994, we performed 179 partial duodenopancreatectomies (Fig. 1). In 127 cases, surgery was performed for malignant diseases including carcinoma of the head of the pancreas (74 cases), papillary carcinoma (20 cases), carcinoma of the distal biliary tree (19 cases), and miscellaneous indications (14 cases). In the remaining 52 patients, a benign underlying disease was the reason for resection, and the majority of this group consisted of patients with chronic pancreatitis (47 cases). The detailed diagnoses are depicted in Table 1. From the 74 cases with cancer of the head of the pancreas which were reviewed in this study, 43 patients were female (58.1%) and 31 male (41.9%). The average age at the time of surgery was 60.7 years, ranging from 19 to 81 years.

Surgical Technique

Preoperative diagnostics to define the resectability always included sonography, a CT scan using intravenous contrast medium and, in selected

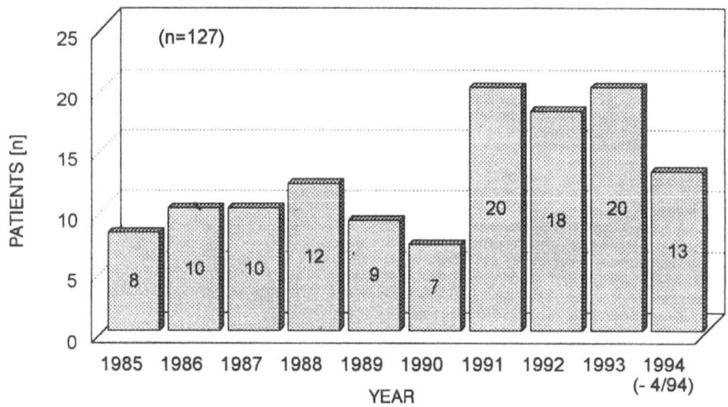

Fig. 1. Number of partial duodenopancreatectomies (Kausch-Whipple procedures) performed per year for all indications

Table 1. Diagnoses of all patients who underwent partial duodenopancreatectomy (Kausch-Whipple procedure) from August 1985 to April 1994

Diagnosis	Patients (*n*)	Frequency (%)
Ca of pancreatic head	74	41.2
Ca of papilla	20	11.2
Ca of dist. common bile duct	19	10.6
Ca of gallbladder	4	2.2
Infiltr. Ca of stomach	3	1.7
APUDom-duodenum	2	1.1
Islet cell Ca	1	0.6
Carcinoid of pancreatic head	1	0.6
Ca of duodenum	2	1.1
solid cystic tumor	1	0.6
Malignant total	127	70.9
Chronic pancreatitis	47	26.2
Adenoma of duodenun	2	1.1
Trauma (stab wound)	1	0.6
Ulcus duodeni	1	0.6
Cyst of bile duct	1	0.6
Benign total	52	29.1
Total (8/85–4/94)	179	100.0

Ca, Carcinoma

cases, when indicated, angiography. Through a transverse laparotomy, with cranial extension if necessary, standard preparation including dissection of the ligamentum gastrohepaticum, mobilization of the flexura coli dextra, Kocher maneuver, and dissection of the ligamentum gastrocolicum was performed,

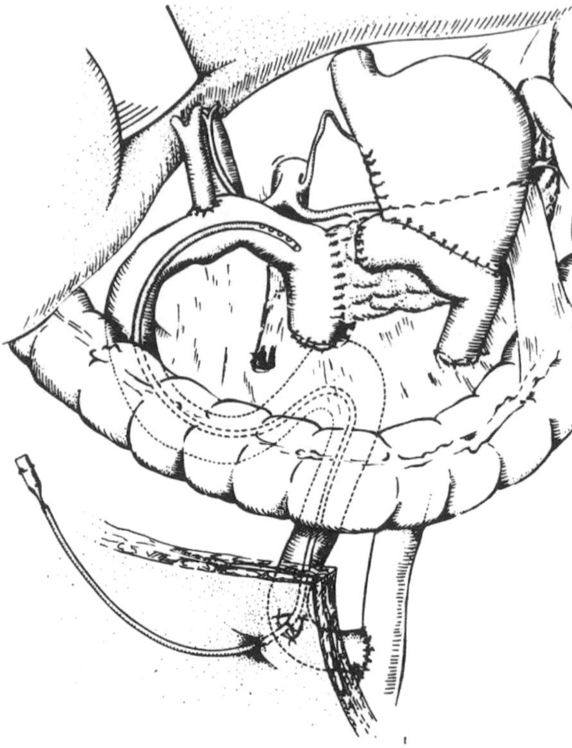

Fig. 2. Operative site and placement of the intraluminal drainage are depicted following reconstruction after resection of the pancreatic head (partial duodenopancreatectomy or Kausch-Whipple procedure)

and after thorough evaluation the head of the pancreas was resected. If possible, lymphadenectomy was performed en bloc in the ligamentum hepatoduodenale, along the cranial and caudal border of the pancreas, including dissection of the celiac trunk, and retropancreatically from the renal capsula to the arteria mesenterica superior.

Drainage of the remaning pancreas was ensured by a second (lower) intestinal Roux-en-Y loop, which was led retrocolically into the right upper abdomen. Both the rest of the pancreatic gland and the common bile duct were separately anastomosed with this loop. The stomach was anastomosed with the upper (first) Roux-en-Y loop, and after completion of the intestinal connection an intraluminal drainage was inserted into the second loop. Reconstruction and placement of intraluminal drainage are shown in Fig. 2. This device relieves both the pancreatic and the biliary anastomosis sufficiently for the early postoperative phase and, after internal fixation of the jejunum, is led out through an incision at the lateral abdominal wall (Keck et al. 1992). The tube was removed on the 12th postoperative day, following radiological proof of sufficient anastomosis.

In 11 patients graded stage III (see below), infiltration of the vena portae or the superior mesenteric vein was detected and a segmental resection of the infiltrated vessel was performed. While end-to-end anastomosis of the resected vessel was feasable in nine patients, prosthetic materials had to be used in two cases to ensure reanastomosis without tension.

Histopathomorphology

Classification of the histopathomorphological findings was performed using the 1987 TMN-classification for malignant tumors of the UICC. In patients who were resected before 1987, the original specimens were classified retrospectively. From the 26 cases (35.2%) classified as stage I, only three patients (4.1%) revealed an "early carcinoma", smaller than 2 cm and limited to the pancreatic gland. In five cases (6.7%) a stage II was detected and the majority of patients (38 cases, 51.4%) showed a stage-III carcinoma upon histologic evaluation. One preoperatively detected solitary liver metastasis, which was therefore determined as stage IV, was resected upon explicit demand of the young female patient. In the remaining four cases (5.4%), a histopathomorphological diagnosis was not obtained for various reasons (Table 2).

Table 2. Histopathological classification of specimens from patients who underwent partial duodenopancreatectomy for carcinoma of the pancreatic head between August 1985 and April 1994

Total (*n*)		74
Sex	male	31
	female	43
Average age		60.7
(years)	range	(19–81)
Stage of tumor	Stage I	*n* (%)
(UICC 1987)	T_1N_0	3 (4.1)
	T_2N_0	23 (31.1)
	Stage II	
	T_3N_0	5 (6.7)
	Stage III	
	$T_{all}N_1$	38 (51.4)
	Stage IV	
	$T_{all}N_{all}M_1$	1 (1.3)
	Not classified	4 (5.4)

Results

Early Complications

The perioperative mortality (30-day mortality) for the 74 patients with carcinomas of the pancreatic head was 1.4% (1/74), whereby it was noted that the one patient who died did not suffer from a surgical complication. The mean hospital stay was 25 days, ranging from 12 to 74 days. Seventeen complications were observed in nine patients (10.9%). One patient (1.4%) developed an insufficiency of the choledochojejunostomy with consecutive peritonits, whereas a leakage of the pancreatojejunostomy was not detected. Application of water-soluble contrast medium through the drain in the lower loop was able to detect and verify the complication. The insufficiency of the choledochojejunostomy was treated with a transhepatic splint. In two cases (2.8%) bleeding from the pancreatic resection plane was detected, necessitating relaparotomy and reresection for successful treatment of the complication. Two cases (2.8%) of intra-abdominal abscesses, responding favorably to conservative treatment, were observed, and one (1.4%) dislocation of the intraluminal drainage occurred. Additionally, four (5.5%) wound infections and four (5.5%) general cardiopulmonary complications were observed, all of which did not require surgery or intensive care. In the patients with vessel resections, perioperative complications were not observed (Table 3).

Table 3. Early complications (30 days postoperatively) following partial duodenopancreatectomy (Kausch-Whipple procedure) for cancer of the pancreatic head

Complications ($n = 17$) in nine patients	n	%
Anastomotic insufficiencies:		
– Pancreatojejunostomy	0	0
– Choledochojejunostomy with consecutive peritonitis	1	1.4
Bleeding from resection site necessitating relaparotomy	2	2.8
Intra-abdominal abscess	2	2.8
Dislocation of the intraluminal drainage	1	1.4
Wound infection	4	5.5
Cardiopulmonary	4	5.5
After vessel resection ($n = 18$)		
– Bleeding	0	0
– Stenosis	0	0
– Thrombosis	0	0
Hospital mortality (30 days)	1	1.4

Survival

The median survival of all 74 patients with carcinomas of the pancreatic head (stages I–IV) was 19.6 months, ranging from 1 to 84 months. The actuarial survival at 5 years for the entire patient population was 20%.

When the survival rates were evaluated according to the TNM classification, we observed that the 26 patients with stage I (T1N0/T2N0) had a median survival of 21.1 months and an actuarial survival of 29% at 5 years (Fig. 3). Patients with TNM-stage II (T3N0) showed a median survival of 18 months and an actuarial survival at 5 years of 25%; however, since only five patients

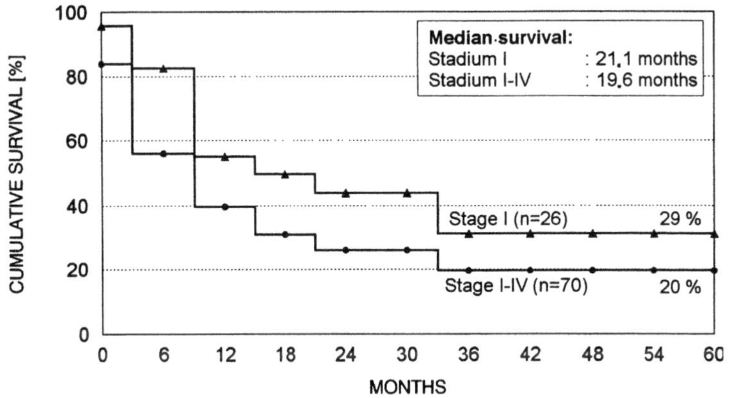

Fig. 3. Cumulative survival of patients with neoplasms of the pancreatic head undergoing partial duodenopancreatectomies (Kausch-Whipple procedures) according to histological grading

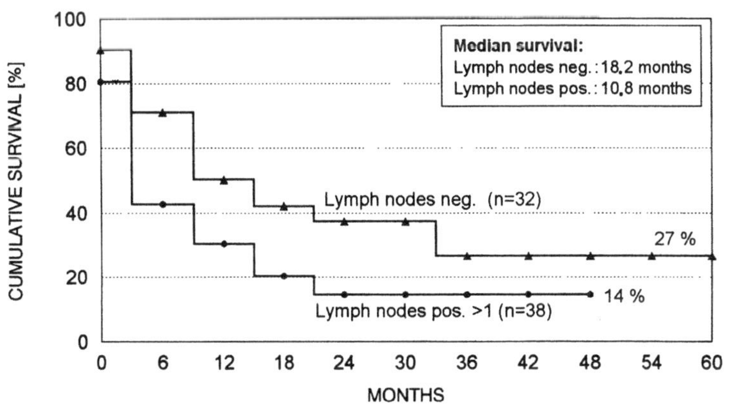

Fig. 4. Cumulative survival of patients with neoplasms of the pancreatic head undergoing partial duodenopancreatectomies (Kausch-Whipple procedures) according to lymph node status

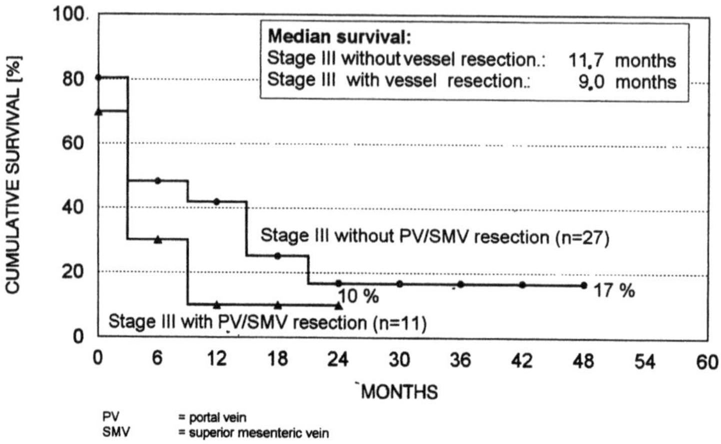

Fig. 5. Cumulative survival of patients with histological stage-III neoplasms of the pancreatic head undergoing partial duodenopancreatectomies (Kausch-Whipple procedures) with an without vessel resection

fell into this group, statistical analysis is limited. When the patient group with positive lymph nodes was assessed (stage III), we found a median survival of 10.8 months and an actuarial survival at 5 years of 14%. Comparing the stage III patients with those without positive lymph nodes (stages I + II), we detected a median survival of 18.2 months and an actuarial survival at 5 years of 27% in the latter group ($p < 0.05$) (Fig. 4). Patients with stage III ($T_{all}N1$) without vessel resection ($n = 27$) had a median survival of 11.7 months and an actuarial survival at 4 years of 17%. The 11 patients with stage III and additional resected vessels showed a median survival of 9 months and an actuarial survival at 3 years of 0% (Fig. 5).

Discussion

Indication and Surgical Technique

For neoplasms of the pancreatic head, careful and thorough preoperative diagnosis is crucial to determine the right therapeutic approach for the patient. All available diagnostic measures, such as sonography, CT scan, angiography, endoscopic retrograde cholangiopancreaticography (ERCP), and, in some cases, even laparoscopy, may be employed to gain as much information as possible. If infiltration of the mesenteric root or the celiac trunk has already taken place, the tumor is considered not resectable. In these cases only selected indications, e.g., severe jaundice when ERCP has failed, may be treated surgically. In contrast, infiltration of the portal or the superior mesenteric vein does not represent a contraindication for resection, since recent communications, including our own herein reported experience, underline the feasability of surgical measures for this condition without an increased complication rate (Trede 1994). Furthermore, with currently advanced anesthesia and perioperative intensive care, age also does not constitute a contraindication (Büchler et al. 1993). However, in patients above 70 years of age cardiovascular and pulmonary risk factors have to be considered during preparation for surgery. The partial duodenopancreatectomy, or Kausch-Whipple procedure, is the standard surgical concept for malignancies of the head and the corpus of the pancreas. Performed by an experienced surgeon, this procedure ensures a safe resection of the tumor-bearing part of the gland and good postoperative endocrine function of the organ in the majority of cases. Total pancreatectomy is considered obsolete by many, since the postoperative quality of life for these patients is poor (Van Heerden et al. 1981). Developed based on the oncologic concept of resecting as radically as possible with wide, tumor-free margins, this procedure produces a complete exocrine and endocrine pancreatic deficiency and, for unknown reasons, is often followed by an intractable diabetes mellitus (Brooks et al. 1989). The second reason for performing total pancreatectomy is that a pancreatojejunostomy is not necessary and therefore the feared complications of such an anastomosis can be avoided. However, recent reports have underlined the fact that with modern suture materials, insuffiencies of the pancreatojejunostomy occur only rarely. Therefore, we do not perform primary pancreatectomies.

A modification of the Kausch-Whipple procedure is the pylorus-preserving duodenopancreatectomy described by Traverso and Longmire (1976). This technique is supposed to yield a better postoperative digestive capacity; however, long-term studies comparing this procedure with the Kausch-Whipple operation are controversial and scarce, and further prospective studies are needed to assess the long-term outcome. We employed the Traverso-Longmire modification only in one case of a young woman with a semimalignant, solid cystic head tumor and therefore cannot estimate its benefits or pitfalls. If, because of the anatomical situation, in rare instances a carcinoma of the pancreatic tail is resectable, the left-sided approach is selected and the Mallet-Guy procedure or the subtotal resection described by Child is performed (Child 1964; Traverso and Longmire 1976).

While a clear concept, as described above, exists for the operative procedure, the question of whether and how a lymphadenectomy should be performed is a matter of controversy (Böttger et al. 1989; Cubilla et al. 1978; Gall and Zirngibl 1986; Roder and Siewert 1992). Different from the periampullary carcinoma, where lymph nodes staging has been proven to be a significant prognostic factor (Roder et al. 1992; Roldan et al. 1988), some authors have denied this fact for the pancreas tumor (Edis et al. 1980). In contrast, several other investigators have supplied statistical evidence for the fact that, as in other carcinomas, the lymph node status has prognostic value (Cameron et al. 1991; Geer and Brennan 1993; Reber 1990). We believe that a prospective multicenter trial should be performed to clarify this important issue.

Perioperative Complications and Survival

Until recently, many surgeons still adhered to the old principle in pancreatic surgery of "noli me tangere". This was especially true for neoplasms of the pancreatic gland, since not only the difficult surgery with its possible grave complications were feared, but also the inacceptably low 5-year survival of below 1% led many surgeons to recommend nonsurgical treatment modalities (Gudjonsson 1987).

Improvements in surgical technique, perioperative intensive care, and suture material, as well as the increasing experience of surgeons with the pancreas, have brought about a reduction of the earlier reported perioperative mortality from 20–25% (Fish and Cleveland 1964; Gall and Zirngibl 1984; Hermann 1979; Shapiro 1975) to less than 5% (Braasch et al. 1986; Büchler et al. 1993; Cameron et al. 1991; Grace et al. 1986; Keck et al. 1991, 1992; Siedeck 1988; Van Heerden 1984). This development is confirmed by our 8-year experience with resections for malignant disease of the pancreatic head, yielding a perioperative mortality of 1.4%. Furthermore, it is also reflected by the increase of procedures performed per year over the study period. Since other centers have also reported much improved results in regard to perioperative mortality, today pancreatic resection for malignant disease can be considered a safe procedure, despite the extensive surgery necessary (Büchler et al. 1993; Cameron et al. 1991; Trede 1985). Concomitant with the reduction of perioperative mortality, the overall results, reflected by the 5-year survival rates, have improved considerably. While in the 1960s and 1970s most patients did not survive longer than 2 years, and 5-year survival was the exception, today 5-year survival rates of approximately 20% are reported from many centers (Hiraoka et al. 1990; Ishikawa et al. 1988). This improvement is even more pronounced when patients are stratified according to their TNM stage. For example, recent studies have shown that in patients with "early cancer" (stage I, tumor smaller than 2 cm and free lymph nodes) surgical therapy can reach 5-year survival rates of almost 60% (Cameron et al. 1991; Trede et al. 1990; Tsuchiya et al. 1986). As for other carcinomas, the importance of early detection of pancreatic cancer becomes obvious when one compares such impressive results with 5-year survival rates from 15 to 25% in patients with stages II or III. In addition, a similar relationship is detected when the 5-year survival rates of patients with or without positive lymph nodes are compared. Furthermore, today the resection of tumor-infiltrated venous vessels (portal vein, superior mesenteric vein) may be part of the standard duodenopancreatectomy, as at our institution. This technical advance (no bleeding or other complication after vessel resection, as described above) gives the surgeon the possibility to ensure a considerable quality of life, even for patients who would have been considered unresectable in the recent past.

Comparing the survival rates with surgical therapy with the results of standard oncologic conservative treatment modalities, it becomes evident that resection of the tumor is still the only treatment which holds not only the chance of cure, but also the chance for long-term survival. In conclusion, considering the low rate of perioperative morbidity and mortality, the moderate length of hospital stay, and the good results even in elderly patients, surgical therapy for carcinomas of the pancreatic head should be considered today for every patient suffering from this entity.

References

Arbuck SG (1990) Overview of chemotherapy for pancreatic cancer. Int J Pancreatol 7:209–222

Beger HG, Bittner R (eds) (1986) Das Pankreaskarzinom. Springer, Berlin Heidelberg New York

Böttger T, Zeck J, Weber W (1989) Prognostisch relevante Faktoren beim duktalen Pankreaskarzinom. Chirurg 60:512–528

Braasch JW, Rossi RL, Watkins E, Deziel DJ, Winter PF (1986) Pyloric and gastric preserving pancreatic resection. Experience with 87 patients. Ann Surg 204:411–418

Brooks JR, Brooks DC, Levine JD (1989) Total pancreatectomy for ductal cell carcinoma of the pancreas. An update. Ann Surg 209:405–410

Büchler M, Ebert M, Beger HG (1993) Grenzen chirurgischen Handelns beim Pankreaskarizinom. Langenbecks Arch Chir [Suppl II] (Kongreßber.):460–464

Cameron Jl, Crist DW, Sitzmann JV, Hruban RH, Boitnott JK, Seidler AJ, Coleman J (1991) Factors influencing survival after pancreaticoduodenectomy for pancreatic cancer. Am J Surg 161:120–124

Child CG (1964) Subtotal pancreatectomies. In: Cooper P (ed) The craft of surgery. Little Brown, Boston, pp 1149–1167

Connolly MM, Dawson PJ, Michelassi F, Moosa AR, Lowenstein F (1987) Survival in 1001 patients with carcinoma of the pancreas. Ann Surg 206:366–373

Cubilla AL, Fortner J, Fitzgerald PJ (1978) Lymph node involvement in carcinoma of the head of the pancreas area. Cancer 41:880

Cullinan SA, Moertel CG, Wieand H (1989) A phase-III evaluation of drug combinations in the therapy of advaced pancreatic cancer. Proc Am Soc Clin Oncol 8:124

Edis AJ, Kierman PD, Taycok WF (1980) Attemted curative resection of the ductal carcinoma of the pancreas. Mayo Clin Proc 55:531–536

Farrow DC, Davis S (1990) Risk of pancreatic cancer in relation to medical history and the use of tobacco, alcohol and coffee. Int J Cancer 45:816–820

Fish JC, Cleveland BR (1964) Pancreaticoduodenectomy for periampullary carcinoma. Ann Surg 159:469

Fisher WE, McCullough PJ, Ramo OJ, Bell RH (1990) Further studies of enhanced growth of pancreatic carcinoma in diabetes. J Surg Res 48:403–407

Gall FP, Zirngibl H (1984) Chirurgische Therapie der Pankreastumoren. In: Gebhardt C (ed) Chirurgie des exokrinen Pankreas. Thieme, Stuttgart, pp 235–268

Gall FP, Zirngibl H (1986) Maligne Tumoren des Pankreas und der periampullären Region, In: Gall FP, Hermanek P, Tonak J (eds) Chirurgische Onkologie: Histologie und stadiengerechte Therapie maligner Tumoren. Springer, Berlin Heidelberg New York

Geer RJ, Brennan MF (1993) Prognostic indicators for survival after resection of pancreatic adenocarcinoma. Am J Surg 165:68–72

Glaser K, Bodner E, Klinler A (1993) Adjuvant intraoperative radiation therapy during duodenopancreatectomy. In: Beger HG, Büchler M, Malfertheimer M (eds) Standards in pancreatic surgery. Springer, Berlin Heidelberg New York, p 676

Grace PA, Pitt HA, Tompkins RK, Den Besten L, Longmire WP (1986) Decreased morbidity and mortality after pancreatoduodenectomy. Am J Surg 151:141–149
Gudjonsson B (1987) Cancer of the pancreas. 50 years of surgery. Cancer 60:2284–2303
Gunderson LL, Martin JK, Kvols LK, Nagorney DM, Fiek JM, Wieand HS, Martinez A, O'Conell MJ, Earlie JD, McIlrath DC (1987) Intraoperative and external beam irradiation ± 5-fluorouracil for locally advanced pancreatic cancer. Int J Radiat Oncol Biol Phys 13:319–329
Hermann RE (1979) Carcinoma of the pancreas and periampullary region. In: Egdahl RH (ed) Manual of surgery of the gallbladder, bile ducts and exocrine pancreas. (Manuals of surgical specialties). Springer, Berlin Heidelberg New York
Hiraoka T, Uchino R, Kanemitsu K, Toyanaga M, Saitok N, Nahamura I, Tashiro I, Miyauchi Y (1990) Combination of intraoperative radiation with resection of cancer of the pancreas. Int J Pancreatol 7:201–207
Hirayama T (1989) Epidemiology of pancreatic cancer in Japan. Jpn J Oncol 19:208–215
Hurdis C, Kelsen D, Dougherty J et al (1990) A randomized trial of streptozotocin (S), mitomycin (M) and 5-fluorouracil (FU) (SMF) vs cisplatin (P), Ara-C (A) and caffeine (C) (CAC) in advanced pancreas cancer (PC). Proc Am Soc Clin Oncol 9:107
Ishikawa O, Ohhigashi H, Sasaki Y, Kabuto T, Fukuda I, Furukawa H, Imaoka S, Iwanaga T (1988) Practical usefulness of lymphatic and connective tissue clearance for the carcinoma of the pancreas head. Ann Surg 208:215–220
Keck H, Steffen R, Waluja W, Neuhaus P (1991) Anastomosenprotektion durch ein spezielles Drainageverfahren bei der Kausch-Whipple-Operation. Chirurg 62:561–565
Keck H, Steffen R, Neuhaus P (1992) Protection of pancreatic and biliary anastomosis after duodenopancreatectomy by external drainage. Surg Gynecol Obstet 174:329–331
Klinkenbijl JHG, Schelling GP, Hop WCJ, Pel R et al (1992) The advantages of pylorus-preserving pancreatoduodenectomy in malignant disease of the pancreas and the periampullary region. Ann Surg 216:142–145
Lowenfels AB, Maisonneuve P, Cavallini G et al (1993) Pancreatitis and the risk of pancreatic cancer. N Engl J Med 328:1433–1437
Moertel CG, Frytak S, Hahn RG et al (1981) Therapy of unresectable pancreatic carcinoma: a randomized comparison of high dose (6000 rads) radiation alone, moderate dose radiation (4000 rads + 5-fluorouracil), and high dose radiation + 5-fluorouracil: the gastrointestinal study group. Cancer 48:1705–1711
Nagai H, Kuroda A, Morioka Y (1986) Lymphatic and local spread of T1 and T2 pancreatic cancer. A study of autopsy material. Ann Surg 204:65–71
National Cancer Institute: Annual cancer statistics review 1973–1988. NIH publication no. 91-2789. Department of Health and Human Services, Bethesda
Offerhaus GJA, Tersmette AC, Tersmette KWF, Tytgat GNJ (1988) Gastric, pancreatic and colorectal carcinogenesis following remote peptic ulcer surgery. Mod Pathol 1:352–356
Reber HA (1990) Lymph node involvement as a prognostic factor in pancreatic cancer. Int J Pancreatol 7:125–127
Roder JD, Siewert JR (1992) Analyse prognoseassoziierter Faktoren beim Pankreaskopf- und periampullären Carcinom. Chirurg 63:410–415
Roder JD, Seebauer L, Ungeheuer A, Lange J, Siewert JR (1992) Beeinflußt der Lymphknotenstatus die Prognose beim kurativ resezierten duktalen Pankreaskopf- bzw. Papillenkarzinom? In: Trede M, Saeger HD (eds) Aktuelle Pankreaschirurgie. Springer, Berlin Heidelberg New York, p 81

Roder JD, Stein HJ, Hüttl W, Siewert JR (1992) Pylorus-preserving versus standard pancreatico-duodenectomy: an analysis of 110 pancreatic and perimapullary carcinomas. Br J Surg 79:152–155

Roldan GE, Gunderson LL, Nagorney DM, Martin JK, Ilstrup DM, Holbrook MA, Kvols LK, McIlrath DC (1988) External beam versus intraoperative and external beam irradiation for locally advanced pancreatic cancer. Cancer 61:1110–1116

Shapiro TM (1975) Adenocarcinoma of the pancreas: a statistical analysis of biliary bypass vs. Whipple resection in good-risk patients. Ann Surg 182:715

Siedeck M (1988) 3-Jahres-Überlebenszeit nach Resektion wegen Pankreaskopf-Ca bei erhöhter Resektionsrate. Langenbecks Arch Chir [Suppl II] (Kongreßber.): 574

Traverso LW, Longmire WP (1976) Preservation of the pylorus during pancreticoduodenectomy. A following evaluation. Surg Gynecol Obstet 6:959–962

Trede M (1985) The surgical treatment of pancreatic carcinoma. Surgery 97:28–35

Trede M (1987) Treatment of pancreatic carcinoma: the surgeon's dilemma. Br J Surg 74:79–80

Trede M, Schwall G, Saeger HD (1990) Survival after pancreatoduodenectomy. Ann Surg 211:447–458

Trede M (1994) Technik der Duodenopankreatektomie nach Whipple. Chirurg 65:232–240

Tsuchiya R, Noda T, Harada N, Miyamoto T, Tomioka T, Yamamoto K, Yamaguchi T, Izawa K, Tsundoa T, Yoshino R, Eto T (1986) Collective review of small carcinomas of the pancreas. Ann Surg 203:77–81

Tuckson WB, Goldson AL, Ashayeri E, Hayard-Richardson M, DeWitty RL, Leffall LD Jr (1988) Intraoperative radiotherapy for patients with carcinoma of the pancreas. Ann Surg 207:648–654

Van Heerden JA, ReMine WH, Weiland LH, McIlrath DC, Ilstrup DM (1981) Total pancreatectomy for ductal adenocarcinoma of the pancrease. Am J Surg 142:302–308

Van Heerden JA (1984) Pancreatic resection for carcinoma of the pancreas. Whipple versus total pancreatectomy – an institutional perspective. World J Surg 8:880–888

Warshaw AL, Fernandez-Del Castillo C (1992) Pancreatic carcinoma. N Engl J Med 326:455–465

Wils JA (1989) Current status of chemotherapy in metastatic pancreatic cancer. Anticancer Res 9:1027–1031

Chemotherapy for Patients with Adenocarcinoma of the Pancreas

H. Riess, P. Htun, J. Löffel, and D. Huhn

Medizinische Klinik und Poliklinik, Virchow-Klinikum der Humboldt-Universität, Augustenburger Platz 1, 13353 Berlin, Germany

Abstract

Adenocarcinomas of the pancreas are diagnosed at an advanced, noncurable stage in most patients. In addition to local relapse or progression, distant metastases determine the poor prognosis, resulting in a median survival of less than 6 months in most studies of patients with locally advanced or metastatic pancreatic cancer. None of the cytotoxic drugs available show impressive activity in treatment of this disease. Therefore, chemotherapy is not recommended in pancreatic cancer. In selected cases, 5-fluorouracil-based therapy – with or without simultaneous radiation – may result in tumor responses.

With a once-a-week outpatient protocol of folinic acid and 5-fluorouracil, we observed a progression-free period from 15 to 42 weeks in nine of 19 patients treated without any serious adverse effects, confirming reports of the weak, but well-tolerated activity of this combination.

To alter the prognosis for patients with advanced adenocarcinomas of the pancreas, new drugs with more activity have to be developed and tested in well-designed trials.

Introduction

Adenocarcinomas of the pancreas are generally diagnosed at an advanced stage, when curability by surgery cannot be expected (Brennan et al. 1993; Harvey and Schein 1984). This is due mostly to the fact that the majority of patients are 65 years or older, and that symptoms of early pancreatic cancer are usually missing or nonspecific, such as weight loss, upper abdominal discomfort, or jaundice. Often the diagnosis is made after a period of rapid clinical deterioration. Thus, at the time of diagnosis more than half of the patients have metastases, and less than 25% can be resected. Even after a

Recent Results in Cancer Research, Vol. 142

potentially curative (R0) resection, most of the patients relapse locally or with distant metastases. Taken together, the prognosis of pancreatic cancer is discouraging, with less than 5% of patients surviving for more than 5 years. For the majority, those with unresectable disease, prognosis is even worse, with a median survival of less than 4 months.

Because the typical patient with pancreatic cancer has a poor performance status as well as evidence of malabsorption, bowel dysmotility, hepatic dysfunction, and effusions, he probably will not tolerate intensive chemotherapy. Indeed, studies of chemotherapy in these patients are often limited by the small size of – sometimes highly selected – patients groups and by the rarity of measurable disease necessary to document tumor response accurately (Brennan et al. 1993; Meyer et al. 1987). On the other hand, considering that adenocarcinomas of the pancreas – unlike endocrine pancreatic tumors (Eriksson and Oberg 1993) – is one of the large cancer killers in adults, more vigorous eeforts should be undertaken to define subgroups that might benefit from systemic therapy, especially in terms of quantity and quality of life.

Single-agent Chemotherapy

There have been many attempts to identify drugs that may be active in patients with advanced and metastatic pancreatic cancer. None resulted in an appreciable number of complete responses, long-term partial responders, long-term survivors or an acceptable survival benefit for the whole treated group. Several agents were studied in more than 30 patients. With regard to response rates above 20% obtained in phase-II studies (Table 1), there are only a few drugs that can be considered active in this disease to date (Brennan et al. 1993). Most of them have not been evaluated sufficiently in prospective and randomized trials.

As with other gastointestinal adenocarcinomas, 5-fluorouracil (5-FU) is the best-studied drug, with response rates reported from 0 to 50% and median

Table 1. Single-agent chemotherapy in pancreatic cancer

Drug	Response rate (%) in phase-II studies	Response rate (%) in phase-III studies
5-Fluorouracil	0–28	7–21
Mitomycin C	21–33	n.a.
Ifosfamide	3–60	n.a
Streptozotocin	11–36	n.a.
4-Epirubicin	0–24	n.a.
5-Fluorouracil + folinic acid	0–50	n.a.
5-Fluorouracil + PALA	5–18	n.a.
5-Fluorouracil + PALA + folinic acid	7–80	n.a.
5-Fluorouracil + interferon alpha	13–12	n.a.

n.a., Not available

survival ranging from 12 to 25 weeks. In contrast to colorectal cancer, the influence of methods of 5-FU administration, e.g., weekly versus 5-day schedules and bolus versus prolonged infusion, has not been extensively studied, and a survival benefit for 5-FU has not been shown yet in cancer of the pancreas (Table 2).

Biochemical modulation of 5-FU, thought to result in clinical benefit for patients with colorectal cancer, by folinic acid, PALA, or interferons has not been shown convincingly to improve results in cancer of the pancreas (Table 1) (Bernhard 1993; Bruckner et al. 1988; Buroker et al. 1994; Crown et al. 1991; De Caprio et al. 1989; Morrell et al. 1991; Wadler et al. 1991). New drugs such as gemcitabine, paclitaxel and taxotere seem to have some activity against pancreatic cancer and merit further evaluation.

Multiagent Chemotherapy

Based to the results reported with single-agent therapy, 5-FU became an important component in trials of two-, three-, or complex multiagent chemotherapy. In phase-II studies of combination chemotherapy response rates up to 50% and median survivals in the range of 12–27 weeks have been reported (Andersen et al. 1981; Brennan et al. 1993; Bukowski et al. 1983; Dougherty et al. 1989; Gastrointestinal Tumor Study Group 1986; Loehrer et al. 1987; Mallinson et al. 1980; Scheitauer et al. 1990; Sporn et al. 1993), results not clearly superior to those for single-agent 5-FU.

Table 2. Some phase-III trials of chemotherapy in pancreatic cancer

Group A	Group B	Group C	*n*	Survival (months) A/B/C
5-Fluorouracil + BCNU	Observation		40	3.0/3.3/–
5-Fluorouracil + CCNU	Observation		152	3.0/3.9/–
5-Fluorouracil + cyclophosphamide + vincristine + methotrexate	Observation		40	10.3/2.1/–
5-Fluorouracil	BCNU	5-Fluorouracil + BCNU	82	6.0/6.0/6.0
5-Fluorouracil	5-Fluorouracil + adriamycin	5-Fluorouracil + adriamycin + mitomycin C	144	4.7/4.7/4.7
5-Fluorouracil	5-Fluorouracil adriamycin + cisplatin	5-Fluorouracil + cyclophosphamide + vincristine + methotrexate	184	/3.5/3.5/4.5
5-Fluorouracil + adriamycin + mitomycin C	5-Fluorouracil + adriamycin + streptozotocin		184	6.1/4.2/–

Phase-III studies (Table 2) demonstrated no survival benefit for – frequently more toxic – 5-FU-based combination therapy as compared with single-agent 5-FU or for one combination versus another.

Hormonal Therapy

There are several lines of evidence suggesting that pancreatic cancer may be influenced by hormones, especially estrogen (Greenway et al. 1981; Korc 1990; Szende et al. 1990). However, the improved survival as compared with historical controls observed in early clinical trials with tamoxifen was not confirmed in prospective, randomized studies (Tonnesen and Kamp-Jensen 1986; Wong et al. 1987).

Biological Response Modifiers

In phase-II studies interferon alpha or interferon gamma showed no objective responses in pancreas cancer. Furthermore, and in contrast to the initial favorable responses by patients with colon cancer (Wadler et al. 1991), the combination of 5-FU with interferon in pancreatic cancer patients showed response rates below 15% (Table 1) (Bernhard 1993; Sporn et al. 1993; Wadler et al. 1991). On the other hand other cytokines (Young 1993) may demonstrate some activity in pancreatic cancer.

Radiochemotherapy

Because 5-FU is active in cancer of the pancreas as well as believed to be an important radiation sensitizer, several studies evaluated the role of this drug in proeperative (neoadjuvant) (Moertel et al. 1994), postoperative (adjuvant) (Gastrointestinal Tumor Study Group 1987), and palliative (Gastrointestinal Tumor Study Group 1979, 1985, 1988; Klassen et al. 1985; Moertel et al. 1981; Whittington et al. 1984) radiotherapy (Table 3). These randomized trials suggest an increased activity of the combined approach as compared with radiotherapy, chemotherapy, or supportive therapy.

Single-Institution Experience with Folinic Acid and 5-FU for Outpatients

Between April 1992 and May 1994, 19 outpatients with progressive metastatic pancreatic carcinoma (Table 4) where treated by chemotherapy in our institution. In this 26-month period 36 patients with metastatic cancer of the pancreas without previous chemotherapy were seen. After an individual evaluation, chemotherapy was offered only to patients (n = 24) with signs of tumor

Table 3. Radiochemotherapy in pancreatic cancer (important studies)

Setting	*n*	Radiation median survival (months)	Radiation +5-FU median survival (months)	5-Fluorouracil median survival (months)	*p*
Not resectable, no distant metastases	64	6.3	10.4	n.d.	s
Not resectable, no distant metastases	55	5.3	9.4	n.d.	s
Not resectable, no distant metastases	91	n.d.	8.3	8.2	ns
Not resectable, no distant metastases	43	n.d.	9.7	7.4 (+ mitomycin + streptotozocin)	ns
Adjuvant	43	11	21	n.d.	s
Neoadjuvant	31	n.d.	>29 (+ mitomycin C)	n.d.	

n.d., Not done; *s*, significant; *ns* not significant

Table 4. Patients characteristics [median (and range)]

Sex	12 female, 7 male
Age (years)	58 (42–69)
Primary tumor resected	8
Time between resection and relapse (weeks)	13 (4–28)
Inclusion criteria	
Increase in tumor marker	8
New metastases	14
Progressive metastases	2
WHO performance status 0	4
WHO performance status 1	12
WHO performance status 2	3

progression within the past 8 weeks. Tumor progression was defined as more than a 20% increase in serum concentrations of tumor marker (CEA, CA 19-9), new metastases, or more than a 20% increase in previously diagnosed measurable disease (e.g., CT scans, X-ray of the thorax, ultrasound).

Chemotherapy consisted of 50 mg folinic acid weekly, followed by 600 mg 5-FU/m^2. Patients were monitored weekly including body weight and performance status assessment, and every 4–6 weeks with ultrasound or radiological tests as needed. CT scans were repeated routinely every 6–10 weeks and when indicated by findings on ultrasound or by physical examination. After start of the treatment, the 5-FU dose was adjusted according to toxicity. Dose was reduced by 10% or 20% when WHO toxicity grade II or grade III, respectively, was reported; 5-FU dose was escalated (+10%) every 4–6 weeks when no gastrointestinal, hematological, or dermal toxicity (grade II) occurred.

Four patients refused therapy because of long distances between their home and hospital; one patient considered alternative therapeutic options. Responses were assessed according to WHO criteria. In addition, decreases and stabilization (increase <10%) of tumor markers were considered "free of progression" when not contradicted by ultrasound or radiological tests.

Results

Gastrointestinal toxicity resulted in dose reductions for 2/19 patients. Doses of 5-FU were increased to 660 mg/m² in 4/19 and to 730 mg/m² in 2/19. No grade-III toxicity occurred.

Early progress within the first 6 weeks was stated in 5/19 patients. No complete remission, but three partial remissions in 11 patients with measurable disease were documented. In addition, according to the course of tumor markers and modern imaging techniques, tumor progression was delayed for 15–42 weeks in 9/19 patients; 2/14 patients (1 PR, 1 SD) survived longer than a year (13 and 15 months). Median survival duration (Kaplan-Meier) for the whole group is 27 weeks.

During therapy, body weight temporarily increased (>3 kg) in 5/12 progression-free patients and was stable (decrease <2 kg) in another eight, including two patients with tumor progression. Performance status stabilized in 11 patients for 18–51 weeks.

Discussion

These results are in agreement with the experience in colorectal cancer, showing that weekly folinic acid and 5-FU is a well-tolerated regimen with acceptable toxicities for outpatients. Furthermore, these data confirm an active principle of 5-FU-based chemotherapy in pancreatic cancer. In spite of the small number of patients and a missing control group, these data support a palliative role of well-tolerated chemotherapy in the management of pancreas cancer. The observed response rate and the observed survival are in the range of results reported from other phase-II and phase-III studies.

Not very different from the situation in advanced colorectal cancer, a clear-cut recommendation of chemotherapy in pancreatic cancer has to be founded on well-designed and well-performed prospective studies in hundreds of patients. Unless these data are available, and unless the significance of disease stabilization ("free of progression") for an individual patient with far advanced cancer of the pancreas has been shown, the decision for the physician facing a patient with advanced pancreatic cancer to offer or to withold chemotherapy in addition to supportive strategies is difficult. Considering the usual rapid deterioration, with a median survival of a few weeks in untreated patients with metastatic pancreas cancer, prolongation for some weeks and/or stabilization of the performance status – suggestive of stabilization of quality of life – in some patients may be worthwhile, at least when therapy can easily be offered on an outpatient basis and harmful side effects are unlikely.

Conclusion

The situation of chemotherapy in cancer of the pancreas basically resembles that in colon cancer some years ago. There are many data suggestive of a positive effect of 5-FU given alone or in combinations, but convincing studies demonstrating or ruling out a substantial benefit are missing. Thus, a general recommendation to treat patients with pancreatic cancer with chemotherapy cannot be given. Only in unresectable, locally advanced disease does radiochemotherapy seem to have proven effective, not only in terms of pain reduction but also in prolonging the patients' survival.

On the other hand, patients with cancer of the pancreas may profit in several additional settings from the kind of chemotherapy available. Among others, the following situations may prove to benefit from chemotherapy in the future:

- Adjuvant after an R0 resection, where more than 80% will relapse
- After a non-R0 resection (with radiation)
- Neoadjuvant to achieve potential curative (R0) resection (with radiation)
- In the palliation of metastatic disease

To test or reject these hypotheses, great numbers of patients with pancreatic cancer have to be entered in well-designed multicenter trials. As prognosis in pancreatic cancer is determined by local and distant relapse, a multimodal strategy combining the efficacy of radiation in local tumor control with systemic therapy may be recommended.

To alter the prognosis more profoundly for patients with cancer of the pancreas, the growing understanding of the molecular basis of cancer biology (Korc 1990; Shibata et al. 1990) must result in new treatment strategies, in addition to new cytotoxic drugs and dose intensification (Brown et al. 1993), including regional therapy (Aigner et al. 1990; Christ et al. 1991), treatment with antibodies (Tempero et al. 1990), new cytokines (Young 1993), and efforts directed against the molecular defect in pancreatic carcinoma cells, to mention some directions of research. Patients with advanced cancer of the pancreas should be offered the option of entering such investigational phase-I/II studies. Until definite benefits from chemotherapy can be expected for patients with cancer of the pancreas, we should bring into focus the possibilities of optimal supportive therapy for an individual patient in order to improve or maintain the quality of his live.

References

Aigner KR, Muller H, Bassermann R (1990) Intra-arterial chemotherapy with MMC, CDDP, and 5-FU for nonresectable pancreatic cancer – a phase II study. Reg Cancer Treat 3:1–6

Andersen JR, Friis-Moller A, Hancke S, Roder O, Steen J, Baden H (1981) A controlled trial of combination chemotherapy with 5-FU and BCNU in pancreatic cancer. Scan J Gastroenterol 16:973–976

Bernhard H (1993) Treatment of advanced pancreatic cancer with 5-fluorouracil, folinic acid and interferon-alpha-2A. Am Soc Clin Oncol 12:210

Brennan MF, Kinsella TJ, Caspar ES (1993) Cancer of the pancreas. In: DeVita VT, Hellman S, Rosenberg SA (eds) Cancer: principles and practice of oncology. Lippincott, Philadelphia, pp 849–882

Brown T, Tangen C, Fleming T, MacDonald J (1993) A phase-II trial of taxol and granulocyte colony-stimulating factor (G-CSF) in patients with adenocarcinoma of the pancreas. Am Soc Clin Oncol 12:200

Bruckner HW, Crown J, McKenna A, Hart R (1988) Leucovorin and 5-fluorouracil as a treatment for disseminated cancer of the pancreas and unknown primary tumors. Cancer Res 48:5570–5572

Bukowski RM, Balcerzak SP, O'Bryan RM, Bonnet JD, Chen TT (1983) Randomized trial of 5-fluorouracil and mitomycin C with or without streptozotocin for advanced pancreatic cancer. A Southwest Oncology Group Study. Cancer 52:1577–1582

Buroker TR, O'Connell MJ, Wieand HS, Krook JE, Gerstner JB, Mailliard JA, Schaefer PL, Levitt R, Kardinal CG, Gesme DH Jr (1994) Randomized comparison of two schedules of fluorouracil and leucovorin in the treatment of advanced colorectal cancer. J Clin Oncol 12:14–20

Christ KA, Arredondo MA, Chaudhuri B, Thomford NR, Chaudhuri PK (1991) Pharmacokinetic and toxicity of isolated perfusion of human pancreas-duodenum with mitomycin-C. Reg Cancer Treat 3:305–307

Crown J, Casper ES, Botet J, Murray P, Kelson DP (1991) Lack of efficacy of high-dose leucovorin and fluorouracil in patients with advanced pancreatic adenocarcinoma. J Clin Oncol 9:1682–1686

De Caprio JA, Arbuck SG, Mayer RJ (1989) Phase-II study of weekly 5-fluorouracil (5-FU) with folinic acid (FA) in previously untreated patients with unresectable measurable pancreatic adenocarcinoma. Proc Am Soc Clin Oncol 8:388

Dougherty JB, Kelsen D, Kemeny N, Magill G, Botet J, Niedzwiecki D (1989) Advanced pancreatic cancer: a phase I–II trial of cisplatin, high-dose cytarabine, and caffeine. J Natl Cancer Inst 81:1735–1738

Eriksson B, Oberg K (1993) An update of the medical treatment of malignant endocrine pancreatic tumors. Acta Oncol 32:203–208

Gastrointestinal Tumor Study Group (1979) A multi-institutional comparative trial of radiation therapy alone and in combination with 5-FU for locally unresectable pancreatic cancer. Ann Surg 189:205–211

Gastrointestinal Tumor Study Group (1987) Further evidence of effective adjuvant combined radiation and chemotherapy following curative resection of pancreatic cancer. Cancer 59:2006–2010

Gastrointestinal Tumor Study Group (1986) Phase-II studies of drug combinations in advanced pancreatic carcinoma: fluorouracil plus doxorubicin plus mitomycin C and two reglimens of streptozotocin plus mitomycin C plus fluorouracil. J Clin Oncol 4:1794

Gastrointestinal Tumor Study Group (1985) Radiation therapy combined with adriamycin or 5-fluorouracil for the treatment of locally unresectable pancreatic carcinoma. Cancer 56:2563–2568

Gastrointestinal Tumor Study Group (1988) Treatment of locally unresectable carcinoma of the pancreas: comparison of combined modality therapy (chemotherapy plus radiotherapy) to chemotherapy alone. J Natl Cancer Inst 80:751–755
Greenway B, Iqbal MJ, Johnson PJ, Williams R (1981) Oestrogen receptor proteins in malignant and fetal pancreas. Br Med J 283:751–753
Harvey JH, Schein PS (1984) The pancreatic cancer problem. World J Surg 8:935–939
Klaasen DJ, MacIntyre JM, Catton GE, Engstrom PF, Moertel CG (1985) Treatment of locally unresectable cancer in the stomach and pancreas: a randomized comparison of 5-fluorouracil alone with radiation plus concurrent and maintenance 5-fluorouracil. An Eastern Cooperative Group study. J Clin Oncol 3:373–378
Korc M (1990) Autocrine regulation in human pancreatic cancer cells. Proc Am Assoc Cancer Res 31:477
Loehrer PJ Sr, Williams SD, Sichols CR (1987) Ifosfamide plus 5-fluorouracil for treatment of adenocarcinoma of the pancreas. Cancer Treat Rep 71:1115–1116
Mallinson CN, Rake MO, Cocking JB, Foc CA, Cwynarski MT, Diffey BL, Jackson GA, Hanley J, Wass VJ (1980) Chemotherapy in pancreatic cancer: results of a controlled prospective randomized multicentre trial. Br Med J 281:1589–1596
McCracken JD, Olson M, Cruz AB Jr, Leichman L, Oishi N (1982) Radiation therapy combined with intra-arterial 5-FU chemotherapy for treatment of localized adenocarcinoma of the pancreas. A Southwest Oncology Group study. Cancer Treat Rep 66:549–551
Meyer J, Sulkowski U, Preusser P, Bünte H (1987) Therapieergebnisse beim Papillen- und Pankreaskarzinom. Tumor Diagn Ther 8:54–58
Moertel CG, Frytak S, Hahn RG et al (1981) Therapy of locally unresectable pancreatic carcinoma: a randomized comparison of high dose (600 rads) radiation alone, moderate dose radiation (4000 rads + 5-fluorouracil) and high dose radiation + 5-fluorouracil. Cancer 48:1705–1710
Moertel CG, Gunderson LL, Mailliard JA, McKenna PJ, Martenson JA Jr, Burch PA, Stephen S (1994) Early evaluation of combined fluorouracil and leucovorin as a radiation enhancer for locally unresectable, residual, or recurrent gastrointestinal carcinoma. J Clin Oncol 12:21–27
Morrell LM, Bach A, Richmann SP, Goodmann P, Fleming TR, MacDonald JS (1991) A phase-II multi-institutional trial of low-dose N-(phosphonacetyl)-L-asparate and high dose 5-fluorouracil as a short-term infusion in the treatment of adenocarcinoma of the pancreas. Cancer 67:363–366
Scheitauer W, Funovics J, Mueller C, Ludwig H (1990) Sequential high-dose methotrexate, 5-fluorouracil and doxorubicin for treatment of advanced pancreatic cancer. J Cancer Res Clin Oncol 116:132–133
Shibata D, Almoguera C, Forrester K, Dunitz J, Martin SE, Cosgrove MM, Perucho M, Arnheim N (1990) Detection of c-K-ras mutations in fine-needle aspirates from human pancreatic adenocarcinoma. Cancer Res 50:1279–1283
Sporn JR, Buzaid A, Slater D, Greenberg BR (1993) Treatment of advanced pancreatic cancer with cisplatin, 5-FU, leucovorin, and interferon-alfa-2B. Am Soc Clin Oncol 12:207
Szende B, Srkalovic G, Schally AV, Lapis K, Groot K (1990) Inhibitory effects of analogs of luteinizing hormone-releasing hormone and somatostatin on pancreatic cancer in hamsters. Cancer 65:2279–2290
Tempero MA, Sivinski C, Steplweski Z, Harvey E, Klassen L, Kay HD (1990) Phase-II trial of interferon gamma and monoclonal antibody 17-1A in pancreatic cancer: Biologic and clinical effects. J Clin Oncol 8:2019–2026
Tonnesen K, Kamp-Jensen M (1986) Antiestrogen therapy in pancreatic carcinoma: a preliminary report. Eur J Surg Oncol 12:69–70
Wadler S, Lembersky B, Atkins M, Kirkwood J, Petrelli N (1991) Phase-II trial of fluorouracil and recombinant interferon alfa-2a in patients with advanced colorectal

carcinoma: an Eastern Cooperative Oncology Group study. J Clin Oncol 9:1806–1810

Whittington R, Solin L, Mohiuddin M, Cantor RI, Rosato FE, Biermann WA, Weiss SM, Pajak TF (1984) Multiomodal therapy of localized unresectable pancreatic adenocarcinoma. Cancer 54:1991–1998

Wong A, Chan A, Arthur K (1987) Tamoxifen therapy in unresectable adenocarcinoma of the pancreas. Cancer Treat Rep 71:7

Young RI (1993) Phase-I study of recombinant interleukin-6 (RHIL-6) in patients with advanced colon or pancreatic cancer. Ann Hematol 67:145

Phase II Data on Paclitaxel and Docetaxel in Gastrointestinal Malignancies

M.S. Aapro

Division of Medical Oncology, European Institute of Oncology, via Ripamonti 435, 20141 Milano, Italy

Abstract

From the contributions in this volume, it is apparent that in spite of promising chemotherapy combinations and new multidisciplinary approaches, the treatment of advanced gastrointestinal malignancies remains a difficult task. New agents have recently been developed with either a better therapeutic ratio (fluoropyrimidine analogs or modulators of the metabolic pathway of those agents) or a better activity due to a different mechanism of action. Among the latter agents, the topoisomerase I inhibitors (especially irinotecan, also known as CPT-11) and new antimetabolities (difluorodeoxycytidine, also known as gemcitabine) are of interest for difficult tumors, such as colon and pancreatic cancer. This short review describes the phase II studies on the activity of taxoids, agents that promote tubulin assembly in microtubules and inhibit their depolymerization.

Preclinical Data

The two representatives of the taxoid family which have been introduced into clinical practice are paclitaxel (Taxol) and docetaxel (Taxotere). They have different preclinical characteristics (Pazdur et al. 1993) which may or may not result in clinical differences. Docetaxel is more myelotoxic in vitro than paclitaxel, although in some models it is considerably more cytotoxic than paclitaxel (Braakhuis et al. 1994), giving it a potential advantage. However, there are also preclinical indications in some instances that paclitaxel may be more active than docetaxel (Hanauske et al. 1992). In the data of Hanauske et al. (1992) it is interesting to note that the lack of clinical activity of taxoids in colon cancer was predicted, since at relevant in vitro concentrations the growth of tumor colonies was rarely inhibited. These data which were obtained with fresh human tumor material contrast with the animal data summa-

Recent Results in Cancer Research, Vol. 142

rized by Lavelle et al. (1995) which demonstrate the activity of docetaxel in human colon xenograft models and also a synergism between 5-fluorouracil and docetaxel in a murine colon cell line.

Esophageal Cancer

While there are no data on the activity of docetaxel in esophageal cancers, Ajani et al. (1994) have conducted a trial with paclitaxel in 52 patients suffering from esophageal cancer (Table 1). Patients with either metastatic or locoregional unresectable tumors, who had not been previously treated, were included in the study. The patients were given premedication to avoid allergic reactions and received paclitaxel at an initial dose of 250 mg/m^2 over 24 h, followed by granulocyte colony-stimulating factor, which was repeated every 21 days. The median age of the patients was 58, with a median performance status of 1. A median of four courses was administered and dosage reductions were carried out in 23% of the 227 courses; dosage increases were carried out in 7% of these courses.

Among the 32 patients with adenocarcinoma there were 11 responses (one complete, ten partial; response rate of 34%). Five partial responses were observed among the 18 patients with evaluable squamous cell carcinoma (reponse rate of 28%). The responses in both groups lasted a median of 17 weeks. These data are very encouraging and highly active combinations of paclitaxel, cisplatin and 5-fluorouracil are currently being investigated (initial results were presented by T. Javed et al. and J.A. Ajani et al. at the American Society for Clinical Oncology meeting in May 1995).

Gastric Cancer

Although the exact location of the adenocarcinomas is somewhat unclear, we may assume that the majority of the patients in the paclitaxel study of Einzig et al. (1993) had a gastric or gastroesophageal adenocarcinoma. The study

Table 1. Treatment of esophageal cancer with paclitaxel (no data for docetaxel)

Dose (mg/m^2)	Patients (n)	CR/PR (%)	Duration of response (median)	Comment	Reference
250	32	3/31	17 weeks	Adenocarcinoma	Ajani et al. 1994
250	18	0/28	17 weeks	Squamous cell carcinoma	Ajani et al. 1994

CR, complete response; PR, partial response

included 25 previously untreated patients, 20 of whom had been evaluated at the time of abstract publication (Table 2). Paclitaxel was administered in a way similar to that in the above-mentioned study by Ajani et al.; however, colony-stimulating factor was not used routinely. One partial response lasting more than 12 weeks was observed in a patient with liver metastases. Docetaxel was used in all but one of the phase II studies cited at a dosage of 100 mg/m^2 over 1 h every 3 weeks. In all except one of the initial phase II studies described in this chapter, no routine antiallergic premedication was used. Sulkes et al. (1994) have reported on 42 patients with previously untreated, advanced, and measurable gastric carcinoma. The median age was 59 years, with a median performance status of 1, and 34% of the patients had liver metastases. Among the 37 eligible patients a 19% response rate was observed (eight partial remissions), and this rate increases to 24% if only the 33 fully evaluable patients are taken into account (Table 2). Taguchi (1994) has reported on 15 patients treated with 60 mg/m^2 every 3–4 weeks (the standard Japanese phase II dosage) and found a similar response rate of 20% (Table 2). Finally, the Eastern Cooperative Oncology Group (Einzig 1995) reported one complete and two partial responses among the 22 evaluable patients (Table 2), out of the 29 who were registered for the study (six patients had not been in the study long enough and one refused further therapy after one cycle). Studies using combinations of docetaxel with other agents active in gastric cancer are underway; however, no results are yet available.

Pancreatic Cancer

A study of the Southwest Oncology Group (SWOG) has been reported by Brown et al. (1993) in preliminary form (Table 3). A total of 44 patients were

Table 2. Treatment of gastric cancer with paclitaxel and docetaxel

Dose (mg/m^2)	Patients (*n*)	CR/PR (%)	Duration of response (median)	Comment	Reference
P 250	20	0/5	12 weeks	Upper gastrointestinal adenocarcinoma	Einzig et al. 1993
D 100	42	0/19	30 weeks	24% RR among evaluable tumors	Sulkes et al. 1994
D 60	15	0/20	?	Low dose	Taguchi 1994
D 100	22	5/9	?	Preliminary report	Einzig et al. 1995

P, paclitaxel; D, docetaxel; CR, complete response; PR, partial response; RR, response rate

Table 3. Treatment of pancreatic cancer with paclitaxel and docetaxel

Dose (mg/m²)	Patients (*n*)	CR/PR (%)	Duration of response (median)	Comment	Reference
P 250	23	0/13	?	Preliminary report	Brown et al. 1993
D 100	30	0/20	17 weeks	Local + liver metastases	Rougier et al. 1995
D 100	12	0/25	?	Local	Rougier et al. 1995
D 100	10	0/20	?	Preliminary report	Abruzzese et al. 1995

P, paclitaxel; D, docetaxel; CR, complete response; PR, partial response

registered according to the abstract, and 23 were evaluated at the time of presentation. All patients were treated with the same regimen as in the study by Ajani et al. with esophageal cancer patients described above. These patients had not previously been treated with chemotherapy. The response rate was 13%.

Docetaxel has been studied in histologically or cytologically proven unresectable pancreatic cancer patients by Rougier et al. (1994). The final data after extramural review have since then been presented at the Second International Conference on Biology, "Prevention and Treatment of Gastrointestinal Malignancies," in Cologne, Germany, in January 1995 (Table 3). Of the 43 patients registered, one could not be evaluated. The authors divided their patients into two groups: 30 patients with metastatic pancreatic carcinoma and 12 patients with locally advanced disease. Among the 30 patients with metastatic disease they observed six partial responses, and there were three clear improvements among the 12 patients with locally advanced disease. All of these responses were accompanied by a decrease in the tumor marker CA 19.9. The median time of tumor progression was 17 weeks. Preliminary results from a North American study (Abruzzese et al. 1995; Table 3) seem to confirm the results obtained by Rougier et al. (1994), since two responses have been observed among ten patients treated for pancreatic cancer in that study. From these data it appears that further evaluation of docetaxel in pancreatic cancer is warranted.

Colorectal Cancer

Despite attempts to vary the mode of drug administration, and the careful selection of patients, neither paclitaxel nor docetaxel have any therapeutic benefits in colorectal cancer patients (Table 4). A study including 19 patients has been reported as showing no responses, with a paclitaxel regimen of

Table 4. Treatment of colorectal cancer with paclitaxel and docetaxel

Dose (mg/m^2)	Patients (n)	CR/PR (%)	Duration of response (median)	Comment	Reference
P 250	19	0/0	NA		Rowinsky et al. 1992
P 120	10	0/0	NA	96-h infusion	Vaughn et al. 1995
D 100	40	3/6	NA		Sternberg et al. 1994
D 100	18	0/0	NA		Clark et al. 1994
D 100	19	0/0	NA		Pazdur et al. 1994

P, paclitaxel; D, docetaxel; CR, complete response; PR, partial response; NA, not applicable or not available

250 mg/m^2 over 24 h every 3 weeks (Rowinsky et al. 1992). Vaughn et al. (1995) have described the initial results of a phase II trial of 96-h infusional paclitaxel at 120 mg/m^2 in ten patients; no response was observed.

A total of 77 patients with advanced colorectal cancer, all previously untreated, have received docetaxel, with premedication in only one study (Clark et al. 1994); the response rate was found to be minimal (Pazdur et al. 1994; Sternberg et al. 1994; Clark et al. 1994).

Conclusion

Esophageal cancer, and possibly gastric and pancreatric cancer, are responsive to taxoids. In some instances there are no data with one of the agents, and in others the different response rates may be simply due to patient selection. In all of these diseases further studies with taxoids are currently being done, and we shall soon have further single-agent and combination phase II data. Colorectal carcinoma is not sensitive to taxoids as they are currently being used; preclinical data did however suggest some activity in animal models. Phase III studies are necessary to assess the role of taxoids in gastrointestinal malignancies.

References

Abruzzese JL, Evans D, Gravel D et al (1995) Docetaxel, a potentially active agent for patients with pancreatic adenocarcinoma. Proc Am Soc Clin Oncol 14:221

Ajani JA, Ilson DH, Daugherty K et al (1994) Activity of taxol in patients with squamous cell carcinoma and adenocarcinoma of the esophagus. J Natl Cancer Inst 86:1086–1091

Braakhuis BJM, Hill BT, Dietel M et al (1994) In vitro antiproliferative activity of docetaxel, paclitaxel and cisplatin against human tumors and normal bone marrow cells. Anticancer Res 14:205–208

Brown T, Tangen C, Fleming T et al (1993) A phase II trial of Taxol and granulocyte colony stimulating factor in patients with adenocarcinoma of the pancreas. Proc Am Soc Clin Oncol 13:200

Clark T, Kemeny N, Conti JA et al (1994) Phase II trial of docetaxel in previously untreated patients with advanced colorectal cancer. Proc Am Soc Clin Oncol 13:212

Einzig AI, Wiernik PH, Lipsitz S et al (1993) Phase II trial of taxol in patients with adenocarcinoma of the upper gastrointestinal tract: the Eastern Cooperative Group results. Proc Am Soc Clin Oncol 12:194

Einzig AI, Lipshitz S, Wiernik PH et al (1995) Phase II trial of taxotere in patients with adenocarcinoma of the upper gastrointestinal tract previously untreated with chemotherapy. The ECOG results. Proc Am Soc Clin Oncol 14:191

Hanauske A, Degen D, Hilsenbeck SG et al (1992) Effects of taxotere and taxol on in vitro colony formation of freshly explanted tumor cells. Anticancer Drugs 3:121–124

Lavelle F, Bissery MC, Combeau C et al (1995) Preclinical evaluation of docetaxel (taxotere). Semin Oncol 22:2 [Suppl 4]:3–16

Pazdur R, Kudelka AP, Kavanagh JJ et al (1993) The taxoids: Paclitaxel and docetaxel. Cancer Treat Rev 19:351–356

Pazdur R, Lasserre Y, Soh LT et al (1994) Phase II trial of docetaxel in metastatic colorectal carcinoma. Ann Oncol 5:468–470

Rougier P, de Forni M, Adenis A et al (1994) Phase II study of Taxotere (RP 56976, docetaxel) in pancreatic adenocarcinoma. Proc Am Soc Clin Oncol 13:200

Rowinsky EK, Onetto N, Canetta RM et al (1992) Taxol: the first of the taxanes, an important class of antitumor agents. Semin Oncol 19:646–662

Sternberg CN, ten Bokkel Huinink WW, Smyth JF et al (1994) Docetaxel, a novel taxoid, in the treatment of advanced colorectal carcinoma: an EORTC Early Clinical Trials Group study. Br J Cancer 70:376–379

Sulkes A, Smyth J, Sessa C et al (1994) Docetaxel (Taxotere) in advanced gastric cancer: results of a phase II clinical trial. Br J Cancer 70:380–383

Taguchi T (1994) An early phase II study of RP 56976 (docetaxel) in patients with cancer of the gastrointestinal tract. Gan To Kagaku Ryoho 21:2431–2437

Vaughn DJ, Shaw LM, Recio A et al (1995) A phase II trial of 96-hour infusional paclitaxel with pharmacokinetic analysis in metastatic colorectal cancer. Proc Am Soc Clin Oncol 15:530

Subject Index

MIX
Papier aus verantwortungsvollen Quellen
Paper from responsible sources
FSC® C105338

If you have any concerns about our products,
you can contact us on
ProductSafety@springernature.com

In case Publisher is established outside the EU,
the EU authorized representative is:
Springer Nature Customer Service Center GmbH
Europaplatz 3, 69115 Heidelberg, Germany

Printed by Libri Plureos GmbH
in Hamburg, Germany